Springer Proceedings in Mathematics & Statistics

Volume 320

Springer Proceedings in Mathematics & Statistics

This book series features volumes composed of selected contributions from workshops and conferences in all areas of current research in mathematics and statistics, including operation research and optimization. In addition to an overall evaluation of the interest, scientific quality, and timeliness of each proposal at the hands of the publisher, individual contributions are all refereed to the high quality standards of leading journals in the field. Thus, this series provides the research community with well-edited, authoritative reports on developments in the most exciting areas of mathematical and statistical research today.

More information about this series at http://www.springer.com/series/10533

Somnath Bhattacharyya · Jitendra Kumar ·
Koeli Ghoshal
Editors

Mathematical Modeling and Computational Tools

ICACM 2018, Kharagpur, India, November 23–25

Springer

Editors
Somnath Bhattacharyya
Department of Mathematics
Indian Institute of Technology Kharagpur
Kharagpur, West Bengal, India

Jitendra Kumar
Department of Mathematics
Indian Institute of Technology Kharagpur
Kharagpur, West Bengal, India

Koeli Ghoshal
Department of Mathematics
Indian Institute of Technology Kharagpur
Kharagpur, West Bengal, India

ISSN 2194-1009 ISSN 2194-1017 (electronic)
Springer Proceedings in Mathematics & Statistics
ISBN 978-981-15-3614-4 ISBN 978-981-15-3615-1 (eBook)
https://doi.org/10.1007/978-981-15-3615-1

Mathematics Subject Classification (2010): 92-08, 92-10, 65-XX, 68Uxx, 97Mxx

This Springer imprint is published by the registered company Springer Nature Singapore Pte Ltd.
The registered company address is: 152 Beach Road, #21-01/04 Gateway East, Singapore 189721, Singapore

Contents

Stochastic Modelling and Machine Learning

Electrokinetic Transport Phenomenon

An Overview on Analytic Expressions for Electrophoretic Velocity of Rigid Colloids

Partha P. Gopmandal, Saurabh K. Maurya and Somnath Bhattacharyya

Abstract Electrophoresis is a process by which a charged colloid is propelled in a polar media under the action of an externally imposed electric field. This has been recognized as a useful tool to characterize macromolecules such as DNA, microorganisms, biocolloids or synthetic nanoparticles. Electrophoresis is also found to be an efficient method in separating, sorting and purification process. The microfluidic technology to address problems in biology, medical technology, such as controlled drug delivery and disease diagnostic are based on the electrophoresis phenomena. Thus, a correct relation between the electrostatic parameters and the electrophoretic velocity constitutes an important research topic. In this chapter, we have elaborated some of the existing simplified models for electrophoretic velocity. The shortcomings of these linear models or models based on weak-field consideration are illustrated in this chapter. An account of improved theory on electrophoresis is provided. The electrophoresis of a hydrophobic colloid is also addressed in the present chapter.

Keywords Rigid colloid · Surface charge · Debye–Huckel parameter · Hydrophobicity · Electrophoretic velocity

---

P. P. Gopmandal
Department of Mathematics, National Institute of Technology Durgapur, Durgapur 713209, India

S. K. Maurya
Department of Mathematics, National Institute of Technology Patna, Patna 800005, India

S. Bhattacharyya (✉)
Department of Mathematics, Indian Institute of Technology Kharagpur, Kharagpur 721302, India
e-mail: somnath@maths.iitkgp.ernet.in

S. Bhattacharyya et al. (eds.), *Mathematical Modeling and Computational Tools*, Springer Proceedings in Mathematics & Statistics 320,
https://doi.org/10.1007/978-981-15-3615-1_1

1 Introduction

When a charged colloidal particle is exposed to an external electric field, the particle moves toward the electrode of opposite polarity and the counterion cloud surrounding the particle opposes the particle motion. Such electrokinetic phenomena are termed as electrophoresis. It was first observed by Reuss [1] for the clay particles dispersed in water under the influence of electric field. Electrophoresis in the present day is established to be important phenomena in the context of microfluidics, colloid science, separation and purification technology. Over the years, a large body of literature is devoted to establish a relation between the electrophoretic velocity, the velocity by which a charged particle translates under the action of an applied electric field, and the strength of the applied field.

The theory of electrophoresis is based on the concept of the electric double layer (EDL) formed along the rigid surface-electrolyte solution interface. Under the application of electric field, the net mobile charge within the diffuse part of the EDL induces Columbic force. At the same time, the viscous forces exerted by the liquid on the particles tend to retard the particle motion. At steady state, both the force balances each other and the charged particle moves with a uniform velocity known as electrophoretic velocity (U_{E}). It is interesting to note that, from the electrophoretic velocity, one can easily measure the surface ζ-potential, which is the indicator of electrical charge carried by the surface.

The first mathematical approach to consider the electrophoresis of colloidal particle is made by von Smoluchowski [2] under thin double layer assumption valid for electrolyte with high concentration. Later, Huckel [3] derived the theoretical description of electrophoretic phenomena of rigid colloid for a dilute electrolyte for which the characteristic length scale (i.e., particle radius a, say) is much smaller than the thickness of the EDL (κ^{-1}). Henry [4] further extends the study of electrophoresis of rigid colloids to consider the effect of Debye–Huckel parameter κa on the particle motion. Besides the theory proposed by Henry, later Ohshima [5] made a similar study based on linear perturbation analysis to obtain the closed-form analytical expression for the particle's velocity.

All the aforementioned theoretical studies are based on weak electric field and low potential assumption for which the EDL around the charged particle remains concentric. However, for higher values of surface potential (i.e., ζ-potential) and strong electric field, the EDL may distort from its spherical shape due to strong fluid convection. Such a nonlinear phenomenon is termed as double layer polarization (DLP) or relaxation effect. O'Brien and White [6] studied electrophoresis of highly charged particle by considering the DLP effect and have shown that the DLP effect has a prominent role for moderate values of Debye–Huckel parameter (κa). Subsequently, several authors studied the effects of DLP on the particle electrophoresis—Hsu et al. [7], Hsu and Chen [8], Sang et al. [9], Bhattacharyya and Gopmandal [10], Khair [11]—under various electrokinetic conditions.

The above-mentioned studies have considered the particle surface is hydrophilic in nature. However, there are various practical situations where the particle may exhibit hydrophobicity and the conventional no-slip velocity boundary condition may not valid across the rigid surface, e.g., for the fabricated engineered micro/nano-particle, the fluid can slip over the surface of the particle (Tretheway and Meinhart [12], Moyano et al. [13]). For such a particle, the fluid velocity along the particle surface can be modeled by Navier boundary condition (Lauga et al. [14]), which state that the slip velocity is proportional to the rate of strain at the rigid surface. The proportionality constant is often known as slip length and it may vary from several nanometer to micrometer (Bocquet and Barrat [15]). Hence, for typical colloidal dispersion, where the characteristic length scale is of the order of hydrodynamic slip length, the particle velocity is influenced greatly by the hydrophobic nature of the particle surface.

Several authors attempt to study the effect of hydrodynamical slippage on the electrophoresis of hydrophobic rigid colloids. Khair and Squires [16], Park [17] studied the electrophoresis problem for hydrophobic rigid colloid. Later, based on low charge and weak-field assumption, Gopmandal et al. [18] derived a closed-form analytical expression for electrophoretic velocity. In their study, they have also established a similarity between charged hydrophobic particle and charged droplet. Subsequently, Bhattacharyya and Majee [19] studied the nonlinear effects on the electrophoresis of highly charged hydrophobic colloids by considering the fluid convection on the ion distribution. Recently, Ohshima [20] studied the electrophoresis and sedimentation of charged hydrophobic particle under low surface potential and weak electric field assumptions.

In the current study, the concept of particle electrophoresis along with the full set of governing equations for the electrohydrodynamics of charged colloids are illustrated rigorously. In this review, we focus on the pioneering theoretical works on electrophoresis provided by Henry [4] and Ohshima [5] for hydrophilic rigid colloids. In addition, we have also discussed two limiting situations where the characteristic length scale is much smaller or much larger than the EDL thickness. We have further considered the electrophoresis of charged hydrophobic rigid colloid. The detailed steps for the derivation of electrophoretic velocity of charged colloids under weak electric field and low potential limits are discussed for each individual case.

2 Governing Equations

In this chapter, we have presented the mathematical theory of electrophoresis of charged rigid colloids subject to the following assumptions. (i) The motion is slow enough for which the inertia term in the fluid flow equation can be neglected. (ii) The liquid is incompressible in nature. (iii) The applied electric field $\mathbf{E}$ is weak enough so that the particle velocity U_{E} is proportional to the electric field strength E_0 $(= |\mathbf{E}|)$. (iv) The slipping plane is located on the particle surface. (v) The rigid surface of the colloidal particle is impenetrable to the mobile electrolyte ions. In addition, we have also assumed that the surface potential of the particle is small so that the potential drop across the EDL is lower than the thermal voltage drop. For such a case, we may invoke the Debye-Huckel approximation to linearize the governing equations for electrophoresis. It is interesting to note that all the assumptions mentioned above are almost certainly valid for the electrokinetics of rigid colloids.

From the classical electrophoresis problem, the particle moves with an uniform electrophoretic velocity U_E under the applied electric field $\mathbf{E}$. We have considered a reference frame where the particle is kept fixed and the liquid at far-field moves with far-stream velocity $-U_\mathrm{E}$. In order to study the problem, we have employed a spherical polar coordinate (r, θ, φ) with the origin is at the center of particle and z-axis is along the migration direction (Fig. 1). The governing equations for electrophoresis are as follows

$$\nabla^2\phi = 0 \tag{1}$$

$$\varepsilon_\mathrm{e}\nabla^2\psi = -\rho_\mathrm{e} \tag{2}$$

$$\eta\nabla \times (\nabla \times \mathbf{v}) + \nabla P = -\rho_\mathrm{e}\nabla(\phi + \psi) \tag{3}$$

$$\nabla.\mathbf{v} = 0 \tag{4}$$

where ϕ and ψ are the potential due to the applied electric field and double layer potential, respectively. Here, $\mathbf{v} = (v_\mathrm{r}, v_\theta, v_\varphi)$ is velocity vector, P is pressure and η is the viscosity. The net charge density is given by $\rho_\mathrm{e} = e\Sigma z_i n_i$, where z_i and n_i are valance and ionic concentration of mobile ions, respectively, and e is the elementary charge. The permittivity of the electrolyte medium is given by $\varepsilon_\mathrm{f} = \varepsilon_\mathrm{r}\varepsilon_0$, where ε_r is the relative permittivity and ε_0 is the permittivity of vacuum. It may be noted that for

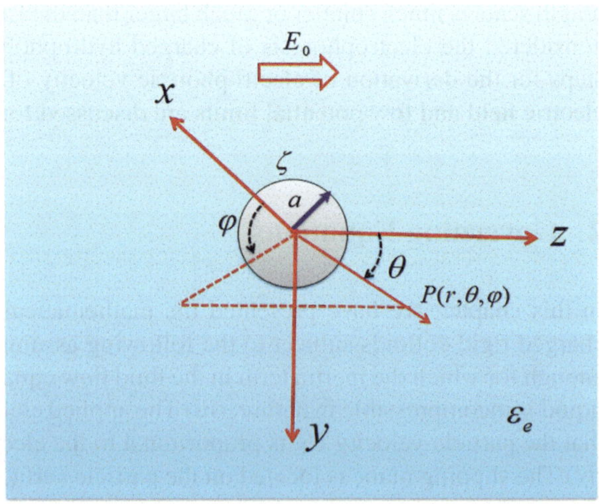

Fig. 1 Schematic illustrations depicting the electrophoresis of charged rigid colloid with radius a and surface potential ζ. A spherical polar coordinate system with the origin at the center of the particle is adopted to study the problem. Here, the applied electric field with a strength E_0 is applied along the z-direction along which the suspension moves with constant electrophoretic velocity U_E

liquid motion within low Reynolds number regime, the velocity components v_r, v_θ along radial and cross-radial direction does not depends on the azimuthal coordinate φ with $v_\varphi = 0$.

Under a low potential limit, we may assume the Boltzmann distribution for the spatial distribution of contribution of ionic species, given as

$$n_i = n_0 \exp\left(-\frac{z_i e\psi}{K_B T}\right) \tag{5}$$

where K_B and T are the Boltzmann constant and absolute temperature, respectively, and n_0 is the bulk value of the concentration where the effect of EDL-induced potential is absent. Under low electric field assumption, the deviation of n_i, ψ and ρ_e from their equilibrium values are small. It may be noted that equilibrium values correspond to the value of the respective variables in the absence of the electric field **E**. In fact under these assumptions, i.e., weak electric field and low surface potential, the fluid convection is low enough to create the distortion of EDL and is remains always spherically concentric, and hence the DLP and relaxation effects are insignificant.

3 Electrophoresis of Hydrophilic Rigid Colloid

Below we have provided the classical theories for electrophoresis provided by Smoluchowski [2], Huckel [3], Henry [4] and Ohshima [5] for hydrophilic rigid colloids.

3.1 Smoluchowski Equation for Thin EDL

In the year 1921, Smoluchowski [2] derive the velocity expression under thin double layer approximation, i.e., $\kappa a \gg 1$ where κ^{-1} is the EDL thickness and a is the particle radius. With this assumption, the electric field can have only the components along the particle surface and the particle surface may be considered as planner, and the applied electric field **E** is set parallel to the surface of the particle (Fig. 2). This reasonable assumption for a particle with dielectric constant much lower than that of the aqueous media (Hunter [21]). For such a typical situation, the governing equation for fluid flow can be written as

$$\eta \frac{d^2 u}{dx^2} = -\rho_e E_0 = \varepsilon_e \frac{d^2 \psi}{dx^2} E_0 \tag{6}$$

Integrating Eq. (6) subject to no-slip boundary condition along the particle surface ($x = a$) and far-field condition $u \to -U_E$ as $x \to \infty$; we can write the velocity field as

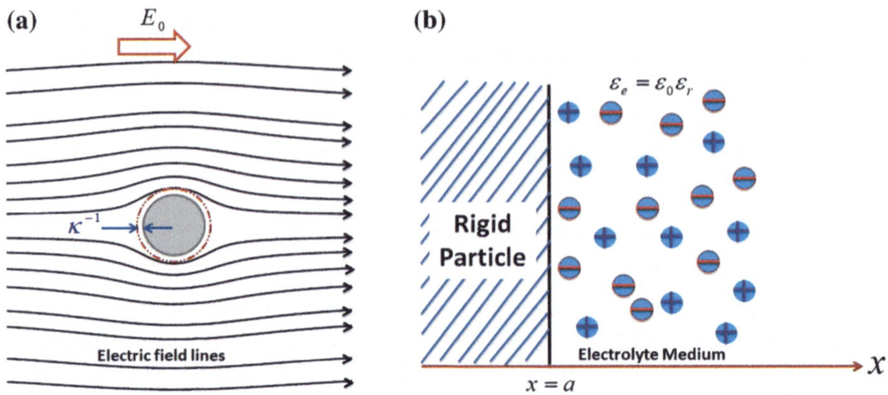

Fig. 2 **a** Schematic illustrations depicting the electric field lines. The red dashed line represents the edge of the EDL with thickness κ^{-1}. **b** Schematic illustrations depicting plate-like rigid particle

$$u(x) = \frac{\varepsilon_e E_0}{\eta}(\psi - \zeta) \tag{7}$$

where ψ is the EDL-induced potential and ζ is the surface potential. It may be noted that far from the particle the induced potential $\psi \to 0$ where $u \to -U_E$. Hence, the electrophoretic velocity may be derived as

$$U_E = \frac{\varepsilon_e \zeta}{\eta} E_0 \tag{8}$$

3.2 *Huckel's Limit for Thick EDL*

Another limiting situation for dilute electrolyte is considered by Huckel [3]. For such a case, the EDL is thick and its thickness is much larger than the particle radius, i.e., $\kappa^{-1} \gg a$. For such a situation, the deflection of the electric field lines due to the presence of the particle is almost negligible (Fig. 3). Here, the neutralization of particle charge due to counterion present in the aqueous media is almost negligible. Hence, the net electric force experienced by charged particle within aqueous medium is given by

$$F_e = QE_0 \tag{9}$$

where Q is the net surface charge of the particle and is given by $Q = 4\pi a^2 \sigma$ where σ is surface charged density. For a spherical particle, the potential equation under spherical symmetry and low potential limit can be written as

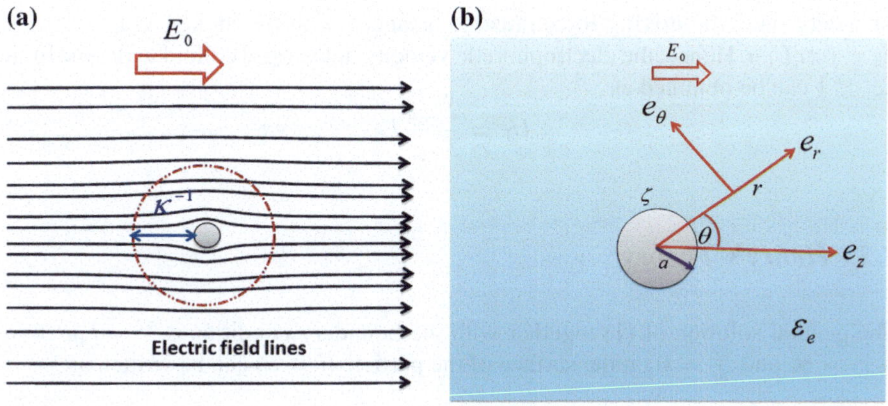

Fig. 3 **a** Schematic illustrations depicting the electric field lines. The red dashed line represents the edge of the EDL. **b** Schematic illustrations spherical polar coordinate system with axisymmetry. Here, the applied electric field E_0 is applied along the z-direction along which the suspension moves with constant electrophoretic velocity U_{E}

$$\frac{\mathrm{d}^2\psi}{\mathrm{d}r^2} + \frac{2}{r}\frac{\mathrm{d}\psi}{\mathrm{d}r} = \kappa^2\psi \tag{10}$$

Here, r is the radial coordinate. The solution of Eq. (10) subject to the boundary conditions on the particle surface and along the far-field, given by $\psi = \zeta$ at $r = a$ and $\psi \to 0$ as $r \to \infty$, respectively, may be derived as follows

$$\psi(r) = \zeta\left(\frac{a}{r}\right)\mathrm{e}^{-\kappa(r-a)} \tag{11}$$

The surface charge density σ can be obtained from the following relation

$$\sigma = -\varepsilon_{\mathrm{e}}\frac{\mathrm{d}\psi}{\mathrm{d}r}\,|_{r=a} = \varepsilon_{\mathrm{e}}\frac{(1+\kappa a)\zeta}{a} \tag{12}$$

Hence, the net electric experienced by the particle may be derived as

$$F_{\mathrm{e}} = 4\pi a^2\varepsilon_{\mathrm{e}}\frac{(1+\kappa a)\zeta}{a}E_0$$

Under the limit $\kappa a \ll 1$ in which the aqueous medium contain no free charge, the net electric force is given by

$$F_{\mathrm{e}} = 4\pi a^2\left(\frac{\varepsilon_{\mathrm{e}}\zeta E_0}{a}\right)$$

At steady state, the driving force must be balanced with the Stokes' drag given by $F_{\mathrm{h}} = 6\pi\eta U_{\mathrm{E}}a$. Hence, the electrophoretic velocity of the rigid colloid under the limit $\kappa a \ll 1$ can be obtained as

$$U_{\mathrm{E}} = \frac{2}{3}\frac{\varepsilon_{\mathrm{e}}\zeta}{\eta}E_0 \tag{13}$$

3.3 *Henry's Theory*

The general solution of (1) together with the boundary condition $\phi \to -E_0 r\cos\theta$ as $r \to \infty$ and $\frac{\mathrm{d}\phi}{\mathrm{d}r} = 0$ on the surface of the particle ($r = a$) can be written as

$$\phi = -E_0\left(r + \frac{1}{2}\frac{a^3}{r^2}\right)\cos\theta \tag{14}$$

Let $p_1 = P - \int_{\infty}^{r}\rho_{\mathrm{e}}\left(\frac{\partial\psi}{\partial r}\right)\mathrm{d}r$. With this we may write

$$\nabla P = \nabla p_1 + \nabla\left[\int_{\infty}^{r}\rho_{\mathrm{e}}\left(\frac{\partial\psi}{\partial r}\right)\mathrm{d}r\right] = \nabla p_1 + \rho_{\mathrm{e}}\nabla\psi$$

and hence the Stokes' equation further reduces to

$$\eta\nabla\times(\nabla\times\mathbf{v}) + \nabla p_1 = -\rho_{\mathrm{e}}\nabla\phi \tag{15}$$

Taking divergence on both sides of Eq. (15) we get

$$\nabla^2 p_1 = -\nabla.(\rho_{\mathrm{e}}\nabla\phi) = -\frac{\partial\phi}{\partial r}\frac{\partial\rho_{\mathrm{e}}}{\partial r}$$

Using (2) and (14), we may write

$$\nabla^2 p_1 = -\nabla.(\rho_{\mathrm{e}}\nabla\phi) = -\epsilon_{\mathrm{e}}\left(1 - \frac{a^3}{r^3}\right)\cos\theta\frac{\partial}{\partial r}\left(\nabla^2\psi\right) \tag{16}$$

Following Henry [4], we may write the pressure filed using (2) and (14), we may write

$$p = \int_{\infty}^{r}\rho_{\mathrm{e}}\frac{\partial\psi}{\partial r}\mathrm{d}r - \epsilon_{\mathrm{e}}E_0\cos\theta\left[\frac{\partial\psi}{\partial r} - a^3 r\int_{\infty}^{r}\frac{1}{r^4}\nabla^2\psi\mathrm{d}r\right] \tag{17}$$

Again taking curl of the Eq. (15), we may write

$$\eta\nabla \times \nabla \times (\nabla \times \mathbf{v}) = -\nabla \times (\rho_{\mathrm{e}}\nabla\phi) \tag{18}$$

Assuming $\Omega = \nabla \times v$ and hence the reduced form of the fluid flow equation can be written in simplified form as

$$\eta\nabla \times \nabla \times \Omega = -\nabla \times (\rho_{\mathrm{e}}\nabla\phi) \tag{19}$$

It may be noted that for two-dimensional steady axisymmetry flow past spherical particle, the velocity vector **v** has a zero azimuthal component, and it leads to a zero radial and cross-radial components of Ω and $\nabla \times \Omega$. The nonzero azimuthal component of Ω can be written as

$$\Omega_{\varphi} = \frac{1}{r}\left\{\frac{\partial}{\partial r}(rv_{\theta}) - \frac{\partial v_{\mathrm{r}}}{\partial v_{\theta}}\right\} \tag{20}$$

In addition azimuthal component of $\nabla \times \nabla \times \Omega$ is given as

$$(\nabla \times \nabla \times \Omega)_{\varphi} = -\frac{1}{r}\left\{\frac{\partial^2}{\partial r^2}(r\Omega_{\varphi}) + \frac{1}{r}\frac{\partial}{\partial\theta}\left[\frac{1}{\sin\theta}\frac{\partial}{\partial\theta}(\Omega_{\varphi}\sin\theta)\right]\right\} \tag{21}$$

On the other hand, only the nonzero azimuthal component of $\nabla \times (\rho_{\mathrm{e}}\nabla\phi)$ is given by

$$\nabla \times (\rho_{\mathrm{e}}\nabla\phi)_{\varphi}\frac{1}{r}\frac{\partial\rho_{\mathrm{e}}}{\partial r}\frac{\partial\phi}{\partial\theta} \tag{22}$$

Thus, (21) can be written in component form as

$$\eta(\nabla \times \nabla \times \Omega)_{\varphi} = -\frac{1}{r}\frac{\partial\rho_{\mathrm{e}}}{\partial r}\frac{\partial\phi}{\partial\theta} \tag{23}$$

Using Eqs. (2) and (14), one can write Eq. (23) as

$$(\nabla \times \nabla \times \Omega)_{\varphi} = \frac{\varepsilon_{\mathrm{e}}E_0}{\eta}\sin\theta\left(1 + \frac{1}{2}\frac{a^3}{r^3}\right)\frac{\partial}{\partial r}\nabla^2\psi \tag{24}$$

The solution of Eq. (24) can be obtain as (Henry [4])

$$\Omega_{\varphi} = -\frac{\varepsilon_{\mathrm{e}}E_0}{\eta}\sin\theta\left\{\frac{\partial\psi}{\partial r} + \frac{1}{2}a^3 r\int\limits_{\infty}^{r}\frac{1}{r^4}\nabla^2\psi\mathrm{d}r\right\} \tag{25}$$

Consider

$$\xi = \frac{\partial \psi}{\partial r} + \frac{a^3 r}{2} \int\limits_{\infty}^{r} \frac{1}{r^4} \nabla^2 \psi \mathrm{d}r \quad (26)$$

With this we may write

$$\Omega_\varphi = -\frac{\varepsilon_\mathrm{e} E_0 \xi}{\eta} \sin\theta \quad (27)$$

Using (20), we may write

$$\frac{1}{r}\left\{\frac{\partial}{\partial r}(r v_\theta) - \frac{\partial v_\mathrm{r}}{\partial v_\theta}\right\} = -\frac{\varepsilon_\mathrm{e} E_0 \xi}{\eta} \sin\theta \quad (28)$$

In addition, the continuity equation for two-dimensional incompressible axisymmetric flow can be written as

$$\frac{1}{r^2}\frac{\partial}{\partial r}\left(r^2 v_r\right) + \frac{1}{r\sin\theta}\frac{\partial}{\partial\theta}(\sin\theta v_\theta) = 0 \quad (29)$$

Solving Eqs. (28) and (29), we may write the velocity components along the radial and cross-radial directions, respectively, as

$$\left.\begin{aligned} v_r &= \tfrac{2}{3}\epsilon_\mathrm{e} E_0 \cos\theta \left(\int^{r} \xi \mathrm{d}r - \tfrac{1}{r^3}\int^{r} r^3 \xi \mathrm{d}r\right) \\ v_\theta &= -\tfrac{2}{3}\epsilon_\mathrm{e} E_0 \sin\theta \left(\int^{r} \xi \mathrm{d}r + \tfrac{2}{r^3}\int^{r} r^3 \xi \mathrm{d}r\right) \end{aligned}\right\} \quad (30)$$

Here, the lower limit of integration appears in Eq. (30) can be determined from the appropriate velocity condition. It may be noted that Eqs. (17) and (30) are the particular solution of the Stokes' equation (3) along with the continuity condition (4). The complete solution may be obtained by adding these solutions with the general solution of

$$\left.\begin{aligned} &\eta\nabla \times \nabla\mathbf{v} + \nabla P = 0 \\ &\nabla.\mathbf{v} = 0 \end{aligned}\right\} \quad (31)$$

By using the boundary conditions for velocity components and EDL potential, given as

$$\left.\begin{aligned} &r \to \infty;\ v_\mathrm{r} = -U_\mathrm{E}\cos\theta,\ v_\theta = U_\mathrm{E}\sin\theta;\ \psi = 0 \\ &\text{and}\ \ v_\mathrm{r} = v_\theta = 0;\ \psi = \zeta;\ \text{on r = a} \end{aligned}\right\} \quad (32)$$

The complete solution of the fluid flow Eqs. (3) and (4) can be obtained as

$$\begin{cases} v_{\mathrm{r}} = \cos\theta \left\{ -\left(1 - \frac{3}{2}\frac{a}{r} + \frac{a^3}{2r^3}\right) U_{\mathrm{E}} - \left(\frac{a}{r} - \frac{a^3}{3r^3}\right) \frac{\varepsilon_{\mathrm{e}} E_0}{\eta} \int\limits_{\infty}^{r} \xi \mathrm{d}r \right. \\ \left. -\frac{2}{3}\left(\int\limits_{\infty}^{r} \xi \mathrm{d}r - \frac{1}{r^3}\int\limits_{a}^{r} r^3 \xi \mathrm{d}r\right)\right\} \\ v_\theta = \sin\theta \left\{ \left(1 - \frac{3}{4}\frac{a}{r} - \frac{a^3}{4r^3}\right) + \left(\frac{a}{r} + \frac{a^3}{6r^3}\right) \frac{\varepsilon_{\mathrm{e}} E_0}{\eta} \int\limits_{\infty}^{r} \xi \mathrm{d}r \right. \\ \left. -\frac{2}{3}\left(\int\limits_{\infty}^{r} \xi \mathrm{d}r + \frac{1}{2r^3}\int\limits_{a}^{r} r^3 \xi \mathrm{d}r\right)\right\} \\ v_\varphi = 0 \\ P = \int\limits_{\infty}^{r} \rho_{\mathrm{e}} \frac{\partial \psi}{\partial r} \mathrm{d}r + \cos\theta \left\{ \frac{3\eta a}{2r^2} U_{\mathrm{E}} - \frac{a}{r^2} \varepsilon_{\mathrm{e}} E_0 \int_{\infty}^{a} \xi \mathrm{d}r - \varepsilon_{\mathrm{e}} E_0 \left(3 \frac{\partial \psi}{\partial r} \xi\right)\right\} \end{cases} \tag{33}$$

The electrophoretic velocity can be obtained from the force balance for a steady-state migration of the charged particle. The hydrodynamic drag force exerted by the fluid on the particle is given by

$$F_{\mathrm{h}} = 2\pi a^2 \int\limits_{0}^{\pi} [-\tau_{rr}\cos\theta + \tau_{r\theta}\sin\theta]_{r=a} \sin\theta \mathrm{d}\theta \tag{34}$$

with

$$\tau_{rr} = -P + 2\eta \frac{\partial v_{\mathrm{r}}}{\partial \theta}, \quad \tau_{r\theta} = \mu \left\{ \frac{\partial v_\theta}{\partial r} - \frac{v_\theta}{r} + \frac{1}{r}\frac{\partial v_{\mathrm{r}}}{\partial \theta} \right\}.$$

Using the velocity components and pressure field given in (33), one can obtain the hydrodynamic drag force experienced by the particle. On the other hand, the electric driving force experienced by the charged colloid of radius a can be obtained form

$$F_{\mathrm{e}} = -2\pi a^2 \int\limits_{0}^{\pi} \varepsilon_{\mathrm{e}} \left[E_{\mathrm{z}} \frac{\partial \psi}{\partial r} \right]_{r=a} \mathrm{d}\theta \tag{35}$$

where E_{z} is the component of total electric field along migration direction of the particle and can be obtained form

$$E_{\mathrm{z}} = \frac{\sin\theta}{r}\frac{\partial}{\partial \theta}(\phi + \psi) - \cos\theta \frac{\partial}{\partial r}(\phi + \psi) \tag{36}$$

It may be noted that the electric double layer potential ψ depends only on r and $\frac{\partial \phi}{\partial r} = 0$, where ϕ is potential due to applied electric field. It results

$$E_{\mathrm{z}} = \frac{1}{r}\frac{\partial \psi}{\partial \theta}\sin\theta - \frac{\partial \psi}{\partial r}\cos\theta \tag{37}$$

Under Debye–Huckel limit-induced electric potential (ψ) is given in (11). Using EDL potential ψ and potential due to applied electric field (ϕ) from (14), one can obtain the net electric force F_e experienced by the particle. From the force balance at steady state (i.e., $F_h = F_e$), the expression for the electrophoretic velocity can be written as

$$U_E = \frac{2}{3}\frac{\varepsilon_e E_0}{\eta}\left[\zeta + \frac{1}{2}a^3\left\{3a^2\int\limits_{\infty}^{a}\frac{1}{r^5}\frac{\partial\psi}{\partial r}dr - 2\int\limits_{\infty}^{a}\frac{1}{r^3}\frac{\partial\psi}{\partial r}dr\right\}\right] \tag{38}$$

Using the value of $\psi(r)$ given in Eq. (12), Eq. (38) takes the following form

$$U_E = \frac{2}{3}\frac{\varepsilon_e E_0 \zeta}{\eta}\left\{1 + \frac{3}{2}e^{\kappa a}[E_7(\kappa a) + \kappa a E_6(\kappa a)] - e^{\kappa a}[E_5(\kappa a) + \kappa a E_4(\kappa a)]\right\} \tag{39}$$

where n^{th} order exponential integral is given by

$$E_n(\kappa a) = \int\limits_{1}^{\infty}\frac{e^{-\kappa a.r}}{r^n}dr \tag{40}$$

Using the following recurrence relation for exponential integrals

$$e^{\kappa a}E_n(\kappa a) = \frac{1}{\kappa a} - \frac{n}{\kappa a}e^{\kappa a}E_{n+1}(\kappa a) \tag{41}$$

we may further simplify the expression for electrophoretic velocity U_E as

$$U_E = \frac{\varepsilon_e E_0 \zeta}{\eta}\left[1 - e^{\kappa a}\left(5E_7(\kappa a) - 2E_5(\kappa a)\right)\right] \tag{42}$$

In terms of Henry function, the general expression for electrophoretic velocity can be written as

$$U_E = \frac{\varepsilon_e E_0 \zeta}{\eta} f_H(\kappa a) \tag{43}$$

where the Henry function is defined as

$$f_H(\kappa a) = 1 - [5E_7(\kappa a) - 2E_5(\kappa a)]e^{\kappa a} \tag{44}$$

Using the series expansion of $E_n(x)$ as

$$E_n(x) = x^{n-1}\Gamma(1-n) + \left[-\frac{1}{1-n} + \frac{x}{2-n} - \frac{x^2}{2(3-n)} + \frac{x^3}{6(4-n)} - \cdots\right] \tag{45}$$

we may write the expression for electrophoretic velocity as

$$U_{\mathrm{E}} = \frac{2}{3}\frac{\varepsilon_{\mathrm{e}} E_0 \zeta}{\eta}\left[1 + \frac{(\kappa a)^2}{16} - \frac{5}{48}(\kappa a)^3 - \frac{(\kappa a)^4}{96} + \frac{(\kappa a)^5}{96} - \frac{11}{96}\int\limits_{\infty}^{\kappa a} \frac{\mathrm{e}^{-t}}{t}\mathrm{d}t\right] \tag{46}$$

For extremely dilute electrolyte solution (i.e., when $\kappa a \to 0$), the electrophoretic velocity U_{E} approaches to

$$U_{\mathrm{E}} = \frac{2}{3}\frac{\varepsilon_{\mathrm{e}} E_0}{\eta}\zeta$$

which is well known as Huckel result. On the other hand, using the following asymptotic expansion of $E_n(x)$

$$E_n(x) = \frac{\mathrm{e}^{-x}}{x}\left[1 - \frac{n}{x} + \frac{n(n+1)}{x^2} + \frac{n(n+1)(n+2)}{x^3} + \cdots\right] \tag{47}$$

we may write the expression for electrophoretic velocity as

$$U_{\mathrm{E}} = \frac{\varepsilon_{\mathrm{e}} E_0}{\eta}\zeta\left[1 - \frac{3}{\kappa a} + \frac{25}{(\kappa a)^2} - \frac{220}{(\kappa a)^3} + \cdots\right] \tag{48}$$

For strong electrolyte solution (i.e., $\kappa a \to \infty$), the electrophoretic velocity U_{E} approaches to the corresponding Smolchowski's result as follows

$$U_{\mathrm{E}} = \frac{\varepsilon_{\mathrm{e}} E_0 \zeta}{\eta}$$

These are two extreme situation and the electrophoretic velocity lies between the Huckel's results (i.e., $U_{\mathrm{E}} = 2\varepsilon_{\mathrm{e}} E_0 \zeta / 3\eta$) and Smolchowski's results (i.e., $U_{\mathrm{E}} = \varepsilon_{\mathrm{e}} E_0 \zeta / \eta$).

3.4 Ohshima's Model

A modified model on electrophoresis is introduced by Ohshima [5], which differs from that by Henry [4]. In order to understand the new technique, one need to consider the motion of mobile ions present into the system along with the flow fluid equations associated with the EDL-induced as well as externally applied electric field. The electrokinetic flow equation at low Reynolds number is given as

$$\eta \nabla \times (\nabla \times \mathbf{v}) + \nabla P = -\rho_{\mathrm{e}} \nabla \Psi \tag{49}$$

$$\nabla . \mathbf{v} = 0 \tag{50}$$

Here, Ψ is the total potential that includes the equilibrium double layer potential, potential due to applied electric field and potential due to polarization of particle and electric double layer (EDL). The governing equation for the total electric potential is as follows

$$\varepsilon_{\mathrm{e}} \nabla^2 \psi = -\rho_{\mathrm{e}} \tag{51}$$

The ionic velocity caused by the liquid flow and the gradient of the electrochemical equation is given by

$$v_i = \mathbf{v} - \frac{1}{\lambda_i} \nabla \mu_i \tag{52}$$

where the electrochemical potential μ_i is given as

$$\mu_i = \mu_i^{\infty} + z_i e \psi + \kappa_{\mathrm{B}} T \ln n_i \tag{53}$$

Here, μ_i^{∞} is the equilibrium electrochemical potential. The continuity equation for the mobile ions is given as

$$\nabla.(n_i v_i) = 0 \tag{54}$$

Introducing the osmotic pressure,

$$P_{\mathrm{osmotic}} = \kappa_{\mathrm{B}} T \Sigma_i n_i(r) \tag{55}$$

one may write the Stokes' equation (49) as

$$\eta \nabla \times \nabla \times \mathbf{v} + \nabla \{P - P_{\mathrm{osmotic}}\} + \Sigma_i n_i(r) \nabla \mu_i = 0 \tag{56}$$

Under the weak electric field assumption, we may assume the deviation of n_i, ψ, μ_i, ρ_{e} from their equilibrium values are quit small. With this we may write

$$\left.\begin{aligned} n_i &= n_i^0 + \delta n_i \\ \psi &= \psi^0 + \delta \psi \\ \mu_i &= \mu_i^0 + \delta \mu_i \\ \rho_{\mathrm{e}} &= \rho_{\mathrm{e}}^0 + \delta \rho_{\mathrm{e}} \end{aligned}\right\} \tag{57}$$

where the quantities with superscript '0' denotes the corresponding equilibrium values and are follows from the given relations as

$$n_i^0 = n_i^{\infty} \exp\left(-\frac{z_i \psi^0 e}{\kappa_{\mathrm{B}} T}\right) \tag{58}$$

$$\varepsilon_{\mathrm{e}} \nabla^2 \psi^0 = -\rho_{\mathrm{e}}^0 \tag{59}$$

$$\rho_{\mathrm{e}}^0 = \Sigma_i z_i e n_i^0 \tag{60}$$

$$\nabla \mu_i^0 = 0 \tag{61}$$

In addition the perturbs terms, due to the presence of applied voltage drop, may be written as

$$\delta \mu_i = z_i e \delta \psi + \kappa_B T \frac{\delta \mu_i}{n_i^0(r)} \tag{62}$$

$$\delta \rho_e = \Sigma_i z_i e \delta n_i \tag{63}$$

$$\nabla^2 \delta \psi = -\frac{1}{\varepsilon_e} \Sigma_i z_i e \delta n_i \tag{64}$$

Subsisting the first and third relations of (57) into the (56) and neglecting the products of small quantities, one can obtain the linearized equation for fluid flow equation as

$$\eta \nabla \times \nabla \times \mathbf{v} + \nabla \{ P - k_B T \Sigma n_i^0(r) - k_B T \Sigma \delta n_i \} + \Sigma_i n_i^0(r) \nabla \delta \mu_i = 0 \tag{65}$$

To eliminate the second term involving the pressure field, we take curl operator on both sides of Eq. (65) and it leads the simplified form of the fluid flow equation as

$$\eta \nabla \times \nabla \times \nabla \times \mathbf{v} = \Sigma_i \nabla \delta \mu_i \times \nabla n_i^0 \tag{66}$$

In a similar manner, we can obtain the linearized form the conservation equation for ionic species (54), as

$$\nabla . \left(n_i^0 \mathbf{v} - \frac{1}{\lambda_i} n_i^0 \nabla \delta \mu_i \right) = 0 \tag{67}$$

The particle surface is ion impenetrable and no slip in nature and it bears surface potential ζ, which lead to the following boundary conditions on the variables appears in Eqs. (66) and (67) as

$$\left. \begin{array}{l} \frac{\partial \mu_i}{\partial r} \mid_{r=a} = 0 \\ v_r = 0, \ v_\theta = 0 \text{ on } r = a \\ \psi^0 \mid_{r=a} = \zeta \end{array} \right\} \tag{68}$$

The far away of the particle is not affected by the presence of the particle which leads the far away boundary condition as

$$\left. \begin{array}{l} \psi = -E_0 r \cos\theta \ \text{ as } r \to \infty \\ n_i \to n_i^\infty \ \text{ as } r \to \infty \end{array} \right\} \tag{69}$$

Using the relations (68) and (69), the boundary conditions for the perturb terms can be written as

$$\left.\begin{array}{l} \frac{\partial \delta\mu_i}{\partial r} \mid_{r=a} = 0 \\ \delta\psi = -E_0 r\cos\theta \;\; \text{as } r \to \infty \\ \delta n_i \to 0 \;\; \text{as } r \to \infty \\ \delta\mu_i \to -z_i e E_0 r \cos\theta \;\; \text{as } r \to \infty \end{array}\right\} \tag{70}$$

Introducing $\phi_i(r)$, we may write

$$\delta\mu_i = -z_i e \phi_i(r) E \cos\theta \tag{71}$$

From the first equation of relation (68), and last equation of the relation (70), one may write

$$\left.\begin{array}{l} \frac{d\phi_i(r)}{dr} \mid_{r=a} = 0 \\ \phi_i(r) \to r \text{ as } r \to \infty \end{array}\right\} \tag{72}$$

Introducing $h(r)$, the spherical symmetry permits us to write the velocity field as

$$\mathbf{v} = \left(-\frac{2}{r}h(r)E_0\cos\theta, \frac{1}{r}\frac{d}{dr}(rh)E_0\sin\theta, 0\right) \tag{73}$$

It may be noted that the velocity field (73) automatically satisfies the equation of continuity for incompressible fluid. Using (73), we may write

$$\nabla \times \nabla \times \nabla \times \mathbf{v} = (0, 0, -L(Lh)E\sin\theta) \tag{74}$$

where the differential operator L is given as

$$L = \frac{d^2}{dr^2} + \frac{2}{r}\frac{d}{dr} - \frac{2}{r^2} \tag{75}$$

Using Eqs. (58), (71) and (74), we may write the governing equation for $h(r)$ may be written as

$$L(Lh(r)) = G(r) \tag{76}$$

where

$$G(r) = -\frac{e}{\eta r}\frac{dy}{dr}\Sigma z_i^2 n_i^{\infty} e^{-z_i y}\phi_i \tag{77}$$

with $y(r) = \psi^0/\phi_0$ is the scaled EDL potential, scaled by $\phi_0 = k_B T/e$. It may be noted that Eq. (77) involves ϕ_i. Using the equation of continuity for incompressible fluid, we may write

$$\nabla.\left(u - \frac{1}{\lambda_i}\nabla\delta\mu_i\right) = -\frac{1}{\lambda_i}\nabla^2\delta\mu_i \tag{78}$$

Using the relation (71), the above equation further reduces to

$$\nabla.\left(u-\frac{1}{\lambda_i}\nabla\delta\mu_i\right)=\frac{1}{\lambda_i}z_ie(\mathcal{L}\phi_i)E_0\cos\theta \tag{79}$$

With the help of Eq. (79), we may write Eq. (67) in terms of $\phi_i(r)$ and $h(r)$ as

$$\mathcal{L}\phi_i=\frac{\mathrm{d}y}{\mathrm{d}r}\left\{z_i\frac{\mathrm{d}\phi_i}{\mathrm{d}r}-\frac{2\lambda_i}{e}\frac{h}{r}\right\} \tag{80}$$

The electrophoretic problem is now reduced to the boundary value problem for $h(r)$ and $\phi_i(r)$ constituting Eqs. (76) and (80). To solve the above the set of differential equations, we need to specify the boundary conditions on the particle surface ($r = a$) and along the far-field ($r \to \infty$). The boundary conditions for $\phi_i(r)$ are already provided in (72). The boundary conditions for $h(r)$ may be obtained from the corresponding velocity boundary conditions. It may be noted that the rigid surface is considered to be non-slip in nature and at steady state the particle migrates with the uniform electrophoretic velocity U_E which leads to the boundary conditions for $h(r)$ on the particle surface and along the far-field as

$$\left.\begin{array}{l} h=\frac{dh}{dr}\,|_{r=a}=0 \\ \frac{h}{r}\to\frac{U}{2E}\ \text{as}\ r\to\infty \end{array}\right\} \tag{81}$$

Solving the boundary value problem (BVP) constituting Eqs. (76) and (80) subject to the boundary conditions given in Eqs. (72) and (81), the general expression for electrophoretic velocity per unit field strength (i.e., electrophoretic velocity) is given as

$$\frac{U_\mathrm{E}}{E_0}=\lim_{r\to\infty}\frac{2h(r)}{r}=\frac{a^2}{9}\int_a^\infty\left(1-\frac{3r^2}{a^2}+\frac{2r^3}{a^3}\right)G(r)\mathrm{d}r \tag{82}$$

where the reduced form of $G(r)$ is given by

$$G(r)=-\frac{\varepsilon_\mathrm{e}\kappa^2}{\eta}\left(1+\frac{a^3}{2r^3}\right)\frac{\mathrm{d}\psi^0}{\mathrm{d}r} \tag{83}$$

where

$$\psi^0=\zeta\frac{a}{r}\mathrm{e}^{-\kappa(r-a)} \tag{84}$$

Substituting Eq. (83) into (82), the expression for electrophoretic velocity may be written as

$$U_\mathrm{E}=-\frac{\varepsilon_\mathrm{e}E_0\kappa^2a^2}{9\eta}\int_a^\infty\left(1-\frac{3r^2}{a^2}+\frac{2r^3}{a^3}\right)\left(1+\frac{a^3}{2r^2}\right)\frac{\mathrm{d}\psi^0}{\mathrm{d}r} \tag{85}$$

Using the EDL potential given in (84), we may derive the expression for electrophoretic velocity as

$$U_{\mathrm{E}} = \frac{\varepsilon_{\mathrm{e}}\zeta E_0}{\eta} f_{\mathrm{H}}(\kappa a) \tag{86}$$

with

$$f_{\mathrm{H}}(\kappa a) = 1 - \mathrm{e}^{\kappa a}(5E_7(\kappa a) - 2E_5(\kappa a)) \tag{87}$$

The function $f_{\mathrm{H}}(\kappa a)$ is known as Henry function. Ohshima [5] further introduced a simple approximate formula for Henrys function $f_{\mathrm{H}}(\kappa a)$, given as

$$f_{\mathrm{H}}(\kappa a) \approx \frac{2}{3}\left[1 + \frac{1}{2(1 + (2.5/\kappa a\{1 + 2\exp(-\kappa a)\}))^3}\right] \tag{88}$$

It may be noted that such a function can approximate the Henry function with relative error is less than 1%.

4 Electrophoresis of Hydrophobic Rigid Colloid

In this section, we have provided the theories for electrophoresis of rigid colloids with charged hydrophobic surface. We adopt a similar linear perturbation technique due to Ohshima as discussed earlier. It may be noted that for hydrophobic particle, the linearized form of the governing equations and boundary conditions are the same as illustrated in the earlier section, except for the velocity boundary condition along the particle's surface ($r = a$). For a hydrophobic rigid colloid, the radial and cross-radial velocity components along the particle's surface are given by

$$u_{\mathrm{r}} = 0 \text{ and } u_\theta = \beta r \frac{\mathrm{d}}{\mathrm{d}r}\left(\frac{u_\theta}{r}\right) \text{ on } r = a \tag{89}$$

where β is the slip length. In term of electrokinetic variable $h(r)$, introduced earlier for velocity components, we may write above boundary conditions as follows

$$\left.\begin{array}{l} h(r) \mid_{r=a} = 0 \\ \frac{\mathrm{d}h}{\mathrm{d}r} \mid_{r=a} = \beta \frac{\mathrm{d}^2 h}{\mathrm{d}r^2} \mid_{r=a} \end{array}\right\} \tag{90}$$

Using the boundary condition given in Eq. (90), and after some lengthy algebra, we may derive expression for electrophoresis velocity as follows

$$U = \frac{\epsilon_{\mathrm{e}} E_0 \zeta}{\eta} f_{\mathrm{H}}^{M}(\kappa a) \tag{91}$$

where the modified Henry function for hydrophobic rigid colloid is given as

$$f_{\mathrm{H}}^{M}(\kappa a) = [1 + 2\mathrm{e}^{\kappa a} E_5(\kappa a) - 5\mathrm{e}^{\kappa a} E_7(\kappa a)] + \frac{2\beta}{3(a+2\beta)}\left[1 + \kappa a + \frac{(\kappa a)^2}{2}\mathrm{e}^{\kappa a} E_5(\kappa a)\right] \tag{92}$$

It may be noted that under thick and thin EDL for which $\kappa a \ll 1$ and $\kappa a \gg 1$, respectively, the limiting value of electrophoretic velocity may be obtained as

$$U_{\mathrm{E}}(\kappa a \ll 1) = \frac{2}{3}\frac{\epsilon_{\mathrm{e}} E_0 \zeta}{\eta}\left(\frac{a+3\beta}{a+2\beta}\right) \tag{93}$$

and

$$U_{\mathrm{E}}(\kappa a \gg 1) = \frac{\epsilon_{\mathrm{e}} E_0 \zeta}{\eta}\left\{\left(\frac{a+3\beta}{a+2\beta}\right) + \left(\frac{\beta\kappa a}{(a+2\beta)}\right)\right\} \tag{94}$$

5 Conclusion

In this chapter, we have illustrated the existing simplified models for electrophoresis of a rigid colloid suspended in an aqueous media. We have provided an outline on the derivation of the Henry formula for the velocity. The improved theory of Ohshima to determine the velocity is also illustrated. These models neglect the polarization and relaxation of the Debye layer, which may become pronounced for a stronger applied field as well as high surface charge density. The velocity based on Ohshima's model agrees well with the experimental results when the voltage drop created by the applied electric field is lower than the thermal potential. However, the nonlinear effects arise due to the stronger surface conduction, polarization and relaxation of the double layer become inevitable on electrophoresis for moderate range of applied field and surface charge density. The velocity of the hydrophobic colloids for the limiting situations of the Debye layer is derived. The surface hydrophobicity, characterized by the slip length, produces a large enhancement in the effective ζ-potential and hence the electrophoretic velocity of a charged colloid.

The linear models or the simplified models under the weak-field consideration are based on the Boltzmann distribution for mobile ions, which neglects the convection and diffusion fluxes. The models based on the Nernst–Planck equations for ions take into account the surface conduction, double layer polarization and relaxation, however, it leads to a set of nonlinear partial differential equations, which can have a seldom analytic solution.

References

1. Reuss, F.: Sur un nouvel effet de le électricité glavanique. Mémoires de la Societé Impériale des Naturalistes de Moscou **2**, 327–337 (1809)
2. von Smoluchowski, M., Elektrische endosmose und strmungsstrme. In: Greatz E (ed) Handbuch der elektrizitt und des magnetismus. Band II Stationre strme, Barth, pp 366–428 (1921)
3. Huckel, E.: Die kataphorese der kugel. Physik. Z. **25**, 204–210 (1924)
4. Henry, D., The cataphoresis of suspended particles. Part 1- The equation of cataphoresis. Proc. Roy. Soc. A, **133**, 106–129 (1931)
5. Ohshima, H.: Electrophoretic mobility of soft particle. J. Colloid Interface Sci. **163**, 474–483 (1994)
6. O' Brien, R.W., White, Lee R., Electrophoretic mobility of a spherical colloidal particle. J. Chem. Soc. Faraday Trans. 2: Molec. Chem. Phys. **74**, 1607–1626 (1978)
7. Hsu, J.P., Ku, M.H.: Boundary effect on electrophoresis: finite cylinder in a cylindrical pore. J. Colloid Interface Sci. **283**, 592–600 (2005)
8. Hsu, J.P., Chen, Z.S.: Electrophoresis of a sphere along the axis of a cylindrical pore: effects of double-layer polarization and electroosmotic flow. Langmuir **23**, 6198–6204 (2007)
9. Sang, W., Joo, W.S., Hou, X., Zhao, H.: Electrophoretic motion of a spherical particle with a symmetric nonuniform surface charge distribution in a nanotube. Langmuir **24**, 5332–5340 (2008)
10. Bhattacharyya, S., Gopmandal, P.P.: Migration of a charged sphere at an arbitrary velocity in an axial electric field. Colloids Surf. A Physicochem. Eng. Aspects **390**, 86–94 (2011)
11. Khair, A.S.: Strong Deformation of the thick electric double layer around a charged particle during sedimentation or electrophoresis. Langmuir **34**, 876–885 (2018)
12. Tretheway, D.C., Meinhart, C.D.: Apparent fluid slip at hydrophobic microchannel walls. Phys. Fluids **14**, L9 (2002)
13. Moyano, D.F., Saha, K., Prakash, G., HaoKong, B., HaoKong, M., Vincent, M.R.: Fabrication of Corona-Free nanoparticles with tunable hydrophobicity. ACS NANO **8**, 6748–6755 (2014)
14. Lauga, E., Brenner, M., Stone, H.A.: Handbook of Experimental Fluid Dynamics, pp. 1219–40. Springer, NY (2007)
15. Bocquet, L., Barrat, J.-L.: Flow boundary conditions from nano-to micro-scales. Soft Matter **3**, 685–693 (2007)
16. Khair, A.S., Squires, T.M.: The influence of hydrodynamic slip on the electrophoretic mobility of a spherical colloidal particle. Phys. Fluids **21**, 042001 (2009)
17. Park, H.M.: Electrophoresis of particles with Navier velocity slip. Electrophoresis **34**, 651–661 (2013)
18. Bhattacharyya, S., Gopmandal, P.P., Ohshima, H.: On the similarity between the electrophoresis of a liquid drop and a spherical hydrophobic particle. Colloid Polym. Sci. **295**, 2077–2082 (2017)
19. Bhattacharyya, S., Majee, P.S.: Electrophoresis of a polarizable charged colloid with hydrophobic surface: a numerical study. Phys. Rev. E **95**, 042605 (2017)
20. Ohshima, H.: Electrokinetic phenomena in a dilute suspension of spherical solid colloidal particles with a hydrodynamically slipping surface in an aqueous electrolyte solution. Adv. Colloid Interface Sci. **272**, 101996 (2019)
21. Hunter, R.J., Foundation of Colloid Science, 2nd edn. Oxford University Press, Oxford (2001)

Solute Transport and Mixing Efficiency on Electrokinetic Flow in a Heterogeneous Microchannel

Subrata Bera and Somnath Bhattacharyya

Abstract The motivation of the present work is to form vortical flow by designing potential heterogeneity in a different manner on both walls of a microchannel. A complete mathematical model of two-dimensional is considered to control the solute transport and mixing efficiency in the combined flow for electroosmotic and pressure gradient. The characteristics equation of this model is governed by simultaneously solving the nonlinear Poisson equation, the Nernst–Planck equations and modified Navier–Stokes equations. The pressure gradient forms in flow direction due to potential heterogeneity of microchannel wall. The vortex forms on patch, increases with ionic concentration and diminishes with the favorable pressure gradient case. The average flow is always increased for pressure-assisted electroosmotic flow. The vortex formation in electroosmotic flow has very much essential for solute mixing. The potential heterogeneity in walls develops a vortex which generates the pressure gradient to promote the mixing efficiency. The mixing performance is compared with the plane channel and several other forms of surface heterogeneity such as patches with symmetric and asymmetric manners and single patch. The mixing performance increases by introducing potential heterogeneity in channel surface. The potential heterogeneity in an asymmetric manner gives maximum mixing performance of a solute. There is no such effective variation on solute mixing between symmetric and asymmetric potential heterogeneity cases. The mixing index decreases with imposed pressure gradient for all forms of surface heterogeneity.

Keywords Electroosmotic-pressure driven flow · Nernst–Planck model · Modified Navier–Stokes equations · Surface heterogeneity · Solute mixing

S. Bera (✉)
Department of Mathematics, National Institute of Technology Silchar, Silchar 788010, India
e-mail: subrata@math.nits.ac.in

S. Bhattacharyya
Department of Mathematics, Indian Institute of Technology Kharagpur, Kharagpur 721302, India

S. Bhattacharyya et al. (eds.), *Mathematical Modeling and Computational Tools*, Springer Proceedings in Mathematics & Statistics 320,
https://doi.org/10.1007/978-981-15-3615-1_2

1 Introduction

The microfluidic technology has large aspect of chemical and biological applications such as solute control and mixing, molecular analysis, pumping and separation [1–5] among many other applications. Studies on transport phenomena of charged species and neutral solute in microchannel have made a great advancement in colloidal and biochemical sciences. Due to its enormous importance, several research groups worldwide are engaged in enlightening the physics behind those physicochemical phenomenons. When an electrolyte comes in contact with channel wall, a layer forms near microchannel wall with nonzero charge is called electric double layer (EDL). The thickness of this layer can be measured by the Debye length. The ζ potential is the potential drop between the liquid–solid interface and the bulk solution outside the EDL. Electroosmosis [6] is the movement of liquid through a channel or capillary under the influence of an external electric field, by interacting with the surplus ion charged in EDL. The electroosmotic flow direction and rate depend upon electric field strength, concentration of electrolytes, surface charge the channel or capillary, viscosity, pressure, temperature, etc. [7].

Different authors investigated the several aspects of EOF in microchannel both theoretically and experimentally. Conlisk and McFerran [8] investigated the electroosmotic flow in a nanochannel with overlapping EDL by applying electric field. Experimental studies of EOF were carried out by Sadr et al. [9] in microchannel where the height and double layer thickness are in same order. Park et al. [10] studied the difference in the linear Nernst–Planck model and the Poisson–Boltzmann model for EOF in microchannel. The parametrical studies were carried out numerically by Červenka et al. [11] to achieve the specified nature of micropumps. Chai and Shi [12] studied the EOF in microchannel with lattice Boltzmann model (LBM). Bera and Bhattacharyya [13] numerically studied the electrokinetic effects near a polarizable material situated on lower wall of a microchannel. Xuan et al. [14] studied theoretically and experimentally about the different aspects of Joule heating on EOF in microcapillary.

The nature of EOF depends upon the magnitude and sign of zeta-potential in microchannel wall. This non-uniformity in potential develops variation on electrokinetic flow and causes the microvortices which are important for mixing performance, ion separation, etc. The formation of microvortices on electroosmotic flow in microchannels with heterogeneous surface potential was studied by Ajdari [15]. Yariv [16] investigated electroosmotic flow in the vicinity of microchannel wall surface charge transitions. They examined the validity on the thin-Debye-layer (TDL) approximation and linearized Boltzmann–Poisson (LBP) model for different circumstances in the neighborhood of charge discontinuity. Ghosal [17] investigated the electroosmotic flow at arbitrary cross-section of a microchannel. Erickson and Li [18] observed the circulation region by introducing potential heterogeneity in channel wall.

Different aspects of mixed electroosmotic flow and pressure driven flow are investigated by different authors, considering the linear Boltzmann distribution. The analytic solutions for mixed flow have been established by Dutta and Beskok [19]. Dutta [20] theoretically studied the separation method of analytes by introducing a pressure gradient combined with EOF. Bera and Bhattacharyya [21] investigated the mixed effects of electroosmotic flow and pressure driven flow and mass transport in a microchannel using the Poisson–Nernst–Plank model. A mathematical model for mixed EO-pressure driven flow has been developed by Mondal et al. [22] for high surface potential and overlapping EDL. Xuan and Li [23] theoretically studied that the solutewall interactions in nanochannel in mixed EO-pressure driven flow.

Species mixing in microchannel and nanochannel becomes challenging task because of small value of Reynolds number. Several authors studied different ways to enhance the mixing performance. The mixing depends on the vortex strength which is induced by the potential patches and surface heterogeneity of the channel. Jain and Nandakumar [24] studied the minimum pattern in heterogeneous potential for improved electrokinetic micromixing performance in three-dimensional microchannel. Alizadeh et al. [25] developed the mixing enhancement method by inserting temperature-patterned walls in microchannels. Loucaides et al. [26] demonstrated the array devices for combined pumping and mixing by alternative current. Tian et al. [27] studied trade-off between solute transport and mixing through heterogeneous microchannels. Dutta [28] investigated the sidewalls' effects for the transport of neutral samples with low zeta-potential within conduits.

In view of the current status, the present work is a great significance as it provides a complete numerical solution by considering the full nonlinear mathematical model. The mathematical model and the numerical tool to simulate the combined EO-pressure driven flow problems are found to be efficient in analyzing the inherent mechanism of the ion dynamics. The fluid convection also plays an important role in the present study. In addition, fluid flow is based on Stokes equation without considering the inertia effects. We considered the Nernst–Planck equations, the modified Navier–Stokes equations and Poisson equation. The investigation has been made to enhance the mixing efficiency by introducing different values of pressure gradient and heterogeneity ζ_p potential. The effective Reynolds number (Re) depends upon height of channel and average flow of mixed EO-pressure driven flow. The external pressure and heterogeneous ζ_p-potential have a strong impact on electroosmotic flow and solutes mixing.

2 Mathematical Model

We have considered a microchannel, filled with an incompressible Newtonian electrolyte. The height of the channel is h and channel width is W where ($h \ll W$). Electrodes are placed at the upstream and the downstream of the channel, and thus, the electric field and pressure gradient ($\mathrm{d}p/\mathrm{d}x$) are acting along axial direction. The surface potential heterogeneity is designed by introducing different zeta-potential of microchannel wall (Fig. 1). The non-dimensional number $\Lambda = E_0 h/\phi_0$ indicates the strength of the electric field E_0.

Fig. 1 Diagram of an asymmetric potential heterogeneous microchannel of length $h = 10\ \mu\text{m}$ and applied electric filed $E_0 = 10^4$ V/m

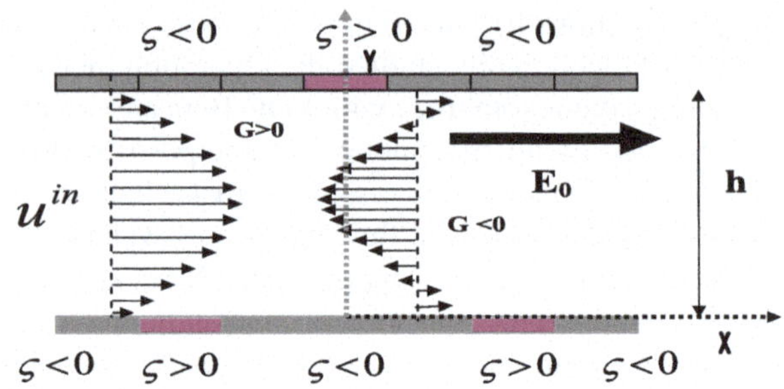

The net-charged density ρ_e^* is expressed as

$$\nabla \cdot (\epsilon_e \mathbf{E}^*) = -\epsilon_e \nabla^2 \Phi^* = \rho_e^* = \sum_i z_i e n_i^* \tag{1}$$

Here, e is the elementary electric charge, Φ^* is the electric potential, z_i are the valance, n_i^* are ionic concentration, and ϵ_e is the permittivity. The parameter $\kappa = [(2e^2 n_0)/(\epsilon_e k_B T)]^{1/2}$ is called the electric double layer thickness. We scale potential Φ^* by $\phi_0\ (= k_B T/e)$ and concentration of the electrolyte n_i^* by bulk value n_0, the coordinates (x, y, z) by $(l,\ h,\ W)$, respectively. Here, T is the absolute temperature, and k_B is the Boltzmann constant. We have taken symmetric electrolyte of valence $z_i = \pm 1$ and denoted them, respectively, as cations (g) and anions (f). The equation of induced potential is given in non-dimensional form as

$$B^2 \frac{\partial^2 \phi}{\partial x^2} + \frac{\partial^2 \phi}{\partial y^2} + C^2 \frac{\partial^2 \phi}{\partial z^2} = -\frac{(\kappa h)^2}{2}(g - f) \tag{2}$$

The distribution of the ion concentration is expressed by the Nernst–Planck equation as

$$\frac{\partial n_i^*}{\partial t^*} + \nabla \cdot \mathbf{N}_i^* = 0 \tag{3}$$

here, $\mathbf{N}_i^*\ (= -D_i \nabla n_i^* + n_i^* \omega_i z_i F \mathbf{E} + n_i^* \mathbf{q}^*)$ is the net ion flux. Here, D_i is the diffusivity, Faraday's constant is F, and ω_i is the mobility of ions. We scale velocity $\mathbf{q}^*\ (= u^*,\ v^*,\ w^*)$ by $U_{HS} (= \epsilon_e E_0 \phi_0 / \mu$ which is called the Helmholtz–Smoluchowski velocity) and time t^* by h/U_{HS}). The Reynolds number, $\mathrm{Re}_{HS} = U_{HS} h/\nu$, Schmidt number, $\mathrm{Sc} = \nu / Di$, and Peclet number, $\mathrm{Pe} = \mathrm{Re}_{HS} Sc$. Here, kinematic viscosity, $\nu = \mu/\rho$; ρ is the density, and μ is the viscosity. We have denoted $B = h/l$ and $C = h/W$. The transport equations for ions can be expressed in dimensionless form as follow

$$\mathrm{Pe}\frac{\partial g}{\partial t} - \left(B^2 \frac{\partial^2 g}{\partial x^2} + \frac{\partial^2 g}{\partial y^2} + C^2 \frac{\partial^2 g}{\partial z^2}\right) + \mathrm{Pe}\left(\mathrm{B}u \frac{\partial g}{\partial x} + v \frac{\partial g}{\partial y} + C w \frac{\partial g}{\partial z}\right)$$

$$+\left[(\Lambda - B\frac{\partial \phi}{\partial x})\frac{\partial g}{\partial x} - \frac{\partial \phi}{\partial y}\frac{\partial g}{\partial y} - C\frac{\partial \phi}{\partial z}\frac{\partial g}{\partial z}\right] + \frac{(\kappa h)^2 g}{2}(g - f) = 0 \tag{4}$$

$$\mathrm{Pe}\frac{\partial f}{\partial t} - \left(B^2\frac{\partial^2 f}{\partial x^2} + \frac{\partial^2 f}{\partial y^2} + C^2\frac{\partial^2 f}{\partial z^2}\right) + \mathrm{Pe}\left(Bu\frac{\partial f}{\partial x} + v\frac{\partial f}{\partial y} + Cw\frac{\partial f}{\partial z}\right)$$

$$-\left[(\Lambda - B\frac{\partial \phi}{\partial x})\frac{\partial f}{\partial x} - \frac{\partial \phi}{\partial y}\frac{\partial f}{\partial y} - C\frac{\partial \phi}{\partial z}\frac{\partial f}{\partial z}\right] - \frac{(\kappa h)^2 f}{2}(g - f) = 0 \tag{5}$$

The fluid transport equation is generated by the Navier–Stokes equations as

$$\nabla \cdot \mathbf{q}^* = 0 \tag{6}$$

$$\rho\left[\frac{\partial \mathbf{q}^*}{\partial t^*} + (\mathbf{q}^* \cdot \nabla)\mathbf{q}^*\right] = -\nabla p^* + \mu\nabla^2\mathbf{q}^* + \rho_e^*\mathbf{E}^* \tag{7}$$

where the $\mathbf{q}^*$ velocity of component u^*, v^* and w^* are, respectively, acting in x, y and z axis. Here, we scaled pressure p^* by $\mu U_{\mathrm{HS}}/h$. The non-dimensional equations for fluid flow are given as,

$$B\frac{\partial u}{\partial x} + \frac{\partial v}{\partial y} + C\frac{\partial w}{\partial z} = 0 \tag{8}$$

$$\begin{aligned}\mathrm{Re_{HS}}\frac{\partial u}{\partial t} + \mathrm{Re_{HS}}\left(\mathrm{Bu}\frac{\partial u}{\partial x} + v\frac{\partial u}{\partial y} + Cw\frac{\partial u}{\partial z}\right)\\ = -B\frac{\partial p}{\partial x} + (g - f)\frac{(\kappa h)^2}{2}\left(\Lambda - B\frac{\partial \phi}{\partial x}\right) + \nabla^2 u\end{aligned} \tag{9}$$

$$\begin{aligned}\mathrm{Re_{HS}}\frac{\partial v}{\partial t} + \mathrm{Re_{HS}}\left(Bu\frac{\partial v}{\partial x} + v\frac{\partial v}{\partial y} + Cw\frac{\partial v}{\partial z}\right)\\ = -\frac{\partial p}{\partial y} - (g - f)\frac{(\kappa h)^2}{2}\frac{\partial \phi}{\partial y} + \nabla^2 v\end{aligned} \tag{10}$$

$$\begin{aligned}\mathrm{Re_{HS}}\frac{\partial w}{\partial t} + \mathrm{Re_{HS}}\left(Bu\frac{\partial w}{\partial x} + v\frac{\partial w}{\partial y} + Cw\frac{\partial w}{\partial z}\right)\\ = -C\frac{\partial p}{\partial z} - C(g - f)\frac{(\kappa h)^2}{2}\frac{\partial \phi}{\partial z} + \nabla^2 w\end{aligned} \tag{11}$$

where $\nabla^2 = B^2\frac{\partial^2}{\partial x^2} + \frac{\partial^2}{\partial y^2} + C^2\frac{\partial^2}{\partial z^2}$. We considered the channel width (W) as order of the length scale, and hence, $C = h/W \ll 1$. Thus, we can consider it as $2D$ flow.

The boundary condition in channel wall is taken as follows

$$\phi = \zeta,\ \mathbf{N}_i \cdot \mathbf{n} = 0,\ u = v = 0, \quad y = 0, 1 \tag{12}$$

where $\mathbf{n}$ is unit normal in outwards direction. The potential along homogeneous part is ζ, and for heterogenous parts, $\zeta = \zeta_p$. The upstream and downstream conditions are followed by the Bera and Bhattacharyya [21] using the Debye–Huckel approximation.

$$\phi = [\zeta_1 \sinh(\kappa h(1-y)) + \zeta_2 \sinh(\kappa h y)]/\sinh(\kappa h) \tag{13}$$

$$u = Gy(1-y) + y(\zeta_1 - \zeta_2) - \zeta_1(1 - \phi/\zeta_1) \tag{14}$$

$$g = \mathrm{e}^{-\phi} \quad \text{and} \quad f = \mathrm{e}^{\phi} \tag{15}$$

Here, ζ_1, ζ_2 are, respectively, the zeta-potential values at $y = 0$ and $y = 1$. The pressure gradient is determined by the scaled quantity as $G = -\frac{1}{\mu}\frac{\mathrm{d}p}{\mathrm{d}x}\frac{h^2}{2}/U_{\mathrm{HS}}$.

2.1 Mass Transport Equation

We have also considered the transport of electrokinetic sample with considering no absorption of sample through channel wall. The solute transport equation is given in non-dimensional form as

$$\frac{\partial c}{\partial t} + (\mathbf{q}.\nabla)c = \frac{1}{\mathrm{Pe_s}}\nabla^2 c \tag{16}$$

Here, $c(x, t)$ is the non-dimensional sample concentration, and Peclet number is defined as $\mathrm{Pe_s} = U_{\mathrm{HS}}h/D$; diffusion coefficient of the sample is D. We assume no mass flux condition at the wall of the microchannel and

$c = c_{\mathrm{in}}$ on the upstream at $x = -L$; $\frac{\partial^2 c}{\partial x^2} = 0$ on the downstream $x = L$ and $\frac{\partial c}{\partial y} = 0$ on the channel wall $y = 0$ and 1
where c_{in} is defined as $c_{\mathrm{in}} = 1$ in lower half of upstream $(0 \le y \le 0.5)$ and $c_{\mathrm{in}} = 0$ in upper half of upstream $(0.5 \le y \le 1)$.

3 Numerical Schemes

These coupled dimensionless governing equations are solved simultaneously in finite volume method over the staggered grid scheme. The discretized form of these equations is calculated by integrating these equations within each control volume. An upwind scheme named as Quadratic Upwind Interpolation Convective Kinemat-

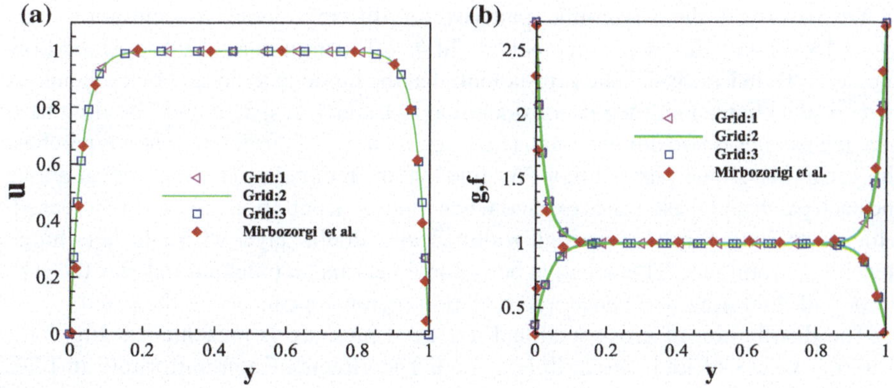

Fig. 2 Comparing the numerical results with Mirbozorgi et al. [31] and considering the grid size effects in pure electroosmotic flow ($G = 0.0$) within a microchannel of height h as 10 μm, Debye–Huckel parameter $\kappa h = 32$ ($\lambda = 0.3125$ μm) and zeta-potential $\zeta = -1$. **a** Axial velocity u and **b** species concentration g, f

ics (QUICK) [29] is used to discretize the convective and electromigration terms. A first-order implicit method is used in time derivative terms. These equations are iteratively solved through the Semi-Implicit Method for Pressure link Equation (SIMPLE) [30]. We have assumed the initial approximation for induced potential ϕ in every cell.

We have taken the non-uniform grid distribution along vertical direction of the channel and uniform grids in horizontal direction (Fig. 2), and δt is considered as 0.001. To validate grid size independency, these computational works have been done in three different meshes as grid 1: 200×240, grid 2: 400×240 and grid 3: 400×500 for pure EOF($G = 0$) and compared with Mirbozorgi et al. [31]. We have taken a non-uniform meshes where δy is varying between 0.005 to 0.01 with δx is either 0.02 (grid 1) or $\delta x = 0.01$ (grid 2). In grid 3, we have taken $\delta x = 0.01$ and $0.0025 \leq \delta y \leq 0.005$. It concludes that the results (Fig. 2a, b) obtained by grid 2 and 3 agree very well and are close with Mirbozorgi et al. [31]. In this away, we consider that the grid 2 is for suitable for our computation.

4 Results and Discussions

We considered that the channel height $h = 10$ μm and electric field $E_0 = 10^4$ V/m, and thus, the scaled parameter for strength of electric field $\Lambda = 4.0$. The zeta-potential (ζ_p) along the modulated surface is taken to be of different sign to that ζ-potential on the other portions of channel wall. The diffusion coefficient is considered to be as equal as $D_{\pm} = 1.3 \times 10^{-10}$ m^2/s.

We described the streamline patterns for different ionic concentration, i.e., $\kappa h = 15$, 40 and 100, when channel height $h = 10\mu m$ in pure electroosmotic flow (i.e., $G = 0$) in Fig. 3a–c. The zeta-potential at the homogeneous and heterogeneous parts of the channel surface is considered as -1 and 1, respectively. The flow field near the patches is two dimensional. However, far away of the heterogeneous patches, the streamline shows parallel flow. We find that the recirculation zones appear above the each patch and these zones expand when ionic concentration, i.e., κh is increased. This electrostatic force is very high within electric double layer where the net-charge density is prominent. The negative body force near patch potential induces the separation of fluid flow, and hence, recirculation region appears above the patch.

The distribution of cross-sectional averaged pressure is presented in Fig. 4 for different values of ionic strength (i.e., κh). The effects of non-uniformity in EDL

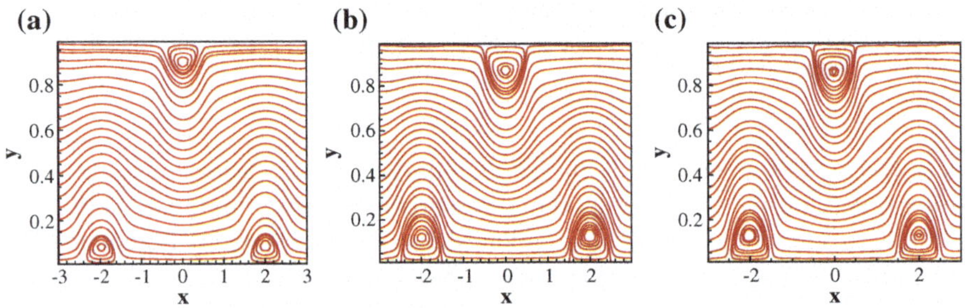

Fig. 3 Streamline profile for different concentration for EOF ($G = 0$) when surface potential $\zeta = -1$, heterogeneous potential $\zeta_p = 1$ and electric field $E_0 = 10^4$ V/m. **a** For $\kappa h = 15$; **b** for $\kappa h = 40$ and **c** for $\kappa h = 100$

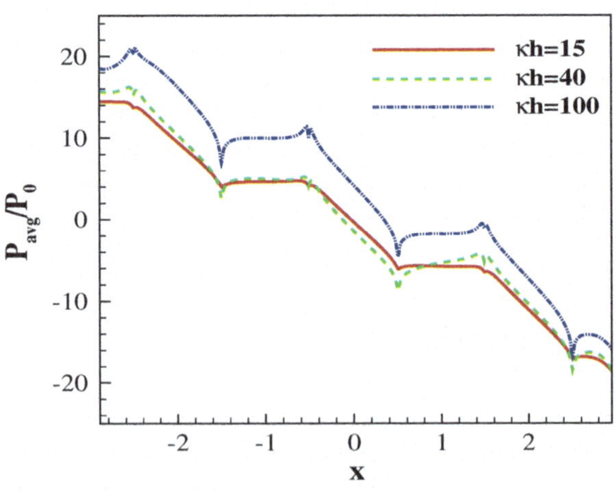

Fig. 4 Variation of averaged pressure (P_{avg}) at various values of ionic strength surface potential $\zeta = -1$, heterogeneous potential $\zeta_p = 1$ and electric field $E_0 = 10^4$ V/m at $G = -5$, 0, 5. Here, $p_0 = 0.018$ Pa

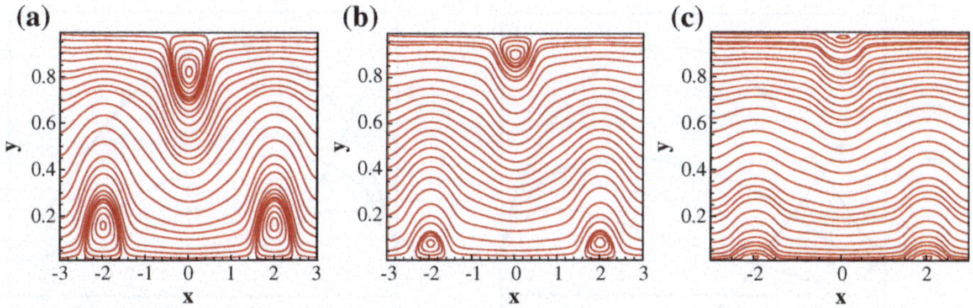

Fig. 5 Streamline profile for different Reynolds number (Re) when surface potential $\zeta = -1$, heterogeneous potential $\zeta_p = 1$ and electric field $E_0 = 10^4$ V/m. **a** For $G = -2$; **b** for $G = 0$ and **c** for $G = 3$

due to the heterogeneity of surface potential lead an important role in vortical flow, and hence, an induced pressure gradient develops close to this region. Figure 4 shows that the pressure distribution becomes strong as the value of ionic concentration is increased.

We now consider the effect of Reynolds number by varying pressure gradient G while U_{HS} is kept constant. Figure 5a–c shows the different patterns of streamline for different positive and negative pressure gradients cases such as $G = -2, 0, 3$. We have presented the streamlines patterns for three different cases mainly pure EOF case ($G = 0$), pressure-assisting EOF ($G = 3$) and pressure-opposing EOF ($G = -2$). The average flow is increased by 60% with comparing between the pure EOF $G = 0$ and favorable pressure gradient $G = 3$. These streamline patterns indicate the occurrence of separation in fluid flow and cause the vortex formation on the heterogeneous potential surface for the low external pressure gradient G. The separation of flow and formation of vortex cannot be expressed by a linear Poisson–Boltzmann model. We observe that vortex increases when the external pressure gradient G acts in opposite direction of electroosmotic flow and vortex shrinks for favorable pressure gradient cases. The electroosmotic forces have a significant impact in the EDL region near the channel wall. The fluid flow away from the wall is dominated by pressure gradient and viscosity.

Velocities' profiles (u, v) for various values of imposed pressure G at $x = -2$ and $x = 0$ are shown in Fig. 6, respectively. There is surface heterogeneity in potential in the lower surface at $-2.5 \leq x \leq -1.5$ and the upper surface at $-0.5 \leq x \leq 0.5$, respectively. Here, we have considered that the value of potential is 1 in heterogeneous surface and -1 in the rest of the channel surface. First column of Fig. 6 shows that both the axial and transverse velocities u and v increase with the increase of pressure gradient G when the potential patch is in the lower surface of the channel at $x = -2$. But at $x = 0$, i.e., where the potential patch is in the upper surface of microchannel, the axial velocity u increases with the pressure gradient G and transverse velocity v decreases with the imposed pressure. The imposed pressure G which is applied along x-direction mainly affects the axial velocity u. There is a small contribution on transverse velocity v in this region. For all the above cases, the

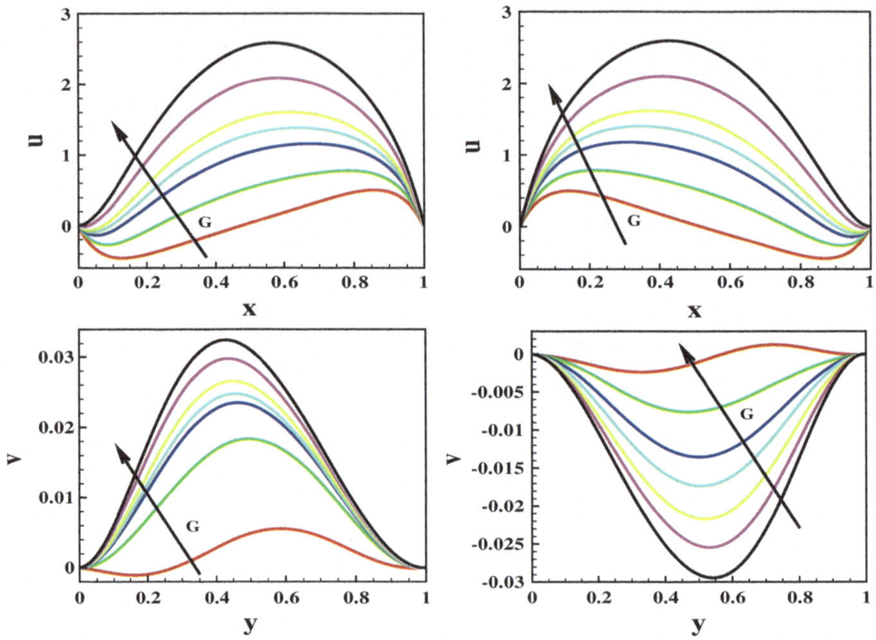

(a) $x = -2.0$ (b) $x = 0$

Fig. 6 Distribution of velocity profiles (u, v) at different Re when $h = 10$ μm, $\lambda = 0.6$ μm, $\zeta = -1$, $\zeta_p = 1$ and $E_0 = 10^4$ V/m at different G. **a** First column corresponds to $x = -2.0$; **b** second column corresponds to $x = 0.0$. Arrows are indicating the increasing direction of G such as $G = -5, -3, -1, 0, 1, 3, 5$. Here, $U_{HS} = 1.8 \times 10^{-4}$ m/s

effect of external pressure gradient G is more prominent in the u velocity profile than v velocity. The general electroosmotic flow characteristic such as plug-like profile and core neutrality happens for pure EOF $G = 0$ with same surface potential cases as pointed in Fig. 2 The electroosmotic forces have great impact in microchannel wall region where electric double layer is formed. This double layer along with potential heterogeneity produces an opposite effect in electroosmotic flow compared to the electric double layer along with homogenous part of microchannel. This non-uniformity in electric double layer is the main cause to develop the vortical flow on potential heterogeneity region. We presented the both positive and negative values of external pressure gradient G in Fig. 6.

4.1 Solute Mixing

We regulated the solute mixing by introducing non-homogeneity in surface potential and imposed pressure gradient. We have considered $C = 1$ at lower half and $C = 0$

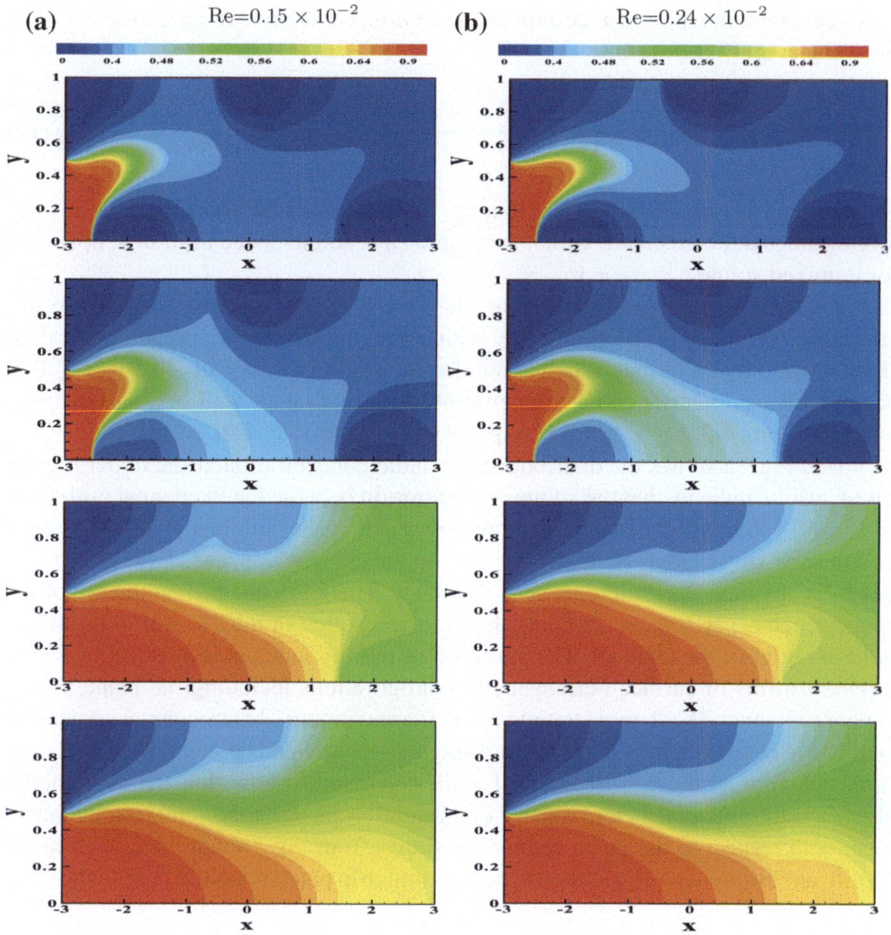

Fig. 7 Distribution of solute concentration within the channel at different times, i.e., $t^* = 0.5, 5.5, 55.6, 556.5$ s, when $h = 10\ \mu$m, $\lambda = 0.6\ \mu$m ($\kappa h = 15$), $\zeta = -2$, $\zeta_p = 2$ and $E_0 = 10^4$V/m. **a** EOF with $G = 0$ and **b** mixed EOF with $G = 3$. Here, $Pe_s = 13.83$

at upper half of upstream of channel. The distribution of solute near the close vicinity of the potential heterogeneity portion is illustrated in Fig. 7a, b for pure EOF and combined favorable pressure gradient ($G = 3$) cases, respectively, for different times. The average flow rate increases for favorable pressure-assisted flow than Pure EOF. In pure electroosmotic flow, solute transport is governed by the diffusion, but the effects of advection are prominent for favorable pressure gradient case $G = 3$.

To calculate the mixing at certain cross-section, we defined mixing efficiency (η) by Wang et al. [32] as follow

$$\eta = \left(1.0 - \frac{\int |c - c_\infty| \mathrm{d}y}{\int |c - c_0| \mathrm{d}y}\right) \times 100\% \tag{17}$$

where c is the concentration distribution, c_∞ is the solute concentration at fully mixing stage at downstream which is 0.5 and c_0 is solute concentration at upstream for unmixed solute, i.e., 0 or 1.

Here, we have compared the mixing efficiency with different forms of surface heterogeneity including the plane channel with homogeneous surface potential. We considered some forms of patch such as single patch at the lower wall $-0.5 \leq x \leq 0.5$, patches with symmetric and asymmetric at lower and upper wall in a unit distance (starting from $-2.5 \leq x \leq 1.5$). A perfect solute mixing can be achieved when $C = 0.5$. Fig. 8a shows the distribution of solute concentration at the outlet region. These results indicate that the solute concentration become flat in channel outlet and close to 0.5 for symmetric and asymmetric patch cases, and hence, the efficiency of solute mixing increases. These circulation zones which appear above the modulated surface increases solute mixing efficiency. The vortices form on the top of the heterogeneous surface and promote the unmixed solute in inlet to shift with mixed fluid in outlet of the channel. The variation of mixing index is shown in Fig. 8b for different forms of surface heterogeneity configurations including the plane homogeneous channel. We demonstrated results for asymmetric heterogeneous potential, symmetric heterogeneous potential and single heterogeneous potential with the constant potential of the rest of channel wall. Our results show that the asymmetric patches with potential heterogeneity configuration produce 12% mixing enhancement with respect to the plane channel. It shows from Fig. 8b that there is no much significant difference for symmetric and asymmetric patch potential cases. The mix-

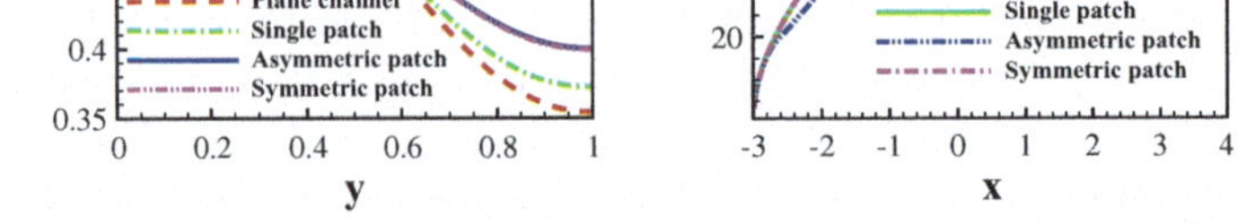

Fig. 8 Profile for **a** non-dimensional solute concentration at outlet ($x = 3$) and **b** mixing efficiency (η) along the channel length for EOF $G = 0$ for different position of the patch when $h = 10\ \mu$m, $\lambda = 0.1\ \mu$m, $\zeta_p = 2$, $\zeta = -2$ and $E_0 = 10^4$V/m

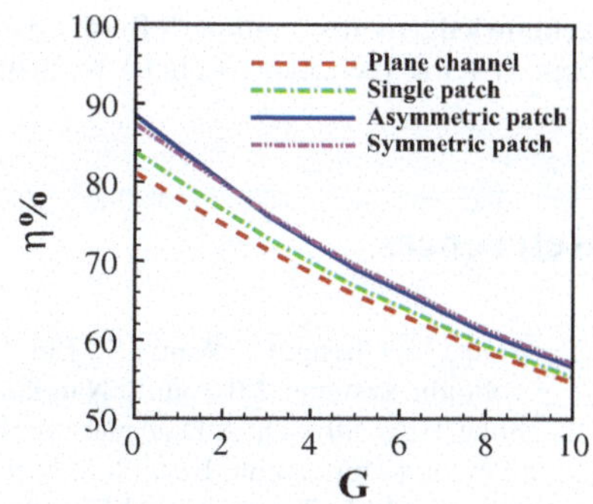

Fig. 9 Variation of mixing efficiency (η) with imposed pressure gradient (G), when $h = 10\ \mu\text{m}$, $\lambda = 0.1\ \mu\text{m}$, $\zeta_P = 2$, $\zeta = -2$ and $E_0 = 10^4$ V/m

ing efficiency is increased for single potential patch case than plane homogeneous channel, and it is maximum for asymmetric patch cases.

Figure 9 presents the pressure gradient effects on the mixing efficiency (η) for various models for potential heterogeneity. The increase of pressure gradient decreases the mixing efficiency for all the above flow configurations. The advection effects increase with Peclet number which leads the reduction of mixing efficacy for all the above cases.

5 Conclusions

The current article presents a numerical study of mixed EO-pressure driven flow and solute mixing in different forms of surface heterogeneity in a rectangular microchannel. A novel model is presented which patterns of surface potential heterogeneous are preferable in order to increase mixing efficacy. Since EOF depends upon the amount and the polarity of surface potential of the wall, a vortex is generated near the adjacent of patch potential. The recirculating vortex forms above the heterogeneous surface, and the average EOF velocity increases with ionic concentration. The nonlinear characteristic is prominent for combined flow on heterogeneity potential region for lower values of external pressure gradient. For large pressure gradient, mixed flow takes the form as Poiseuille flow, but there exists a transverse velocity. The vortex, appeared in heterogeneous region, diminishes for favorable pressure gradient and increases for adverse pressure gradient. The mixed EO-pressure driven flow above the patch indicates nonlinear characteristics for the lower value of external pressure gradient where the electric body force is comparable with this external pressure gradient. Inertial effects on heterogeneous region are not negligible for small values of external pressure gradient. The variation of body force factor is faster in lower value of external pressure gradient. The microvortex formation has very important role in producing solute dispersion and hence promotes mixing. The mixing performance is increased with the potential heterogeneity in the channel wall, and it is maximum for asymmetric surface potential patch cases.

Acknowledgements Author (S.Bera) acknowledges the Science and Engineering Research Board, Dept. of Sci. & Tech., Govt. of India, for financial support through project grant (ECR/2016/000771).

References

1. Wang, X., Cheng, C., Wang, S., Liu, S.: Electroosmotic pumps and their applications in microfluidic systems. Microfluid Nanofluid **6**, 145–162 (2009)
2. Stone, H.A., Stroock, A.D., Ajdari, A.: Engineering flows in small devices: microfluidics toward a lab-on-a-chip. Annu. Rev. Fluid Mech. **36**, 381–411 (2004)
3. Ewinga, M.M., Thompsona, J.M., McLarena, R.S., Purpero, V.M., Thomas, K.J., Dobrowski, P.A., DeGroot, G.A., Romsos, E.L., Storts, D.R.: Human DNA quantification and sample quality assessment: developmental validation of the PowerQuant® system. Forensic Sci. Int. Genet. **23**, 166–177 (2016)
4. Srinivasan, V., Pamula, V.K., Fair, R.B.: An integrated digital microfluidic lab-on-a-chip for clinical diagnostics on human physiological fluids. Lab Chip **4**, 310–315 (2004)
5. Nguyen, N.-T., Wu, Z.: Micromixersa review. J. Micromech. Microeng. **15**, R1–R16 (2005)
6. Masiliyah, J.H., Bhattacharjee, S.: Electrokinetic and Colloid Transport Phenomena. Wiley, Hoboken, New Jersey (2006)
7. Probstein, R.F.: Physicochemical Hydrodynamics: An Introduction, 2nd edn. Wiley Interscssience, New York (1994)
8. Conlisk, A.T., McFerran, J.: Mass transfer and flow in electrically charged micro-and nanochannels. Anal. Chem. **74**, 2139–2150 (2002)
9. Sadr, R., Yoda, M., Zheng, Z., Conlisk, A.T.: An experimental study of electro-osmotic flow in rectangular microchannels. J. Fluid Mech. **506**, 357–367 (2004)
10. Park, H.M., Lee, J.S., Kim, T.W.: Comparison of the Nernst Planck model and the Poisson Boltzmann model for electroosmotic flows in microchannels. J. Colloid Interface Sci. **315**, 731–739 (2007)
11. Červenka, P., Přibyl, M., Šnita, D.: Numerical study on AC electroosmosis in microfluidic channels. Microelectron. Eng. **86**, 1333–1336 (2009)
12. Chai, Z., Shi, B.: Simulation of electro-osmotic flow in microchannel with lattice Boltzmann method. Phys. Lett. A **364**, 183–188 (2007)
13. Bera, S., Bhattacharyya, S.: Electroosmotic flow in the vicinity of a conducting obstacle mounted on the surface of a wide microchannel. Int. J. Eng. Sci. **94**, 128–138 (2015)
14. Xuan, X., Xu, B., Sintonb, D., Li, D.: Electroosmotic flow with Joule heating effects. Lab Chip **4**, 230–236 (2004)
15. Ajdari, A.: Electro-osmosis on inhomogeneously charged surfaces. Phys. Rev. Lett. **75**, 755–758 (1995)
16. Yariv, E.: Electro-osmotic flow near a surface charge discontinuity. J. Fluid Mech. **521**, 181–189 (2004)
17. Ghosal, S.: Lubrication theory for electro-osmotic flow in a microfluidic channel of slowly varying cross-section and wall charge. J. Fluid Mech. **459**, 103–128 (2002)
18. Erickson, D., Li, D.: Influence of surface heterogeneity on electrokinetically driven microfluidic mixing. Langmuir **18**, 1883–1892 (2002)
19. Dutta, P., Beskok, A.: Analytical solution of combined electroosmotic pressure driven flows in two-dimensional straight channels: finite Debye layer effects. Anal. Chem. **73**, 1979–1986 (2001)
20. Dutta, P.: A numerical analysis of nanofluidic charge based separations using a combination of electrokinetic and hydrodynamic flows. Chem. Eng. Sci. **93**, 124–130 (2013)
21. Bera, S., Bhattacharyya, S.: On mixed electroosmotic-pressure driven flow and mass transport in microchannels. Int. J. Eng. Sci. **62**, 165–176 (2013)

22. Mondal, M., Misra, P.R., De, S.: Combined electroosmotic and pressure driven flow in a microchannel at high zeta potential and overlapping electrical double layer. Int. J. Therm. Sci. **86**, 48–59 (2014)
23. Xuan, X., Li, D.: Solute separation in nanofluidic channels: pressure-driven or electric field-driven. Electrophoresis **28**, 627–634 (2007)
24. Jain, M., Nandakumar, K.: Optimal patterning of heterogeneous surface charge for improved electrokinetic micromixing. Comput. Chem. Eng. **49**, 18–24 (2013)
25. Alizadeh, A., Zhang, L., Wang, M.: Mixing enhancement of low-Reynolds electro-osmotic flows in microchannels with temperature-patterned walls. J. Colloid Interface Sci. **431**, 50–63 (2014)
26. Loucaides, N., Ramos, A., Georghiou, G.E.: Configurable AC electroosmotic pumping and mixing. Microelectron. Eng. **90**, 47–50 (2012)
27. Tian, F., Li, B., Kwok, D.Y.: Tradeoff between mixing and transport for electroosmotic flow in heterogeneous microchannels with nonuniform surface potentials. Langmuir **21**, 1126–1131 (2005)
28. Dutta, D.: Solutal transport in rectangular nanochannels under pressure-driven flow conditions. Microfluid Nanofluid **10**, 691–696 (2011)
29. Leonard, B.P.: A stable and accurate convective modelling procedure based on quadratic up-stream interpolation. Comput. Methods Appl. Mech. Eng. **19**, 59–98 (1979)
30. Fletcher, C.A.J.: Computational Techniques for Fluid Dynamics, Vol. I and II. Springer Series in Computational Phyics, 2nd edn. Springer, Heidelberg, New York (1991)
31. Mirbozorgi, S.A., Niazmand, H., Renkrizbulut, M.: Electroosmotic flow in reservoir-connected flat microchannels with non-uniform zeta potential. J. Fluid Eng.-T ASME., **128**, 1133–1143 (2006)
32. Wang, Y., Zhe, J., Dutta, P., Chung, B.T.: A Microfluidic mixer utilizing electrokinetic relay switching and asymmetric flow geometries. J. Fluid Eng.-T ASME., **129**, 395–403 (2007)

Effect of Temperature-Dependent Electrostatic Parameters on Electroosmotic Flow with Hydrophobic Patches

Sirsendu Sekhar Barman and Somnath Bhattacharyya

Abstract Microfluidics has broad utilizations in the field of medical science. The architecture of microfluidic devices desires an improved compassionate of the action of flow and heat transfer attributes in micro- or nano-channel. Electroosmosis is one of the main electrokinetic effects. For the hydrophobic surfaces, a slip boundary condition is established. The present study investigates the effect of temperature-dependent electrostatic parameters on electroosmotic flow with hydrophobic patches. The present study comprises the coupled Poisson–Boltzmann equation, the modified Navier–Stokes equations, the modified Nernst–Planck equation, and the modified energy equation. Governing equations with proper boundary conditions are solved numerically through control volume approach over a staggered grid arrangement. The results are expressed in terms of velocity profiles and surface temperature. Also, we have considered average entropy generation, S_{avg}; average Bejan number, Be_{avg}.

Keywords Debye length · Slip coefficient · Joule number · Average entropy · Average Bejan number

1 Introduction

For the last few years, lab-on-a-chip (or Biochip) technology has a rapid development. Electroosmosis is being broadly exploited as the propulsive forces to control liquid flows in microfluidic devices used for chemical diagnosis and medical diagnosis [1–4]. Electrosmosis is the procedure of moving of an ionized liquid relative to an immobile charged surface under the response of an applied electric field. The rate of flow and direction of electroosmotic flow (EOF) are conducted by many aspects, such as the electric field strength, electrolyte concentration, surface charge density on the surface of the channel or capillary, temperature, pressure, and viscosity. For a negatively charged inner part of the channel wall, the positive charge forms beside to the surface, and thus a diffuse layer of dense charge forms. This layer is termed as an

S. S. Barman (✉) · S. Bhattacharyya
Department of Mathematics, Indian Institute of Technology Kharagpur, Kharagpur 721302, India
e-mail: sirsendu012@maths.iitkgp.ernet.in

S. Bhattacharyya et al. (eds.), *Mathematical Modeling and Computational Tools*, Springer Proceedings in Mathematics & Statistics 320,
https://doi.org/10.1007/978-981-15-3615-1_3

electric double layer (EDL). A wide variety of literature are available regarding EOF in microcapillaries of various geometric shapes such as rectangular microchannel [5], T-shaped structure, and Y-shaped structure [6], cylindrical capillary [7], annulus [8], elliptical pore [9], slit parallel plate [10].

In hydrophilic surfaces, there is no difference between fluid velocity and the wall velocity, and this is shaped by a no-slip boundary condition. On the other hand, for hydrophobic surfaces, the fluid velocity is not the same as wall velocity and it varies with velocity gradient (Navier 1823)

The Navier slip equation defines a slip coefficient β as

$$u = \beta \frac{\partial u}{\partial y} \tag{1}$$

where y is the normal coordinate and $u(y)$ is the velocity of the fluid tangential to the wall. h is the channel height. Recently, many researchers have shown their immense interest toward hydrophobic surfaces. Choi et al. [11] experimentally observed microflows by considering slip and no-slip boundary conditions. Choi et al. [12] calculated effective slip in superhydrophobic microchannel. Devakar et al. [13] obtained analytical derivations of couple stress fluid in hydrophobic surfaces. De et al. [14] studied electroosmotic flow with superhydrophobic boundary in a long channel.

Our main focus is to study the effect of temperature-dependent electrostatic parameters on EOF on a long slit nanochannel with hydrophobic patches. The characteristics of the electrokinetic flows are derived by numerically solving the coupling Poisson–Boltzmann equation, modified Navier–Stokes equation, modified Nernst–Planck equation, and modified energy equation simultaneously.

2 Physical Model

We have considered a slit nanochannel of height h, filled with an incompressible conductive Newtonian (e.g., NaCl with water) electrolyte (Fig. 1). The length of the channel is taken $L = 5$ h. The channel walls consist of hydrophobic patches. We also consider a shift δ between the upper and lower walls as depicted in (Fig. 1). The walls of the channel are non-conductive and a constant heat flux is imposed along

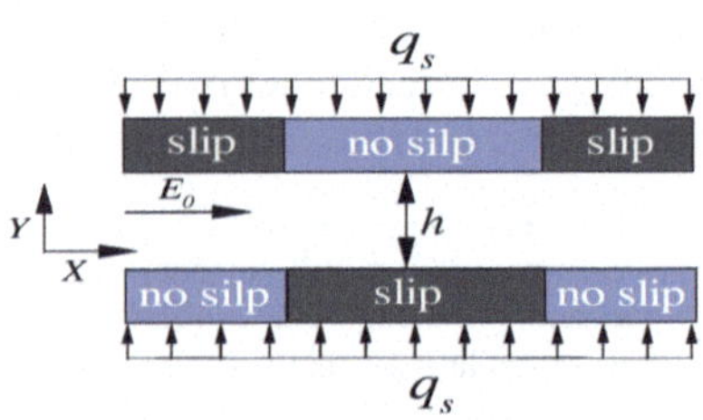

Fig. 1 Schematic diagram of the model geometry in the Cartesian coordinate system

the wall of the channel. The electric field is applied externally along the axis of the channel (Fig. 1).

3 Mathematical Formulation

We have considered X-axis along the length of the channel. The governing equations characterizing the motion of the fluid in the liquid medium are considered to be based on Navier–Stokes equations. The ion transport in liquid is commanded through the Nernst–Planck equation. The electric potential of the applied electric field is governed by the Laplace equation and induced electric potential is conducted by the Poisson equation. The energy equation can be asserted as

$$\rho c_{\mathrm{p}}\left(\frac{\partial T}{\partial t} + (\mathbf{q}.\nabla)T\right) - \nabla.(k(T)\nabla T) - G = 0 \tag{2}$$

where $q = (u; v)$ is the velocity field of the fluid with $(u; v)$ are the velocity component in the X, Y directions, respectively. Here, ρ is the density of the liquid. $\mathbf{E}$ is determined by $-\nabla\varphi$, where φ is the total electric potential.

c_{p} is the specific heat capacity and $k(T)$ is the temperature-dependent thermal conductivity. G is the Joule heating term which is given as

$$G = \frac{(u\rho_{\mathrm{e}} + \mathbf{E}\lambda(T))^2}{\lambda(T)}$$

ρ_{e} is the charge density and furthermore the contribution to the Joule heating due to the convection electric current (i.e., $u\rho_{\mathrm{e}}$) is negligible. Therefore, G can be approximated as

$$G = (\mathbf{E}.\mathbf{E})\lambda(T)$$

The temperature-dependent parameter dynamic viscosity ($\mu(T)$), electrical conductivity ($\lambda(T)$), permittivity ($\epsilon(T)$), diffusivity ($D_i(T)$), and thermal conductivity ($k(T)$) are expressed as follows [15–18]:

$$\begin{aligned}
\mu(T) &= 2.761\mathrm{e}^{(1713/T)} \times 10^{-6}\mathrm{kg/(m\ s)} \\
\lambda(T) &= 126.4[1 + 0.025(T - T_{\mathrm{ref}})] \times 10^{-4}\mathrm{m^2s/mol} \\
\epsilon(T) &= 305.7\mathrm{e}^{(-T/219)}\mathrm{C/V\ m} \\
D_i(T) &= D_{i0} + 0.0309 D_{i0}(T - T_{\mathrm{ref}})\mathrm{m^2s},
\end{aligned}$$

D_{i0} is the diffusion coefficient of corresponding ions at fluid temperature (i.e., 298 K)

$$k(T) = 0.61 + 0.0012(T - T_{\text{ref}})W/(m\ K)$$

We have taken slip boundary condition and temperature jump condition in the hydrophobic surfaces. For hydrophilic surfaces, we have taken no-slip boundary condition and constant heat flux. And also constant ζ-potential is taken in the homogeneous surface of the wall.

4 Numerical Methods

The equations governing the fluid flow, coupled with the equations for ion transport, temperature, and the Poisson equations for electric field, along with the prescribed boundary conditions are solved numerically in a coupled manner through a control volume approach over a staggered grid arrangement. The pressure link between the continuity and momentum equations is accomplished by transforming the discretized continuity equation into a Poisson equation for pressure correction. This procedure is similar to the SIMPLE algorithm, which is based on a cyclic guess-and-correct operation to solve the governing equations.

5 Results and Discussion

In the present analysis, we have considered the height of the channel $h = 100$ nm.

The thermo–physical properties at room temperature, used in this study, have been given in Table 1.

We have taken ζ surface potential along the homogeneous channel walls and the imposed external electric field is $E_0 = 10^4$ V/m.

Table 1 Thermophysical properties

Parameter	Value
Density (kg/m^3)	1000
Specific heat capacity (J/kg K)	4180
Reference viscosity (kg/(m s))	0.001
Reference permittivity (C/V m)	695.39×10^{-12}
Reference diffusivity (m^{2}s)	2.0×10^{-9}
Reference thermal conductivity (W/m K)	0.613
Reference electrical conductivity (m^{2}s/mol)	10^{-2}

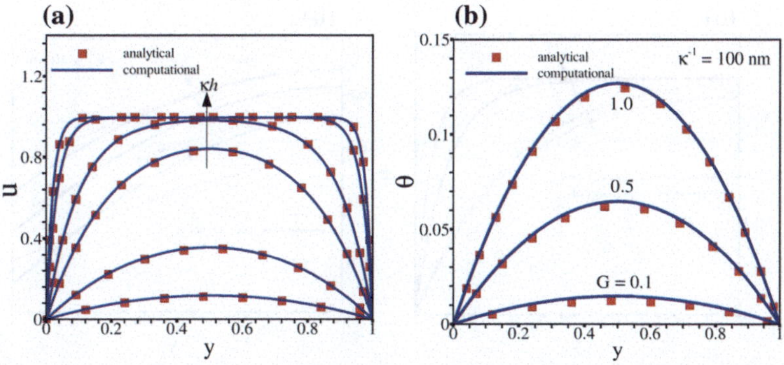

Fig. 2 **a** Numerically (lines) and analytically [19] (symbols) computed velocity profiles in a channel with planar, homogeneously charged walls for $\mathrm{Re} = 0.89 \times 10^{-5}$; $\mathrm{Pe} = 0.44 \times 10^{-2}$; $\zeta = -0.1$. The different curves correspond to $\kappa h = 1; 2; 5; 10; 30; 50$. **b** Comparison of surface temperature along the channel with the analytic results (symbols) presented by Matin and Ohshima [20]. Different curves correspond to $G = 0.1; 0.5; 1.0$

5.1 Comparison with Existing Results

In order to establish our numerical scheme, we have treated the case of EOF in a nanochannel with a hydrophilic surface of a given ζ-potential. We compared our result with the corresponding analytical solution of Masliyah and Bhattacharjee [19]. In Fig. 2a, the numerical and analytical results for the velocity profile are shown for different values of the dimensionless Debye–Huckel parameter κh, which is reciprocal to the electric double layer thickness. We have obtained a good agreement of our computed solutions with the corresponding analytical solutions [19].

In Fig. 2b, the surface temperature for three different Joule heating terms, $G = 0.1; 0.5; 1.0$ for $\kappa h = 1.0$ across the channel has been validated with the result of the analytical expressions given by Matin and Ohshima [20]. They have taken a polyelectrolyte layer on the channel wall. In order to compare with our result, we have neglected the term consisting of the effect of polyelectrolyte layer. The numerical solutions are in good agreement with the analytical estimation of Matin and Ohshima [20].

5.2 Comparison with Slip Model

In Fig. 3, we have compared the velocity and temperature profiles with the results given by Nayak et al. [21]. They have considered a hydrophobic channel and a power-law fluid. Also, they have considered the height of the channel as 2 h and it is symmetric with respect to the centerline of the channel. We have recognized the case for Newtonian fluid. The velocity profiles with different κh have been demonstrated in Fig. 3a, for both the numerical results and the analytical estimation given by Nayak

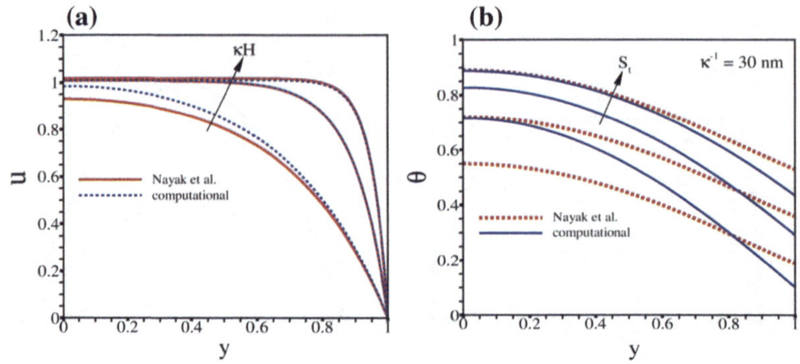

Fig. 3 **a** Comparison of u-velocity along a hydrophobic channel with analytic results presented by Nayak et al. [21] for different $\kappa h = (3; 10; 20)$ with fixed $\beta = 0.001$. **b** Comparison of θ along a hydrophobic channel with analytical results presented by Nayak et al. [21] for different temperature jump factors, S_{T} with fixed β, and Joule heating term

et al. [21]. In their estimation, they have examined fully developed flow with Debye–Huckel linearization technique and also they have contemplated with negligible ζ—potential and slip parameter. For $\kappa h = 10.0$ and 20.0, our numerical results match with the results given by Nayak et al. [21]. But for thick Debye layer, our result deviates from the solution due to the limitation of Debye–Huckel approximation.

In Fig. 3b, we have plotted surface temperature for different temperature jump factors with a fixed Joule heating parameter. We have considered three temperature jump factors as $S_{\mathrm{T}} = 0.1$, 0.3 and 0.5. There is a significant deviation between the results [21] and our results. They have taken the linearized model by considering the linear equations for temperature.

5.3 *Flow and Temperature Field*

In our analysis, the electrostatic parameters are temperature dependent. The velocity distributions are mainly provoked by the change of surface temperature due to the temperature dependency of electrostatic parameters and the EOF field is strongly coupled with the temperature field. The influence of temperature on the EOF velocity is attributed to the dependence of solution viscosity on temperature. Therefore, increment of solution temperature causes a decrease in the solution viscosity and dielectric constant and hence increases the dimensionless EOF velocity than the reference Smoluchowski velocity. In our analysis, we have varied slip coefficient (β) from 0 to 1.

The influence of slip coefficient is studied in Fig. 4. Different values of $\beta = 0.01$; 0.1; 0.5 and 1.0 are considered. De et al. [14] have obtained that the average velocity is maximized when a shift $\delta = L/2$ between the upper and lower surfaces occurs, i.e., a solid-wall segment of one surface is facing a gas–liquid interface segment of the

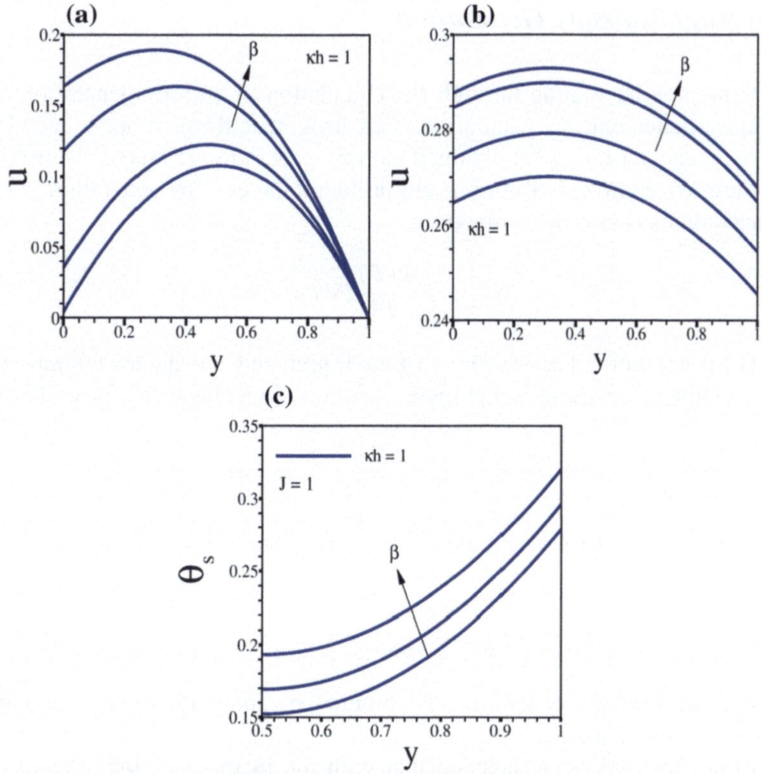

Fig. 4 Variation of velocity profiles along the length of the channel when $\zeta = -0.1$, $\kappa h = 1$, $S_T = 0.5$, $J = 1$ for different ($\beta = 0.01$; 0.1; 0.5; 1.0) **a** for parameters temperature independent; **b** for parameters temperature dependent. **c** variation of surface temperature along the length of the channel when $\zeta = -0.1$, $\kappa h = 1$, $S_T = 0.5$, $J = 1$ for different ($\beta = 0.1$; 0.5; 1.0)

opposite surface. So we have considered $\delta = L/2$. Also previously, many researchers have obtained the hydrophobic problems analytically by considering thin Debye-layer analysis. But here, we have analyzed the thick Debye-layer consideration. In Fig. 4a, b we have plotted the velocity profiles along the length of the channel for different slip coefficients, ($\beta = 0.01$; 0.1; 0.5; 1.0) for both the cases when electrostatic parameters are temperature independent and dependent. As usual, the temperature-dependent velocity is greater than the temperature independent velocity and also the velocity increases with the increase of β.

The normalized surface wall temperature, θ_S, distribution along the channel is plotted in Fig. 4c for different slip coefficients. For positive values of Joule number, J, the surface temperature will increase due to both heat generation in the entire volume and heat addition through the top and bottom walls. In Fig. 4c, we have plotted θ_S along the channel at $J = 1.0$. Here, different curves correspond to $\beta =$ 0.1; 0.5; 1. In both cases, the surface temperature, θ_S, increases along the channel. This is due to the hydrophobic nature of the wall.

5.4 Average Entropy Generation

Many researchers have gone through the calculation of entropy generation. Zhao et al. [22] estimated entropy generation of electrokinetic flows in open- and closed-end microchannels. Matin [23] obtained entropy generation in mixed electrokinetic and pressure-driven flow. For our present problem, the entropy generation [22] rate due to heat conduction is determined as:

$$S'''_{\text{gen},c} = \frac{k(T)}{T^2}(\nabla T)^2 \tag{3}$$

where $k(T)$ is the thermal conductivity of the liquid, and T is the local temperature. The local volumetric entropy generation rate due to Joule heating is described as:

$$S'''_{\text{gen},j} = \frac{G}{T} \tag{4}$$

where $G = (\mathbf{E}.\mathbf{E}).\ \lambda(T)$ is the joule heating. The total entropy generation can be written as:

$$S'''_{\text{gen}} = S'''_{\text{gen},c} + S'''_{\text{gen},j} \tag{5}$$

The average entropy generation is obtained by integrating the total entropy generation into the domain.

From Fig. 5, it has been deduced that with the increase of Joule heating, the average entropy generation increases. The average entropy generation rate always increases with the increase of J. But in the hydrophobic surface, the heat transfer rate increases more. So, for an arbitrary fixed J, the average entropy generation decreases

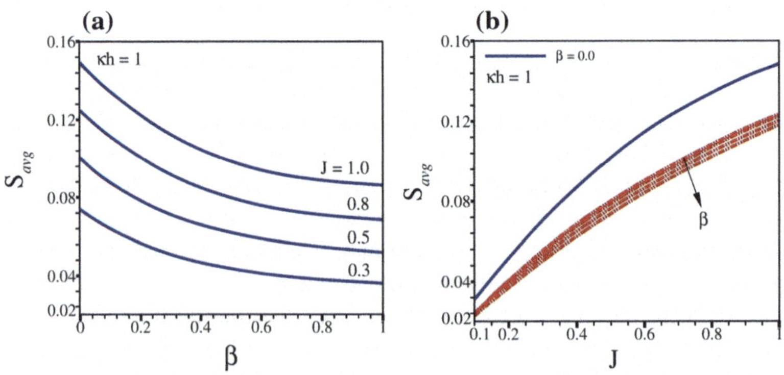

Fig. 5 Variation of average entropy **a** with β for $\zeta = -0.1$, $\kappa h = 1$, $S_T = 0.5$ for different Joule numbers, ($J = 0.3$; 0.5; 0.8; 1.0); **b** with Joule number, J for $\zeta = -0.1$, $\kappa h = 1$, $S_T = 0.5$ for different slip coefficients, ($\beta = 0.0$; 0.1; 0.5; 0.8; 1.0). The red-dashed lines correspond to ($\beta =$ 0.1; 0.3; 0.5; 0.8). The blue solid line corresponds to ($\beta = 0.0$)

with the increase of β. The surface temperature, θ_S, and the fluid temperature, θ, increase with the increase of β. So by using a hydrophobic surface, we can reduce the average entropy generation rate.

5.5 Average Bejan Number

The relative dominance of entropy generation due to heat transfer and Joule heating is determined by the Bejan number Be, which is defined by $\mathrm{Be} = \frac{S'''_{\mathrm{gen},c}}{S'''_{\mathrm{gen}}}$. The average Bejan number $\mathrm{Be_{avg}}$ is obtained by integrating Be in the whole domain. The value of the average Bejan number varies from 0 to 1. At any location of the domain, if $\mathrm{Be_{avg}} > 0.5$, then the heat transfer irreversibility dominates the Joule heating irreversibility and if $\mathrm{Be_{avg}} < 0.5$, it implies that the Joule heating irreversibility dominates the process. If $\mathrm{Be_{avg}} = 0.5$, then both the heat transfer irreversibility and Joule heating irreversibility have equal contributions to the entropy generation.

Now, as J has increased $\mathrm{Be_{avg}}$ decreases (Fig. 6). For $J = 1.0$, $\mathrm{Be_{avg}}$ is always less than 0.5 for varying β, 0 to 1. So for $J = 1.0$ J, heating irreversibility always dominates the heat transfer irreversibility. But as β increases, the dominance of Joule heating reduces at $J = 1.0$. Now for other Source terms (J) as β increases, local entropy generation increases and Be is the ratio of $\mathrm{Be_{avg}}$, also increases. So $\mathrm{Be_{avg}}$ increases with the increase of β. For $0.1 < J < 0.5$, always heat transfer irreversibility dominates the Joule heating irreversibility.

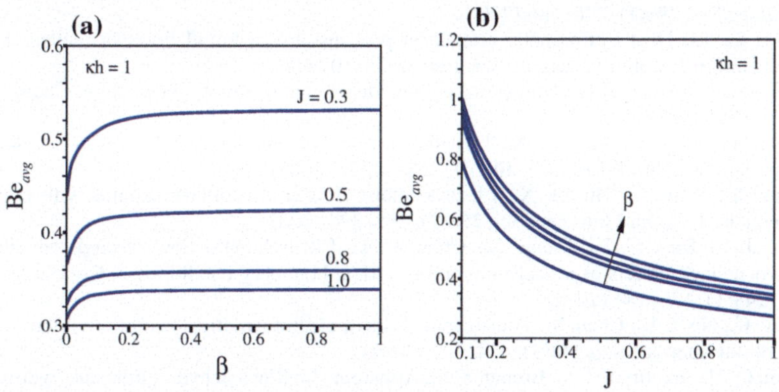

Fig. 6 Variation of average Bejan number $\mathrm{Be_{avg}}$ **a** with β for $\zeta = -0.1$, $\kappa h = 1$, $S_T = 0.5$ for different Joule numbers, ($J = 0.3$; 0.5; 0.8; 1.0); **b** with Joule number, J for $\zeta = -0.1$, $\kappa h = 1$, $S_T = 0.5$ for different slip coefficients, ($\beta = 0.0$; 0.1; 0.5; 1.0)

6 Conclusions

Effect of temperature-dependent electrostatic parameters on EOF is analyzed and also we have considered hydrophobic patches to enhance the velocity. In this article, our aim is to enhance the velocity and also simultaneously to reduce the entropy. The temperature-dependent velocity is much higher than the temperature-independent velocity and also it increases with the increase of slip coefficient and slip length. Finally, our illustration captures an average entropy and it has been observed that entropy is mainly dependent on joule heating and it reduces with the increase of slip coefficient. Also average Bejan number increases with the increase of slip coefficient and simultaneously decreases with the increase of Joule number. For $J = 1.0$, average Bejan number is always <0.5 and for $0.1 < J < 0.5$, always heat transfer irreversibility dominates the Joule heating irreversibility.

References

1. Masliyah, J.: Electrokinetic Transport Phenomena Aostra. Edmonton, Alta., Canada
2. Harrison, D.J., Fluri, K., Seiler, K., Fan, Z., Effenhauser, C.S., Manz, A.: Micromachining a miniaturized capillary electrophoresis-based chemical analysis system on a chip. Science **261**(5123), 895–897 (1993)
3. Bousse, L., Cohen, C., Nikiforov, T., Chow, A., Kopf-Sill, A.R., Dubrow, R., Parce, J.W.: Electrokinetically controlled microfluidic analysis systems. Ann. Rev. Biophys. Biomolec. Struct. **29**(1), 155–181 (2000)
4. Ma, H.C., Keh, H.J.: Diffusioosmosis of electrolyte solutions in a fine capillary slit. J. Colloid Interface Sci. **298**(1), 476–486 (2006)
5. Yang, C., Li, D.: Electrokinetic effects on pressure-driven liquid flows in rectangular microchannels. J. Colloid Interface Sci. **194**(1), 95–107 (1997)
6. Patankar, N.A., Hu, H.H.: Numerical simulation of electroosmotic flow. Anal. Chem. **70**(9), 1870–1881 (1998)
7. Kang, Y., Yang, C., Huang, X.: Dynamic aspects of electroosmotic flow in a cylindrical microcapillary. Int. J. Eng. Sci. **40**(20), 2203–2221 (2002)
8. Kang, Y., Yang, C., Huang, X.: Electroosmotic flow in a capillary annulus with high zeta potentials. J. Colloid Interface Sci. **253**(2), 285–294 (2002)
9. Hsu, J.-P., Kao, C.-Y., Tseng, S., Chen, C.-J.: Electrokinetic flow through an elliptical microchannel: effects of aspect ratio and electrical boundary conditions. J. Colloid Interface Sci. **248**(1), 176–184 (2002)
10. Yang, C., Ng, C.B., Chan, V.: Transient analysis of electroosmotic flow in a slit microchannel. J. Colloid Interface Sci. **248**(2), 524–527 (2002)
11. Choi, C.-H., Westin, K.J.A., Breuer, K.S.: Apparent slip flows in hydrophilic and hydrophobic microchannels. Phys. UIDS **15**(10), 2897–2902 (2003)
12. Choi, C.-H., Ulmanella, U., Kim, J., Ho, C.-M., Kim, C.-J.: Effective slip and friction reduction in nanograted superhydrophobic microchannels. Phys. Fluids **18**(8), 087105 (2006)
13. Devakar, M., Sreenivasu, D., Shankar, B.: Analytical solutions of couple stress fluid flows with slip boundary conditions. Alexandria Eng. J. **53**(3), 723–730 (2014)
14. De, S., Bhattacharyya, S., Hardt, S.: Electroosmotic flow in a slit nanochannel with superhydrophobic walls. Microfluid. Nanofluid. **19**(6), 1465–1476 (2015)
15. Tang, G., Yang, C., Chai, C., Gong, H.: Numerical analysis of the thermal effect on electroosmotic flow and electrokinetic mass transport in microchannels. Anal. Chim. Acta **507**(1), 27–37 (2004)

16. Mukherjee, S., Dhar, J., DasGupta, S., Chakraborty, S.: Patterned surface charges coupled with thermal gradients may create giant augmentations of solute dispersion in electroosmosis of viscoelastic fluids. Proc. R. Soc. A **475**(2221), 20180522 (2019)
17. Tang, G., Yang, C., Chai, J., Gong, H.: Joule heating effect on electroosmotic flow and mass species transport in a microcapillary. Int. J. Heat Mass Transf. **47**(2), 215–227 (2004)
18. Kang, Y., Yang, C., Huang, X.: Joule heating induced transient temperature field and its effects on electroosmosis in a microcapillary packed with microspheres. Langmuir **21**(16), 7598–7607 (2005)
19. Masliyah, J.H., Bhattacharjee, S.: Electrokinetic and Colloid Transport Phenomena. Wiley, New York (2006)
20. Matin, M.H., Ohshima, H.: Thermal transport characteristics of combined electroosmotic and pressure driven flow in soft nanofluidics. J. Colloid Interface Sci. **476**, 167–176 (2016)
21. Nayak, A., Haque, A., Weigand, B.: Analysis of electroosmotic flow and joule heating effect in a hydrophobic channel. Chem. Eng. Sci. **176**, 165–179 (2018)
22. Zhao, L., Liu, L.: Entropy generation analysis of electro-osmotic flow in open—end and closed—end microchannels. Int. J. Thermal Sci. **49**(2), 418–427 (2010)
23. Matin, M.H., Khan, W.A.: Entropy generation analysis of heat and mass transfer in mixed electrokinetically and pressure driven flow through a slit microchannel. Energy **56**, 207–217 (2013)

Influence of Thermophoresis and Brownian Motion on MHD Mixed Convective Chemically Reacting Couple Stress Fluid Flow in Porous Medium Between Parallel Plates

Swapna Jawalkar, Odelu Ojjela and Debasish Pradhan

Abstract In the present chapter, we have investigated an unsteady incompressible laminar electrically conducting heat and mass transfer distributions of couple stress nanofluid flow through parallel plates with porous medium having the thermal slip boundary condition. By applying the suitable similarity transformations, the governing partial differential equations are reduced to nonlinear ordinary differential equations, which are numerically solved by the shooting method along with Runge–Kutta fourth-order scheme. The influence of different non-dimensional numbers on the fluid flow, heat and mass transfer characteristics of the fluid is presented in graphs and discussed in detail. Numerical values of skin friction, Sherwood number and Nusselt number with different parameters are also computed and presented in the form of tables. The Hartmann number, chemical reaction parameter and thermophoresis parameter were having the same result on velocity, concentration and temperature distributions. The data presented are compared with the recent viscous case conditions and are concluded to be in better agreement.

Keywords Couple stress fluid · Mixed convection · Thermophoresis · Brownian motion · MHD · Shooting method

List of Symbols

C	Concentration
$C_1 e^{i\omega t}$	Lower plate concentration
$C_2 e^{i\omega t}$	Upper plate concentration
$T_1 e^{i\omega t}$	Lower plate temperature
$T_2 e^{i\omega t}$	Upper plate temperature
$V_0 e^{i\omega t}$	Lower plate injection velocity

S. Jawalkar · O. Ojjela (✉) · D. Pradhan
Department of Applied Mathematics, Defence Institute of Advanced Technology (Deemed to be University), Pune 411025, India
e-mail: odelu@diat.ac.in

S. Bhattacharyya et al. (eds.), *Mathematical Modeling and Computational Tools*, Springer Proceedings in Mathematics & Statistics 320,
https://doi.org/10.1007/978-981-15-3615-1_4

$V_1 e^{i\omega t}$	Upper plate injection velocity
$T*$	Dimensionless temperature $\frac{T-T_1 e^{i\omega t}}{(T_2-T_1)e^{i\omega t}}$
$C*$	Dimensionless concentration $\frac{C-C_1 e^{i\omega t}}{(C_2-C_1)e^{i\omega t}}$
h	Distance between parallel plate
Ec	Eckert number $\frac{\mu V_1}{\rho h C(T_2-T_1)}$
$\dot{n}_A$	Mass transfer rate
K_1	Permeability parameter
Pr	Prandtl number $\frac{\mu c}{K}$
Sc	Schmidt number
K_2	Non-dimensional chemical reaction parameter
Sh	Sherwood number $\frac{\dot{n}_A}{h\vartheta(C_2-C_1)}$
Gr	Thermal Grashof number $\frac{\rho g \beta_T (T_2-T_1)h^2}{\mu V_1}$
C	Specific heat at constant temperature
A	Suction–injection ratio
Nb	Brownian motion parameter $\frac{D_B(T_2-T_1)}{\alpha T_2}$
Nt	Thermophoresis parameter $\frac{D_2(T_2-T_1)}{\alpha T_2}$
Da	Darcy parameter $\frac{K}{h^2}$
B_0	Magnetic field strength
Ha	Hartmann number $\sqrt{\frac{\sigma}{\mu}} B_0 h$
D_B	Brownian diffusion coefficient
D_T	Thermophoretic diffusion coefficient
Re	Reynolds number $\frac{\rho h \upsilon}{\mu}$
$\bar{q}$	Velocity vector
$u(x, y)$	Primary velocity component
$v(x, y)$	Secondary velocity component

Greek Letters

α^2	Dimensionless couple stress parameter $\frac{\eta}{\mu h^2}$
λ	Non-dimensional y-coordinate $\frac{y}{h}$
ξ	Non-dimensional axial variable, $\left(\frac{U_0}{a} - \frac{V_1 x}{h}\right)$
μ	Fluid viscosity
ρ	Fluid density
η	Couple stress fluid parameters

1 Introduction

Nowadays, many researchers focus on a study of the characteristics of non-Newtonian fluid flows passing between channels because of wide range of applications in industry such as glass fibre production, movement of lubrication, heavy oil recovery, liquid polymer moulding, food preservation, aerodynamic heating, petroleum industry, transpiration cooling, MHD pumps, artificial dialysis and cosmetic industry. Sochi [1] has studied the flow of non-Newtonian fluid in a porous medium and notice that the non-Newtonian fluid was highly complex and they required mathematical modelling for a proper description. Wu et al. [2] developed the one-dimensional non-Newtonian fluid flow through porous medium and described an exact solution for the displacement mechanism. Recently, Huang et al. [3] derived a single-dimensional flow analytical solution based on the Barree–Conway approach that explains the non-Darcy displacement in porous media for a non-Newtonian model. Fayed et al. [4] investigated an incompressible laminar flow using the Carreau model to generalize Newtonian fluid flow in a single pore. Narvaez et al. [5] worked on the porous parallel walls having continuous injected or ejected the conducting fluid which comes out on both sides along the channel. Belhouideg [6] developed the laminar two-dimensional flow model through a porous tube combined with Darcy's law and numerically solved using the finite element method. Sandeep [7] found out for constant wall permeability, and an exact solution is presented for pressure drop in fluid flow in a cylindrical tube and rectangular slit with porous boundaries.

The couple stress fluid described as a special case of non-Newtonian fluids. The concept of couple stresses in fluids developed by Stokes [8] which allows the classical theory the easiest generalization by permitting the existence in the fluid medium of body pairs and couple stresses. The important characteristic of the couple stress fluid flow is the stress tensor as asymmetric, and the normal theory of Newtonian fluid cannot predict its precise flow. The examples of these fluids are blood, electrorheological liquids, lubricants containing small polymer additives and synthetic liquids. Srinivasacharya et al. [9, 10] noted that the incompressible laminar couple stress fluid between porous plates and expanding/contracting walls having continuous injection–suction on upper and lower walls, respectively, and the reduced nonlinear standard equations are solved by quasilinearization method. Eldabe et al. [11] have studied an unsteady laminar that conducts electrically non-Newtonian fluid flow in the presence of couple stresses and external uniform magnetic field in the Eyring–Powell model and accumulated a numerical solution for nonlinear PDEs using a finite differentiation technique. Adesanya et al. [12] have investigated the second law of analysis of the MHD convective flow of couple stress nanofluid through the vertical channel and obtained an exact solution by the technique of homotopy evaluation. Opanuga et al. [13] have investigated the entropy generation through porous medium on an electrically conductive couple stress fluid, and the improved streamflow equations are solved using Adomian decomposition (ADM) technique.

Magnetohydrodynamics (MHD) is an important interdisciplinary field. MHD is a mixture of fluid mechanics theory and electromagnetism. The main assumption behind MHD is that in a moving conductive fluid, the magnetic fields can induce currents that in combination produce the forces on fluid and affect the magnetic field itself. The main applications of MHD are pumps commonly used in astrophysics for extra kinematic treatments, earthquakes, sensors for accurate measurement in metallurgical and nuclear industry, nuclear reactors, geophysics, MHD power generators, etc. Davidson [14] has discussed in detail the fundamental concepts and applications of MHD in his book. Rehaman et al. [15] have been examined the impacts of thermophoresis, Brownian motion on MHD chemically reacting Eyring–Powell nanofluid flow to both cylindrical and flat tilting surfaces with dual stratification and appropriate transformations are regarded to be used to transform flow field equations into ODEs then solved using shooting technique together with Runge–Kutta technique. Dastagiri Babu et al. [16] have examined a laminar unsteady convective flow of non-Newtonian fluid over a semi-infinite moving porous plate with heat absorbing and hall current and obtained an analytical solution with non-harmonic and two-term harmonic functions. Ahmed [17] has researched the effect of Soret and continuous heat source of the laminar incompressible viscous MHD flow between two horizontal isothermal parallel walls. Mateen [18] explored through a horizontal channel with Joule dissipation an electrically conducting incompressible properly developed by the continuous flow of two immiscible fluids.

Thermophoresis is the migration of molecules along with a temperature gradient while Brownian motion is a random movement of tiny colloidal particles suspended in the fluid resulting in rapid and continuous movement of molecules. Ojjela et al. [19] have considered the UCM fluid passing through parallel plates with an inclined magnetic field and the impacts on thermophoresis and Brownian motion. Anbuchezhian et al. [20] have analysed the thermal stratification, Brownian motion and thermophoresis of the nanofluids flow with variable solar-powered stream conditions. Shit et al. [21] have explored the effect of MHD on mixed convective viscoelastic nanofluid flow on a linear stretching sheet, and the issue is numerically resolved by the finite difference technique. Falana et al. [22] have discussed the effects of flow, temperature and concentration through a stretching sheet of Brownian motion and thermophoresis. Michaelides [23] has researched the impact of thermophoresis and Brownian motion using Monte Carlo simulations with several common nanofluids. Mahdi et al. [24] have done an elaborate review on nanofluid flows through porous media along with other properties like inertia coefficient, effective conductivity of heat. Das et al. [25] have experimentally researched thermal conductivity improvements for water-based nanofluids carrying CuO or Al_2O_3 as nanoparticles with temperature from 21 to 51 °C.

Mixed convection is an effect of mixture free and forced convection heat transfer. For improving the cooling effect in engineering, mixed convection flow through parallel plates is of significant value. This involves the contemporary exchange of heat, solar cells, atomic reactor, etc. Khan et al. [26] researched an unsteady laminar incompressible couple stress nanofluid flows through stretching surface with mixed convection and obtained an analytical solution form by reducing governing equations with the help of HAM method. Ojjela and Naresh Kumar [27] have considered MHD chemically reacting radiative flow of couple stress fluid with Soret and Dufour effects through parallel plates. Kaladhar and Srinivasacharya [28] have considered the couple stress fluid flow between the circular annulus with the Dufour, Soret and chemical reaction effects and obtained an analytical by HAM. Yirga and Tesfay [29] have considered the Soret and chemical reaction effects on MHD flow of nanofluid with Ag-water and Cu-water through porous media over a stretching sheet and solved numerically with the Keller-Box technique.

In the present paper, we have investigated the impact of Brownian motion and thermophorosis on an electrically conducting flow of couple stress nanofluid between porous parallel plates with the thermal slip boundary conditions. The reduced ordinary differential equations are solved using shooting technique along with R-K fourth-order method. The results are analysed in detail for different flow properties such as dimensionless axial, radial velocities, concentration and temperature distributions for different fluid and geometric parameters and shown in tables and graphs.

2 Formulation of the Problem

Considered an unsteady incompressible laminar non-Newtonian electrically conducting flow under the effect of couple stresses passing through two parallel porous plates situated at a distance 'h' apart. We have selected X- and Y-axes along and transverse to the plats also assuming $\overline{B}$ as an uniform magnetic field applied perpendicular to the XY-plane as shown in Fig. 1. The upper and lower plates are kept at different temperatures and concentrations $T_2 e^{i\omega t}$, $C_2 e^{i\omega t}$ and $T_1 e^{i\omega t}$, $C_1 e^{i\omega t}$, respectively.

The flow characteristics of couple stress nanofluid in the presence of a magnetic field are described through the governing equations without body forces and couples as follows

$$\nabla.\bar{q} = 0 \tag{1}$$

$$\rho\left[\frac{\partial \bar{q}}{\partial t} + (\bar{q}.\nabla)\bar{q}\right] = -\nabla p + \mu\nabla^2\bar{q} - \eta\nabla^4\bar{q} + J \times B - \frac{\mu}{k_1}\bar{q} + \overline{F}_{\mathrm{b}} \tag{2}$$

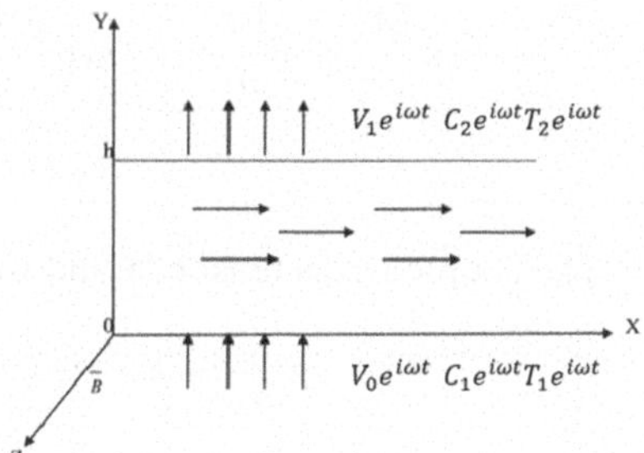

Fig. 1 Fluid geometry for flow through parallel porous plates

$$(\rho c)_f\left[\frac{\partial T}{\partial t}+(\bar{q}.\nabla)T\right]=K\nabla^2 T+\mu\left[(\nabla\bar{q}):(\nabla\bar{q})^{\mathrm{T}}+(\nabla\bar{q}):(\nabla\bar{q})\right]$$
$$+\eta\left[(\nabla\bar{\omega}):(\nabla\bar{\omega})^{\mathrm{T}}\right]+\eta'[(\nabla\bar{\omega}):(\nabla\bar{\omega})]+\frac{J^2}{\sigma}+\frac{\mu}{k_1}\bar{q}^2$$
$$+(\rho c)_p\left[D_{\mathrm{B}}\left(\frac{\partial T}{\partial x}\frac{\partial C}{\partial x}+\frac{\partial T}{\partial y}\frac{\partial C}{\partial y}\right)+\frac{D_{\mathrm{T}}}{T_\infty}\left(\left(\frac{\partial T}{\partial x}\right)^2+\left(\frac{\partial T}{\partial y}\right)^2\right)\right] \quad (3)$$

$$\left[\frac{\partial C}{\partial t}+(\bar{q}.\nabla)C\right]=D_{\mathrm{B}}\left(\frac{\partial^2 C}{\partial y^2}+\frac{\partial^2 C}{\partial x^2}\right)+\frac{D_{\mathrm{T}}}{T_\infty}\left(\left(\frac{\partial T}{\partial x}\right)^2+\left(\frac{\partial T}{\partial y}\right)^2\right)$$
$$-K_2\left(C-C_1\mathrm{e}^{iwt}\right) \quad (4)$$

Here, $\overline{F}_{\mathrm{b}}$ is the buoyancy force given as,

$$\overline{F_{\mathrm{b}}}=\left(\rho g B_{\mathrm{T}}\left(T-T_1\mathrm{e}^{iwt}\right)+\rho B_{\mathrm{c}}(C-C_1\mathrm{e}^{iwt})\right)\hat{i} \quad (5)$$

Convert Eqs. (1)–(4) in u and v, we obtain

$$\rho\left[\frac{\partial u}{\partial t}+u\frac{\partial u}{\partial x}+v\frac{\partial u}{\partial y}\right]=-\nabla p+\mu\nabla^2 u-\eta\nabla^4 u-\frac{\mu}{k_1}u$$
$$+\sigma\beta_0 u+\rho g B_T\left(T-T_1\mathrm{e}^{iwt}\right)+\rho B_c(C-C_1\mathrm{e}^{iwt}) \quad (6)$$

$$\rho\left[\frac{\partial v}{\partial t}+u\frac{\partial v}{\partial x}+v\frac{\partial v}{\partial y}\right]=-\nabla p+\mu\nabla^2 v-\eta\nabla^4 v-\frac{\mu}{k_1}v+\sigma\beta_0 v \quad (7)$$

$$(\rho c)_f\left[\frac{\partial T}{\partial t}+(\overline{q}.\nabla)T\right]=K\nabla^2 T+\mu\left[2\left(\frac{\partial u}{\partial x}\right)^2+2\left(\frac{\partial v}{\partial y}\right)^2+\left(\frac{\partial v}{\partial x}+\frac{\partial u}{\partial y}\right)\right]$$
$$+\eta\left[\left(\frac{\partial^2 u}{\partial x^2}+\frac{\partial^2 u}{\partial y^2}\right)^2+\left(\frac{\partial^2 v}{\partial x^2}+\frac{\partial^2 v}{\partial y^2}\right)^2\right]+\frac{J^2}{\sigma}+\frac{\mu}{k_1}\left(\frac{\partial\bar{u}}{\partial x}+\frac{\partial\bar{v}}{\partial y}\right)^2$$
$$+(\rho c)_p\left[D_B\left(\frac{\partial T}{\partial x}\frac{\partial C}{\partial x}+\frac{\partial T}{\partial y}\frac{\partial C}{\partial y}\right)+\frac{D_T}{T_\infty}\left(\left(\frac{\partial T}{\partial x}\right)^2+\left(\frac{\partial T}{\partial y}\right)^2\right)\right] \quad (8)$$

$$\frac{\partial C}{\partial t}+u\frac{\partial C}{\partial x}+v\frac{\partial C}{\partial y}=D_{\mathrm{B}}\left(\frac{\partial^2 C}{\partial y^2}+\frac{\partial^2 C}{\partial x^2}\right)+\frac{D_{\mathrm{T}}}{T_\infty}\left(\left(\frac{\partial T}{\partial x}\right)^2+\left(\frac{\partial T}{\partial y}\right)^2\right)$$
$$-K_2\left(C-C_1\mathrm{e}^{iwt}\right) \quad (9)$$

The couple stress tensor M and force stress tensor τ are given by

$$M=mI+2\eta\nabla(\nabla\times\bar{q})+2\eta'(\nabla(\nabla\times\bar{q}))^{\mathrm{T}} \quad (10)$$

$$\tau = (-p + \lambda_1 \nabla.\bar{q})I + \mu[\nabla\bar{q} + \nabla\bar{q}^{\mathrm{T}}] + \frac{1}{2}I\,x[\nabla.M + \rho C] \tag{11}$$

The material constants satisfy the inequalities as,

$$\mu \geq 0.3\lambda + 2\mu \geq 0, \quad \eta \geq 0, \quad \eta' \leq \eta \tag{12}$$

The Maxwell and generalized Ohm's law equations after neglecting the displacement currents are,

$$\nabla.\overline{B} = 0, \quad \nabla \times \overline{E} = \frac{\partial \overline{B}}{\partial t}, \quad \nabla \times \overline{B} = \mu' \overline{J}, \quad \text{where } \overline{J} = \sigma\left(\overline{E} + \bar{q} \times \overline{B}\right) \tag{13}$$

$\overline{B} = B_0\hat{k} + \bar{b}$, where $\bar{b}$ is induced magnetic field and
The following similarity transformations have been considered,

$$\begin{aligned}
u(x,\lambda,t) &= \left(\frac{U_0}{a} - \frac{V_1 x}{h}\right) f'(\lambda)\mathrm{e}^{i\omega t} \\
v(x,\lambda,t) &= V_1 f(\lambda)\mathrm{e}^{i\omega t} \\
T(x,\lambda,t) &= \left(T_1 - \frac{\mu V_1}{\rho h c}\left(\phi_1(\lambda) + \left(\frac{U_0}{V_1 a} - \frac{x}{h}\right)^2 \phi_2(\lambda)\right)\right)\mathrm{e}^{i\omega t} \\
C(x,\lambda,t) &= \left(C_1 - \frac{\dot{n}_A}{h\vartheta}\left(g_1(\lambda) + \left(\frac{U_0}{V_1 a} - \frac{x}{h}\right)^2 g_2(\lambda)\right)\right)\mathrm{e}^{i\omega t}
\end{aligned} \tag{14}$$

where U_0 = average entrance velocity, $\lambda = \frac{y}{h}$, $a = 1 - \frac{v_0}{v_1}$, i.e. suction–injection ratio

The boundary conditions are

$$\begin{aligned}
&u = 0;\ V = V_0\mathrm{e}^{i\omega t};\ \nabla \times \bar{q} = 0;\ -K\frac{\partial T}{\partial y} = h_1\left(T - T_1\mathrm{e}^{i\omega t}\right);\ C = C_1\mathrm{e}^{i\omega t} \quad \text{at } y = 0 \\
&u = 0;\ V = V_1\mathrm{e}^{i\omega t};\ \nabla \times \bar{q} = 0;\ T = T_2\mathrm{e}^{\omega t};\ C = C_2\mathrm{e}^{i\omega t} \quad \text{at } y = h
\end{aligned} \tag{15}$$

Substituting (14) in (6)–(9), we obtain

$$\begin{aligned}
\alpha^2 f^{vi} &= \mathrm{Re}\left(f'f'' - ff'''\right)\cos\omega t - f^{iv} - D^{-1}f'' - \mathrm{Ha}^2 f'' + \frac{1}{\xi}\left[\mathrm{Gr\,Ec}\left(\phi_1' + \xi^2\phi_2'\right).\right. \\
&\left. + \mathrm{Sh\,Gm}\left(g_1' + \xi^2 g_2'\right)\right]
\end{aligned} \tag{16}$$

$$\begin{aligned}
\phi_1'' = &\left[\mathrm{Re\ Pr}\left(f\phi_1' - \alpha^2 f''^2 - 4f'^2 - D^{-1}f^2 - \mathrm{Ha}^2 f^2\right)\right. \\
&\left. -\tau\left(\mathrm{Sh\,Nb}(g_1'\phi_1') + \mathrm{Nt\,Ec}(\phi_1'^2)\right)\right]\cos\omega t
\end{aligned} \tag{17}$$

$$\phi_2'' = \left[\mathrm{Re\ Pr}\left(f\phi_2' - f''^2 - 2f'\phi_2 - \alpha^2 f'''^2 - \mathrm{Ha}^2 f'^2 - D^{-1}f'^2\right) - \right.$$

$$\tau\left(\mathrm{Sh\,Nb}(4g_2\phi_2 + g_1'\phi_2' + g_2'\phi_1' + \xi^2 g_2'\phi_2') + \mathrm{Nt\,Ec}(2\phi_2' + \xi^2\phi_2'^2))\right]\cos\omega t \tag{18}$$

$$g_1'' = \mathrm{Re\,Sc}\,\cos\omega t\left(fg_1'\right) - \frac{\mathrm{Nt}}{\mathrm{Nb}}\mathrm{Ec\,Sh}\left(2\phi_2 + \phi_1''\right) - 2g_2 + K_2 g_1 \tag{19}$$

$$g_2'' = \mathrm{Sc\,Re}\,\cos\omega t\left(-2f'g_2 + fg_2'\right) - \frac{\mathrm{Nt}}{\mathrm{Nb}}\mathrm{Ec\,Sh}\left(\phi_2''\right) + K_2 g_2 \tag{20}$$

The boundary conditions in f, ϕ_1, ϕ_2, g_1 and g_2 are given as

$$\begin{array}{ll} f(0) = 1 - a, & f(1) = 1 \\ f'(0) = 0, & f'(1) = 0 \\ f'(0) = 0, & f'(1) = 0 \\ \phi_1'(0) = -\gamma\phi_1(0), & \phi_1(1) = \frac{1}{\mathrm{Ec}} \\ \phi_2'(0) = -\gamma\phi_2(0), & \phi_2(1) = 0 \\ g_1(0) = 0, & g_1(1) = \frac{1}{\mathrm{Sh}} \\ g_2(0) = 0, & g_2(1) = 0 \end{array}$$

The non-dimensional skin friction, the heat transfer rate in terms of the Nusselt number and the mass transfer rate in terms of the number of Sherwood on the plates are given by,

$$\mathrm{Sf} = \left(\frac{2\tau_{k1}}{\rho v_1^2}\right)_{\lambda=0.1} = \left(\frac{2}{\mathrm{Re}}\left(\frac{U_0}{V_1 a} - \frac{x}{h}\right)f'(\lambda)\cos\beta\right)_{\lambda=0.1} \tag{21}$$

$$\mathrm{Nu} = \frac{-\frac{\partial T}{\partial y}}{\frac{(T_2 - T_1)}{h}} = -\left[\mathrm{Ec}\left(\phi_1'(\lambda) + \left(\frac{U_0}{V_1 a} - \frac{x}{h}\right)^2\phi_2'(\lambda)\right)\cos\beta\right]_{\lambda=0.1} \tag{22}$$

$$\mathrm{Sh} = \frac{\frac{\partial C}{\partial y}}{\frac{(C_2 - C_1)}{h}} = \left[\mathrm{Sh}\left(g_1'(\lambda) + \left(\frac{U_0}{V_1 a} - \frac{x}{h}\right)^2 g_2'(\lambda)\right)\cos\beta\right]_{\lambda=0.1} \tag{23}$$

3 Problem Solution

The nonlinear Eqs. (16)–(20) are transformed into first-order differential equations as

$$\left(f, f', f'', f''', f^{iv}, f^{v}, \phi_1, \phi_1^1, \phi_2, \phi_2^1, g_1, g_1^1, g_2, g_2^1\right)$$
$$= (x_1, x_2, x_3, x_4, x_5, x_6, x_7, x_8, x_9, x_{10}, x_{11}, x_{12}, x_{13}, x_{14})$$

$$\frac{dx_1}{d\lambda} = x_2$$

$$\frac{dx_2}{d\lambda} = x_3$$

$$\frac{dx_3}{d\lambda} = x_4$$
$$\frac{dx_4}{d\lambda} = x_5$$
$$\frac{dx_5}{d\lambda} = x_6$$
$$\frac{dx_6}{d\lambda} = \frac{1}{\alpha^2}\left[\mathrm{Re}\,\cos\beta(x_2x_3 - x_1x_4) + x_5 - D^{-1}x_3 - \mathrm{Ha}^2x_3 + \frac{\mathrm{Ec\,Gr}}{\xi}(x_8 + \xi^2x_{10}) + \frac{\mathrm{Sh\,Gm}}{\xi}(x_{12} + \xi^2x_{14})\right]$$
$$\frac{dx_6}{d\lambda} = x_8$$
$$\frac{dx_6}{d\lambda} = \cos\beta\left[\mathrm{Re\,Pr}(x_1x_7 - 4x_2^2 - \alpha^2x_3^2 - \mathrm{Ha}^2x_1^2 - D^{-1}x_1^2) - \tau(\mathrm{Sh\,Nb}\,x_{11}x_8 + \mathrm{Ec\,Nt}\,x_8^2)\right]$$
$$\frac{dx_9}{d\lambda} = x_{10}$$
$$\frac{dx_{10}}{d\lambda} = \cos\beta\begin{bmatrix}\mathrm{Re\,Pr}(x_1x_{10} - 2x_2x_9 - x_3^2 - \alpha^2x_4^2 - \mathrm{Ha}^2x_2^2 - D^{-1}x_2^2) - \\ \tau(\mathrm{Sh\,Nb}\,(4x_9x_{13} + x_{10}x_{12} + x_{14}x_8 + \xi^2x_{10}x_{14}) + \mathrm{Ec\,Nt}\,(2x_{10} + \xi^2x_{10}^2))\end{bmatrix}$$
$$\frac{dx_{11}}{d\lambda} = x_{12}$$
$$\frac{dx_{12}}{d\lambda} = \mathrm{Re\,Sc}\,\cos\beta(x_1x_{12}) - \frac{\mathrm{Nt}}{\mathrm{Nb}}\mathrm{Ec\,Sh}\left(2x_9 + \frac{dx_8}{d\lambda}\right) - 2x_{13} + K_2x_{11}$$
$$\frac{dx_{13}}{d\lambda} = x_{14}$$
$$\frac{dx_{14}}{d\lambda} = \mathrm{Re\,Sc}\,\cos\beta(x_1x_{14} - 2x_2x_{13}) - \frac{\mathrm{Nt}}{\mathrm{Nb}}\mathrm{Ec\,Sh}\frac{dx_{10}}{d\lambda} + K_2x_{11}$$

The boundary conditions in terms of $x_1, x_2, x_3, x_4, x_5, x_6, x_7, x_8, x_9, x_{10}, x_{11}, x_{12}, x_{13}, x_{14}$ are

$$\begin{array}{lllllll} x_1(0) = 1 - a, & x_2(0) = 0, & x_3(0) = 0, & x_7(0) = -\gamma\phi_1(0), & x_9(0) = -\gamma\phi_2(0), & x_{11}(0) = 0, & x_{13}(0) = 0 \\ x_1(1) = 1, & x_2(1) = 0, & x_3(1) = 0, & x_7(1) = \frac{1}{\mathrm{Ec}}, & x_9(0) = 0, & x_{11}(0) = \frac{1}{\mathrm{Sh}}, & x_{13}(1) = 0 \end{array}$$

At this point, the solution depends on 7 initial assumptions; this can be achieved by Newton-Raphson method in such a manner that the boundary conditions are met at $\lambda = 1$. Further, the Runge–Kutta fourth-order method is introduced in order to present at least 10^{-6} convergence criteria.

4 Results and Discussions

The axial and radial velocities, the temperature as well as concentration distributions are plotted having the various values of parameters like ‘a’ (suction–injection ratio), Pr (Prandtl number), Sc (Schmidt number), K (Chemical reaction parameter), Nt (thermophoresis parameter), Ha (Hartmann number) and Nb (Brownian motion parameter). From Fig. 2, it is analysed that the suction–injection ratio increases with the axial velocity, while the secondary velocity, concentration and temperature decrease towards the upper plate. From Fig. 3, it is analysed that as the value of Schmidt number increases, the radial velocity, temperature and concentrations are increased, whereas the primary velocity profiles increase up to the middle of the

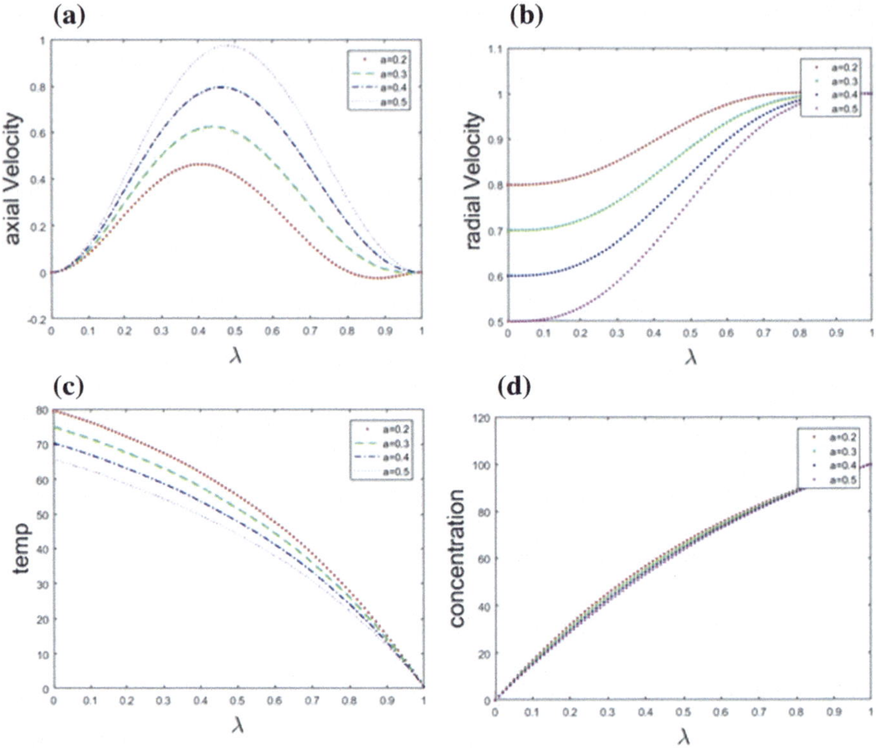

Fig. 2 Variation of a (suction–injection ratio) for **a** axial velocity, **b** radial velocity, **c** temperature and **d** concentration for Re = 2; Pr = 0.5; beta = 10; $G = 0.1$; Ec = 2; $a = 0.2$; $D = 1.2$; Ha = 2; Sc = 1; Gm = 4; Gr = 4; $b = 0.2$; Nt = 0.002; Sh = 0.01; $T = 0.8$; Nb = 3; $\alpha = 0.1$; $K = 0.2$

channel then decrease. Schmidt number is a dimensionless number defined as the ratio of viscosity and mass diffusivity. Hence, the concentration profile increases with Schmidt number. Figure 4 shows that the radial velocity, temperature and concentration also improve with Prandtl numbers. The axial velocity, however, is increased from $\lambda = 0$ to $\lambda = 0.5$ then reduced towards $\lambda = 1$. Figure 5 shows that as the chemical reaction parameter increases, the profiles of temperature, secondary velocity and concentration are decreases towards the upper plate, whereas the primary velocity profiles are decreases up to the middle of the plates then increases. This is because of the relation between the chemical reaction rate and mass diffusivity is inversely proportional to each other. Figure 6 shows the impact of the external magnetic field imposed across the flow. As the magnetic field intensity parameter Ha increases, the temperature, radial velocity and concentration decrease towards the upper plate due to the particle accumulation and retarding action of Lorentz forces. Also, the axial velocity decreases from $\lambda = 0$ to $\lambda = 0.5$ then increases further. Figure 7 depicts that as thermophoresis parameter increases, the profiles of velocity components, temperature and concentration distributions are following the Hartman

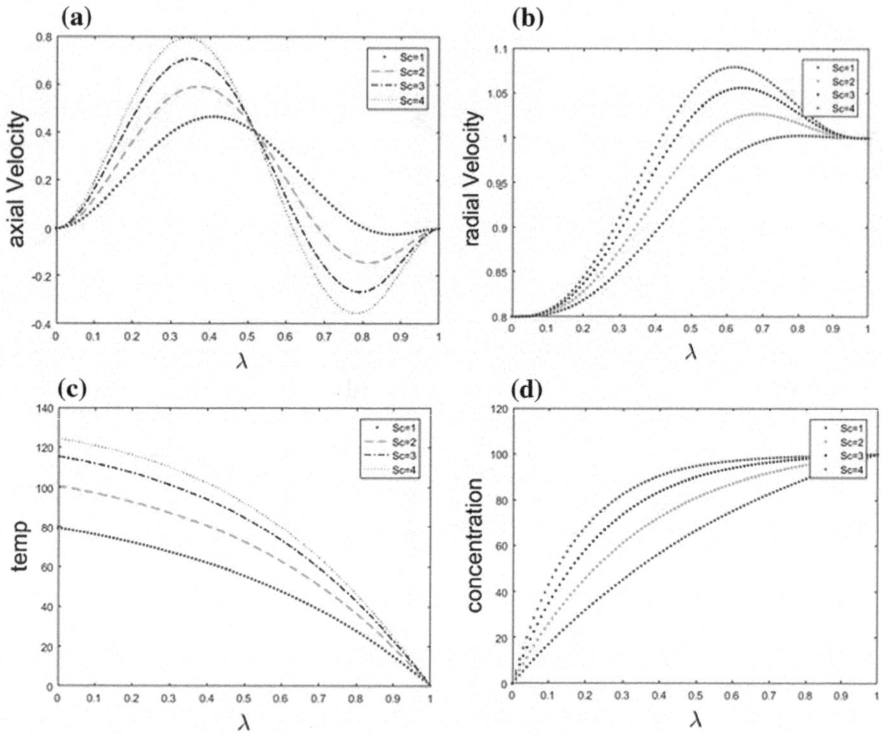

Fig. 3 Variation of Sc (Schmidt number) for **a** axial velocity, **b** radial velocity, **c** temperature and **d** concentration for Re = 2; Pr = 0.5; beta = 10; $G = 0.1$; Ec = 2; $a = 0.2$; Ha = 2; $D = 1.2$; Gm = 4; Gr = 4; $b = 0.2$; Nt = 0.002; Sh = 0.01; $T = 0.8$; Nb = 3; $\alpha = 0.1$; $K = 0.2$

number and the chemical reaction parameter. From Fig. 8, it is understood that as the Brownian motion parameter increases, the profiles of temperature, concentration distributions and velocity components follow the reversed trend of thermophoresis parameter. Brownian motion takes place due to fluid particles random motion; hence, it disturbed the laminar flow of the fluid as given in the graph and it increases the fluid inter-particle collision. That is why when the Brownian motion parameter increases, the temperature profiles of the fluid raises.

Table 1 indicates the heat transfer rate on the plates $\lambda = 0$ and $\lambda = 1$. From this, we noticed that as Ec increases, the Nusselt number also increases at both the plates. As Sc and Pr increase, the heat transfer rate decreases at $\lambda = 0$. Also, as the temperature slip parameter increases, the Nusselt number also increases at the lower plate. Table 2 shows a comparison study for $f'(0)$ for the viscous fluid, and it shows that the present results have good agreement with published work [27, 30].

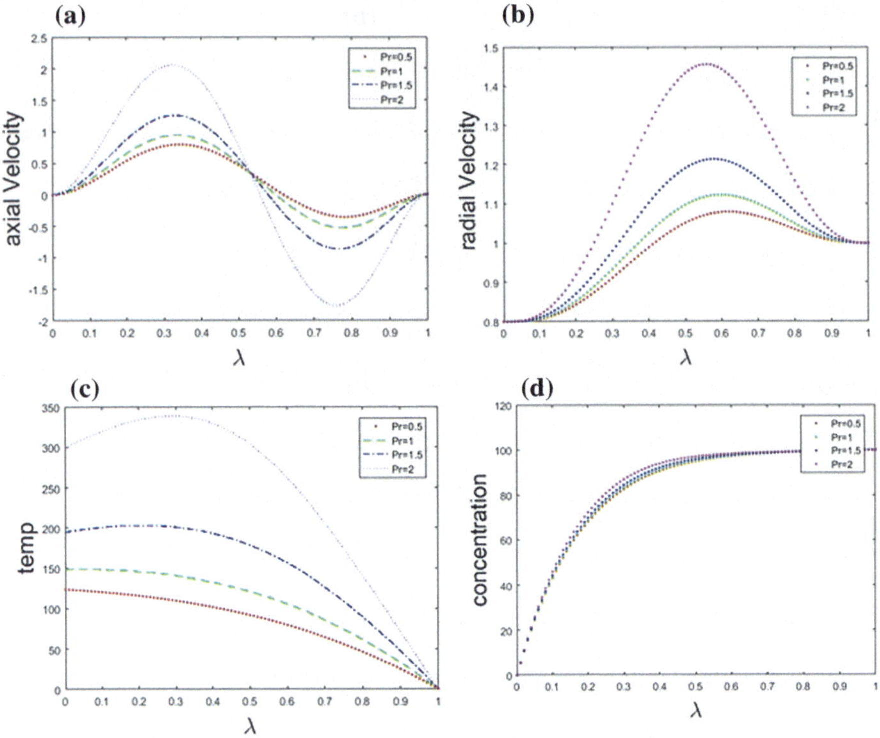

Fig. 4 Variation of Pr (Prandtl number) for **a** axial velocity, **b** radial velocity, **c** temperature and **d** concentration for Re = 2.0; beta = 10; $G = 0.1$; Ec = 2; $a = 0.2$; Ha = 2; $D = 1.2$; Sc = 4; Gm = 4; Gr = 4; $b = 0.2$; Nt = 0.002; Sh = 0.01; $T = 0.8$; Nb = 3; $\alpha = 0.1$; $K = 0.2$

5 Conclusions

In this paper, we have considered an incompressible laminar unsteady MHD mixed convective couple stress flow through porous parallel plates with thermophoresis and Brownian motion. The reduced ODEs are solved using shooting method with R-K fourth-order scheme, and the results are analysed in relation to various geometric and fluid parameters for non-dimensional velocities, concentration and temperature distributions and presented in graphs and tables. We therefore conclude that

- Brownian parameter enhanced the temperature and concentration of the fluid
- The impact of Brownian and thermophoresis parameter is opposite on temperature and concentration.
- The primary velocity of the fluid increases with increasing the suction–injection velocity, while the temperature distribution and concentration reduce from lower to upper plates.

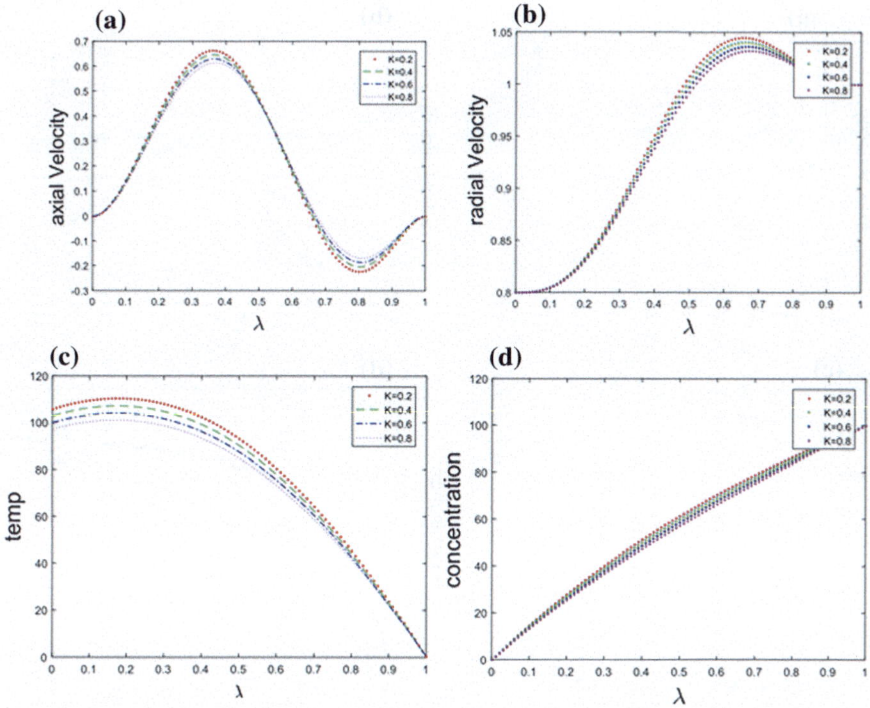

Fig. 5 Variation of K (chemical reaction parameter) for **a** axial velocity, **b** radial velocity, **c** temperature and **d**. concentration for Pr = 2.0; Re = 2.0; beta = 10; $G = 0.1$; Ec = 2; $a = 0.2$; Ha = 1.5; $D = 1.2$; Sc = 0.65; Gm = 4; Gr = 4; $b = 0.2$; Sh = 0.01; $T = 0.8$; Nb = 2; $\alpha = 0.1$; Nt = 0.0025

- The Schmidt number, Prandtl number and Brownian motion parameter show a similar influence on the temperature, concentration and velocity profiles of the fluid.
- The Hartmann number, chemical reaction parameter and thermophoresis parameter were having the same result on velocity, concentration and temperature distributions.
- The present results are compared with previously published work for Newtonian fluid and are found to be in good agreement.

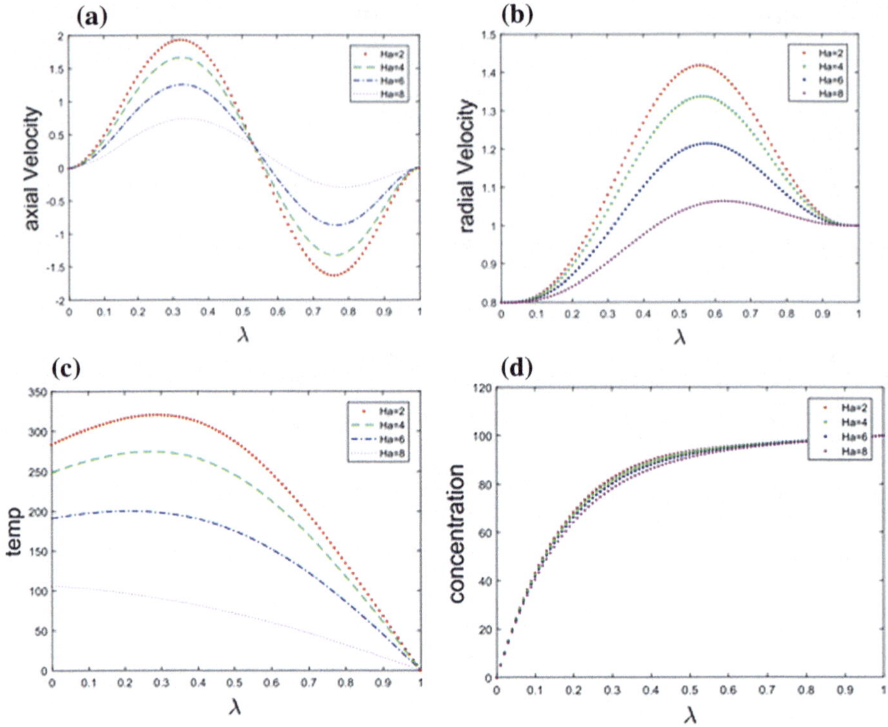

Fig. 6 Variation of Ha (Hartmann parameter) for **a** axial velocity, **b** radial velocity, **c** temperature and **d** concentration for Pr = 2.0; Re = 2.0; beta = 10; $G = 0.1$; Ec = 2; $a = 0.2$; $D = 1.2$; Sc = 4; Gm = 4; Gr = 4; $b = 0.2$; Sh = 0.01; $T = 0.8$; Nb = 3; $\alpha = 0.1$; $K = 0.8$; Nt = 0.002

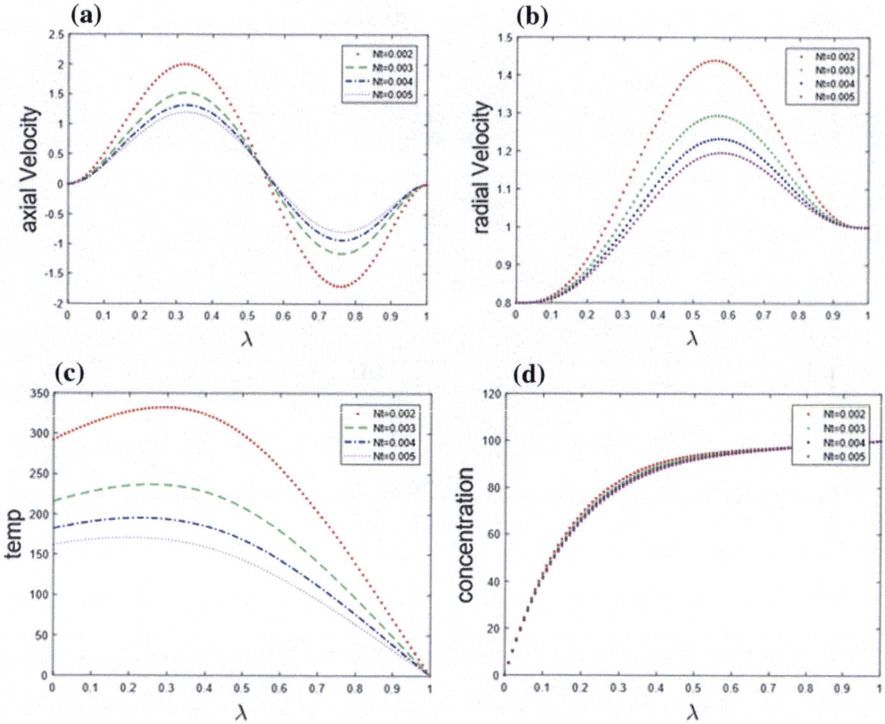

Fig. 7 Variation of Nt (thermophoresis parameter) for **a** axial velocity, **b** radial velocity, **c** temperature and **d** concentration for Pr = 2.0; Re = 2.0; beta = 10; $G = 0.1$; Ec = 2; $a = 0.2$; Ha = 1; $D = 1.2$; Sc = 2; Gm = 4; Gr = 4; $b = 0.2$; Nb = 3; Sh = 0.01; $T = 0.8$; $\alpha = 0.1$; $K = 0.025$

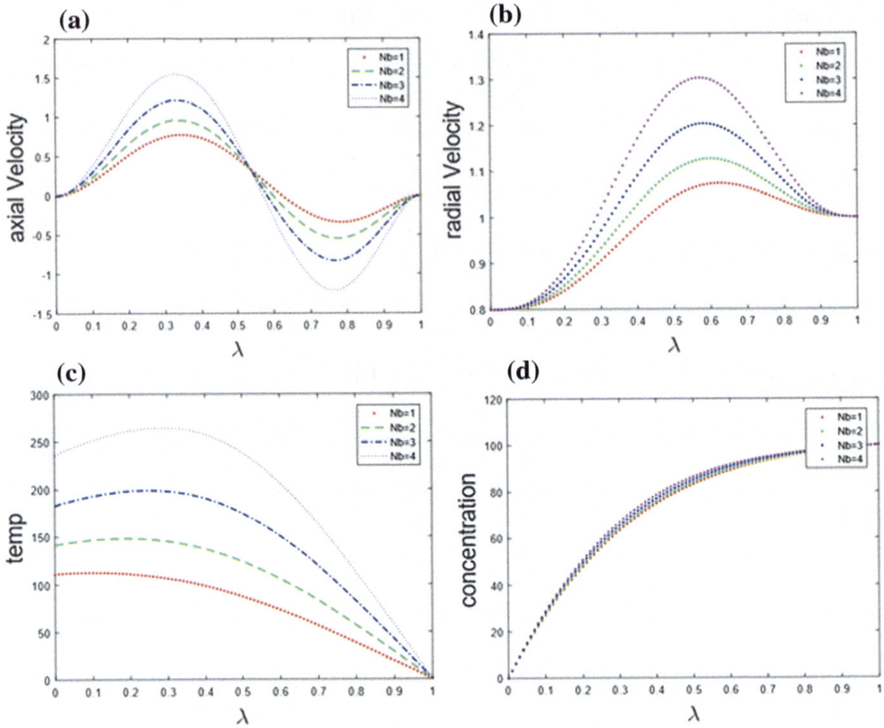

Fig. 8 Variation of Nb (Brownian motion) for **a** axial velocity, **b** radial velocity, **c** temperature and **d** concentration for Pr = 2.0; Re = 2.0; beta = 10; $G = 0.1$; Ec = 2; $a = 0.2$; Ha = 1; $D = 1.2$; Sc = 2; Gm = 4; Gr = 4; $b = 0.2$; Nt = 0.0033; Sh = 0.01; $T = 0.8$; $\alpha = 0.1$; $K = 0.025$

Table 1 Numerical values of Nusselt number with respect to various parameters like Re = 2.0; beta = 10; $a = 0.2$; Ha = 1; D = 1.2; Gm = 4; Gr = 4; $b = 0.2$; Nt = 0.0033; Nb = 3; Sh = 0̇.01; $T = 0.8$; $\alpha = 0.1$; $K = 0.025$

Ec	Sc	Pr	G	Nusselt number (Nu)	
				$\lambda = 0$	$\lambda = 1$
2	**1**	2	0.1	−158.807	−0.5
2	**2**	2	0.1	−222.74	−0.5
2	**3**	2	0.1	−263.303	−0.5
2	**4**	2	0.1	−284.012	−0.5
0.5	2	2	0.1	−417.688	−2
1	2	2	0.1	−335.031	−1
1.5	2	2	0.1	−270.893	−0.67
2	2	**2**	0.1	−222.74	−0.5
2	2	**0.5**	0.1	−93.652	−0.5
2	2	**1**	0.1	−110.034	−0.5
2	2	**1.5**	0.1	−142.045	−0.5
2	2	2	**0.2**	−75.2311	−0.5
2	2	2	**0.3**	−61.7626	−0.5
2	2	2	**0.4**	−51.2232	−0.5

Table 2 Validation of skin friction results with published paper [27, 30] for Newtonian case

Lower plate				
a	Re	Terril and Shresta	Ojjela and Kumar	Present
−0.00505	19.2038	−0.01129	−0.01129	−0.01128
−0.01573	11.8647	−0.03803	−0.03803	−0.03790
−0.12621	10.9454	−0.3220	−0.32224	−0.31267
−0.26170	12.1760	−0.679	−0.68433	−0.64285

Acknowledgements One of the authors (SJ) thanks to the Vice Chancellor, Defence Institute of Advanced Technology, Pune, for providing senior research fellowship for the project DIAT/F/ADM (RCT)/08-2017/P-71.

References

1. Sochi, T.: Non-Newtonian flow in porous media. Polymer **51**, 5007–5023 (2010)
2. Wu, Y.S., Pruss, K., Witherspoon, P.A: Displacement of a Newtonian fluid by a non-Newtonian fluid in a porous medium. Transp. Porous Media **6**, 115–142 (1991)
3. Huang, Z., Zhang, X., Yao, J., Wu, J.: Non-Darcy displacement by a non-Newtonian fluid in porous media according to the Barree-Conway model. Adv. Geo-energ. Res. **1**(2), 74–85 (2017)

4. Fayed, H.E., Sheikh, N.A., Iliev, O.: On laminar flow of non-newtonian fluids in porous media **111**(1), 253–264 (2016)
5. Narvaez, D.M.D., Parra, E.R., Mesa, F.: Conduction of fluids through porous parallel walls. Sci. et Tech. Año XIX **19**(2) (2014)
6. Belhouideg, S.: Modeling and numerical simulation of fluid flow in a porous tube with parietal suction. Contemp. Eng. Sci. **10**(9), 447–456 (2017)
7. Sandeep, K.: Karode: laminar flow in channels with porous walls, revisited. J. Membr. Sci. **191**, 237–241 (2001)
8. Stokes, V.K.: Couple stresses in fluid. Phys. Fluids **9**, 1709–1715 (1966)
9. Srinivasacharya, D., Srinivasacharyulu, N., Odelu, O.: Flow of couple stress fluid between two parallel porous plates. IAENG Int. J. Appl. Math. **41**(2), 1–5 (2011)
10. Srinivasacharya, D., Srinivasacharyulu, N., Odelu, O.: Flow and heat transfer of couple stress fluid in a porous channel with expanding and contracting walls. Int. Comm. Heat Mass Transf. **36**(2), 180–185 (2009)
11. Eldabe, N.T.M., Hassan, A.A., Mohamed, M.A.A.: Effect of couple stresses on the MHD of a Non-Newtonian unsteady flow between two parallel porous plates. Z. Naturforsch. **58**, 204–210 (2003)
12. Adesanya, S.O., Ogunseye, H.A., Falade, J.A., Lebelo, R.S.: Thermodynamic analysis for buoyancy-induced couple stress nanofluid flow with constant heat flux. Entropy **19**, 1–9 (2017)
13. Opanuga, A.A., Gbadeyan, J.A., Lyase, S.A.: Second law analysis of a reactive MHD couple stress fluid through porous medium. Int. J. Appl. Math. Stat. **56**(5), 85–100 (2017)
14. Davidson, P.A.: Introduction to Magnetohydrodynamics. Cambridge University Press, Cambridge (2017)
15. Rehman, K.U., Ali Khan, A., Malik, M.Y.: Magneto-nanofluid numerical modelling of chemically reactive Eyring-Powell fluid flow towards both flat and cylindrical an inclined surfaces: a comparative study. AIP Adv. **7**(6), 1–23 (2017)
16. Dastagiri Babu, D., Venkateswarlu, S., Keshava Reddy, E.: Heat and mass transfer on MHD flow of Non-Newtonian fluid over an infinite vertical porous plate with Hall effects. Int. J. Pure Appl. Math. **119**(15), 87–103 (2018)
17. Ahmed, N.: Heat and mass transfer in Hartmann flow with Soret effect in presence of a constant heat source. Turk. J. Phys. **36**, 446–460 (2012)
18. Mateen, A.: Magnetohydrodynamic flow and heat transfer of two immiscible fluids through a horizontal channel. Int. J. Curr. Eng. Technol. **3**(5), 1952–1956 (2013)
19. Ojjela, O., Kashyap, K.P., Naresh Kumar, N., Das, S.K.: Influence of inclined magnetic field on a mixed convective UCM fluid flow through a porous medium with thermophoresis and Brownian Motion. Int. J. Appl. Comput. Math. **3**(3), 2655–2669 (2017)
20. Anbuchezhian, N., Srinivasan, K., Chandrasekaran, K., Kandasamy, R.: Thermophoresis and Brownian motion effects on boundary layer flow of nanofluid in presence of thermal stratification due to solar energy. Appl. Math. Mech. Engl. Ed. **33**(6), 765–780 (2012)
21. Shit, G.C., Haldar, R., Ghosh, S.K.: Convective heat transfer and MHD viscoelastic nanofluid flow induced by a stretching sheet. Int. J. Appl. Comput. Math. **2**(4), 593–608 (2016)
22. Falana, A., Ojewale, O.A., Adeboje, T.B.: Effect of Brownian motion and thermophoresis on a nonlinearly stretching permeable sheet in a nanofluid. Adv. Nanoparticles **5**, 123–134 (2016)
23. Michaelides, E.E.: Brownian motion and thermophoresis of nanoparticles in liquids. Int. J. Heat Mass Transf. **81**, 79–187 (2015)
24. Mahdi, R.A., Mohammed, H.A., Munisamy, K.M., Saeid, N.H.: Review of convection heat transfer and fluid flow in porous media with nanofluid. Renew. Sustain. Energy Rev. **41**, 715–734 (2015)
25. Das, S.K., Putra, N., Thiesen, P., Roetzel, W: Temperature dependence of thermal conductivity enhancement for nanofluids. J. Heat Transf. **125**(4), 567–574 (2003)
26. Khan, S.U., Shehzad, S.A., Rauf, A., Ali, N.: Mixed convection flow of couple stress nanofluid over oscillatory stretching sheet with heat absorption/generation effects. Results Phys. **8**, 1223–1231 (2018)

27. Ojjela, O., Kumar, N.N.: Unsteady MHD mixed convective flow of chemically reacting and radiating couple stress fluid in a porous medium between parallel plates with Soret and Dufour Effects. Arab. J. Sci. Eng. **41**, 1941–1953 (2016)
28. Kaladhar, K., Srinivasachaya, D.: Mixed convection flow of chemically reacting couple stress fluid in an annulus with Soret and Dufour effects. WSEAS Trans. Heat Mass Transf. **9**, 2224–3461 (2014)
29. Yirga, Y., Tesfay, D.: Heat and mass transfer in MHD flow of nanofluids through a porous media due to a permeable stretching sheet with viscous dissipation and chemical reaction effects. Int. J. Mech. Mechatron. Eng. **9**(5), 709–716 (2015)
30. Terrill, R.M., Shrestha, G.M.: Laminar flow through a channel with uniformly porous walls of different permeability. Appl. Sci. Res. **15**, 440–468 (1965)

Modelling of Fluid Flow

Computational Fluid Dynamics Studies of Effect of Blockage Ratio on Drag

Vishal Kumar, Vivek Kumar Srivastav and Akshoy Ranjan Paul

Abstract There are several real-life problems exist where fluid flows over the heated solid body. In the present work, drag force and Nusselt number are studied for centrally fixed heated sphere. Computational fluid dynamics tool is used to simulate the present problem. The heated sphere is fixed radially at the centre of the cylinder. Total four cases corresponding to Reynolds numbers 100, 200, 300 and 500 are simulated to analyse the effects of blockage ratio of drag. The simulated results show that drag reduction is about 5%. The maximum value of drag coefficient is computed for the blockage ratio 0.8, and it decreases as the Reynolds numbers increases.

Keywords Computational fluid dynamics · Drag force · Blockage ratio · Nusselt number

1 Introduction

Fluid flow over solid bodies frequently occurs in practice, and it is responsible for numerous physical phenomena in which drag force plays an important role. The force of a flowing fluid exerts on a body in the flow track is drag. It is usually an adverse effect, like friction that should be reduced as much as possible. The drag is widely investigating under various conditions. The flow fields and geometries for most of the external flow problems are too complicated to be solved analytically, and therefore, either computer simulation or experiment is the optimum options to know the external flow physics. The scope of such types of design is to underlying various transport phenomena like food processing, fluidization and combustion. In this application, a heated sphere is fixed radially at the centre of the cylinder.

V. Kumar (✉) · V. K. Srivastav
Motihari College of Engineering, Motihari, Bihar, India
e-mail: vishalviswkarma176@gmail.com

A. R. Paul
Motilal Nehru National Institute of Technology Allahabad, Prayagraj, Uttar Pradesh, India

S. Bhattacharyya et al. (eds.), *Mathematical Modeling and Computational Tools*,
Springer Proceedings in Mathematics & Statistics 320,
https://doi.org/10.1007/978-981-15-3615-1_5

Bharti and Chhabra [1] have numerically studied two-dimensional steady Poiseuille flow of power-law fluids across a circular cylinder. They have presented total drag coefficients, surface pressure coefficients and their values at stagnation points and streamline patterns to provide physical insights into the hydrodynamics of the confined power-law fluid flow over a cylinder [1]. Krishnan and Kanan [2] have discussed about effect of blockage ratio on drag and heat transfer from a centrally located sphere in pipe flow. They have found that at higher Re, the drag and Nusselt number values have not attained steady state particularly at lower blockage ratios and Re exceeding 300 [2]. Gupta et al. [3] were presented numerical studied of laminar and steady free convection of power-law fluids from a heated spheroidal particle. They have correlated the average Nusselt number and drag coefficient in simple analytical form based on a general composite parameter proposed for power-law fluids [3]. Golani and Dhiman [4] studied on fluid flow and heat transfer across a circular cylinder in the unsteady flow regime in range of Reynolds number $50 \leq \text{Re} \leq 180$. They have found that the average Nusselt number increases with increasing Reynolds number. As the Reynolds number increases, the drag coefficient increases [4]. Samantaray et al. [5] studied the wall effects for Newtonian fluid flow over a cone and calculated the drag coefficient which increases with increasing the diameter ratio. This effect was more significant in low Reynolds numbers in comparison with higher Reynolds number [5]. The present work is focused on to understand how the drag coefficient is affected by blockage due to the presence of sphere at the centre of cylinder.

2 Geometrical Model

A three-D model of sphere inside a cylinder is created using Ansys Workbench. The diameter of cylinder is fixed to 60 mm, while diameter of sphere varies corresponding to different blockage ratio. The blockage ratio is defined as the ratio of the sphere diameter to that of cylinder diameter. Total five blockage ratio (BR) was used as 0.2, 0.4, 0.5, 0.6 and 0.8. The length of cylinder is divided into upstream (L_u) and downstream (L_d) from the centre of sphere. The length of upstream is $10D_s$ and downstream is $12D_s$ (*where* D_s *is diameter of sphere*). The geometrical model of the flow domain is shown in Fig. 1.

3 Grid Generation

The pre-processor Ansys Workbench is used for the grid generation. The computational fluid domain is divided into three sub-domains, upstream sub-domain, sphere sub-domain and downstream sub-domain. In the upstream and downstream sub-domain, 60 divisions of sweep method are used to make all structural quadrilaterals shape. Patch independent method along with inflation layer of thickness about 0.05 mm is used to make unstructured grid (tetrahedron shape elements) of spherical

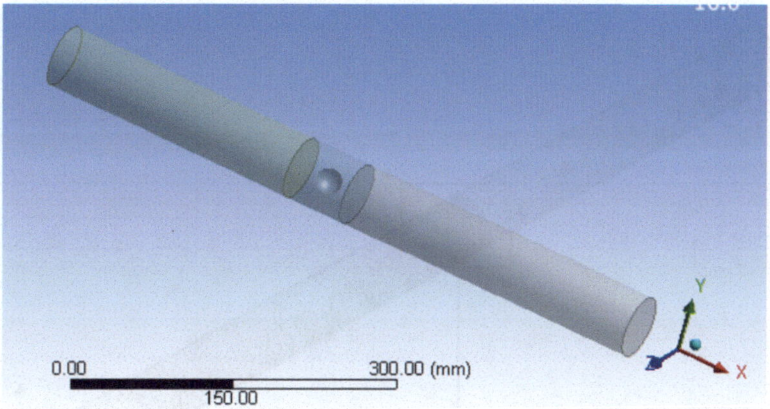

Fig. 1 Isometric view of geometrical model

sub-domain. Total 398,349 unstructured elements are created after grid independency test. The grid generated model of flow domain is shown in Fig. 2.

4 Boundary Conditions

In the present studies, flow has occurred over the sphere which implies external flow, and therefore, the following boundary conditions are used.

Inlet velocity	Parabolic velocity profile
Pressure outlet	0 Gauge pressure
Fluid	Water
Inlet temperature	29 °C
Surface temperature of sphere	32 °C
Density of water	997 kg/m^3
Viscosity of water	7.64×10^{-4} kg/m^{-s}

5 Results and Discussion

5.1 CFD Validation

The present result is validated with the result reported by Krishnan and Kannan [2]. It is found that at the blockage ratio 0.5, drag coefficient (C_d) is computed 0.589 against 0.62 computed by Krishnan and Kannan. Total five percent deviation is found against the C_d reported by Krishnan and Kannan. The comparisons of drag coefficient are summarized in Table 1.

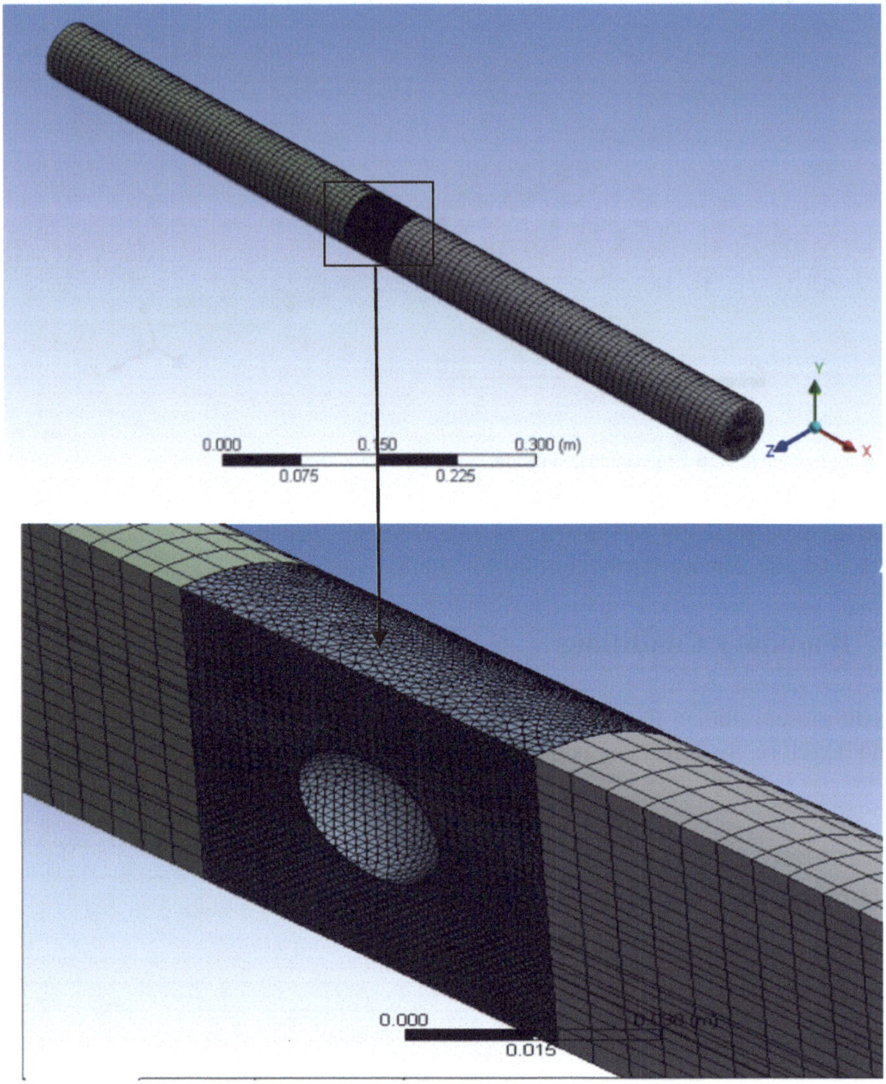

Fig. 2 Grid generation of flow domain

The total pressure on the surface of sphere was compared with the result shown by Krishnan and Kannan [2], which is found good agreement with the present result (Fig. 3).

Table 1 Validation of CFD results

	Clift et al. [6]	Krishnan and Kannan	Present result	Krishnan and Kannan	Present result	Krishnan and Kannan	Present result	Krishnan and Kannan	Present result
Re		BR = 0.1	BR = 0.1	BR = 0.2	BR = 0.2	BR = 0.4	BR = 0.4	BR = 0.5	BR = 0.5
500	0.555	0.56 (0.56)%	0.643 C_{lift} (15.85) paper (14.82)	0.558 (0.54)%	0.475 C_{lift} (−14.41) paper (−14.87)	0.554 (−0.18)%	0.494 C_{lift} (−10.99) paper (−10.83)	0.62 (11.71)%	0.589 C_{lift} (6.12)% paper (−5)%
350	0.63	0.63 (0)%	–	0.62 (−1.58)%	0.548 C_{lift} (−13.01) paper (−11.61)	0.63 (0)%	0.569 C_{lift} (−9.68) paper (−9.68)	0.722 (14.60)%	0.711 C_{lift} (12.85)% paper (−1.52)%

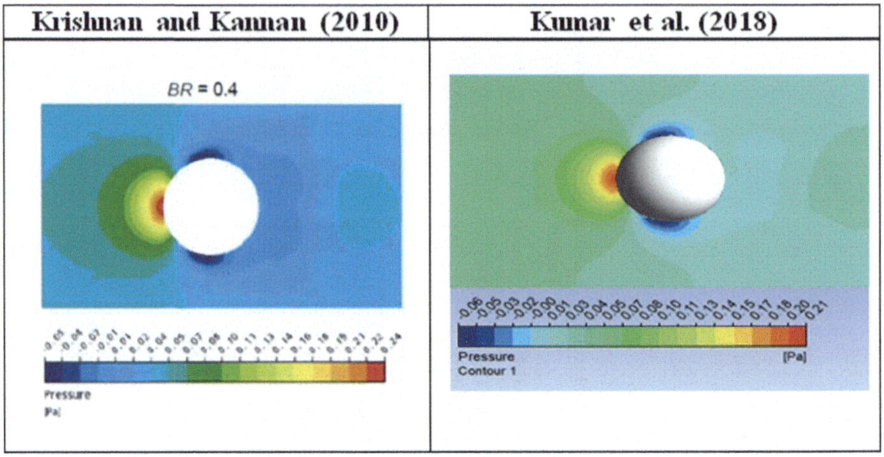

Fig. 3 Total pressure contours of the two models

5.2 *Velocity Contours*

Velocity contours are plotted at different locations of the flow domain. Velocity contours at the centre of cylinder are shown in Fig. 4. Parabolic velocity profile is fixed at the inlet of the cylinder however as the flow proceeds towards the sphere, it

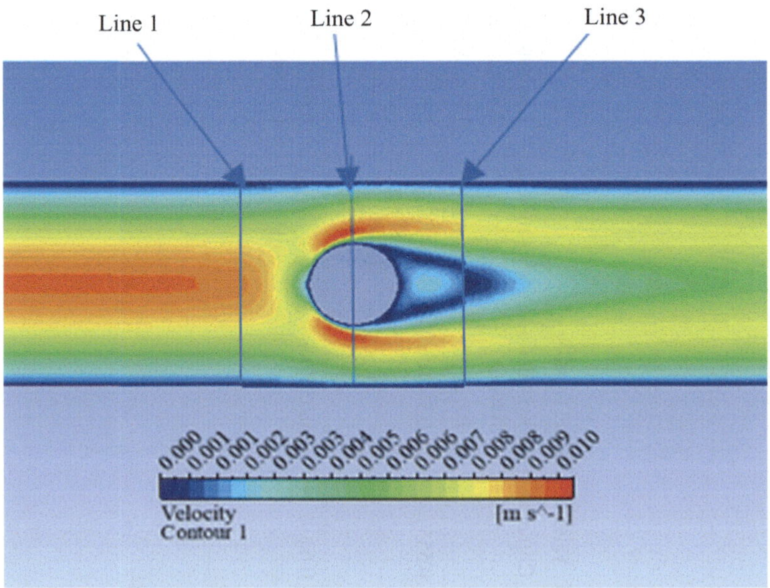

Fig. 4 Velocity contour of BR = 0.4 at Re = 300

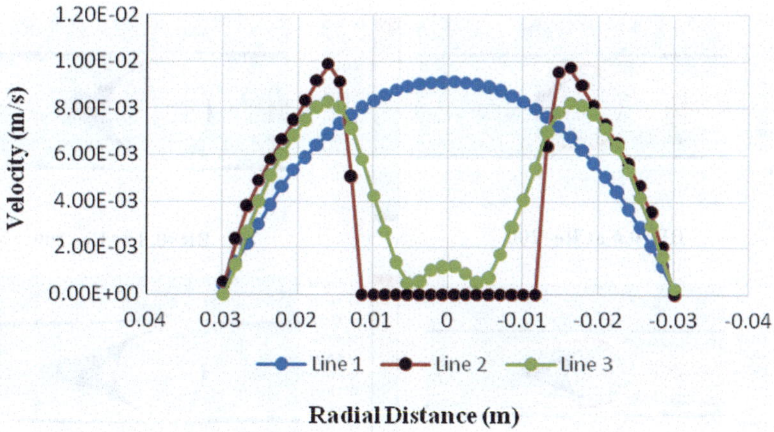

Fig. 5 Velocity profile of Line-1, Line-2 and Line-3

bifurcated into two parts (up and down). This is because of the presence of sphere as the obstruction in the flow path. In this work, the velocity profile was plotted at Line-1, Line-2 and Line-3 for Reynolds number 300 as shown in Fig. 5.

It was observed that the velocity profile at the Line-1 is very smooth but the same at Line-2 and Line-3 is not smooth due to existance of sphere in the flow path. As a result, a large deviation occurs in the velocity profile.

The velocity and pressure contours for blockage ratio 0.6 and 0.8 at Reynolds no. 200 and 300 are plotted. It was seen that an increase in blockage ratio increases the velocity in the pipe, and therefore, the pressure in the pipe is significantly changed as shown in Figs. 6 and 7.

6 Conclusions

In the present study, total four cases corresponding to Reynolds numbers 100, 200, 300 and 500 are simulated to analyse the effects of blockage ratio on drag. The simulated results show that drag reduction is about 5%. Drag coefficient is found to be suddenly increased as BR increases beyond 0.6 for Re = 100. The maximum value of C_d is found to be 11.557 at BR = 0.8, and it decreases as the Reynolds number is increased.

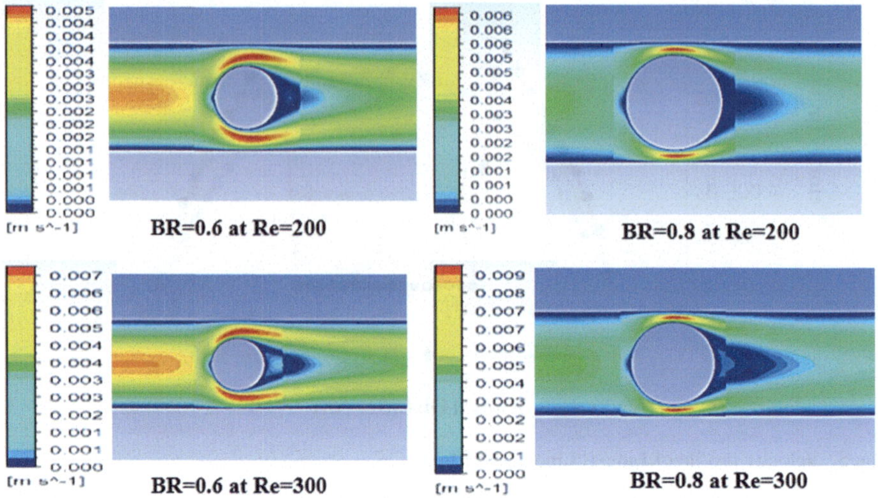

Fig. 6 Velocity contours for blockage ratio (BR) 0.6 and 0.8 at Re number 200 and 300

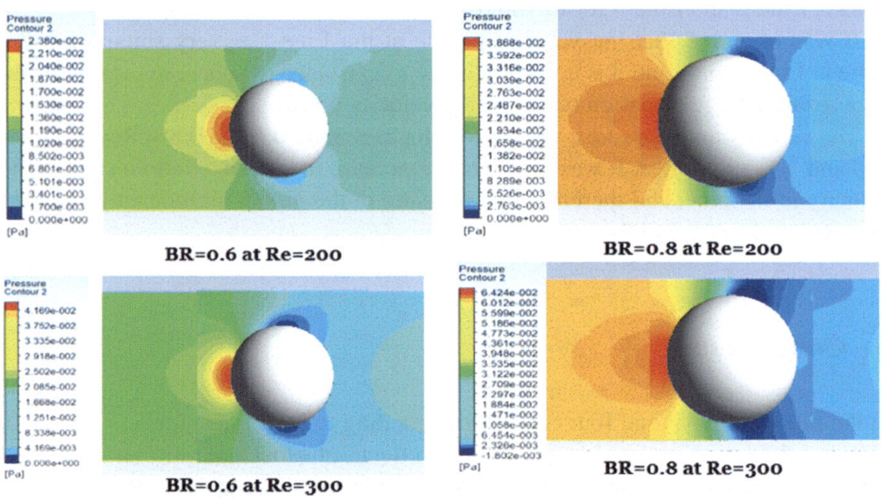

Fig. 7 Pressure contours for BR 0.6 and 0.8 at Re No. 200 and 300

References

1. Bharti, R.P., Chhabra, R.P.: Two-dimensional steady Poiseuille flow of power-law fluids across a circular cylinder in a plane confined channel: wall effects and drag coefficients. Ind. Eng. Chem. Res. **46**(11), 3820–3840 (2007)
2. Krishnan, S., Kannan, A.: Effect of blockage ratio on drag and heat transfer from a centrally located sphere in pipe flow. Eng. Appl. Comput. Fluid Mech. **4**(3), 396–414 (2010)
3. Gupta, A.K., Sasmal, C., Sairamu, M., Chhabra, R.P.: Laminar and steady free convection in power-law fluids from a heated spheroidal particle: a numerical study. Int. J. Heat Mass Transf. **75**, 592–609 (2014)
4. Golani, R., Dhiman, A.K.: Fluid flow and heat transfer across a circular cylinder in the unsteady flow regime. Int. J. Eng. Sci. (IJES). **3**(3), 08–19 (2014)
5. Samantaray, S.K., Mohapatra, S.S., Munshi, B.: A numerical study of the wall effects for Newtonian fluid flow over a cone. Eng. Sci. Tech. Int. J. **20**(6), 1662–1675 (2017)
6. Clift, R., Grace, J.R., Weber, W.R.: Bubbles, Drops and Particles. Academic Press Inc., New York (1978) (International Standard Book Number: 0-486-44580-1)

Distribution of Two-Dimensional Unsteady Sediment Concentration in an Open Channel Flow

Shiv Mohan, Sudip Debnath, Koeli Ghoshal and Jitendra Kumar

Abstract An unsteady two-dimensional transport equation is considered to investigate the distribution of suspended sediment in an open channel turbulent flow, where the mechanism of hindered settling is also taken into account. Due to the consideration of concentration-dependent settling velocity on sediment transportation, the transport equation is a partial differential equation with a highly nonlinear term, which has been solved numerically by using the alternating direction implicit (ADI) finite-difference method. It is found that the sediment concentration increases along the vertical direction due to the inclusion of hindered settling effect.

Keywords Open channel flow · Diffusion equation · Hindered settling mechanism · Suspended sediment concentration

1 Introduction

In an open channel turbulent flow, the study of sediment transport is a challenging task due to the irregular behavior of the turbulence. Sediment transport is mainly classified into two categories: suspended sediment transport and bed-load transport. The transportation of non-equilibrium suspended sediment is one of the important problems in the area of sediment transport.

Hjelmfelt and Lenau [1], Liu and Nayamatullah [2], Liu [3] and Jing et. al. [4] worked on the transportation of non-equilibrium suspended sediments. Hjelmfelt and Lenau [1] and Liu [3] studied the steady two-dimensional suspended sediment transport problem, and Liu and Nayamatullah [2] solved the one-dimensional unsteady non-equilibrium suspended sediment transport problem by GITT technique. The problems of non-equilibrium sediment transport are generally governed by partial differential equations. It is observed by researchers that in high concentrated

S. Mohan · S. Debnath · K. Ghoshal (✉) · J. Kumar
Department of Mathematics, Indian Institute of Technology Kharagpur, Kharagpur 721302, India
e-mail: koeli@maths.iitkgp.ac.in

S. Bhattacharyya et al. (eds.), *Mathematical Modeling and Computational Tools*, Springer Proceedings in Mathematics & Statistics 320,
https://doi.org/10.1007/978-981-15-3615-1_6

flows, the settling velocity of the suspended sediment particles decreases in comparison with that in clear fluid. This physical phenomenon is commonly known as the hindered settling effect. Inclusion of this phenomenon makes the governing equation nonlinear in nature, and hence, the problem becomes more challenging.

In this model, we consider the unsteady two-dimensional non-equilibrium transport problem considering the hindered settling effect and solve the problem by alternating direction implicit (ADI) finite-difference scheme. The obtained results are discussed with figures and based on that important conclusions are drawn.

2 Mathematical Modeling

We consider an unsteady two-dimensional transport equation to describe the distribution of suspended sediment in an open channel (separation width h) turbulent flow. The flow in the axial (stream-wise) and vertical directions is represented by a Cartesian coordinate system, say, x and y. We assume that the flow is uniform in the axial direction and also independent of time; thus, the velocity varies only in the vertical direction. In the following subsections, the problem has been mathematically formulated.

2.1 Governing Equation

The governing equation for the unsteady two-dimensional suspended sediment concentration distribution in a wide open channel flow is given as follows:

$$\frac{\partial c}{\partial t} + u\frac{\partial c}{\partial x} - \frac{\partial}{\partial y}\left(\omega_s c\right) = \frac{\partial}{\partial y}\left(\epsilon_s \frac{\partial c}{\partial y}\right), \tag{1}$$

where c is the volumetric sediment concentration, t denotes time. u is the flow velocity in stream-wise direction, ϵ_s is the sediment diffusivity in the vertical direction, and ω_s is the settling velocity of the sediment particles which is treated as a function of concentration c. In high concentrated flow, the magnitude of ω_s is less than that of ω_0 and the relationship between them is provided by Richarson and Zaki [5] as

$$\omega_s = \omega_0(1-c)^{n_H}, \tag{2}$$

where ω_0 is the settling velocity of the particles in clear fluid and n_H is the exponent of reduction whose value depends on the particle Reynolds number. In the present work, taking the average value of n_H as 4, the governing equation (1) becomes:

$$\frac{\partial c}{\partial t} + u\frac{\partial c}{\partial x} - \omega_0\frac{\partial}{\partial y}\left[c(1-c)^4\right] = \frac{\partial}{\partial y}\left(\epsilon_s \frac{\partial c}{\partial y}\right). \tag{3}$$

2.2 Initial and Boundary Conditions

The boundary conditions at top and bottom surface are considered according to Hjelmfelt and Leanu [1] as follows

$$c = 0 \text{ at } y = h, \tag{4}$$

and

$$c = c_a \text{ at } y = a, \tag{5}$$

respectively, where c_a is the reference concentration at the reference level $y = a$. At the inlet, we consider that there is uniform sediment concentration, i.e.,

$$c = 1 \text{ at } x = 0, \tag{6}$$

and at initial time

$$c = 1 \text{ at } t = 0. \tag{7}$$

2.3 Dimensionless Form of Governing Equation Together with Initial and Boundary Conditions

The governing equation (3) and the boundary conditions (4–7) are non-dimensionalized as per the following scales:

$$C = \frac{c}{c_a}, \quad Y = \frac{y}{h}, \quad X = \frac{x}{h}, \quad T = \frac{tu_*}{h},$$

$$A = \frac{a}{h}, \quad K(Y) = \frac{\epsilon_t}{\beta u_* h}, \quad U(Y) = \frac{u}{u_*}, \quad V_0 = \frac{\omega_0}{u_*},$$

where u_* is the shear velocity and β is the ratio of turbulent diffusivity ϵ_t to sediment diffusivity ϵ_s. Accordingly, the dimensionless form of Eq. (3) and boundary conditions (4–7) becomes:

$$\frac{\partial C}{\partial T} + U(Y)\frac{\partial C}{\partial X} - V_0\frac{\partial}{\partial Y}\left[C(1 - c_a C)^4\right] = \frac{\partial}{\partial Y}\left(K(Y)\frac{\partial C}{\partial Y}\right), \tag{8}$$

$$C(T, X, Y) = 0 \text{ at } Y = 1, \tag{9}$$

$$C(T, X, Y) = 1 \text{ at } Y = A, \tag{10}$$

$$C(T, X = 0, Y) = 1, \tag{11}$$

and

$$C(T = 0, X, Y) = 1, \tag{12}$$

So, finally, we have a PDE with nonlinear term $(1 - c_a C)^4$ given by Eq. (8) together with the boundary conditions (Eqs. 9 and 10) and the initial conditions (Eqs. 11 and 12) which we will solve numerically.

3 Numerical Solution

In the present problem, the concentration distribution of suspended sediment in an open channel flow is described by the two-dimensional unsteady convection-diffusion Eq. (8). Due to the complexity in Eq. (8), we have adopted an alternating direction implicit (ADI) finite-difference scheme [6] to solve Eq. (8) together with initial and boundary conditions (9)–(12). In ADI method, the finite-difference equation can be factored into a multistage process to step ahead one-time increment in such a way that the solution of the nonlinear equations emerging at each time level is very easy to handle computationally.

The whole width of the channel is divided into $(M - 1)$ equal parts, having length ΔX in the axial direction and ΔY in the vertical direction. The time increment is denoted by ΔT. The lengths in the vertical and axial directions are represented by the grid point j and k, whereas time is represented by the grid point i. So the general formulae are: $Y_j = A + (j - 1)^* \Delta Y$, $X_k = (k - 1) \times \Delta X$ and $T_i = (i - 1) \times \Delta T$, respectively.

Utilizing Douglas–Rachford [7] procedure on the convection diffusion equation (8), the finite difference equation splits into two implicit equations, as

$$\left[1 - \Delta T \left\{ \frac{\partial K}{\partial Y} + V_0 (c_a C(i,j) - 1)^3 (5 c_a C(i,j) - 1) \right\} S_Y - K \Delta T S_{YY} \right] C^*(i+1) = (1 - U(Y) \Delta T S_X) C(i), \tag{13a}$$

$$(1 + U(Y) \Delta T S_X) C(i+1) = C^*(i+1, j) + U(Y) \Delta T S_X C(i), \tag{13b}$$

where $S_Y C^* = \frac{C^*(j+1,k) - C^*(j-1,k)}{2\Delta Y}$, $S_{YY} C^* = \frac{C^*(j+1,k) - 2C^*(j,k) + C^*(j-1,k)}{\Delta Y^2}$ and $S_X C = \frac{C(j,k+1) - C(j,k-1)}{2\Delta X}$ are the discretized operators.

Clearly, the process needs two steps: In the first step, we solve C^* from Eq. (13a), and in the next step, we solve C from Eq. (13b) by using the values of C^*. To find the solution, we have considered a mesh size: $\Delta T = 0.00001$, $\Delta Y = (1 - A)/(M - 1)$ and $\Delta X = 1/(M - 1)$ for the present problem, where $M = 500$. Different cases have been considered to investigate the hindered settling effect on the distribution of sediment concentration. In all the cases, we have assumed fixed value of $V_0 = 0.2$, $Y_0 = 0.001$, and $A = 0.05$, respectively. The considered spatial and temporal discretization parameters ensure a precision of 10^{-6} in the results.

4 Results and Discussion

4.1 Input Functions

It is clear from Eq. (8) that to assess the solution, known expression for the functions $K(Y)$ and $U(Y)$ are needed. So, in the present problem we consider the following expressions (Liu [3]):

$$K(Y) = \kappa Y(1 - Y), \tag{14}$$

and

$$U(Y) = \frac{1 - Y_0}{Y_0 - \ln Y_0 - 1} \ln \frac{Y}{Y_0} \quad \text{for } Y_0 \leq Y \leq 1, \tag{15}$$

where κ is the universal von Karman constant ($= 0.41$) and $Y_0 = 0.001$.

4.2 Validation of the Solution

In this section, we validate our obtained solution with the existing models. In Fig. 1a, the concentration profile is the same as the well-known Rouse profile [8], who found the analytical solution for steady transport equation and Fig. 1b agrees with the work of Liu [3] for two-dimensional steady non-equilibrium sediment transport. It is clear from the figure that as one tends toward the surface of the channel from the bottom, concentration profiles decrease and tend to zero which is usual characteristics of sediment concentration profile. It happens because at the surface suspended sediment particles are negligible.

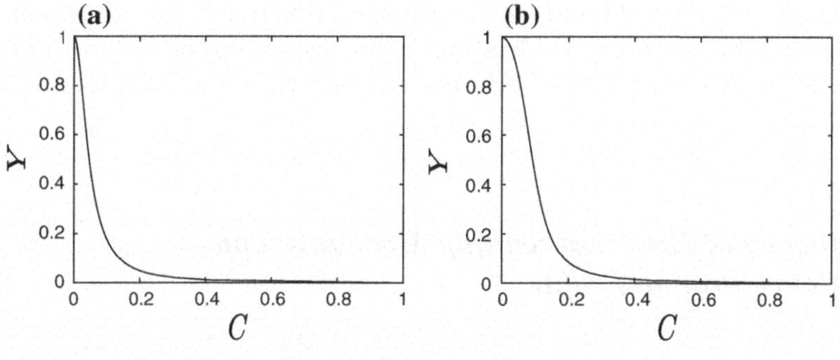

Fig. 1 Vertical distribution of sediment concentration when $c_a = 0.02$, $V_0 = 0.2$, $Y_0 = 0.001$ and $A = 0.05$. **a** For $T \to \infty$, $X \to \infty$; **b** for $T \to \infty$, $X = 2$

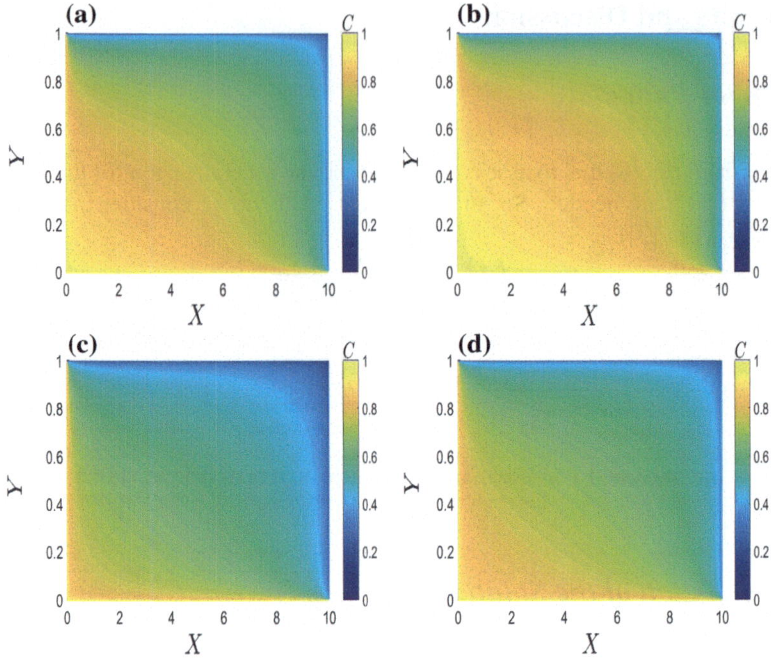

Fig. 2 Concentration contours at time $T = 5$ (1st row) and $T = 10$ (2nd row), when $V_0 = 0.2$, $Y_0 = 0.001$ and $A = 0.05$. **a**, **c** For $c_a = 0.005$; **b**, **d** for $c_a = 0.02$

4.3 Contour Plot of Concentration Profiles

Figure 2 shows the variation of suspended sediment concentration in the stream-wise and vertical directions simultaneously. Figures 2a, b is plotted at a fixed time $T = 5$ with different reference concentration and Figs. 2c, d is plotted for the same but at a fixed time $T = 10$. From Figs. 2a, b it is clear that the area of concentration distribution is higher in Fig. 2b than Fig. 2a because of higher value of reference concentration. A similar kind of behavior can be seen in Fig. 2c, d for large time $T = 10$.

4.4 Impact of Hindered Settling Mechanism on Concentration Profile

The effect of hindered settling mechanism is shown in Fig. 3 where the vertical distribution of sediment concentration is plotted at different time. In Fig. 3a, b, reference concentration is taken as $c_a = 0.005$ and $c_a = 0.02$, respectively, and it can be seen

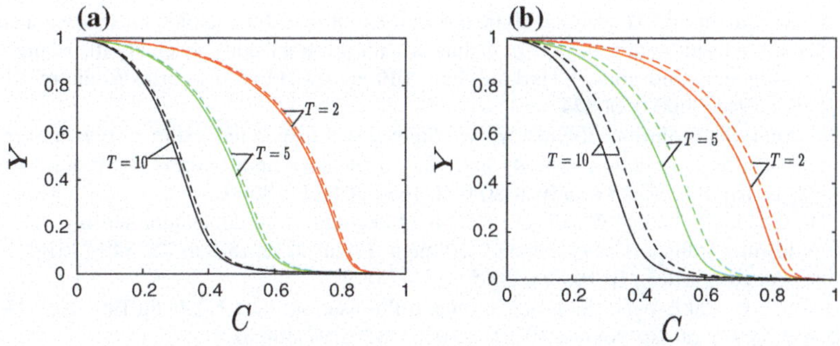

Fig. 3 Vertical distribution of sediment concentration under the effect of settling velocity of particles, when $V_0 = 0.2$, $Y_0 = 0.001$, $A = 0.05$ and $X = 3$. **a** For $c_a = 0.005$, $n_H = 0$ (solid line), $n_H = 4$ (dashed line); **b** For $c_a = 0.02$, $n_H = 0$ (solid line), $n_H = 4$ (dashed line)

from the figures that the effect is more in Fig. 3b comparison with Fig. 3a. It happens because the hindered settling effect is more effective in high concentrated flow due to the presence of surrounding particles.

5 Conclusions

Distribution of suspended sediment is studied in the present work for an unsteady two-dimensional turbulent flow through an open channel. The presence of sediment affect the settling velocity of a particle which is commonly known as the hindered settling effect, and accordingly, the concentration profile is also changed. This phenomenon is taken into account in the governing partial differential equation, and ADI method is adopted to solve the equation numerically. At large time and far from the downstream, the concentration shows similarity with Rouse [8] profile of concentration. Contour plots of concentration at different times are plotted to see the variation of concentration along vertical and axial direction. Also that, at a fixed time and axial direction, concentration is plotted with and without hindered settling effect and it is found that higher the concentration, more is the change in concentration due to inclusion of hindered settling effect.

Acknowledgements The last three authors are thankful to the Science and Engineering Research Board (SERB), Department of Science and Technology (DST), Government of India for providing financial support through Research Project No. EMR/2015/002434.

References

1. Hjelmfelt, A., Lenau, C.W.: Nonequilibrium transport of suspended sediment. In: Journal of the Hydraulics Division: Proceedings of the American Society of Civil Engineers (ASCE), pp. 1567–1587. ASCE, New York (1970). http://www.vliz.be/en/imis?refid=143170

2. Liu, X., Nayamatullah, M.: Semianalytical solutions for one-dimensional unsteady nonequilibrium suspended sediment transport in channels with arbitrary eddy viscosity distributions and realistic boundary conditions. J. Hydraul. Eng. **140**, 04014011 (2014). https://doi.org/10.1061/(ASCE)HY.1943-7900.0000874
3. Liu, X.: Analytical solutions for steady two-dimensional suspended sediment transport in channels with arbitrary advection velocity and eddy diffusivity distributions. J. Hydraul Res. **54**, 389–398 (2016). https://doi.org/10.1080/00221686.2016.1168880
4. Jing, H., Chen, G., Wang, W., Li, G.: Effects of concentration dependent settling velocity on non-equilibrium transport of suspended sediment. Environ. Earth Sci. **77**, 549 (2018). https://link.springer.com/article/10.1007/s12665-018-7731-9
5. Richarson, J.F., Zaki, W.N.: Sedimentation and fluidisation: part 1. Chem. Eng. Res. Des. **75**, S82-S100 (1997). https://doi.org/10.1016/S0263-8762(97)80006-8
6. Peaceman, D.W., Rachford Jr., H.H.: The numerical solution of parabolic and elliptic differential equations. J. Soc. Ind. Appl. Math. **3**, 28–41 (1955). https://doi.org/10.1137/0103003
7. Douglas, J., Rachford Jr., H.H.: On the numerical solution of heat conduction problems in two and three space variables. Trans. Am. Math. Soc. **82**, 421–439 (1956). https://www.jstor.org/stable/1993056
8. Rouse, H.: Modern conceptions of the mechanics of fluid turbulence. Trans ASCE. **102**, 463–505 (1937). https://ci.nii.ac.jp/naid/10029236933/

Solution to One-Dimensional Diffusion Equation with Concentration-Dependent Mixing Length

Punit Jain and Koeli Ghoshal

Abstract The present study focuses on vertical distribution of concentration in a turbulent flow where the swapping of fluid parcels and suspended sediment parcels takes place over a vertical distance l_m, the mixing length and generates a net vertical flux of momentum and sediment. The Fickian diffusivity of sediment has been considered not to be equal to the Fickian diffusivity of momentum, i.e., the eddy viscosity. Also, the study assumes that in the stream-wise direction the velocity of fluid and solid particles is identical, and in the transverse direction, they differ by the particle settling velocity w_s. Apart from these, the study considers the reduction of mixing length due to the presence of suspended solid particles which damp the characteristic oscillation of turbulent flow. The model is solved numerically and is validated by comparing the solution with relevant set of laboratory experimental data.

Keywords Turbulent flow · Mixing length · Sediment suspension · Hindered settling effect · Concentration distribution

1 Introduction

Investigation of concentration distribution along a vertical in a turbulent flow carrying sediment is a topic of research since long. Several models have been developed by researchers to address the vertical distribution of sediment in an open channel flow. The present study is an addition to those studies where the concentration is viewed from the mixing length aspect.

The mixing length theory of turbulent flow was originally developed by Prandtl [1] which proposes that the fluctuating velocity components in the longitudinal and vertical directions are each proportional to $l_0 \frac{du}{dz}$ where l_0 is the mixing length in clear

P. Jain (✉) · K. Ghoshal
Department of Mathematics, Indian Institute of Technology Kharagpur, Kharagpur 721302, India
e-mail: punitjain51@gmail.com

K. Ghoshal
e-mail: koeli@maths.iitkgp.ac.in

S. Bhattacharyya et al. (eds.), *Mathematical Modeling and Computational Tools*, Springer Proceedings in Mathematics & Statistics 320,
https://doi.org/10.1007/978-981-15-3615-1_7

water, and u is the longitudinal velocity of fluid, and z is the vertical distance from channel bed. Bialik [2, 3] explained the mixing length as that small distance which is lump of fluid particles may randomly travel before mixing with the surrounding fluid. Prandtl used a very simple form of mixing length for clear water as $l_0 = \kappa z$ which was used to obtain the universal log-law velocity distribution. Later on, he gave a parabolic form of mixing length as $l_0 = \kappa z \sqrt{1 - \frac{z}{h}}$ for clear water flow. Van Driest [4] suggested that near the wall the mixing must be damped with a damping factor $(1 - e^{\frac{-z}{A^*}})$, A^* being the damping function. Nishioka and Iida [5] proposed a differential equation describing the mixing length. Galbraith et al. [6] showed that when substantial variation of shear stress occurs, the mixing length must be a function of wall shear stress. Umeyama and Gerritsen [7] proposed a mixing length for sediment-laden flow as $l_0 = \kappa z \left(1 - \frac{z}{h}\right)^{\alpha}$ where α is a function of sediment concentration; but they were unable to justify why the form of α should be like that. Kovacs [8] formulated the mixing length including a damping factor $D(C)$ where $D = 1 - C^{1/3}$. He gave a proper justification for such type of damping factor. The explanations are like this—the suspended particles in a fluid–sediment mixture occupy a volume given by their concentration C. If a little cube is imagined to be occupied by sediments, then the cube has a length proportional to $C^{1/3}$ and the mixing length l_m will be reduced by the length taken by the particles in suspension. Consequently, the damping function takes the above-mentioned form. The present study takes into account the mixing length formulated by Kovacs [8] as it is a function of concentration which can be used to study sediment-laden flow and also as the form of mixing length was proposed with a proper physical justification.

The governing equations to study vertical concentration distribution were given by Rouse [9] and Hunt [10] and since then these equations were widely used by the researchers in the study of sediment transport. Nielsen and Teakle [11] looked at the same problem through mixing length concept where they developed the governing equation for concentration by considering the turbulent mixing in terms of interchanging fluid–sediment mix parcels over a vertical distance, which is the mixing length in a sediment carrying fluid. They expressed the sediment flux density in terms of concentration and mixing length and developed the governing equation of time-averaged concentration of suspended sediment by balancing the upward mixing flux with downward settling flux. But for solving the governing equation, they did not take the mixing length and settling velocity of sediment as function of concentration. The present study takes the governing equation of concentration from [11] and solves it numerically taking into account the mixing length and settling velocity both as function of concentration. It has been shown graphically the changes in concentration values for the inclusion of the above-mentioned effects, and at the end, comparison of the model with laboratory data has been made to check the validity of the model.

2 Mathematical Model

A steady uniform flow is considered where the swapping of fluid parcels with sediment occurs between different levels (Fig. 1). As a result, a net vertical flux of momentum is generated. The lower parcel has the sediment concentration $C\left(z-\frac{l_m}{2}\right)$, and the upper parcel has $C\left(z+\frac{l_m}{2}\right)$. If the parcels travel vertically with equal and opposite velocities $\pm w_m$, the resulting sediment flux density is [11]

$$q_m = w_m\left[C\left(z-\frac{l_m}{2}\right)-C\left(z+\frac{l_m}{2}\right)\right] \tag{1}$$

and the Taylor series expansion of $C\left(z\pm\frac{l_m}{2}\right)$ up to 2 terms gives

$$q_m = -l_m w_m \frac{dC}{dz} \tag{2}$$

where l_m is the mixing length in a sediment mixed fluid. In a sediment-laden flow, a balance between an upward mixing flux and downward settling flux occurs and result in time-averaged concentration of suspended sediment. Mathematically, it can be written as

$$q_m - w_s C(z) = 0 \tag{3}$$

where w_s is the settling velocity of sediment. After putting the expression of sediment flux density q_m from Eq. (2) in Eq. (3), we can rewrite Eq. (3) as

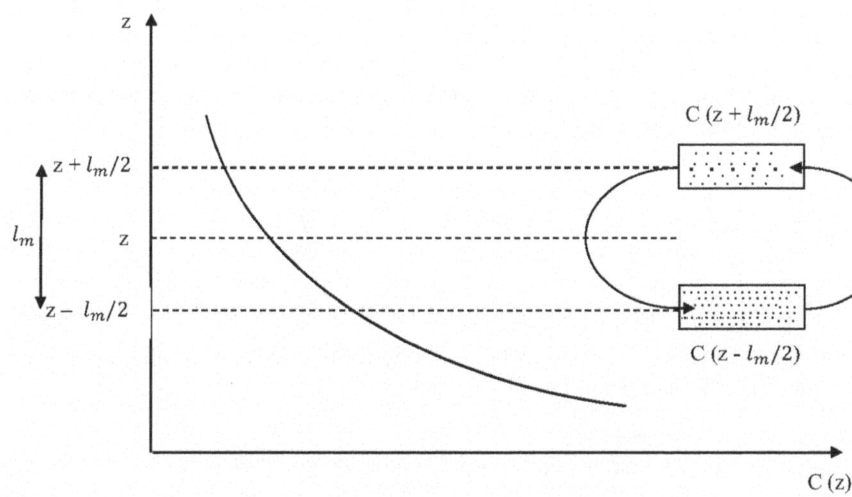

Fig. 1 Swapping of fluid parcels (including suspended sediment) over a vertical distance l_m, the mixing length. (Fig. from [11])

$$l_{\mathrm{m}} w_{\mathrm{m}} \frac{\mathrm{d}C}{\mathrm{d}z} + w_{\mathrm{s}} C = 0 \tag{4}$$

As mentioned previously, in this study, we take mixing length l_{m} as a function of suspended sediment concentration C and vertical distance z which is given as follows [8]

$$l_{\mathrm{m}} = l_0(1 - C^{1/3}) \tag{5}$$

where $l_0 = \kappa z\sqrt{1 - \frac{z}{h}}$ is the mixing length in clear water flow [8]. In a sediment-laden flow, it was observed by the experiment that the flow around the neighboring settling particles exhibits a larger drag as compared to the clear water flow. Due to this, the settling velocity w_{s} of sediment in sediment-laden flow is less than the settling velocity w_0 in clear fluid, which is known as hindered settling. In this study, expression of w_{s} is chosen from Richardson and Zaki [12] which is given as follows:

$$w_{\mathrm{s}} = w_0(1 - C)^{\eta} \tag{6}$$

where that η is the exponent of reduction of settling velocity that depends on the particle Reynolds number Out of several expressions available for η in the literature, we choose the expression of Richardson and Zaki [12] in this study, which is given as

$$\eta = \begin{cases} 4.65 & \text{when Re} < 0.2 \\ 4.4\mathrm{Re}^{-0.03} & \text{when } 0.2 < \text{Re} < 1 \\ 4.4\mathrm{Re}^{-0.1} & \text{when } 1 < \text{Re} < 500 \\ 2.4 & \text{when Re} > 500 \end{cases} \tag{7}$$

where $\mathrm{Re} = \frac{w_0 D_{\mathrm{p}}}{\nu_{\mathrm{f}}}$, D_{p} is the particle diameter and ν_{f} denotes the kinematic viscosity of clear fluid. Here settling velocity of particle in clear fluid is calculated from the widely used formula given as [13]

$$w_0 = \frac{\nu_{\mathrm{f}}}{D_{\mathrm{p}}}\left(\sqrt{25 + 1.2D_*^2} - 5\right)^{1.5} \tag{8}$$

where $D_*\left(= \left(\frac{\Delta g}{\nu_{\mathrm{f}}^2}\right)^{1/3} D_{\mathrm{p}}\right)$ is the dimensionless particle diameter, g is the gravitational acceleration and $\Delta = s - 1$, s being the specific gravity of sediment particle. After using Eqs. (5) and (6) in Eq. (4), we get

$$\kappa z\sqrt{1 - \frac{z}{h}}(1 - C^{1/3}) w_{\mathrm{m}} \frac{\mathrm{d}C}{\mathrm{d}z} + w_0 C(1 - C)^{\eta} = 0 \tag{9}$$

The non-dimensionalization of Eq. (9) gives

$$\kappa\hat{z}\sqrt{1-\hat{z}}\left(1-C^{\frac{1}{3}}\right)\frac{\mathrm{d}C}{\mathrm{d}\hat{z}}+\overline{w_0}C(1-C)^{\eta}=0 \quad (10)$$

where $\hat{z}=\frac{z}{h}$, h being the flow depth, and $\overline{w_0}=\frac{w_0}{w_\mathrm{m}}$. In this study, we take $w_\mathrm{m}=u_*$, u_* being the shear velocity. Equation (10) represents the one-dimensional distribution equation which is solved numerically to obtain the concentration distribution along a vertical. A reference concentration C_a at a reference level a is taken as the boundary condition for the numerical solution.

3 Result and Discussion

3.1 Variation of Concentration Profile with η

Two concentration profiles of suspended sediment particles are plotted in Fig. 2 with and without hindered settling. It can be seen from the figure that the concentration values are more in the main flow region due to the presence of hindered settling. Effect of hindered settling can be seen only in main flow but not near the bed and surface; this may be due to the reason that the particles are not present near the water surface and not in suspension near the bed. The difference in concentration values in the main flow region with and without hindered settling says the importance of including this effect in the mathematical model of concentration.

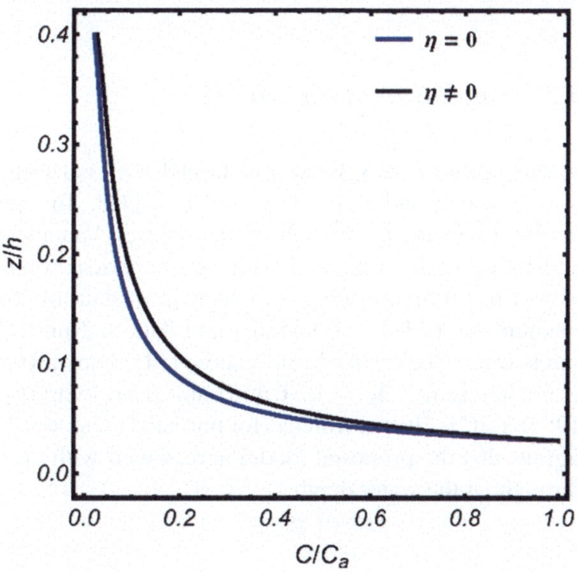

Fig. 2 Effect of η on the vertical concentration of suspended particles

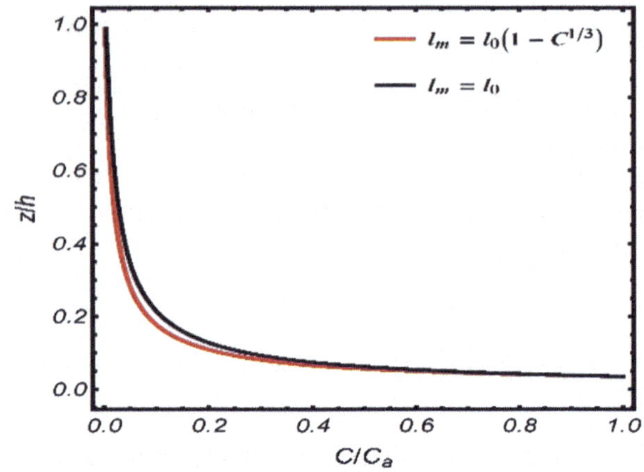

Fig. 3 Effect of mixing length with and without function of concentration on vertical concentration distribution

3.2 Variation of Concentration Profile with l_m and l_0

In Fig. 3, two concentration profiles of suspended particles are displayed. Black curve stands for concentration profile with mixing length as a function of concentration $l_\mathrm{m} = l_0(1 - C^{1/3})$ and red curve stands for concentration profile with mixing length as clear water mixing length ($l_\mathrm{m} = l_0$). From the figure, it can be observed that the for a fixed height say $z = z_0$, value of concentration is less when mixing length is taken as function of concentration, i.e., mixing length is damped in the presence of sediments.

3.3 Validation of the Model

In this section, we validate our model with existing experimental data of Vanoni [14], Einstein and Chien [15] and Lyn [16]. To check the accuracy of proposed model, two runs from each of the data of Vanoni [14], Einstein and Chien [15] and Lyn [16]are compared with the numerical solution and displayed in Figs. 4, 5, and 6. From Einstein and Chien [15], data of Run-S6 is chosen which is for medium sand ($D_{50} = 0.94$ mm) and data of Run-S12 is chosen which is for fine sand ($D_{50} = 0.27$ mm). From Vanoni [14], data of Run-4 and Run-6 is chosen which is for fine sand ($D_{50} = 0.16$ mm) and from Lyn [16] data of Run-1957ST-2B and 1957ST-2C is chosen which is for fine sand ($D_{50} = 0.19$ mm). It can be seen from the figures that the proposed model agrees well with observed values of concentration throughout the water depth.

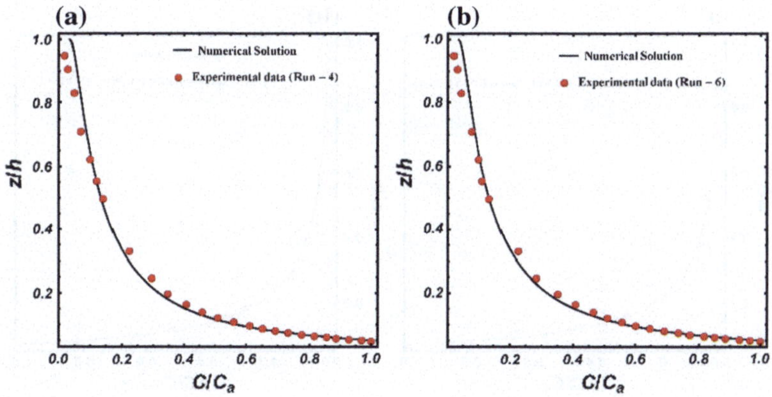

Fig. 4 Comparison between computed particle concentration profile and observed data of Vanoni [14] **a** Run-4 and **b** Run-6

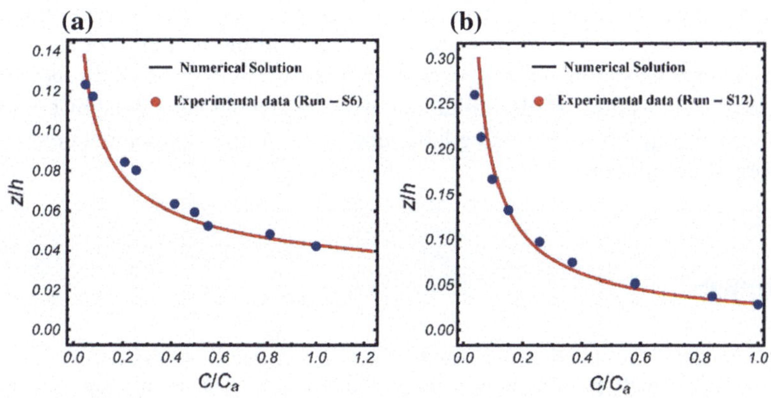

Fig. 5 Comparison between computed particle concentration profile and observed data of Einstein and Chien [15] **a** Run-S6 and **b** Run-S12

4 Conclusions

The present study derives a model for vertical concentration distribution in a sediment carrying fluid using the governing equation from Nielsen and Teakle [11] who derived it using a finite mixing length theory. Unlike most of the researchers, the study uses the mixing length as a function of concentration from Kovacs [8] where the mixing length has been derived with a proper physical justification. Apart from that, the settling velocity of sediment particles has been taken as a function of concentration. The modified governing equation which is a nonlinear first-order ordinary differential equation is solved numerically. The changes in the concentration values for including the above-mentioned effects are shown graphically. It is found that the hindered

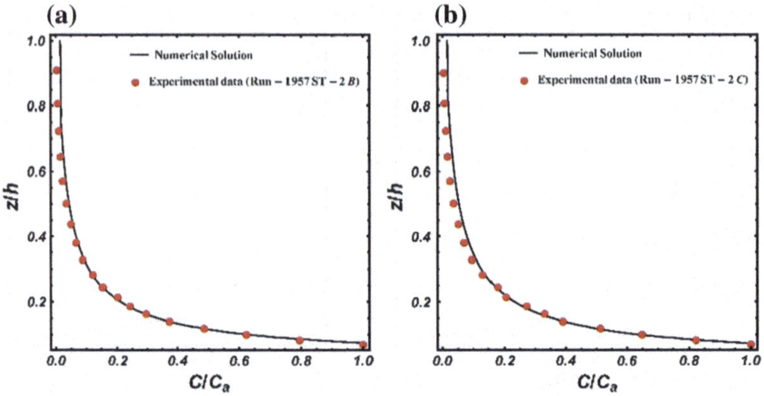

Fig. 6 Comparison between computed particle concentration profile and observed data Lyn (1988) **a** Run-1957-2B and **b** Run-1957-2C

settling effect can be seen only in the main flow region, and the concentration values are higher when hindered settling effect is present in the model, and also that the presence of concentration in the expression of mixing length makes the concentration values to be less. At the end, the validation of the model has been done by comparing the numerical solution with existing laboratory data. A good agreement confirms the efficiency of the model.

References

1. Schlichting, H., Gersten, K.: Boundary-layer theory. Springer, New York (2016)
2. Bialik, R.J.: Particle–particle collision in lagrangian modelling of saltating grains. J. Hydraul. Res. **49**(1), 23–31 (2011)
3. Bialik, R.J.: Numerical study of near-bed turbulence structures influence on the initiation of saltating grains movement. J. Hydrol. Hydromech. S. **61**(3), 202–207 (2013)
4. Van Driest, E.R.: The problem of aerodynamic heating. Institute of the Aeronautical Sciences (1956)
5. Nishioka, M., Iida, S.: The mixing length derived from k´arm´ans similarity hypothesis. Aeronaut. Q. **24**(1), 71–76 (1973)
6. Galbraith, R.M., Sjolander, S., Head, M.: Mixing length in the wall region of turbulent boundary layers. Aeronaut. Q. **28**(2), 97–110 (1977)
7. Umeyama, M., Gerritsen, F.: Velocity distribution in uniform sediment-laden flow. J. Hydraul. Eng. **118**(2), 229–245 (1992)
8. Kovacs, A.: Prandtl's mixing length concept modified for equilibrium sediment-laden flows. J. Hydraul. Eng. **124**(8), 803–812 (1998)
9. Rouse, H.: Modern conceptions of the mechanics of turbulence. Trans. ASCE **102**, 463–543 (1937)
10. Hunt, J.: The turbulent transport of suspended sediment in open channels. Proc. R. Soc. Lond. A **224**(1158), 322–335 (1954)
11. Nielsen, P., Teakle, I.A.: Turbulent diffusion of momentum and suspended particles: a finite-mixing-length theory. Phys. Fluids **16**(7), 2342–2348 (2004)

12. Richardson, J., Zaki, W.: Sedimentation and fluidisation: part 1. Trans. Inst. Chem. Eng. **32**, 35–53 (1954)
13. Cheng, N.S.: Simplified settling velocity formula for sediment particle. J. Hydraul. Eng. **123**(2), 149–152 (1997)
14. Vanoni, V.A.: Transportation of suspended sediment by water. Trans. of ASCE **111**, 67–102 (1946)
15. Einstein, H., Chien, N.: Effects of heavy sediment concentration near the bed on velocity and sediment distribution. Missoury river division, corps of engineers. US Army (1955)
16. Lyn, D.: A similarity approach to turbulent sediment-laden flows in open channels. J. Fluid Mech. **193**, 1–26 (1988)

A Study on the Effect of Various Fluid, Flow and Mechanical Parameters on the Flow of Newtonian Fluid in an Expanding and Contracting Pipe

A. Karthik, K. Sashank and T. S. L. Radhika

Abstract In this paper, a study has been carried out to understand the effect of the fluid, flow and the mechanical parameters on a pulsatile flow of a Newtonian fluid in an expanding and contracting pipe. The fluid parameters considered are the viscosity and the density, flow parameters are the amplitude of the pressure gradient and the frequency of oscillations, and the mechanical parameter considered is the radius of the pipe. A mathematical model is constructed in the cylindrical polar coordinate system with the fluid flow assumed to be axisymmetric. Further, the fluid is taken to be incompressible, and the radius of the pipe to vary with time. Navier–Stokes equations are used to describe this fluid flow problem. The resulting nonlinear coupled system of equations together with an appropriate boundary and initial conditions is solved using the homotopy perturbation method. The model is then applied to the human circulatory system, and the effect of the three sets of parameters on wall shear stress and volumetric flux is studied. Data for the model parameters are taken from literature on human blood, and human circulatory system and graphs have been plotted to understand their effect on the flow.

Keywords Expanding and contracting pipe · Newtonian fluid · Homotopy perturbation method

1 Introduction

Unsteady flow of viscous fluids in pipes produced by a simple contraction or expansion of the walls has applications in biological systems [1, 2]. This study was initiated by Uchida and Aoki, who considered the flow of Newtonian fluid in a semi-infinite contracting and expanding circular pipe [3]. They derived an exact solution to the Navier–Stokes equation using similarity transformation. Secomb [4] extended the work done by Uchida to understand the flow in a channel with pulsating walls. In his work, the wall motion was taken to be sinusoidal with the amplitude of oscillations

A. Karthik · K. Sashank · T. S. L. Radhika (✉)
BITS Pilani Hyderabad Campus, Hyderabad, India
e-mail: radhikatsl@hyderabad.bits-pilani.ac.in

S. Bhattacharyya et al. (eds.), *Mathematical Modeling and Computational Tools*, Springer Proceedings in Mathematics & Statistics 320,
https://doi.org/10.1007/978-981-15-3615-1_8

being small. Ohki, in his work [5], discussed the flow in a semi-infinite porous pipe with expanding and contracting radius in the axial direction. Recently, Si et al. [6] calculated multiple solutions for the contracting or expanding porous pipe using the singular perturbation method.

As is seen, the focus of most of these studies was on the study of the effect of the parameter representing the expansion/contraction of the pipe on the flow of fluid under a constant pressure gradient, and however, in some biological systems, e.g.. human circulatory system, the flow of fluid, i.e. the blood, is under a pulsatile pressure gradient which is due to the pulsatile pumping of the heart. Also, the walls of the pipes, i.e. the blood vessels, contract and expand to enable the blood to flow through them. Thus, a study on the effect of the expanding/contracting parameter on pulsatile flows is of interest in these studies. Hence, in this work, the effect of pulsatile flow parameters, i.e. the amplitude of pressure gradient and the frequency of oscillations, the fluid parameters, precisely, the density and the viscosity, and the mechanical parameters, i.e. the radius of the pipe is studied.

2 Construction of Mathematical Model

To describe the contracting and expanding nature of the blood vessel, the expression for the radius of the vessel is taken as considered by Uchida and Aoki (for circular pipes) [3]. The flow is further assumed to be pulsatile, as described by Shankar and Lee [7]. Under the assumption that the fluid is incompressible and the flow axisymmetric, fluid flow equations have been derived using the Navier–Stokes equations. These equations are then solved using homotopy perturbation method [8] for the radial and the axial velocity components. These approximations are then used to compute expressions for wall shear stress and volumetric flux. The model is then applied for the blood flow in the human circulatory system by assigning data to the flow parameters, fluid and mechanical parameters taken from published results. Graphs have been plotted to understand the effect of these parameters on wall shear stress and volumetric flux, and the results have been discussed.

3 Problem Formulation

Consider the flow of a Newtonian fluid in a pipe whose radius varies with time as described in Uchinda [3]. Cylindrical polar coordinate system (r, θ, z) (where r and z are the radial and the axial coordinates, respectively, and θ is the azimuthal angle) is taken to describe the geometry of the problem, and it is assumed that the fluid flow is in the z-direction. Further, the fluid is considered to be incompressible, and the flow axisymmetric so that the velocity vector, and the pressure, denoted by $\bar{q}$ and p, respectively, are functions of r, z and time t only. Assume that the non-vanishing components of the velocity vector are in radial and axial directions so that the velocity vector is $\bar{q}(r, z, t) = (u(r, z, t), 0, w(r, z, t))$. Also, let the thermodynamic pressure p be $p(r, z, t)$.

Now, the continuity equation and momentum equations take the form [9, 10]:

Continuity equation:

$$\frac{\partial u}{\partial r} + \frac{u}{r} + \frac{\partial w}{\partial z} = 0. \tag{1}$$

Momentum equation:

$$\frac{\partial u}{\partial t} + u\frac{\partial u}{\partial r} + w\frac{\partial u}{\partial z} = -\frac{1}{\rho}\frac{\partial p}{\partial r} - \frac{1}{\rho}\left(\frac{1}{r}\frac{\partial}{\partial r}(r\tau_{rr}) + \frac{\partial}{\partial z}(\tau_{rz})\right), \tag{2}$$

$$\frac{\partial w}{\partial t} + u\frac{\partial w}{\partial r} + w\frac{\partial w}{\partial z} = -\frac{1}{\rho}\frac{\partial p}{\partial z} - \frac{1}{\rho}\left(\frac{1}{r}\frac{\partial}{\partial r}(r\tau_{rz}) + \frac{\partial}{\partial z}(\tau_{zz})\right). \tag{3}$$

Here, ρ is the density of the blood, and τ_{ij} are the components of the deviatoric stress tensor.

Under the assumption that the radial flow velocity and the convective acceleration terms are, respectively, of a smaller order of magnitude for the axial flow velocity, and the local acceleration terms, the radial momentum Eq. (2) reduces to

$$-\frac{\partial p}{\partial r} = 0. \tag{4}$$

Thus, it can be seen that the pressure is independent of r. The pressure gradient is taken to be a function of t as

$$-\frac{\partial p}{\partial z} = A\cos\omega t, \tag{5}$$

where A is the amplitude of the pressure gradient and $\omega = 2\pi f_1$, f_1 being the frequency of oscillations [7].

The fluid is taken to be Newtonian whose constitutive equation is [9]

$$\tau_{ij} = -p\delta_{ij} + 2\mu e_{ij}, \tag{6}$$

where p is the thermodynamic pressure, μ is the viscosity and e_{ij} is the rate of deformation tensor.

The contraction and expansion of the walls of the pipe is described as in [3] as

$$R(t) = R_0(1 - \omega\alpha t)^{1/2}, \tag{7}$$

where R_0 is the radius of the pipe when $t = 0$, and α is the parameter that describes the behavior of the wall. Positive values of α indicate contraction while negative values of this parameter describe the expansion of the walls of the pipe.

Using the constitutive equation (6), Eqs. (1) and (3) take the form

$$\frac{\partial u}{\partial r} + \frac{u}{r} + \frac{\partial w}{\partial z} = 0, \tag{8}$$

$$\rho\left(\frac{\partial w}{\partial t} + u\frac{\partial w}{\partial r} + w\frac{\partial w}{\partial z}\right) = -\frac{\partial P}{\partial z} + \mu\left(\frac{1}{r}\frac{\partial}{\partial r}\left(r\frac{\partial w}{\partial r}\right) + \frac{\partial^2 w}{\partial z^2}\right). \tag{9}$$

Now, the problem is to solve the above coupled system of partial differential equations together with the boundary conditions given by

$$\begin{array}{ll} w = 0 \,\text{on}\, r = R(t), & \text{(No} - \text{slip boundary condition)} \\ u = \frac{dR}{dt} \text{on}\, r = R(t), & \text{(Velocity of the fluid matches with wall velocity)} \\ \frac{\partial w}{\partial r} = 0 \,\text{at}\, r = 0, & \text{(Velocity is finite at the center of the pipe)} \end{array} \tag{10}$$

4 The Solution to the Problem

The above system of partial differential equations together with the initial and boundary conditions is solved using the homotopy perturbation method (HPM) [8]. For this, we take

$$\begin{aligned} u(r,z,t) &= u_0(r,z,t) + pu_1(r,z,t) + p^2u_2(r,z,t) + \cdots \\ w(r,z,t) &= w_0(r,z,t) + pw_1(r,z,t) + p^2w_2(r,z,t) + \cdots \end{aligned} \tag{11}$$

Also, the initial approximation satisfying the conditions (10) is taken as $w_0(r,z,t) = r^2 - R(t)^2$, $u_0(r,z,t) = \frac{dR}{dt}$. The subsequent approximations for $u(r,z,t)$, and $w(r,z,t)$ are found by defining homotopy functions as,

$$H_1(p) = (1-p)\left(\frac{\partial u}{\partial r} - \frac{\partial u_0}{\partial r}\right) + p\left(\frac{\partial u}{\partial r} + \frac{u}{r} + \frac{\partial w}{\partial z}\right), \tag{12}$$

for Eq. (8), and that for Eq. (9) as

$$\begin{aligned} H_2(p) = (1-p)\left(\frac{\partial^2 w}{\partial r^2} - \frac{\partial^2 w_0}{\partial r^2}\right) + p\left(\rho\left(\frac{\partial w}{\partial t} + u\frac{\partial w}{\partial r} + w\frac{\partial w}{\partial z}\right)\right. \\ \left. + \frac{\partial p}{\partial z} - \mu\left(\frac{1}{r}\frac{\partial w}{\partial r} + \frac{\partial^2 w}{\partial r^2} + \frac{\partial^2 w}{\partial z^2}\right)\right), \end{aligned} \tag{13}$$

Comparing the coefficient of p, we get the equations governing $u_1(r,z,t)$ and $w_1(r,z,t)$ as

$$\frac{\partial u_1}{\partial r} = -\left(\frac{\partial w_0}{\partial z} + \frac{\partial u_0}{\partial r} + \frac{u_0}{r}\right), \tag{14}$$

$$\frac{\partial^2 w_1}{\partial r^2} = -\left(\frac{\partial p}{\partial z} + \rho\left(\frac{\partial w_0}{\partial t} + u_0\frac{\partial w_0}{\partial r} + w_0\frac{\partial w_0}{\partial z}\right)\right.$$
$$\left.-\mu\left(\frac{1}{r}\frac{\partial w_0}{\partial r} + \frac{\partial^2 w_0}{\partial r^2} + \frac{\partial^2 w_0}{\partial z^2}\right)\right). \tag{15}$$

And the conditions are

$$u_1 = 0 \,\text{on}\, r = R(t)$$
$$w_1 = 0 \,\text{on} = R(t), \frac{\partial w_1}{\partial r} = 0 \,\text{at}\, r = 0 \tag{16}$$

Solving these equations, the expressions for the first approximation of the velocity components can be obtained. Similarly, the coefficient of p^2, and higher powers have been collected to find the next approximations.

5 Results and Discussions

A code has been developed in Mathematica to compute approximations for the radial and axial components of the velocity and wall shear stress (WSS) and volumetric flux are evaluated. The effect of the fluid parameters, flow parameters, mechanical parameters and the contracting/expanding parameter, on these quantities, has been studied, and the results are presented and discussed. Data related to all parameters except for the contracting/expanding parameter, which is given the set of values −0.05, −0.01, 0, 0.01, and 0.05 has been taken from data published [11–14] related to the human blood, and the human circulatory system. The following table shows the set of values of the parameters taken for study (Table 1).

5.1 Effect of the Fluid Parameters on the Flow

5.1.1 Effect of the Density of the Fluid (ρ) on WSS and Volumetric Flux

The plots of wall shear stress (WSS) with time for different values of density (ρ), with other parameters fixed, are shown in Figs. 1 and 2, respectively, for expanding pipe (α negative) and contracting pipe (α positive). From expression (7), it is seen that positive values of α indicate an increase in radius with time 't' while negative values of α show decrease in radius with time.

It is known that WSS increases with an increase in the radius of the pipe, and the model developed in this study can be seen to predict the same in both expanding and

Table 1 Values of the parameters taken from literature for the study

Density (ρ) (in kg m^{-3})	1055
	1058.1
	1061.2
Viscosity (μ) (in Pa s)	0.00552
	0.00619
	0.00686
Pulse difference (A) (in mmHg)	42
	43
	44
Heart rate (in bpm)	72
	75
	76

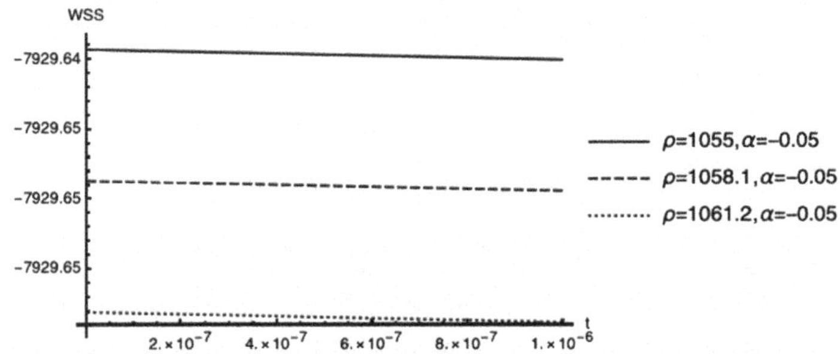

Fig. 1 Plot of WSS versus time when $\omega = 2\pi{*}72/60\ \mathrm{s}^{-1}$, $\mu = 0.00552$ Pa s, $A = 41$ mmHg, $\alpha = -0.05$

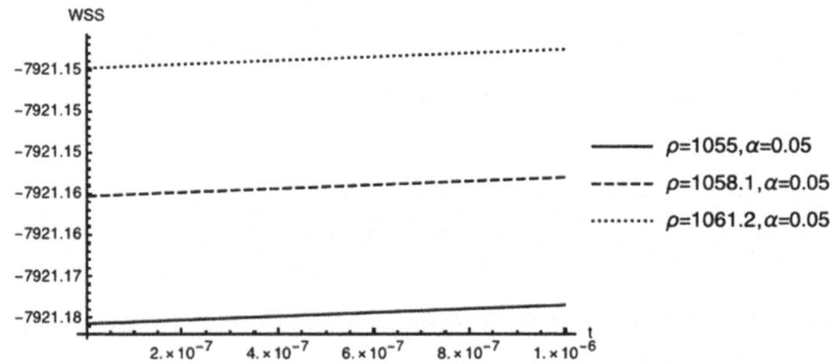

Fig. 2 Plot of WSS versus time when $\omega = 2\pi{*}72/60\ \mathrm{s}^{-1}$, $\mu = 0.00552$ Pa s, $A = 41$ mmHg, $\alpha = 0.05$

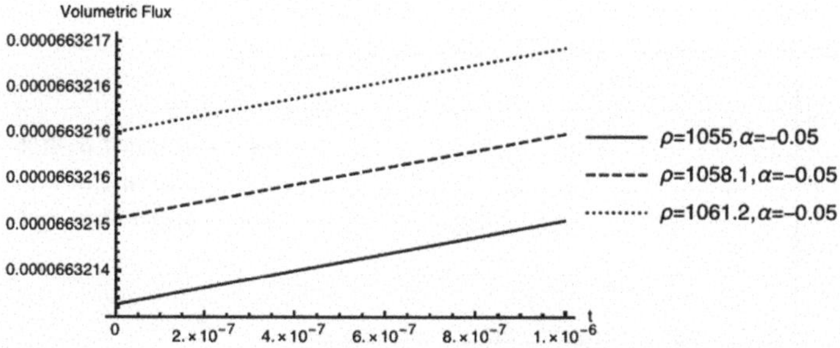

Fig. 3 Plot of volumetric flux versus time when $\omega = 2\pi{*}72/60\ \text{s}^{-1}$, $\mu = 0.00552$ Pa s, $A =$ 41 mmHg, $\alpha = -0.05$

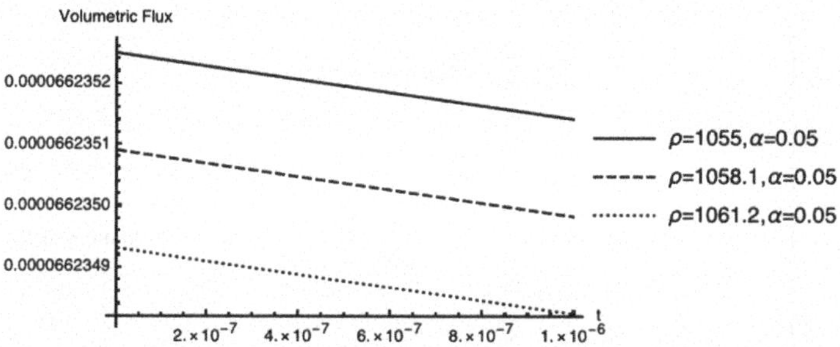

Fig. 4 Plot of volumetric flux versus time when $\omega = 2\pi{*}72/60\ \text{s}^{-1}$, $\mu = 0.00552$ Pa s, $A =$ 41 mmHg, $\alpha = 0.05$

contracting pipes. Further, in expanding pipes, denser fluids are found to experience greater WSS, while in contracting pipes, denser fluids are found to experience lesser WSS.

Figures 3 and 4 show the plots of volumetric flux with time for different values of density ρ in expanding and contracting pipes, respectively. As is seen in the plots, an increase in radius increases the volumetric flux in both expanding and contracting pipes. In case of expanding pipe, denser fluids are seen to have higher volumetric flux, while in contracting pipes, they are seen to have lesser volumetric flux.

5.1.2 Effect of the Viscosity of the Fluid (μ) on WSS and Volumetric Flux

The plots of WSS with time for different values of viscosity are shown in Figs. 5 and 6. In expanding as well as contracting pipes, fluids with higher viscosity are seen to experience greater WSS. Further, for a particular value of μ, WSS increases with time in case of expanding pipes while it decreases for contracting pipes.

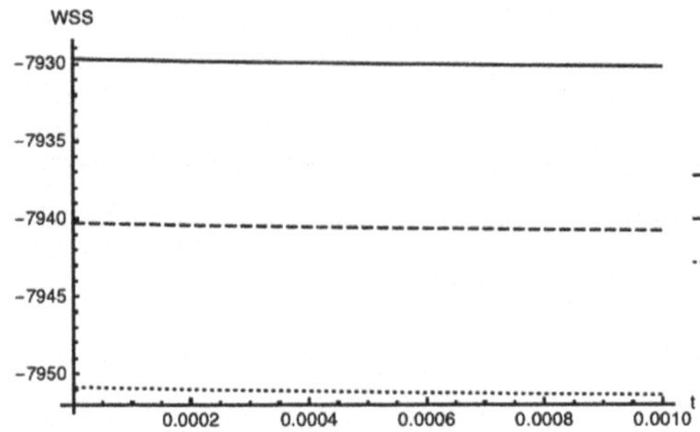

Fig. 5 Plot of WSS versus time when $\omega = 2\pi{*}72/60\ \text{s}^{-1}$, $\rho = 1055\ \text{kg m}^{-3}$, $A = 41$ mmHg, $\alpha = -0.05$

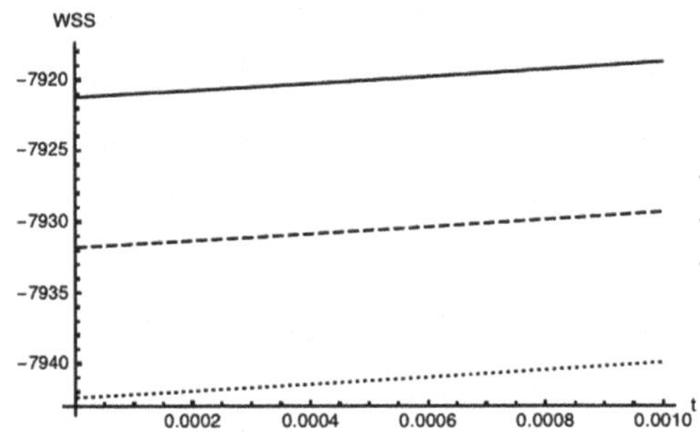

Fig. 6 Plot of WSS versus time when $\omega = 2\pi{*}72/60\ \text{s}^{-1}$, $\rho = 1055\ \text{kg m}^{-3}$, $A = 41$ mmHg, $\alpha = 0.05$

Figures 7 and 8 show the variation of volumetric flux with μ. It is seen that volumetric flux is greater for more viscous fluids in both expanding and contracting pipes while not much significant effect on it is seen with time.

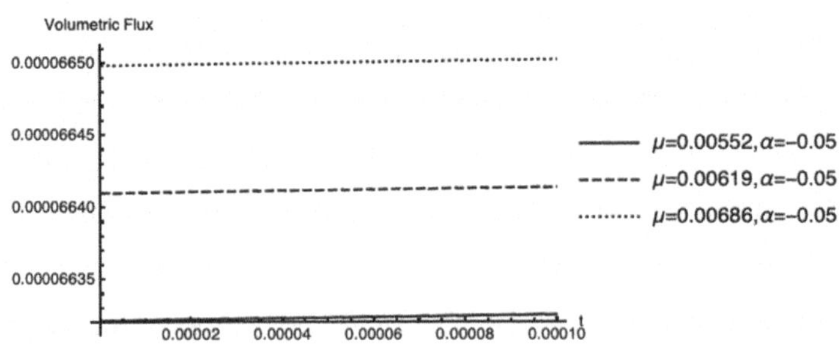

Fig. 7 Plot of volumetric flux versus time when $\omega = 2\pi{*}72/60\ \text{s}^{-1}$, $\rho = 1055\ \text{kg m}^{-3}$, $A = 41$ mmHg, $\alpha = -0.05$

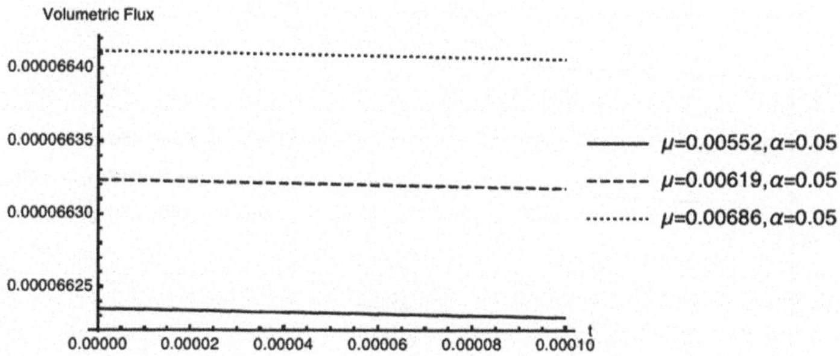

Fig. 8 Plot of volumetric flux versus time when $\omega = 2\pi*72/60\ \mathrm{s}^{-1}$, $\rho = 1055\ \mathrm{kg\ m}^{-3}$, $A =$ 41 mmHg, $\alpha = 0.05$

5.2 *Effect of the Flow Parameters on the Flow*

5.2.1 Effect of the Amplitude (A) on WSS and Volumetric Flux

Variation of WSS with the amplitude of oscillations is depicted in Figs. 9 and 10. WSS is seen to be more at higher amplitudes than that at a lesser. Further, at a particular amplitude, WSS is seen to decrease with time.

Figures 11 and 12 show the variation of volumetric flux with the amplitude of oscillation. Greater amplitudes resulted in higher flux in both expanding and contracting pipes. Further, for a given amplitude, it can be seen that flux is increasing with time in expanding pipes, whereas it is decreasing in contracting pipes.

5.2.2 Effect of the Frequency of Oscillations (ω) on WSS and Volumetric Flux

Figures 13 and 14 depict the variation of WSS with the frequency of oscillations. In expanding pipes, higher frequency resulted in greater WSS, whereas greater values

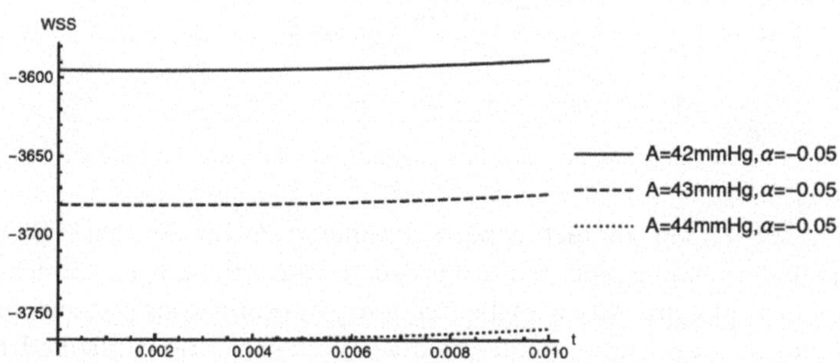

Fig. 9 Plot of WSS versus time when $\omega = 2\pi*72/60\ \mathrm{s}^{-1}$, $\rho = 1055\ \mathrm{kg\ m}^{-3}$, $\mu = 0.00552$ Pa s, $\alpha = -0.05$

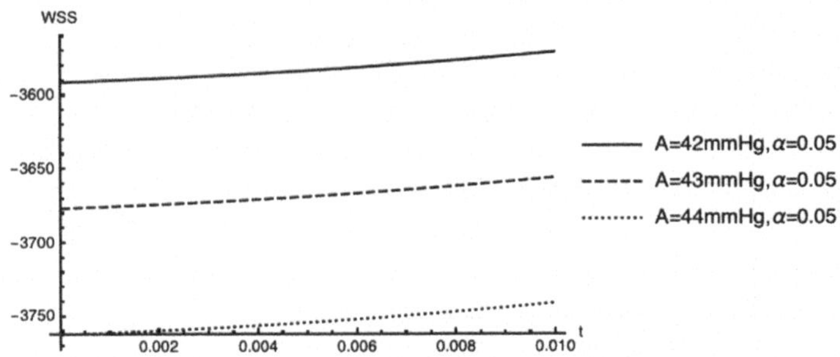

Fig. 10 Plot of WSS versus time when $\omega = 2\pi*72/60\ \text{s}^{-1}$, $\rho = 1055\ \text{kg m}^{-3}$, $\mu = 0.00552$ Pa s, $\alpha = 0.05$

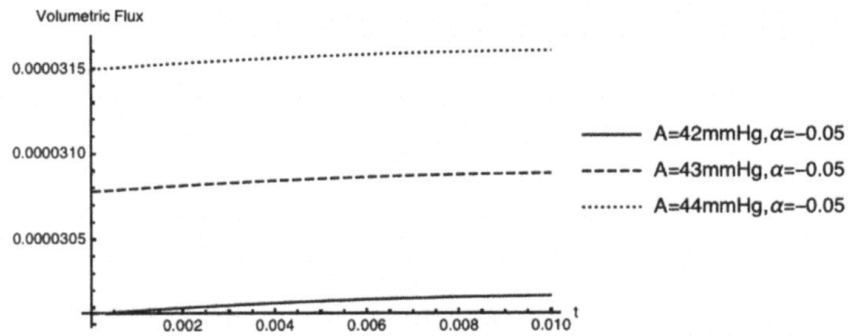

Fig. 11 Plot of volumetric flux versus time when $\omega = 2\pi*72/60\ \text{s}^{-1}$, $\rho = 1055\ \text{kg m}^{-3}$, $\mu = 0.00552$ Pa s, $\alpha = -0.05$

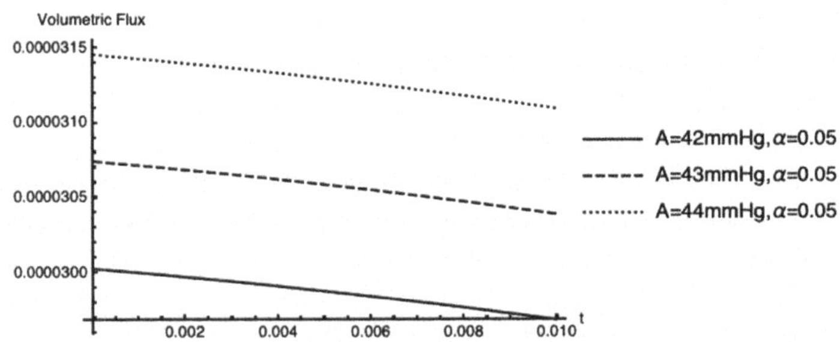

Fig. 12 Plot of volumetric flux versus time when $\omega = 2\pi*72/60\ \text{s}^{-1}$, $\rho = 1055\ \text{kg m}^{-3}$, $\mu = 0.00552$ Pa s, $\alpha = 0.05$

resulted in lesser WSS in contracting pipes. Further, it can be seen that WSS increases with time in the expanding pipes while it is decreasing with time in contracting pipes.

Variation of volumetric flux with the frequency of oscillations is shown in Figs. 15 and 16. It can be seen that a greater frequency of oscillations resulted in higher volumetric flux in expanding pipes while it resulted in lower flux in contracting pipes.

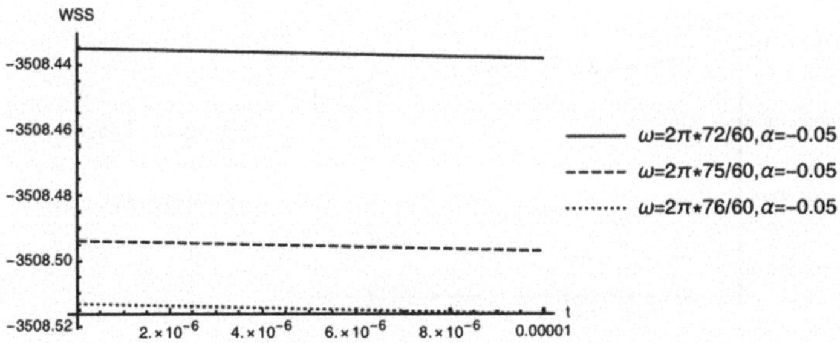

Fig. 13 Plot of WSS versus time when $\rho = 1055$ kg m^{-3}, $\mu = 0.00552$ Pa s, $A = 41$ mmHg, $\alpha = -0.05$

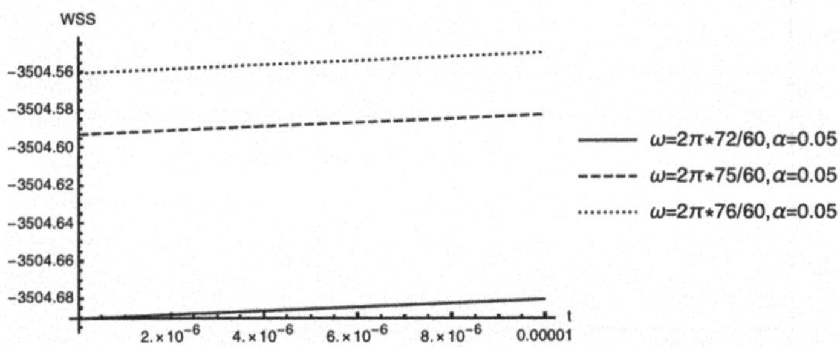

Fig. 14 Plot of WSS versus time when $\rho = 1055$ kg m^{-3}, $\mu = 0.00552$ Pa s, $A = 41$ mmHg, $\alpha = 0.05$

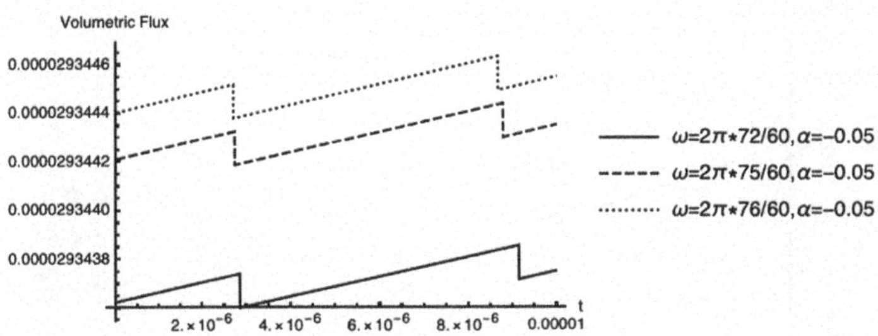

Fig. 15 Plot of volumetric flux versus time when $\rho = 1055$ kg m^{-3}, $\mu = 0.00552$ Pa s, $A = 41$ mmHg, $\alpha = -0.05$

5.3 *Effect of the Material Parameters on the Flow*

5.3.1 Effect of Contracting/Expanding Parameter (α) on WSS and Volumetric Flux

An increase in α indicates a decrease in radius, which results in a decrease in the WSS. Also, a decrease in volumetric flux as is seen in Figs. 17 and 18.

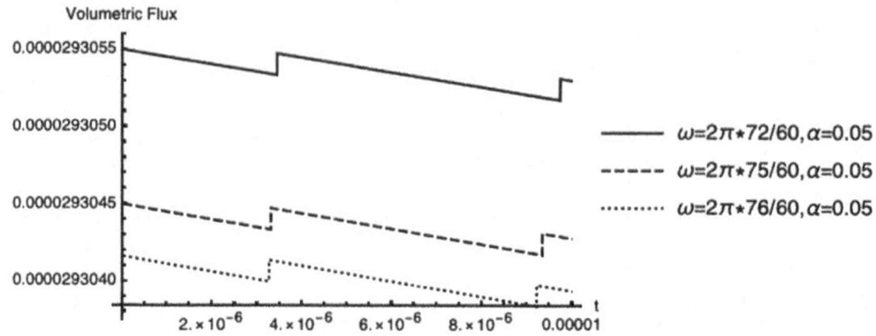

Fig. 16 Plot of volumetric flux versus time when $\rho = 1055$ kg m^{-3}, $\mu = 0.00552$ Pa s, $A =$ 41 mmHg, $\alpha = 0.05$

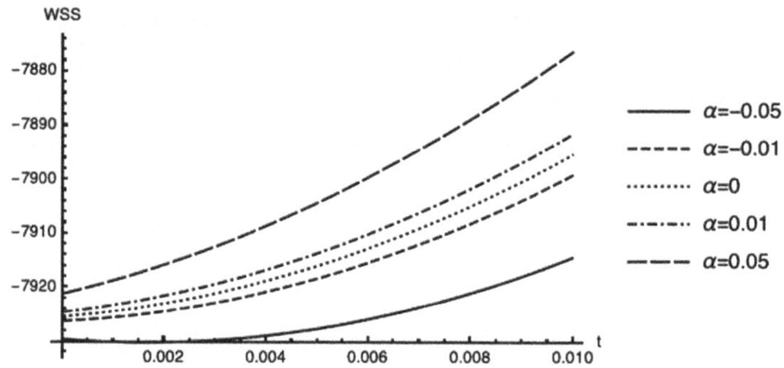

Fig. 17 Plot of WSS versus time when $\omega = 2\pi*72/60$ s^{-1}, $\rho = 1055$ kg m^{-3}, $\mu = 0.00552$ Pa s, $A = 41$ mmHg

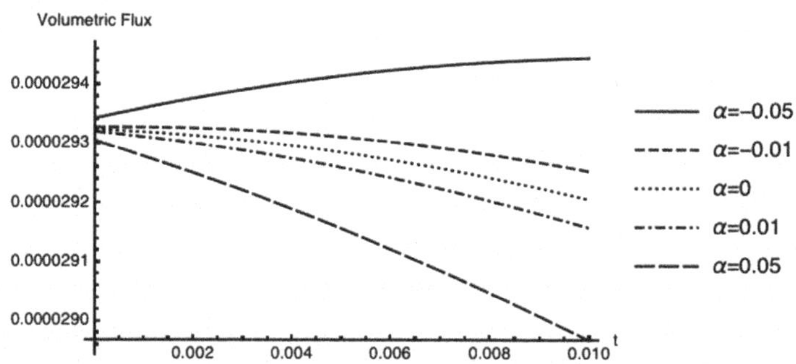

Fig. 18 Plot of volumetric flux versus time when $\omega = 2\pi*72/60$ s^{-1}, $\rho = 1055$ kg m^{-3}, $\mu =$ 0.00552 Pa s, $A = 41$ mmHg

6 Conclusions

In the present work, the pulsatile flow of the Newtonian fluid in an expanding and contracting pipe has been studied. HPM has been used to find approximate solutions to the fluid flow equations developed in the model. The expressions for the velocity components derived are then used to derive expressions for wall shear stress and volumetric flux. Graphs have been plotted to visualize the effect of the flow, fluid and mechanical parameters on these quantities computed. Some interesting observations of this study are as follows: In expanding pipes, denser fluids are found to experience greater WSS and had higher volumetric flux, while in contracting pipes, they are found to experience lesser WSS and had less volumetric flux. The study also reveals that, in the case of both expanding and contracting pipes, an increase in viscosity increases WSS and volumetric flux under the pulsatile pressure gradient with a given amplitude and frequency. Also, an increase in the amplitude of oscillations resulted in an increase in WSS as well as the volumetric flux in case of both expanding and contracting pipes. In expanding pipes, higher frequency of oscillations resulted in greater WSS, whereas they resulted in lesser WSS in contracting pipes. It is also seen that a higher frequency of oscillations produced greater volumetric flux in expanding pipes while it produced lower values in contracting pipes.

Acknowledgements The authors thank DST—FIST for providing computational facilities at the Department of Mathematics, BITS-Pilani, Hyderabad Campus.

References

1. Bertram, C.D., Pedley, T.J.: A mathematical model of unsteady collapsible tube behaviour. J. Biomech. **15**, 39–50 (1982)
2. Walawender, W.P., Tien, C., Cerny, L.C.: Experimental studies of blood flow through tapered tubes. Int. J. Eng. Sc. **10**, 1123–1135 (1972)
3. Uchida, S., Aoki, H.: Unsteady flows in a semi-infinite contracting or expanding pipe. J. Fluid Mech. **82**, 371–387 (1977)
4. Secomb, T.W.: Flow in a channel with pulsating wall. J. Fluid Mech. **88**(2), 273–287 (1978)
5. Ohki, M.: Unsteady flow in a porous, elastic, circular tube—I. The wall contracting or expanding in an axial direction. Bull. JSME **23**(179), 679–686 (1980)
6. Si, X., Zheng, L., Zhang, X., Li, M., Yang, J., Chao, Y.: Multiple solutions for the laminar flow in a porous pipe with suction at slowly expanding or contracting wall. Appl. Math. Comput. **218**(7), 3515–3521 (2011)
7. Shankar, D.S., Lee, U.: Mathematical modelling of pulsatile flow of non-Newtonian fluid in stenosed arteries. Commun. Non-Linear Sci. Numer. Simul. **74**(7), 2971–2981 (2009)
8. He, Ji-Huan: Homotopy perturbation method: a new nonlinear analytical technique. Appl. Math. Comput. **135**(1), 73–79 (2003)
9. Bird, R.B., Stewart, W.E., Lightfoot, E.N.: Transport Phenomena, 2nd edn. Wiley, Hoboken (2005)
10. Mazumdar, J.N.: Bio-Fluid Mechanics. World Scientific Publishing, Singapore (2004)
11. Carallo, C., Irace, C., De Franceschi, M.S., Coppoletta, F., Tiriolo, R., Scicchitano, C., Scavelli, F., Gnasso, A.: The effect of aging on blood and plasma viscosity. An 11.6 years follow-up study. Clin. Hemorheol. Microcirc. **47**, 67–74 (2011)

12. Trudnowski, R.J., Rico, R.C.: Specific gravity of blood and plasma at 4 and 37 °C. Clin. Chem. **20**(5), 615–616 (1974)
13. Resting heart rate chart: Factors that influence heart rate in elderly. https://www.belmarrahealth.com/resting-heart-rate-chart-factors-influence-heart-rate-elderly/. Last Accessed 18 Sep 2019
14. Understanding blood pressure readings key to overall well-being. https://www.belmarrahealth.com/understanding-blood-pressure-readings-is-key-to-overall-well-being/. Last Accessed 18 Sep 2019

Unsteady Stagnation Point Nanofluid Flow Over a Stretching Sheet with Thermal Radiation

B. Kumar and G. S. Seth

Abstract This research work is done to investigate the magnetohydrodynamic unsteady stagnation point nanofluid flow and the heat transfer influenced by the thermal radiation. The suitable transformations give rise to ordinary differential equations. A similar form of differential equations is solved numerically by successive linearization method (SLM). The influence of various active flow parameters, such as thermal radiation parameter, and stagnation parameter on the flow field, concentration field, and temperature field are plotted graphically and described in detail. Various critical outcomes are uncovered in this investigation. The outcome indicates that increment in stretching parameter increases the fluid velocity but it decreases fluid temperature and nanoparticle concentration.

Keywords Successive linearization method (SLM) · Unsteady flow · Brownian and thermophoretic diffusions

Nomenclature

a	Constant
A	Unsteadiness parameter
B	Magnetic field
B_0	Constant magnetic field
D_B	Brownian diffusion (coefficient)
D_T	Thermophoretic diffusion (coefficient)
g	Gravitational acceleration
k	Thermal conductivity
k^*	Rosseland mean absorption coefficient
M	Magnetic parameter
Nb	Brownian motion parameter

B. Kumar (✉) · G. S. Seth
Department of Applied Mathematics, IIT (ISM), Dhanbad, Jharkhand, India
e-mail: chauhanbhuvan6@gmail.com

S. Bhattacharyya et al. (eds.), *Mathematical Modeling and Computational Tools*, Springer Proceedings in Mathematics & Statistics 320,
https://doi.org/10.1007/978-981-15-3615-1_9

T	Temperature
t	Time
u	Velocity along x direction
v	Velocity along y direction
λ	Stretching parameter
$(\rho c)_{\mathrm{f}}$	Specific heat capacity of the base fluid
σ	Electrical conductivity
ρ_{f}	Density
ρ_{p}	Nanoparticle mass density
$\rho_{\mathrm{f}\infty}$	Base fluid density in free stream
$\tau = (\rho c)_{\mathrm{p}} / (\rho c)_{\mathrm{f}}$	Ratio of nanoparticles specific heat capacity to fluid specific heat capacity
Nt	Thermophoresis parameter
N_r	Buoyancy ratio parameter
Pr	Prandtl number
Pr_{eff}	Effective Prandtl number
R_a	Mixed convection parameter
Re_x	Local Reynolds number
Sc	Schmidt number
α_{nf}	Thermal diffusivity
β^*	Thermal expansion coefficient
C	Nanoparticle concentration
θ	Dimensionless temperature
ν	Kinematic coefficient of viscosity
σ^*	Stefan Boltzmann constant

1 Introduction

Nanofluid is envisioned to expound a fluid in which the nanometer-sized particles are suspended in base fluids like ethylene glycol, oil, water, and so forth. The main aim for suspending nanometer-size particle in base fluid is to get a strange increment in the thermal conductivity. This kind of act assists the heat transfer rate of the fluid astoundingly by changing its thermophysical properties. Choi [1] was the first who noticed that how the thermal conductivity of fluid enhances with the suspension of nanoparticles into it. Eastman et al. [2] found that when copper nanoparticles disperse into ethylene glycol, then its thermal conductivity anomalously enhanced. Recently, some studies regarding nanofluid flow are due to Kumar et al. [3] and Hayat et al. [4].

Thermal radiation plays an exceptionally huge job in the heat exchange when there is a very small convection heat transfer. The wide uses of it are in nuclear plant, different drive gadgets for aircraft, satellites, and space vehicle. The thermal radiation is used immensely in the processes in which high temperature is required.

Rahman and Eltayeb [5] used convective boundary condition to analyze radiative heat transfer in nanofluid. Rashidi et al. [6] studied the thermal radiation and convection effect on nanofluid flow adjacent to stretching surface. This study is dedicated to find flow behavior of nanofluid adjacent to linearly stretching sheet but there are several situations in which stretching sheet velocity cannot be linear, for example, in the metallurgical and production of plastic sheets. Keeping this in mind, Mabood et al. [7] numerically studied nanofluid flow adjacent to a nonlinear stretching surface by considering the effect of viscous dissipation. They noticed that thermophoresis phenomenon enhances the fluid temperature.

Unsteady flow occurs in many situations. Therefore, Ahmed et al. [8] described axisymmetric unsteady flow of nanofluid. Reddy and Chamkha [9] studied the Dufour and Soret effect on unsteady flow of nanofluid by taking thermophoresis and heat absorption/generation into account. Recently, Shen et al. [10] considered Maxwell viscoelastic nanofluid to observe unsteady flow with different shapes of particles and Cattaneo heat flux.

The investigation of the flow near stagnation point is likewise an essential subject in fluid dynamics. It occurs when fluid collides on the solid material. It has pulled legitimate concerns of various researchers because of its applications in industry, submarines, aircrafts, etc. Stagnation point flow is usually noticed in the blowing and spinning of fiber glass. Lok et al. [11] studied non-orthogonal flow near stagnation point of a micropolar fluid over a vertical stretching surface. Recently, Hayat et al. [12] studied the internal heat generation and melting heat effect on stagnation point Jeffrey fluid flow over a stretchable surface with variable thickness.

In the present article, we have investigated the unsteady stagnation point nanofluid flow over a stretching sheet with Brownian motion, thermophoresis, and thermal radiation. For numerical solution of governing equations, we have used a spectral technique, in particular successive linearization method.

2 Formulation of the Problem

In the present model, we have considered two-dimensional, unsteady, electrically conducting, and viscous stagnation point flow of a nanofluid adjacent to stretching surface. Figure 1 represents the geometry of the problem. The stretching sheet velocity is taken as $u_w(x, t)$ and the fluid velocity in free stream, i.e., far from the sheet, is taken as $u_e(x, t)$. The nanofluid temperature and concentration at the sheet are, respectively, T_w, and C_w. The constant concentration and temperature of fluid in free stream are, respectively, C_∞ and T_∞. The magnetic field having strength B is exerted perpendicular to the sheet. Induced magnetic field is neglected.

Using these assumptions, the governing equations are

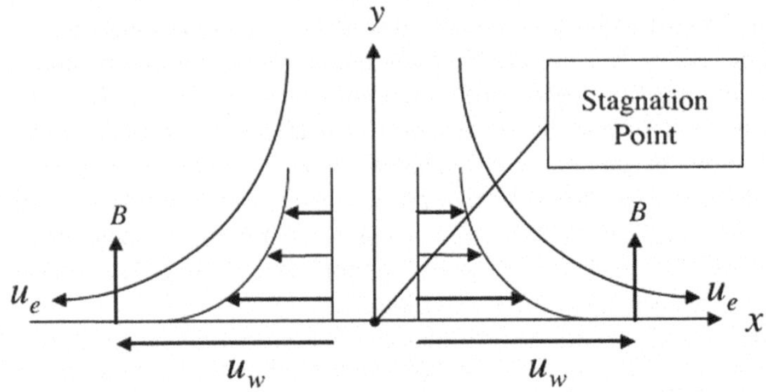

Fig. 1 Boundary layer flow model

$$\frac{\partial v}{\partial y}+\frac{\partial u}{\partial x}=0, \tag{1}$$

$$u\frac{\partial u}{\partial x}+v\frac{\partial u}{\partial y}+\frac{\partial u}{\partial t}=\upsilon\frac{\partial^2 u}{\partial y^2}+\frac{\partial u_{\mathrm{e}}}{\partial t}+u_{\mathrm{e}}\frac{\partial u_{\mathrm{e}}}{\partial x}+\frac{\sigma B^2}{\rho_{\mathrm{f}}}(u_{\mathrm{e}}-u) + \frac{g}{\rho_{\mathrm{f}}}\left[-(\rho_{\mathrm{p}}-\rho_{\mathrm{f}\infty})(C-C_\infty)+(1-C_\infty)\rho_{\mathrm{f}\infty}\beta^*(T-T_\infty)\right], \tag{2}$$

$$u\frac{\partial T}{\partial x}+v\frac{\partial T}{\partial y}+\frac{\partial T}{\partial t}=\alpha_{\mathrm{nf}}\frac{\partial^2 T}{\partial y^2}+\frac{1}{(\rho c)_{\mathrm{f}}}\frac{16\sigma^* T_\infty^3}{3k^*}\frac{\partial^2 T}{\partial y^2}+\tau\left[D_{\mathrm{B}}\frac{\partial C}{\partial y}\frac{\partial T}{\partial y}+\frac{D_{\mathrm{T}}}{T_\infty}\left(\frac{\partial T}{\partial y}\right)^2\right], \tag{3}$$

$$u\frac{\partial C}{\partial x}+v\frac{\partial C}{\partial y}+\frac{\partial C}{\partial t}=\frac{D_T}{T_\infty}\frac{\partial^2 T}{\partial y^2}+D_{\mathrm{B}}\frac{\partial^2 C}{\partial y^2}. \tag{4}$$

The initial and boundary constraints are assumed as

$$t\le 0:\{T=T_{\mathrm{w}},\, C=C_{\mathrm{w}},\, v(x,t)=0,\, u(x,t)=0, \tag{5}$$

$$t>0:\begin{cases} T=T_{\mathrm{w}},\, C=C_{\mathrm{w}},\, v=0,\quad u=\lambda u_{\mathrm{w}}(x,t), & \text{at } y=0,\\ C\to C_\infty,\, T\to T_\infty,\, u\to u_{\mathrm{e}}(x,t), & \text{as } y\to\infty \end{cases} \tag{6}$$

For getting similarity solutions of Eqs. (2)–(4) with initial and boundary constraints (5) and (6), we have taken $u_{\mathrm{e}}(x,t)$, $u_{\mathrm{w}}(x,t)$ and $B^2(t)$ as

$$B^2(t)=\frac{B_0^2}{(1-\beta t)},\; u_{\mathrm{e}}(x,t)=\frac{ax}{(1-\beta t)},\; u_{\mathrm{w}}(x,t)=\frac{ax}{(1-\beta t)}.$$

The similarity transformations for Eqs. (2)–(4) are

$$\psi(x, y, t) = \sqrt{\frac{a\upsilon}{(1-\beta t)}}xf(\eta), \eta = y\sqrt{\frac{a}{\upsilon(1-\beta t)}}, \phi(\eta) = \frac{C - C_\infty}{C_\mathrm{w} - C_\infty}, \theta(\eta) = \frac{T - T_\infty}{T_\mathrm{w} - T_\infty}, \tag{7}$$

here ψ is a stream function and

$$(u, v) = \left(\frac{\partial\psi}{\partial y}, -\frac{\partial\psi}{\partial x}\right). \tag{8}$$

Here η, $\phi(\eta)$, $\theta(\eta)$ correspond to independent similarity variable, nanoparticle concentration, and temperature, respectively.

Using Eqs. (7) and (8) in Eqs. (2)–(6), we get

$$f''' + 1 - f'^2 + ff'' + M(1 - f') - A\left(f' - 1 + \frac{\eta}{2}f''\right) + R_\mathrm{a}[\theta - N_\mathrm{r}\phi] = 0, \tag{9}$$

$$\frac{1}{\mathrm{Pr}_\mathrm{eff}}\theta'' + Nb\theta'\phi' + (f - A\eta)\theta' + Nt\theta'^2 - 2(A + f')\theta = 0, \tag{10}$$

$$\phi'' + Sc\left[f - \frac{A\eta}{2}\right]\phi' - 2Sc[f' + A]\phi + \frac{Nt}{Nb}\theta'' = 0. \tag{11}$$

Subject to boundary constraints:

$$\left.\begin{array}{ll} \theta(\eta) = 1, f(\eta) = 0, \phi(\eta) = 1, f'(\eta) = \lambda, & \text{at } \eta = 0, \\ \theta(\eta) \to 0, \phi(\eta) \to 0, f'(\eta) \to 1, & \text{as } \eta \to \infty, \end{array}\right\} \tag{12}$$

where $R_\mathrm{a} = \frac{g(1-C_\infty)(T_\mathrm{w}-T_\infty)\beta^*\rho_{\mathrm{f}\infty}}{\rho_\mathrm{f}a^2}$, $N_\mathrm{R} = \frac{(\rho_\mathrm{p}-\rho_{\mathrm{f}\infty})(C_\mathrm{w}-C_\infty)}{(1-C_\infty)(T_\mathrm{w}-T_\infty)\beta^*\rho_{\mathrm{f}\infty}}$, $M = \frac{\sigma B_0^2}{\rho_\mathrm{f}a}$, $A = \frac{\beta}{a}$, $\mathrm{Pr} = \frac{\upsilon}{\alpha_\mathrm{nf}}$, $\mathrm{Pr}_\mathrm{eff} = \frac{\mathrm{Pr}}{(1+R)}$, $Nt = \frac{\tau D_\mathrm{T}(T_\mathrm{w}-T_\infty)}{T_\infty\upsilon}$, $R = \frac{16T_\infty^3\sigma^*}{3kk^*}$, $Nb = \frac{\tau D_\mathrm{B}(C_\mathrm{w}-C_\infty)}{\upsilon}$ and $Sc = \frac{\upsilon}{D_\mathrm{B}}$.

The local Nusselt number Nu_x and skin friction coefficient C_{f_x} are as follows

$$\mathrm{Nu}_x = \frac{-x(1-\beta t)^{1/2}}{(T_\mathrm{w} - T_\infty)}\left(\frac{\partial T}{\partial y}\right)_{y=0}, C_{f_x} = \frac{\upsilon(1-\beta t)^{-1/2}}{u_\mathrm{w}^2}\left(\frac{\partial u}{\partial y}\right)_{y=0}, \tag{13}$$

Using Eqs. (7) and (8), Eq. (13) reduced to

$$C_{f_x}\mathrm{Re}_x^{1/2} = f''(0), \mathrm{Nu}_x\mathrm{Re}_x^{-1/2} = -\theta'(0). \tag{14}$$

where $\mathrm{Re}_x = \frac{u_r(x)x}{\upsilon}$ is local Reynolds number with $u_r(x) = ax$.

3 The Numerical Solution

Successive linearization method is utilized to solve coupled nonlinear Eqs. (9)–(11) with boundary conditions (12). This spectral scheme is briefly explained in the article by Motsa and Sibanda [13]. The initial guesses which we have chosen for using this method are as follows

$$f_0 = -e^{-\lambda\eta} + e^{-\eta} + \eta, \quad \theta_0 = e^{-\eta}, \quad s_0 = e^{-\eta}.$$

4 Results and Discussion

To give the physical knowledge of the present flow problem, complete numerical calculations are performed for various appropriate parameters and the results are explained graphically. The default values of parameters for this computation are $A = 0.5$, $\mathrm{Pr} = 1$, $\lambda = 0.5$, $M = 0.5$, $\mathrm{Ra} = 0.5$, $Nr = 0.5$, $R = 0.5$, $Nt = 1$, $Nb = 1$, and $Sc = 1$.

Figures 2, 3, 4, and 5 show the effect of some active parameters on fluid velocity. The effect of parameter M on velocity profile for $\lambda = 0.5$ and $\lambda = 1.5$ is presented in Fig. 2. It is perceived here that in case of $\lambda = 1.5$, velocity profile depreciates with the increasing values of magnetic parameter. This event may be the reason of Lorentz force which reduces the velocity of the fluid. When $\lambda = 0.5$, magnetic parameter has tendency to enhance fluid velocity and increase boundary layer thickness. Figure 3 shows the sway of parameter Nr on velocity profile. It can be observed here that velocity profiles diminish as parameter Nr rises. Figure 4 shows the effect of mixed

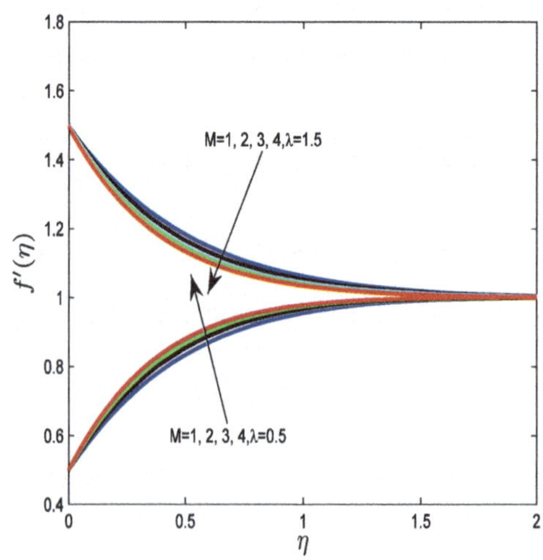

Fig. 2 Velocity distribution for M

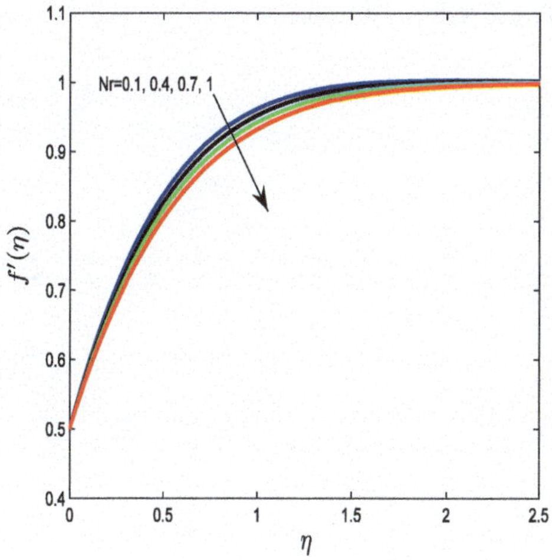

Fig. 3 Velocity distribution for Nr

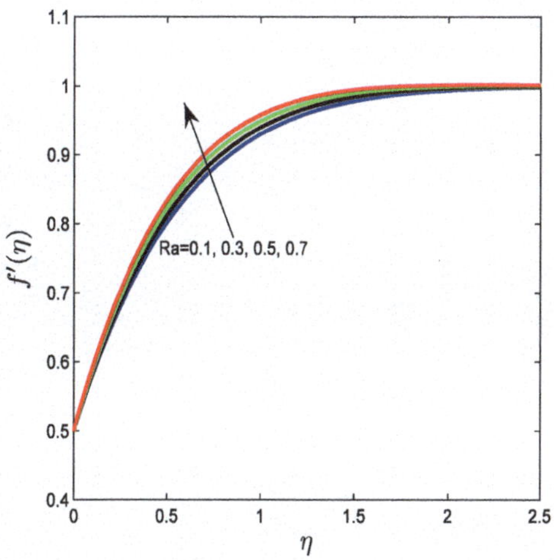

Fig. 4 Velocity distribution for Ra

convection parameter Ra on fluid velocity. It is worthy to note here that velocity distribution enhances with rising values of Ra. This event is contribution of buoyancy force acting on it. Figure 5 shows the effect of parameter λ on fluid velocity and it indicates that as we increase parameter λ, fluid velocity increases and boundary layer width also tends to increase.

Temperature profile for different parameters is shown from Figs. 6, 7, 8, 9, and 10. The variation of temperature distribution corresponding to parameter λ is depicted via Fig. 6, which indicates that temperature decreases with enhancement in parameter λ. The behavior of temperature of nanofluid due to variation in unsteadiness parameter is explained via Fig. 7. It is observed here that temperature distribution decrease near the sheet as increment in parameter A but as going away from the sheet, temperature profiles rise up. Influence of parameter R on temperature of fluid is displayed in

Fig. 5 Velocity distribution for λ

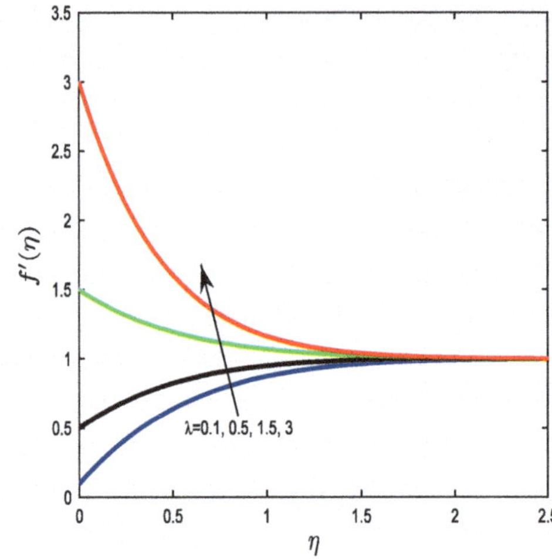

Fig. 6 Temperature distribution for λ

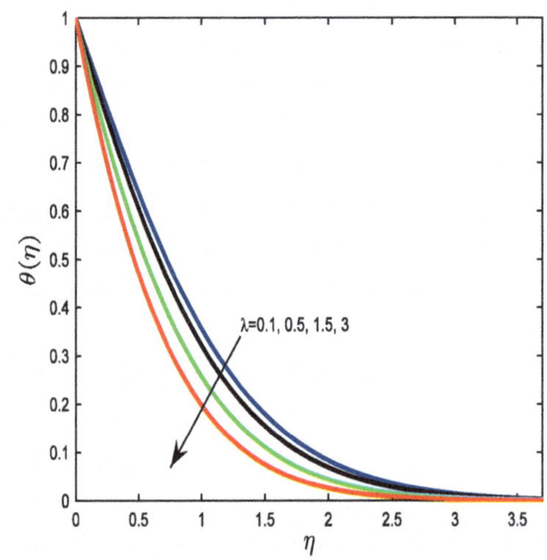

Fig. 8, which indicates that the thermal radiation parameter enhances the temperature profile. It is very obvious because in the presence of thermal radiation, more heat is absorbed by the fluid; therefore, enhancement in temperature profile is found. Figure 9 shows the nature of temperature profile against parameter Nb and it is observed that parameter Nb has tendency to enhance temperature since Brownian motion is the particle analogue phenomenon; therefore, heat is produced due to direct collisions of fluid particles and hence enhancement in temperature is found. The influence of parameter Nt on temperature distribution is presented by Fig. 10. It indicates that temperature increases with increment in parameter Nt because thermophoresis force tends to push nanoparticles from hot area to cold area.

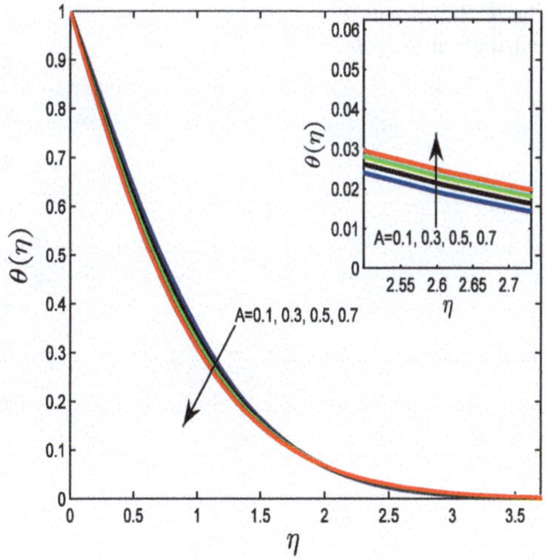

Fig. 7 Temperature distribution for A

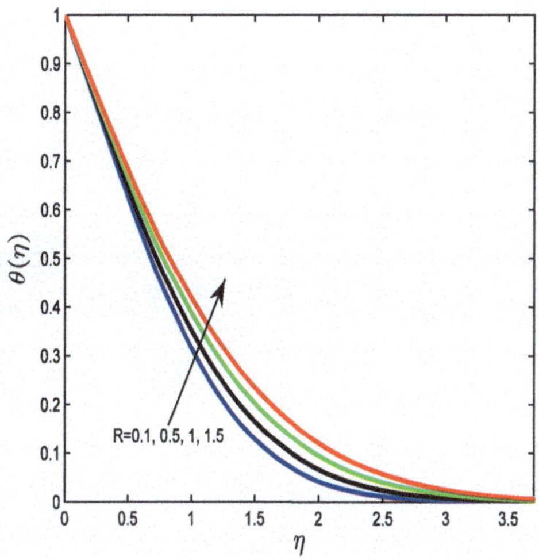

Fig. 8 Temperature distribution for R

Figures 11, 12, 13, and 14 are plotted to understand the behavior of nanoparticle concentration corresponding to some parameters. Figure 11 shows the effect of parameter A on nanoparticle concentration. It is evident here that increment in unsteady parameter reduces the nanoparticle distribution throughout the boundary layer. Figure 12 represents the influence of parameter λ on concentration profile which indicates that reduction in concentration profile is found as we increase parameter λ. The influence of Brownian motion parameter on concentration distribution can be seen from Fig. 13, which indicates that concentration profiles impede with enhancement in parameter Nb. This event occurs because parameter Nb represents random motion of nanoparticles. As Nb increases, random motion of nanoparticles increases and they collide each other very frequently. Influence of parameter Nt

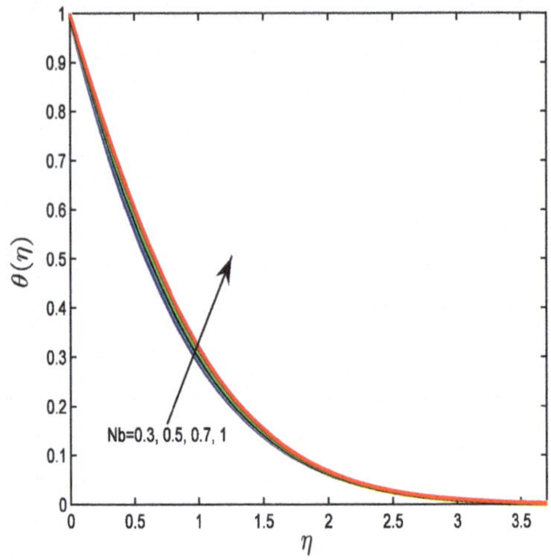

Fig. 9 Temperature distribution for Nb

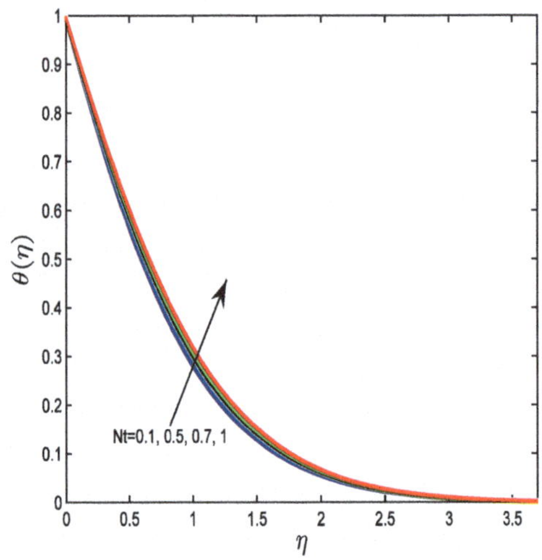

Fig. 10 Temperature distribution for Nt

is displayed in Fig. 14. It is visible here that concentration profiles increase with enhancement in parameter Nt because of thermophoresis force.

Table 1 is presented to explain that how skin friction and local Nusselt number vary with variation in different parameters. It is visible here that enhancement in parameters A, Ra and Nb lead to enhance skin friction at the surface while parameters Nr, Nt and λ do the vice versa. On the other hand, parameters Nr, Nb and Nt have tendency to boost local Nusselt number, while parameters A, Ra and λ reduce it significantly.

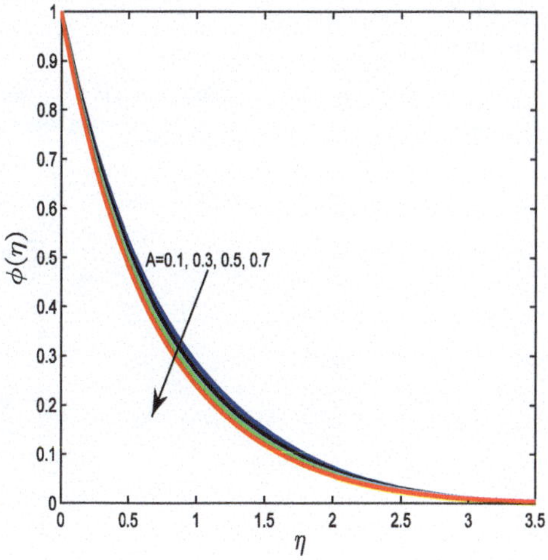

Fig. 11 Concentration distribution for A

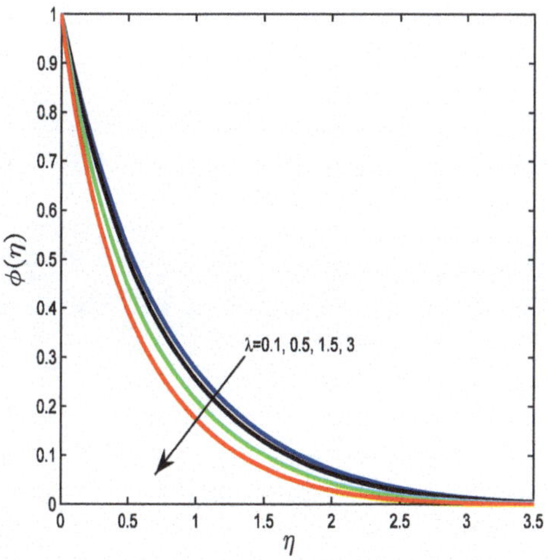

Fig. 12 Concentration distribution for λ

5 Outcomes of the Investigation

The important outcomes of the present investigation include:

i. Velocity of nanofluid increases with increment in parameters R and λ, while parameter Nr decreases it. Parameter M has tendency to enhance fluid velocity for $\lambda < 1$, however, for $\lambda > 1$, this effect is reversed.
ii. With the enhancement in parameters R, Nb, and Nt, nanofluid temperature increases while parameter λ does the vice versa. The parameter A decreases it near the sheet but increases it as going away from the sheet.
iii. Nanoparticle concentration is decreased with the enhancement in parameter λ, A and Nb, while parameter Nt increases it significantly.

Fig. 13 Concentration distribution for Nb

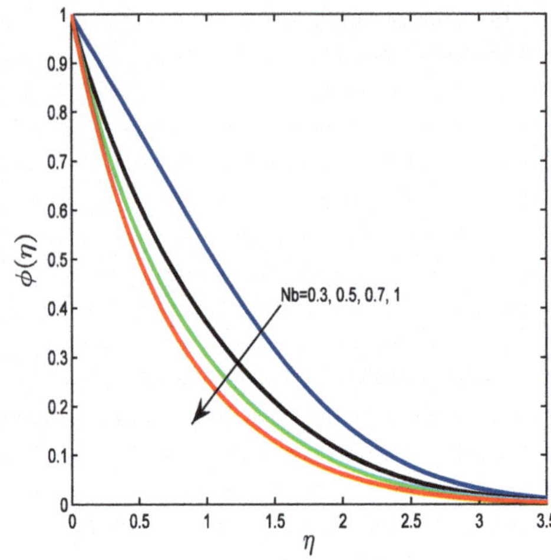

Fig. 14 Concentration distribution for Nt

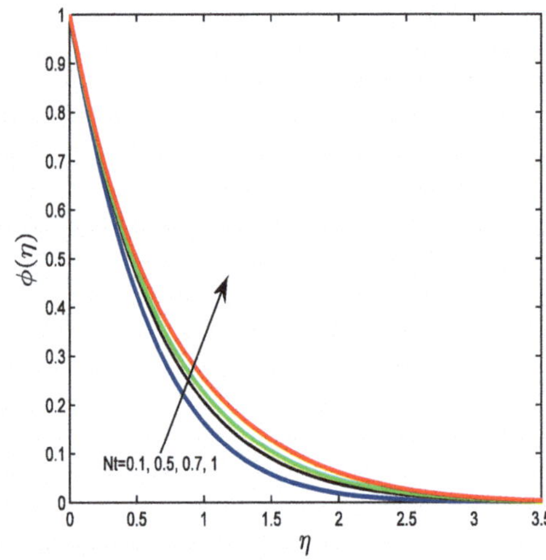

iv. The parameters A, Ra, and Nb lead to enhance skin friction at the surface while parameters Nr, Nt, and λ do the vice versa. On the other hand, parameters Nr, Nb and Nt have tendency to boost local Nusselt number, while parameters A, Ra, and λ reduce it significantly.

Table 1 The values of $f''(0)$ and $\theta'(0)$ for different parameters

A	Ra	Nr	Nb	Nt	λ	$f''(0)$	$-\theta'(0)$
0.1						0.918385	0.7276
0.3						0.936408	0.78976
0.5						0.954249	0.84862
	0.1					0.870652	0.84401
	0.3					0.912565	0.84633
	0.5					0.954249	0.84862
		0.1				1.020451	0.85195
		0.4				0.970844	0.84946
		0.7				0.920966	0.84693
			0.1			0.833371	1.06019
			0.5			0.936604	0.96518
			0.7			0.945795	0.91683
				0.1		0.954487	0.97346
				0.5		0.954133	0.91393
				0.7		0.954111	0.88667
					0.1	1.531376	0.73332
					0.5	0.954249	0.84862
					1.5	−0.89935	1.09297

References

1. Choi, S.U.S.: Enhancing thermal conductivity of fluids with nanoparticles. Proc. ASME Int. Mech. Eng. Cong. Exposition **66**, 99–105 (1995)
2. Eastman, J.A., Choi, S.U.S., Li, S., Yu, W., Thompson, L.J.: Anomalously increased effective thermal conductivities of ethylene glycol-based nanofluids containing copper nanoparticles. Appl. Phys. Lett. **78**(6), 718–720 (2001)
3. Kumar, R., Kumar, R., Shehzad, S.A., Sheikholeslami, M.: Rotating frame analysis of radiating and reacting ferro-nanofluid considering Joule heating and viscous dissipation. Int. J. Heat Mass Transf. **120**, 540–551 (2018)
4. Hayat, T., Aziz, A., Muhammad, T., Alsaedi, A.: An optimal analysis for Darcy-Forchheimer 3D flow of nanofluid with convective condition and homogeneous–heterogeneous reactions. Phys. Lett. A **382**(39), 2846–2855 (2018)
5. Rahman, M.M., Eltayeb, I.A.: Radiative heat transfer in a hydromagnetic nanofluid past a non-linear stretching surface with convective boundary condition. Meccanica **48**(3), 601–615 (2013)
6. Rashidi, M.M., Ganesh, N.V., Hakeem, A.A., Ganga, B.: Buoyancy effect on MHD flow of nanofluid over a stretching sheet in the presence of thermal radiation. J. Mol. Liq. **198**, 234–238 (2014)
7. Mabood, F., Khan, W.A., Ismail, A.M.: MHD boundary layer flow and heat transfer of nanofluids over a nonlinear stretching sheet: a numerical study. J. Magn. Magn. Mater. **374**, 569–576 (2015)
8. Ahmed, J., Mahmood, T., Iqbal, Z., Shahzad, A., Ali, R.: Axisymmetric flow and heat transfer over an unsteady stretching sheet in power law fluid. J. Mol. Liq. **221**, 386–393 (2016)

9. Reddy, P.S., Chamkha, A.J.: Soret and Dufour effects on unsteady MHD heat and mass transfer from a permeable stretching sheet with thermophoresis and non-uniform heat generation/absorption. J. Appl. Fluid Mech. **9**(5) (2016)
10. Shen, M., Chen, S., Liu, F.: Unsteady MHD flow and heat transfer of fractional Maxwell viscoelastic nanofluid with Cattaneo heat flux and different particle shapes. Chin. J. Phys. **56**(3), 1199–1211 (2018)
11. Lok, Y.Y., Pop, I., Ingham, D.B., Amin, N.: Mixed convection flow of a micropolar fluid near a non-orthogonal stagnation-point on a stretching vertical sheet. Int. J. Numer. Meth. Heat Fluid Flow **19**(3/4), 459–483 (2009)
12. Hayat, T., Saif, R.S., Ellahi, R., Muhammad, T., Alsaedi, A.: Simultaneous effects of melting heat and internal heat generation in stagnation point flow of Jeffrey fluid towards a nonlinear stretching surface with variable thickness. Int. J. Therm. Sci. **132**, 344–354 (2018)
13. Motsa, S.S., Sibanda, P.: A linearisation method for non-linear singular boundary value problems. Comput. Math Appl. **63**(7), 1197–1203 (2012)

New Universal Classification of Fluid Flows Structural Components

Yuli D. Chashechkin

Abstract New classification of fluid flow components which includes ligaments describing fine filaments or interfaces, together with waves and products of their nonlinear interactions is proposed. The classification is based on total solutions of the linearized system of the fundamental equations taking into account the compatibility condition. General analysis of periodic motion structures is illustrated by numerical calculations and schlieren visualizations of flow fields generated by uniform motion of a vertical plate in a stratified medium. Both the numerical and laboratory visualization results show that the flow patterns, which contain complex systems of internal waves, including upstream and attached waves, as well as thin interfaces, such as ligaments, formed due to the combined influence of the stratification and dissipation effects. The observation and calculation results are in good qualitative and quantitative agreement. Visualization of ligaments in a flow induced by a drop impact in targeted fluid presents to support the universality of classification.

Keywords Stratified flow · Fundamental equations · Complete solutions · Ligaments · Waves · Vortices · Drop · Visualization

1 Introduction

The attempts of an intuitive classification of fluid flow components can be traced throughout the history of civilized humanity, starting with the oldest rock carvings where systems of a wavy line are commonly thought of as waves and spirals—as vortices. Beautiful sketches of waves and vortices in fluid flows are presented in many renaissance paintings (widespread drawings by Leonardo da Vinci). The development of mathematics contributed to the formalization of the process and giving the clearly marked content of selected components.

Analysis of the properties of the solutions of the first closed system of equations allowed Euler and D'Alembert to introduce the concepts of potentials and stream

Y. D. Chashechkin (✉)
Ishlinsky Institute for Problems in Mechanics, Russian Academy of Sciences, Moscow, Russia
e-mail: yulidch@gmail.com

S. Bhattacharyya et al. (eds.), *Mathematical Modeling and Computational Tools*, Springer Proceedings in Mathematics & Statistics 320,
https://doi.org/10.1007/978-981-15-3615-1_10

functions—scalar functions whose derivatives display the components of the velocity vector, as a consequence, establish the properties of potential waves, and define the vorticity as a differential property of the velocity fields [1].

The Industrial Revolution in Europe was accompanied by the intensive development of mathematics in general and the theory of fluid flows, respectively. The derivation of the C. Navier equation, which contains a term describing the viscous friction, has been carefully analyzed and justified in the framework of the theory of continuous functions by G. G. Stokes [1]. He constructed a number of particular solutions to the problems of linear and nonlinear waves propagation, calculated the flow around a sphere and in a channel, together with a number of other problems.

At the same time, the physical limits of the obtained solutions validity, the mismatch of which with experiment grew with increasing a flow velocity, were experimentally found. A narrow range of parameters for the consistency of the calculations C. Navier and G. G. Stokes results with Hagen and Poiseuille experiments questioned the validity of proposed theory to solve the practically important problems. Among developed alternative models were equations of nonlinear waves proposed by Russell, Rayleigh, Korteweg, de Vries, and many others, as well as the constitutive models, among which the theory of turbulence proposed by O. Reynolds, based on visualization of flow patterns in tube, became the most widespread.

Only with the publication of Lamb's treatise [2], the Navier–Stokes equations were finally accepted as the fundamental basis of fluid mechanics, which was subsequently confirmed by Landau and Lifshitz, Batchelor, Müller, Vallis, and in many other monographs [3–6] devoted to the study of the dynamics and thermodynamics of fluids and gases flows.

Simultaneously with the construction of solutions of the fundamental equations system and the study of their properties, the development of specialized models describing the dynamics of specific structural components continued. One of the most widely spread models is the theories of the boundary layer [7], as well as the theories of various waves—acoustic, surface and internal gravity, inertial, and hybrid, each one is connected with real physical properties of the environment—heterogeneity in composition and density, compressibility, general rotation [8], as well as for separate vortices [9]. Correspondingly, the experiment is developed by mainly focusing on the study of boundary layers, waves, vortices, jets or wakes, and other flow components. At the same time, different forms of the theory of stability were developed to define the conditions for the occurrence and duration of the existence of separate structural components of flows. Due to technical difficulties, many calculations were characterized by relatively low accuracy, and the experiments were incomplete. The creation of every group of models was accompanied by the formulation of a new classification of forms or components of flows based on some mathematical or geometric features of selected models.

L. Euler was the first who investigated the flows and the velocity $\mathbf{v}$ fields in which are described by scalar φ ($\mathbf{v} = \nabla\varphi$) or vector $\mathbf{A}$ potential ($\mathbf{v} = \operatorname{rot}\mathbf{A}$). The properties of both irrotational ($\operatorname{rot}\operatorname{grad}\varphi = 0$) and vortex flows ($\operatorname{rot}\mathbf{v} = \operatorname{rot}\operatorname{rot}\mathbf{A} = \operatorname{grad}\operatorname{div}\mathbf{A} - \Delta\mathbf{A}$, ∇ is Hamilton and $\Delta = \frac{\partial^2}{\partial x_i^2}$ is the Laplace operators) continue to be actively studied in the theory of an actually homogeneous fluid (with identically constant density). In the actually homogeneous fluid, the velocity and momentum, which are the measures of the kinematics of the velocity field and the physical motions of liquid particles, became identical. Experimental and theoretical verifications of some conclusions of the homogeneous fluid theory are difficult due to the unreality of hypothesis of density constancy and the absence of proof for the 3D Navier–Stokes equations solution (6th Millennium problem [10]).

The popular method uses the geometric separation of the flow on the "boundary layer" near the obstacle [7], which is described by the own set of equations, and the external flow, for which the equations of Euler and Navier–Stokes are used. The formalization of the description is difficult due to the absence of a criterion for determining the position of outer frontier of the boundary layer.

The most common classification includes laminar flow, which is described by different versions of the Navier–Stokes equations, and turbulent flow, which assumes a high level of fluctuations and active mixing. The boundary between the two regimes is determined by the values of characteristic parameters ("numbers" of Reynolds and others). The most common disadvantage is that the definition of "turbulence" is not proposed and, as a result, a variety of mathematical models is used in practice. The scale invariance of the equations of fluid mechanics was emphasized by G. G. Stokes in a review of the manuscript of the first experimental paper by O. Reynolds: "In one part the language seems to imply (which was not perhaps intended) that he discovered new dimensional properties of fluids, and might even lead to the supposition that he supposed that he had shown that another constant beyond those recognized was necessary in order to define a fluid mechanically. This certainly is not the case, the dimensional properties are already obviously involved in the equations of motion; and there is absolutely nothing to prove that he has discovered the necessity of an additional constant to define a fluid" (G. G. Stokes, 19 April 1883, reproduced in [11]).

The situation began to change significantly in the second half of the twentieth century, when with the creation of satellites, pronounced structures of the global pattern of flows began to be recognized in the Earth atmosphere, in the ocean, in the atmospheres of other planets and stars, and in the interstellar medium on galactic scales [12], as well as in small-scale laboratory flows, both slow [13] and fairly fast, initiated by immersion a free-falling drop into a liquid [14], where the pattern of the matter is not described by common theory of flows.

At the same time, the intensive development of computing and programming provided the room for implementing previously developed complex algorithms, and realization new ones, more efficient, for calculating the dynamics and structure of flows, both stratified (strongly for laboratory and weakly for natural systems) and homogeneous—potentially (extremely weak) and actually (identically homogeneous liquids [15]). The emergence of theoretical models, the results of which are consistent with experiment in general properties, and in fine details of the flow [16], justify the need to analyze the criteria for choosing the system of equations and the properties of complete solutions, which give a room to formulate universal requirements for the methods of calculations and experiments that are consistent with the completeness and consistency criteria.

2 Determination of Fluid State

In classical hydrodynamics, it is accepted to state that the properties of a fluid motion completely determine the density together with one of the thermodynamic parameters, for example, pressure, and indicator of a fluid flow is velocity [3, 4]. However, the recent development of theoretical and experimental studies of the structures of the flows has led to a radical change in the ideas about the nature of the flows and the properties of the fluid. The changes are related to the reassessment of the role of energy as an independent parameter describing the complex nature of flows patterns in truly multicomponent, thermally and concentration inhomogeneous media with free surfaces due to a variety of energy transport mechanisms.

Basing on ideas of interrelations of atomic physics and macroscopic hydrodynamics, the International Association for Water and Steam recommended to select one of the thermodynamic potentials, namely the free enthalpy, or the Gibbs potential, as the main parameter of the fluid state [17]. Derivatives of the Gibbs potential $dG = -sdT + VdP - S_{\mathrm{d}}d\sigma + \mu_i dn_i$ determine the entropy s, the specific volume V and density $\rho = \frac{1}{V} = \left(\frac{\partial G}{\partial P}\right)^{-1}_{T,S_{\mathrm{d}},n_i}$, the surface tension coefficient σ and the chemical potential component μ_i due to the presence of the ith dissolved impurity with concentration n_i (here T is the temperature, S_{d} is the area of the free surface).

Relations between thermodynamic quantities determining the equation of state of the medium usually are represented in the form of the dependence of density ρ on other thermodynamic quantities—in temperature T pressure P,, and salinity S_i

$$\rho = \rho(T,\ P,\ S_i) \tag{1}$$

It should be noted that free enthalpy, like other types of thermodynamic potentials, is a natural macroscopic parameter that takes into account the anisotropy of atomic–molecular interactions in structured multicomponent fluids with a free surface. Due to the non-uniform distribution of internal energy in a fluid and the intrinsic features of its structure, transport of the energy can occur with different characteristic time intervals.

Energy is transported rather slowly in the processes of molecular diffusion and dissipation; more quickly together with the velocity of macroscopic flows, at special celerity characterizing propagation of a wave and very fast for directly atomic–molecular processes during chemical reactions, the elimination of the free surface or the release of chemical energy. The processes of transfer of the energy in fluid flows are not fully understood.

Therefore, thermodynamic parameters, such as density or temperature, can change in flows quite slowly and extremely rapidly. The diversity of the intrinsic scales of the structural components of fluids, including molecular clusters with a size from 10^{-7} to 10^{-6} cm, and larger macroscopic structural components, characterizing by different rates of energy exchange, provides the necessary conditions for the formation of macroscopic flow structures of various scales. Among them, the separate scales of the studied phenomena, the magnitude of which is determined by the governing equations, initial and boundary conditions, are well distinguished.

3 The System of Governing Equations

One of the key achievements of theoretical physics is the discovery of a relation between symmetries of the space and time as well as the governing equations system and the laws of conservation of physical quantities. Selection of basic conserved quantities that are mass, momentum, energy predetermined the choice of the system of governing equations of fluid mechanics, which, in addition to the equations of state, contains the equations of continuity and of momentum, entropy or temperature, and substances transport [3, 5, 6].

The behavior of the angular momentum is not studied in flows due to the absence of stability of an inertia tensor, which is the characteristic physical parameter of a medium in description of a body rotation. Due to the continuous variation of the forms of the components and the complex three-dimensional structure of real flows, as well as irregular variations of "liquid particles" positions, the tensor of inertia of a rotating fluid is not constant and continuously changes unpredictably.

The conventional system of fluid mechanics equations has the form [3, 5, 6]

$$\begin{cases} G = G(\mathbf{x}, t) \\ \rho(\mathbf{x}, t) = \rho(T, P, S_i) \\ \frac{\partial \rho}{\partial t} + \nabla \cdot (\rho \mathbf{v}) = Q_M \\ \frac{\partial S_n}{\partial t} + \nabla \cdot (S_n \mathbf{v} + \mathbf{I}_n) = Q_n \\ \frac{\partial (\rho v^i)}{\partial t} + \nabla_j \Pi^{ij} = \rho g^i + Q^i \\ \frac{\partial E}{\partial t} + \nabla_i (E v^i) + \nabla_i \left(q^i + P v^i - \sigma^{ij} v_j + \frac{\partial w}{\partial S_n} I_n^i \right) = Q_e \end{cases} \tag{2}$$

where $\mathbf{x}$ is the absolute coordinate frame, t is time, $\mathbf{v}$ is the velocity field, S_n, $\mathbf{I}_\mathrm{n}$ are the mass concentration and the vector of the specific diffusion flux for the nth impurity, respectively, $\Pi^{ij} = \rho v^i v^j + P\delta^{ij} - \sigma^{ij}$ is the specific momentum flux, $\sigma^{ij} = \mu\left(\frac{\partial v^i}{\partial x^j} + \frac{\partial v^j}{\partial x^i} - \frac{2}{s}\delta^{ij}\frac{\partial v^k}{\partial x^k}\right) + \zeta_2 \delta^{ij}\frac{\partial v^k}{\partial x^k}$ is the symmetric tensor of viscous stresses, δ^{ij} is the Kronecker metric tensor, μ, ζ_2 are the first and second dynamic viscosities, $E = \rho\left(\frac{v^2}{2} + \varepsilon + \Phi\right)$ is the specific total energy, ε is the specific internal energy, $w = \varepsilon + \frac{P}{\rho}$ is the specific enthalpy, Φ is the gravity potential, $\mathbf{g} = -\nabla\Phi$ is the acceleration of gravity, $\mathbf{q}$ is the vector of the heat flux, Q_M, Q_n, Q^i, Q_e are the density of sources of mass—impurity, momentum and energy—respectively, ∇, Δ are Hamilton and Laplace operators.

The combination of the equations of the system (2) is used to transform the energy transport equation into the evolution equation for the temperature field

$$\rho\, c_{\mathrm{P}}\left(\frac{\mathrm{d}T}{\mathrm{d}t} - \Gamma\frac{\mathrm{d}P}{\mathrm{d}t}\right) = -\nabla_i q^i + \frac{1}{2}\sigma^{ij} e_{ij} + I_{\mathrm{n}}^i \nabla_i \frac{\partial w}{\partial S_{\mathrm{n}}} + Q_T \tag{3}$$

where c_{P} is heat capacity at constant pressure, Γ is adiabatic temperature gradient, $e_{ij} = \frac{1}{2}\left(\frac{\partial v_i}{\partial x_j} + \frac{\partial v_j}{\partial x i_j}\right)$ is the strain rate tensor, Q_{T} is density of the source of temperature.

The system of Eqs. (2) is considered taking into account the compatibility condition, which determines its rank, the order of the linearized version, and the degree of the characteristic equation (dispersion) equation in the case of a solution represented by periodic functions [16]. The system (2) determines the flow of fluids as forced fluxes of momentum and energy, accompanied by self-consistent changes in the thermodynamic parameters of the medium fields that are density, temperature, pressure, and concentration of components.

The intrinsic parameters of a fluid include the coefficients in the equations of state for thermodynamic quantities—thermal expansion, salt contraction, adiabatic compressibility, and kinetic coefficients in transport equations that are dynamic μ or kinematic $\nu = \mu/\rho$ viscosity, temperature κ_{T} or thermal κ_{q} conductivity, and diffusion of a substance κ_i that are parameters of molecular diffusion of momentum, energy, and impurities.

Since the medium is, in most cases, bounded either solid boundaries or a free surface, the equations of motion (2) must also be supplemented by boundary conditions.

On solid impermeable boundaries, the conditions for fluid flow and absence of impurity and heat fluxes (in the absence of sources of corresponding thermodynamic variables at the boundary) are

$$\mathbf{v}\cdot\mathbf{n}\,|_{\Sigma} = \mathbf{I}_{\mathrm{n}}\cdot\mathbf{n}\,|_{\Sigma} = \mathbf{q}\cdot\mathbf{n}\,|_{\Sigma} = 0 \tag{4}$$

where $\mathbf{n}$ is the normal to the boundary surface.

In a viscous fluid, the boundary condition for the velocity is transformed into no-slip condition

$$\mathbf{v}\,|_{\Sigma} = 0 \tag{5}$$

If temperature or impurity sources with known values are placed on solid boundaries, conditions (4) for thermal $\mathbf{q}$ and density $\mathbf{I}_{\mathrm{n}}$ fluxes change

$$\kappa_{\mathrm{T}}\frac{\partial T}{\partial n} + \gamma_{\mathrm{T}} T = \phi_{\mathrm{T}}, \quad \kappa_{\mathrm{n}}\frac{\partial S_{\mathrm{n}}}{\partial n} + \gamma_{S_{\mathrm{n}}} S_{\mathrm{n}} = \phi_{S_{\mathrm{n}}} \tag{6}$$

where $\gamma_{\mathrm{T}}, \gamma_{S_{\mathrm{n}}}$ are coefficients of heat and mass transfers (temperature and mass transfers), $\kappa_{\mathrm{T}}, \kappa_{\mathrm{n}}$ are temperature diffusivity and diffusion coefficients of this impurity, $\phi_{\mathrm{T}}, \phi_{S_{\mathrm{n}}}$ are given source functions.

The boundary conditions on the free surface $\zeta(\mathbf{r}, t)$ are derived from the integral formulations of the laws of conservation for the mass of the medium and impurities supplemented by the conditions of the momentum and energy transfer. They are conventionally divided into three types that are kinematic, dynamic, and energetic.

The kinematic boundary conditions describe the motion of a free surface and the transport processes on it

$$\frac{\partial \zeta}{\partial t} + \mathbf{u} \cdot \nabla \zeta = b|\nabla \zeta|, \quad \mathbf{I}_{\mathrm{n}} \cdot \nabla \zeta = -bS_{\mathrm{n}}|\nabla \zeta| \tag{7}$$

where b is the flow of pure water caused by evaporation, precipitation, formation, and melting of ice (there is no impurity fluxes from outside).

Dynamic boundary conditions are the formulation of the condition for mutual compensation of all forces acting on the surface [3]

$$\left(P_1 - P_2 + \alpha\left(\frac{1}{R_1} + \frac{1}{R_2}\right)\right)n^i = \left(\sigma_1^{ij} - \sigma_2^{ij}\right)\nabla_j \zeta + \nabla_i \alpha \tag{8}$$

where P_1, P_2 and σ_1^{ij}, σ_1^{ij} are the pressures and tensors of viscous stresses in media separated by a free surface, α is the surface tension coefficient, R_1, R_2 are the principal radii of curvature of the free surface.

The energetic boundary condition describes the influx of heat into the medium from outside

$$\mathbf{q} \cdot \nabla \zeta = Q\,|\nabla \zeta| \tag{9}$$

where Q is the total heat flux.

Until now, the properties of a high-rank nonlinear system (2), with deep multilevel internal connections between physical quantities, have not been studied. In practice, reduced versions of the system of fundamental equations are considered. Usually, due to the high heat capacity of water and aqueous solutions, the effect of dissipation on medium parameters and momentum transfer is usually neglected; the energy transfer equation is excluded from consideration in hydrodynamics.

To simplify the analysis, nonlinear functions of several variables in the equations of state and transport equations are replaced by constant coefficients and the system of Eqs (2) in the Boussinesq approximation and incompressibility takes the form [3, 16]

$$\begin{cases} \rho = \rho_0 + \rho_{00} \cdot s, \\ \operatorname{div} \mathbf{v} = 0, \\ \frac{\partial s}{\partial t} + \nabla \cdot (s\,\mathbf{v}) = \nabla \cdot (\kappa_S \nabla s) + \frac{v_z}{\Lambda} \\ \frac{\partial \mathbf{v}}{\partial t} + \nabla \cdot (\mathbf{v}\,\mathbf{v}) = -\frac{1}{\rho_{00}} \nabla P + \nabla \cdot (\nu \nabla \mathbf{v}) - s \cdot \mathbf{g} \end{cases} \tag{10}$$

Physically valid no-slip and no-flux boundary conditions have the following form,

$$\begin{aligned} &\mathbf{u}|_{t\le 0} = 0,\ s|_{t\le 0} = 0,\ P|_{t\le 0} = 0, \\ &u_x|_\Sigma = u_z|_\Sigma = 0, \quad \left[\frac{\partial s}{\partial \mathbf{n}}\right]\Bigg|_\Sigma = \frac{1}{\Lambda}\frac{\partial z}{\partial \mathbf{n}}, \\ &u_x|_{x,z\to\infty} = U,\ u_z|_{x,z\to\infty} = 0. \end{aligned} \tag{11}$$

The unperturbed medium, which is selected as the initial state, is supposed to be salinity stratified $\rho_0 = \rho_0(S_0(z))$, where $\rho_{00} = \rho_0(z = 0)$ is reference density. The density is described by a linearized equation of state, which permits to include the coefficient of salt contraction in the definition of salinity. The exponential profile of density over height $\rho_0 = \rho_{00}\exp(-z/\Lambda)$ is characterized by a constant values of the stratification length scale $\Lambda = \left|\frac{1}{\rho}\frac{d\rho}{dz}\right|^{-1}$, buoyancy frequency $N = \sqrt{\frac{g}{\Lambda}}$ and period $T_b = \frac{2\pi}{N}$. In practice, calculations are carried out in the approximation of strong stratification (for laboratory conditions $N_b \sim 1\ s^{-1}$), weak stratification (in the earth environment $N_b \sim 10^{-2}\ s^{-1}$), potentially homogeneous ($N_b \sim 10^{-5}\ s^{-1}$), and actually homogeneous ($N = 0$) liquids [15].

Basic flow components, described by the complete solution of the fundamental equations system (2) or (10) for given initial and boundary conditions, which consist of several independent functions, exist in the whole space; however, their relative intensity can be distinguished in different domains of flows. Due to the nonlinearity of the basic Eqs. (2), all the distinguished flow components, both large, and small, interact with each other and produce new components. Existence of multiple components with different incommensurable scales is manifested in the spatial heterogeneity of the flow pattern, as well as, and its evolution and fast variations over time.

Of practical interest is the determination of the minimum number of independent functions that make up the complete solution of the system (10). To carry out such a classification, it is necessary to consider a complete solution of the linearized problem for describing periodic flows in viscous fluids. The analysis of periodic solutions is usually limited to the investigation of the waves representing large-scale regular components which are only a part of a general set of solutions [3].

4 Classification of Components of Periodic Fluid Flows

With the action of each physical factor, such as the general rotation, stratification, surface tension, compressibility of the fluid, the existence of a characteristic type of waves is associated. General properties of inertial, gravitational surface or internal, capillary, acoustic, and hybrid waves are analyzed, as a rule, separately in specified frequency ranges, and for clarifying the physical sense, in approximation of an ideal fluid. However, elementary waves do not fully describe the properties of periodic motions in a real dissipative medium, where all the above-mentioned factors act simultaneously and waves are described by complex dispersion relations. Detailed analysis shows that all types of waves coexist with the fine dissipative components of the flows, caused by the viscosity, thermal diffusivity, and diffusion effects.

Traditionally, the heat conductivity and diffusion effects on wave properties are neglected, and the effect of viscosity is taken into account phenomenologically, by introducing attenuation factors that ensure damping of motions, with the exception of thin regions near the boundaries where the boundary layers, described by own specified equations, are formed [3]. However, the dissipation effects lead to an increase in the order and change in the type of the system of governing equation, and, accordingly, the degree of the dispersion equation. In practically important case of weak dissipation, the system (10) belongs to the class of singularly perturbed equations [18], whose solutions describe various forms of fluid motions. In this section, a complete classification of the components of three-dimensional infinitesimal periodic flows inside a continuously stratified fluid and examples of some total solutions of dispersion equations are presented.

Three-dimensional periodic flows with a constant positive frequency ω and a complex wave number $\mathbf{k} = \left(k_x, k_y, k_z\right), \mathbf{k} = \mathbf{k}_1 + i\mathbf{k}_2$ are considered. The imaginary part of the wave vector characterizes the spatial attenuation of the wave fields. The motions themselves are assumed to be low-intensity, allowing linearization of the governing equations. Stratification is considered to be weak, and dissipative factors (kinematic viscosity and diffusion coefficients) are small.

The analysis is carried out in a Cartesian coordinate frame (x, y, z) in which the axis z is vertical and oriented against the direction of the gravity acceleration. In the linear approximation, the system of fundamental Eq. (2.1) in traditional variables takes the form [3, 5, 19]

$$\begin{cases} \frac{\partial \rho}{\partial t} + \mathrm{div}\rho\mathbf{v} = 0 \\ \frac{\partial \mathbf{v}}{\partial t} = -\nabla P + \rho\nu\Delta\mathbf{v} + \left(\zeta + \frac{1}{3}\rho\nu\right)\nabla\mathrm{div}\mathbf{v} + \mathbf{g} \\ \frac{\partial \rho S_i}{\partial t} = \kappa_{S_i}\Delta\rho S_i \end{cases} \quad (12)$$

with the no-slip boundary conditions for velocity and no-flux for the substance concentration or temperature.

5 Dispersion Equation of the Linearized Fundamental Equations System

The equations of system (12), in which the small coefficients stand for terms with the highest derivatives with respect to spatial variables, belong to the class of singularly perturbed equations [18]. To obtain complete solutions of such equations, it is necessary to use both converse and reverse expansions in the small parameter of the form

$$k = k_0 + \varepsilon\, k_1 + \varepsilon^2 k_2 + \ldots \tag{13}$$

$$k_z = \varepsilon^{-\gamma}\left(k_0 + \varepsilon k_1 + \varepsilon^2 k_2 + \ldots\right), \quad \gamma > 0 \tag{14}$$

The value of the coefficient γ is determined by substituting (14) into the system of equations under consideration from the precedence condition of the resulting principal term of the expansion.

When studying small periodic motions with a real frequency ω and a complex wave vector $\mathbf{k}$, all the variables are chosen in the form [19]

$$\mathbf{v} = \mathbf{v}_0 \tau(r,t),\, \bar{p} = p_0 \tau(r,t),\, \bar{\rho} = \rho_0 \tau(r,t),\, \tau(r,t) = \exp(i(\mathbf{kr} - \omega t)) \tag{15}$$

The solution of the linearized system (12) in the unlimited space is searched in the form of expansions in plane waves

$$A = \sum_j \int_{-\infty}^{+\infty} \int_{-\infty}^{+\infty} a_j(k_x, k_y) \exp\left(i\left(k_{zj}(k_x, k_y) z + k_x x + k_y y - \omega t\right)\right) \mathrm{d}k_x \mathrm{d}k_y \tag{16}$$

where A are components of velocity, density, pressure, and salinity.

The summation in the expansion (16) is carried out over all the roots of the dispersion equation expressing the condition for the solvability of the linearized system (12), which satisfy the boundary conditions of the problem or the radiation condition in an infinite distance from the source (or attenuation of all perturbations at infinity).

Substituting expansions of functions for all physical variables into the system (12) and taking into account the compatibility condition for equations, one can find the dispersion relation, which has the form

$$D_\nu(k, \omega) \cdot F(k, \omega) = 0 \tag{17}$$

where

$$F(k, \omega) = -D_\nu(k, \omega) D_{\kappa_S}(k, \omega)\left(k^2 + i\frac{k_z}{\Lambda}\right) + D_{\kappa_S}(k, \omega)\left(\frac{\omega\, k_z}{\Lambda_T} D_\nu(k, \omega) - N_T^2 k_\perp^2\right)$$

$$D_\nu(k,\omega) = -i\omega + \nu k^2,\ D_{\kappa_S}(k,\omega) = -i\omega + \kappa_S k^2,$$
$$k^2 = k_x^2 + k_y^2 + k_z^2,\ k_\perp^2 = k_x^2 + k_y^2.$$

Disregarding the dissipative effects, the dispersion equation of the eighth degree (17) goes into a quadratic equation describing the internal and surface gravitational waves in an ideal fluid.

The spectral components in which $|\mathbf{k}_1| \gg |\mathbf{k}_2|$, and the damping factor is proportional to the kinetic coefficients (here $\gamma = i(\nu + \kappa_T + \kappa_S)k^2$), are regular perturbed components of flow which describe the large-scale wave components of periodic flows. Regularly perturbed solutions of the algebraic equation correspond to the system of differential Eq. (12) solutions of which, satisfying to the boundary conditions, determine the conical beams of periodic internal waves.

The remaining six roots of Eq. (17), the imaginary part of which is not small ($|\mathbf{k}_1| \sim |\mathbf{k}_2|$) and inversely proportional to the kinetic coefficients, define ligaments—singular perturbed components, characterizing the fine structure of flows. In the case of an infinite medium, four of them, which do not satisfy the damping boundary condition at infinity, were discarded. The remaining solutions form two distinct groups.

From the form of Eq. (17), in which the multiplier $D_\nu(k,\omega) = 0$ is present, it follows that all fluid flows are structured and the waves always coexist with ligaments—fine singularly perturbed components. They are similar to the periodic Stokes boundary layer on an oscillating surface in a viscous liquid [3, 4]. However, they are located not only near the boundaries, but also inside the fluid volume involved in the wave motion. The transverse length scale (thickness) of such components are determined by the kinematic viscosity and frequency of the wave $\delta_\omega^\nu = \sqrt{\nu/\omega}$ (or buoyancy frequency $\delta_N^\nu = \sqrt{\nu/N}$).

Simultaneously, the viscosity effects determine the existence of other flow components whose properties are described by the second terms in (17). Their transverse sizes depend on the frequencies or and the values of the kinetic coefficients, as well as on the direction of wave propagation. In case of internal waves, they are oriented along the direction of the group velocity vector. Ligaments are linear precursors of vortices, vortex systems, and shock waves in fluid flows [19].

All solutions of the set (10), which are regularly and singularly perturbed, form a single family described by the functions of the unique form (16), which differ in the magnitude of the ratios of the real and imaginary parts. All of them are formed, transferred, and disappear simultaneously, despite the differences in characteristic length scales. Each of the flows components impacts on the transport of energy, matter, and vorticity. Mechanical energy is transported mainly by slow large-scale components. Dissipation of the motion energy occurs both in largescale and in fine-structure components, which are characterized by large derivatives of all quantities. The pressure distribution in the fine-structure fast components is hydrostatic that is the pressure perturbations are absent inside ligaments. From analysis of the solutions properties follow the next definitions of periodic flows components.

Definitions.

Waves are large-scale periodic flow components, whose characteristic of local temporal evolution (real positive frequency ω) is connected by functional (dispersion) relation $\omega = \omega(\mathbf{k}, \mathbf{k}^2, \ldots \mathbf{k}^n)$ with instantaneous parameters of spatial flow pattern that are wavelength λ or wave vector $\mathbf{k} = (k_x, k_y, k_z)$. The imaginary part of complex wave number $\mathbf{k} = \mathbf{k}_1 + i\mathbf{k}_2$ is small with respect to the real part $|\mathbf{k}_2| \ll |\mathbf{k}_1|$.

Ligaments are thin in the transverse direction but extended in other directions 2D (interfaces) or 3D (trickles or filaments) components of periodic flows with the same frequency of variations ω, in which real and imaginary parts of the wave numbers are equal or of the same order on magnitude $|\mathbf{k}_1| \cong |\mathbf{k}_2|$.

As rectilinear motion is a limiting case of circular flows with an infinite radius of a fluid particle trajectory, the ligaments fill the rectilinear flow pattern as well. Their thickness is defined by Prandtl's scale $\delta_U^\nu = \nu/U$.

Transient ligaments also are formed in the process of beginning or restructuring of the flow. In this case, their transverse length scale $\delta_{\Delta t}^\nu$ is determined by the temporal variability parameter Δt whose order of magnitude is the duration of the interval for formation or restructuring the flow pattern.

To reduce the system of equations for periodic motions (10) of an incompressible homogeneous fluid in the phase space $(\omega, \ \mathbf{k})$

$$(\omega + i\nu)v_{i0} + k_i P_0 = 0, \quad k_x v_{x0} + k_y v_{y0} + k_z v_{z0} = 0 \tag{18}$$

Corresponds to the next dispersion equation

$$\mathbf{k}^2(\omega + i\nu\mathbf{k}^2)^2 = 0 \tag{19}$$

The first multiplier $\mathbf{k}^2 = 0$ in Eq. (19) with the solution in the form $k_z = \pm i\sqrt{k_x^2 + k_y^2}$ represents in a collapsed form all kinds of wave processes caused by the effects of compressibility, stratification, rotation, and other physical factors in inhomogeneous liquids in external force fields.

The second multiplier in the dispersion Eq. (19) defines a pair of identically singular perturbed solutions of the boundary layer type $(\omega + i\,\nu\,k^2)^2 = 0$. Since $\mathbf{k} \neq 0$, from (18) it follows) that $P = 0$. The solution has the character of a degenerate internal thin layer, in the plane of whose centers $v_z = 0$, and the values v_x, v_y depend on the local normal coordinate z.

In a compressible medium, the dispersion equation corresponding to the reduced part of the complete system, which includes only Eq. (10), has the form

$$\left(k^2\left(1 - \frac{i\omega\,\tilde{\nu}}{c_s^2}\right) - \frac{\omega^2}{c_s^2}\right)(\omega + i\nu\,k^2)^2 = 0 \tag{20}$$

where $\tilde{\nu} = \zeta + 4\nu/3$; ν, ζ are shear (first) and convergence (second) kinematic viscosity, c_s is the sound velocity.

The first multiplier in (20) is the classical dispersion relation for a sound wave in a dissipative medium [3], which describes waves with a frequency ω and wave vector **k** propagating with a velocity c_s. The second multiplier is twice degenerated singularly perturbed solution of the Stokes type. Consequently, the account of compressibility does not remove the degeneracy of the equations set for a homogeneous fluid. The system of equations of motion for a viscous inhomogeneous incompressible fluid is usually written in the form [3, 8]

$$\frac{\partial \tilde{\rho}}{\partial t} - \frac{v_z}{\Lambda} = 0, \quad \operatorname{div} \mathbf{v} = 0$$
$$\rho_0(z)\frac{\partial v_i}{\partial t} = -\frac{\partial \tilde{p}}{\partial x_i} + \nu\, \rho_0(z)\Delta\, v_i - \delta_{i3}\tilde{\rho}\, g \tag{21}$$

where $\rho = \rho_0(z) + \tilde{\rho}(\mathbf{x},\ t)$, $P = P_0(z) + \tilde{P}(\mathbf{x},\ t)$.

The dispersion equation for system (21) has the form

$$\left(\omega^2\mathbf{k}^2 - N^2\mathbf{k}_\perp^2 + i\omega\nu\,\mathbf{k}^4\right)\left(\omega + i\nu\,\mathbf{k}^2\right) = 0 \tag{22}$$

Regular solutions (22) describe internal waves whose oscillations occur in the direction of the wave propagation and group velocity of the waves. They are supplemented by two kinds of different singularly perturbed solutions describing the fine-structure components of the flows in the volume and on the boundary of the medium.

It should also be noted, that from the no-slip boundary condition on the fixed reflecting wave plane, it follows that the oscillations in the internal waves (incident and reflected) and in fine flow components are in antiphase.

In one-dimensional and two-dimensional formulations, all the considered model equations are solvable. In the three-dimensional case, in a homogeneous compressible and incompressible fluid, the complete solution of the linear system is degenerated with respect to the singular components.

Stratification ensures the existence of two different types of singularly perturbed solutions, which removes second-order degeneracy in problems of radiation, propagation, or reflection of internal waves from an inclined surface. More detailed descriptions of periodic internal wave beams of various types and accompanying fine-structure components are given in [20].

Incorporating into analysis of all singular perturbed components gives a room to construct exact in the linear approximation solutions for problems of generation, propagation and reflection of periodic internal wave beams from a solid wall or a critical level where frequencies of the wave and buoyancy equal, without application of additional hypothesis or constants. Results of calculations for 2D periodic internal waves beams generation by oscillating plate [21] and 3D conical wave beams, produced by vertically oscillating horizontal disk [22], as well as propagation of plane periodic wave beams in a stratified fluid with an arbitrary profile of density [23], are in good agreement with schlieren visualization and PIV measurements of wave velocities patterns even near the critical level where frequencies of the wave and buoyancy equal [24]. In generally posed problems, nonlinear interactions between waves and ligaments create new flow components including waves, ligaments, and vortices. Due to complex status and co-existence of components, which are characterized by different spatio-temporal scales, all fluid flows are nonstationary and have no stationary limit in time and space.

Because, as noted by G. G. Stokes, the system of fundamental equations is scale-invariant and applicable for any parameter values, the proposed classification, including an estimation of the scales of linear components for unsteady, uniform, or periodic flow is universal as well. Accordingly, nonlinear components such as nonlinear and shock waves or vortices, which are the product of the nonlinear interaction of primary components, conserve in their structures the traces of all primary components, including ligaments forming their fine internal structure.

6 Nonlinear Effects: Example of Complete Solutions of the Basic System

Progress in the construction of high-performance computers and programming techniques has enabled the solution of systems of Eqs. (2) and (10) in complete nonlinear, physically sound statements. The evolution of diffusion-induced flow patterns, which is formed on an impermeable obstacle, which was introduced without a disturbance into a stably stratified fluid at rest and a fixed, was studied in [25]. Both calculated and observed schlieren images of diffusion-induced flows on a horizontal and inclined plate are in good agreement with each other.

The solutions obtained are used as initial conditions for solving the problem of flow formation by a body starts moving at a constant velocity from a rest. The calculations were performed in a wide range of 2D obstacle shapes [26] at different orientation relative to the trajectory of motion [27], the values of velocities and the buoyancy frequency [28], which corresponds to the range of Reynolds numbers from 1 to 100,000 [27]. The numerical codes were written taking into account the condition of the observability for large components (internal wavelengths), which determine the size of the calculation region or observation field and the resolution of thin ligaments with thickness $\delta_{\mathrm{U}}^{\nu}$ and $\delta_{\mathrm{N}}^{\nu}$, which are defining the fine structure of the flow.

Comparison of calculations data on high-resolution observations of the flow pattern, conducted by the schlieren instrument IAB-458 at the LMT stand of the URF "HPC IPMech RAS," presented in Fig. 1 shows a good qualitative and quantitative agreement. The experiments were conducted using a vertical slit illumination diaphragm and a flat vertical Foucault knife [29]. Changes in illumination are proportional to variations in the horizontal component of refraction index gradient.

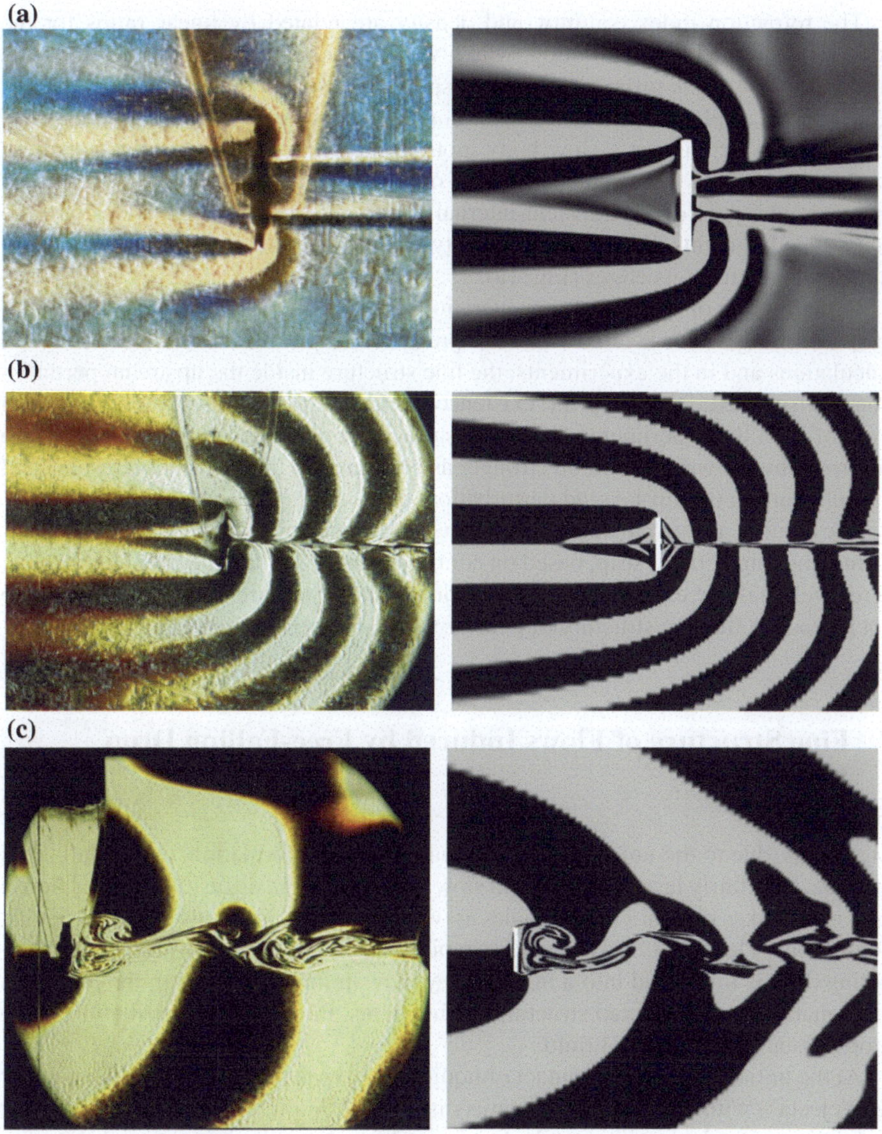

Fig. 1 Comparison of schlieren images (gradient of light refraction index) and calculated flow patterns (horizontal component of density gradient) around a vertical plate (h = 2.5 cm, T_b = 12.5 s): **a–c** U = 0.03, 0.18, 0.75 cm/s

The refraction index, salinity, and density are related by linear ratios for the aqueous sodium chloride solution, which was used to create the stratification. The coloring is due to the pronounced light dispersion in such a medium [28].

The vertical plate was moving with constant velocity from right to left. In the creeping flow regime, at a slow body motion, the schlieren image of flow pattern is characterized by the existence of a set of flow structural components, including upstream oblique rays of transient internal waves, attached internal waves past the body. Fine ligaments, bounding the density wake, touch the rear side of the plate at some distance from its edges (Fig. 1a).

In the regime of intense wave generation, both waves and a rich family of ligaments forming a thin-layered wake are presented (Fig. 1b). Moreover, both in the calculations and in the experiments, the fine structure inside the upstream perturbation is visualized, indicating the existence of ligaments both past the body and in front of it. In the experiments, the phase surfaces of the attached internal waves are deformed by the wake flow a bit stronger as compared to the calculation results, and the split pattern of thin-layered perturbations is more pronounced (Fig. 1c).

The numerically calculated large-scale wave components of the flow around a uniformly moving vertical strip, based on common versions of the theory of turbulence, agree well with the experimental observation of the flow pattern, but calculations do not reproduce the fine structure of density wake and its boundary [30].

7 Fine Structure of Flows Induced by Free-Falling Drop Impact

Ligaments, due to the universality of the nature of their formation, exist in all types of flows, both fairly large and small, in slow (for example in diffusion-induced flows) and in the wakes past moving obstacles as well as in fast compact flows. In particular, nonstationary ligaments are formed in a rapidly varying flow that forms when a freely falling drop is immersed into a liquid. They play an important role in the processes of formation of the selected structural components, transfer, and distribution of the drop substance in the target fluid.

At the initial stage of the contact of liquids, the expanding thin sheet-like circular jet ("ejecta") with narrow edge streamers is formed. In the initial stage of the drops immersion, the plane of jet is tilted at a small angle to the horizon and the most part of forming small droplets fly outside from the domain of the fluids confluence. First droplets fly out at small angles, and with time at more steep. Moreover, even in the early stages of the cavity and crown formation, some of the droplets fly inwards and fall onto the surface of the immersing drop [31]. Photographs of typical impact markers produced by the shock of small droplets at surface of the immersing drop surrounded by short capillary waves are shown in Fig. 2.

The formation of fibers and thin trickles is a result of the spatial inhomogeneity of an internal energy distribution. The energy takes different values at and near the

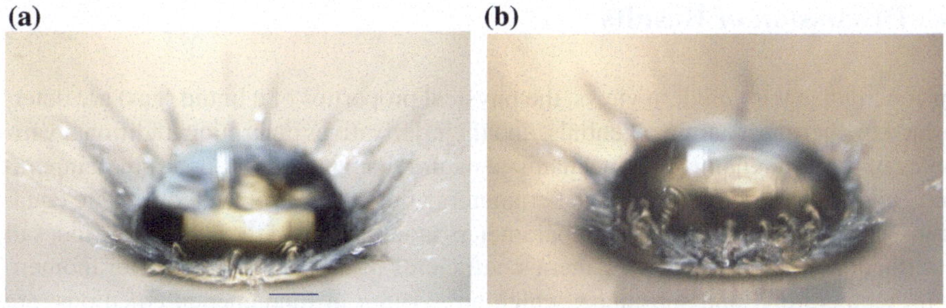

Fig. 2 Capillary waves on the surface of immersing drop produced by small hitting droplets: **a** drop of water with a diameter of $D = 0.42\,\text{cm}$ falling into water at a velocity $U = 2.5\ \text{m/s}$; **b** drops of brine are immersing in water, $D = 0.5\,\text{cm}$, $U = 2.5\,\text{m/s}$

surface of a liquid, where the effects of surface tension are manifested, and in the bulk of the liquid. Excessive surface potential energy is quickly released when the free surfaces of confluent liquids are eliminated. Released energy is transformed into other forms, including the energy of mechanical motion of thin layers of liquids.

The thin fibrous structure of the flow is observed at all stages of the rapid evolution of the flow pattern. With beginning of the fluid confluence, the ligaments, which appear in the form of thin jets containing the drop matter, form a fairly regular-ruled pattern on the crown [14] and netted at the bottom of the cavity (Fig. 3a).

Separately isolated radially directed colored jets with vortex tips, which are also observed at later stages of the flow evolution, in the mode of a thick ascending (cumulative) jet formation, are shown in Fig. 3b.

Slow ring vortices, propagating inside the targeted fluid at the final stage of flow evolution, also have a thin fibrous structure, which was noted in the first experiments of Rogers [32] and Thomson and Newall [33], performed in the nineteenth century and stably reproduced in many experiments [34].

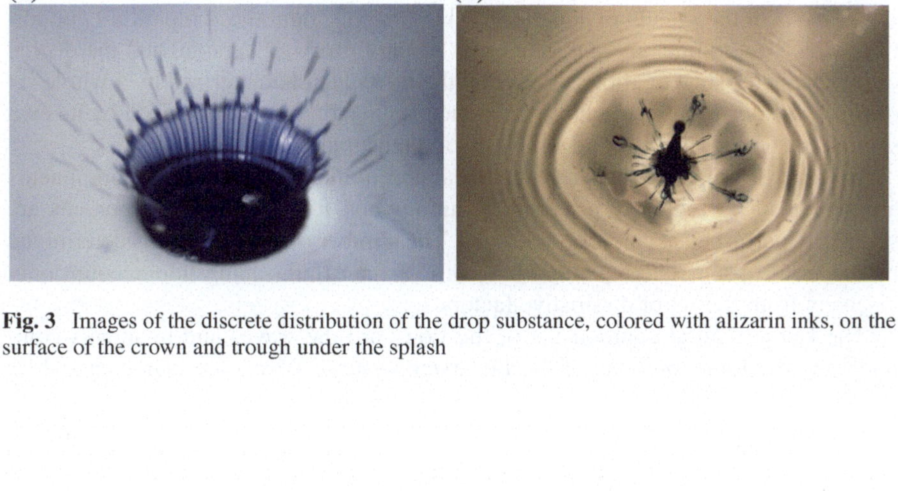

Fig. 3 Images of the discrete distribution of the drop substance, colored with alizarin inks, on the surface of the crown and trough under the splash

8 Discussion of Results

In accordance with modern views, the physical properties of a liquid (gas) are determined by thermodynamic potentials, and their derivatives determine traditional variables of thermodynamic and mechanistic nature that are density, pressure, temperature, and concentration of solutes. Parameters of media are connected by state equations, containing their own sets of parameters (coefficients of thermal expansion, salt contraction, compressibility). Kinetic coefficients of molecular transfer for momentum, temperature, and substance, which are written in fundamental equations, are important parameters of studied media as well.

An important role in the structuration of flows plays the energy, whose distribution in a medium with boundaries and contact surfaces is non-uniform and includes thin interfaces and filaments with high density (in particular, in the vicinity of the free surface and in areas of high gradients of thermodynamic quantities). Energy exchange in flows can occur slowly in dissipative processes with molecular transfer rates, more quickly in flows with transport velocity, with characteristic group velocity in waves, and extremely quickly under the influence of direct atomic-molecular interactions.

Changes in the state of the investigated medium are described by the traditional system of fundamental partial differential equations that characterize the transport of matter (the density of the medium as a whole and its constituent components), momentum, and energy. The equations are supplemented by physically reasonable initial and boundary conditions. The variety of forms of energy distribution and the difference in exchange rates provides the possibility of the formation and existence of complex evolving flow structures.

A complete system of equations of fluid mechanics, including the equations of state, which is scale-invariant, closed, self-consistent and solvable, was selected as the basis for determining the flow of liquids as:

Flows are a forced flux of momentum and energy, accompanied by self-consistent changes in the fields of other physical quantities—density, temperature, pressure, impurity concentration, and physical parameters (velocity of sound, index of refraction, specific conductivity, and others).

Analysis of the system of equations, taking into account the compatibility condition, which determines its rank, the order of the linearized version, and the degree of the characteristic equation, shows that the flows are characterized by a whole set of functions describing structural components, each one is characterized by its own spatial and temporal scales, generally incommensurable.

In weakly dissipative media, in the linear approximation, large-scale components are described by regularly perturbed solutions and fine-structure components are singularly perturbed asymptotic solutions. The number of components is determined by the form of the state equation, but not less than four, taking into account only viscosity from the set of dissipative factors.

The key structural components of the flows are the waves and ligaments compounding the total solutions of the linearized system. Waves are characterized by dispersion relations connecting real positive frequency ω with instantaneous parameters of spatial flow pattern (wavelength λ or wave vector $\mathbf{k}$). Ligaments are thin in the transverse direction but extended in other directions 2D (interfaces) or 3D (trickles or filaments) components of periodic flows with the same frequency variations ω, in which real and imaginary parts of the wave numbers are equal or of the same order on magnitude $|\mathbf{k}_1| \cong |\mathbf{k}_2|$.

Ligaments exist in all types of flows—in nonstationary, translational, vortex, wave, and creeping. Their transverse spatial scales are determined by dissipative coefficients and a characteristic time interval that is by the duration of the flow formation, inverse frequency of a wave, or ratio of length scale to the flow velocity.

In the nonlinear description, all the components of the flows interact with each other and generate new ones, both with large and small length scales including vortices, jets interfaces, fibers, shock waves, and others. In practice, ligaments are observed as high-gradient surfaces and fibers in all the spatial scales are available for observation, from molecular cluster size to galactic scales. Due to complex status and co-existence of components, which are characterized by different spatio-temporal scales, all fluid flows are nonstationary and have no stationary limit in time and space.

The solutions of the fundamental system of equations, chosen as the basis of analytical, numerical, and laboratory modeling techniques, provide the ability to directly compare the results and determine the error of the data.

9 Conclusion

The system of fundamental governing equations for transport of substance, momentum, and energy together with equations of state for thermodynamics potential and density is used as basis for compatible analytical, numerical, and experimental study of a stratified fluid flow. The system is analyzed taking into account the compatibility conditions which define its rank, power of linearized version, and degree of the characteristic (dispersion) relation. The total solutions of the system contain several independent functions characterized by their individual spatial and temporal scales, generally incommensurable.

New classification of fluid flows components including ligaments (fine interfaces and filaments) as precursors supplementing all conventional flows components that are waves, vortices, jets, wakes is proposed basing on total solutions of linearized system of fundamental fluid dynamics equations. The thickness of ligaments is defined by dissipative factors and characteristic time interval or frequency, the length—by boundary condition and prehistory of the flow.

High-resolution visualization of stratified flows past obstacles in the laboratory tank was performed on the stand of Unique Research Facility "Hydrophysical complex IPMech RAS (HPC IPMech RAS)" and numerically calculated within the frame of the open-source CFD utility OpenFOAM using computing resources of cluster systems and supercomputers SRCC Lomonosov Moscow State University.

Both in the calculated and visualized patterns of flow perturbations formed by uniform movement of a vertical plate, systems of internal waves, including advanced, attached and short ones, and thin interfaces such as ligaments, formed due to the combined influence of the stratification and dissipation effects, are distinguished. The observation and calculation results are in good qualitative and quantitative agreement with each other.

Acknowledgements The experiments were conducted at the stand of the Unique Research Facility "Hydrophysical complex IPMech RAS (HPC IPMech RAS)." The work was supported by the Russian Scientific Fund (Grant 19-19-00598). The experiments were performed on the stands of the URF "HPC IPMech RAS." The computations were performed using the equipment of the shared research facilities of HPC computing resources at Lomonosov Moscow State University and the computing resources of the Federal Collective Usage Center at NRC "Kurchatov Institute."

References

1. Darrigol, O.: Worlds of Flow. A History of Hydrodynamics from the Bernoullis to Prandtl. Oxford University Press, Oxford (2005)
2. Lamb, H.: Hydrodynamics. Cambridge University Press, Cambridge (1879)
3. Landau, L.D., Lifshitz, E.M.: Course of theoretical physics. In: Fluid Mechanics, vol. 6, 2nd edn. Pergamon Press, Oxford (1987)
4. Batchelor, G.K.: An Introduction to Fluid Dynamics. Cambridge University Press, Cambridge (1967)
5. Müller, P.: The Equations of Oceanic Motions. Cambridge University Press, Cambridge (2007)
6. Vallis, G.K.: Atmospheric and Oceanic Fluid Dynamics. Cambridge University Press, Cambridge (2007)
7. Schlichting, H.: Boundary-Layer Theory. McGraw-Hill, New York (1955)
8. Lighthill, M.J.: Waves in Fluids. Cambridge University Press, Cambridge (2001)
9. Lugt, H.J.: Introduction to Vortex Theory. Vortex Flow Press, Potomac, MD, USA (1996)
10. Ladyzhenskaya, O.: Sixth problem of the millennium: Navier-Stokes equations, existence and smoothness. Russ. Math. Surv. **58**(2), 251–328 (2003)
11. Jackson, D., Launder, B.: Osborne Reynolds and the publication of his papers on turbulent flow. Annu. Rev. Fluid Mech. **39**, 19–35 (2007)
12. Hubble sees Red Giant blow a bubble. https://www.nasa.gov/multimedia/imagegallery/image_feature_2302.html
13. Chashechkin, YuD, Bardakov, R.N.: Formation of texture in residue of a drying drop of a multicomponent fluid. Dokl. Phys. **55**(2), 68–72 (2010)
14. Chashechkin, YuD, Ilinykh, AYu.: Banded structures in the distribution pattern of a drop over the surface of the host liquid. Dokl. Phys. **63**(7), 282–287 (2018)
15. Zagumennyi, Ya.V., Chashechkin Yu.D.: Pattern of unsteady vortex flow around plate under a zero angle of attack (two-dimensional problem). Fluid Dyn. **51**(3), 53–70 (2016)
16. Chashechkin, YuD: Differential fluid mechanics—harmonization of analytical, numerical and laboratory models of flows. In: Neittaanmäki, P., Repin, S., Tuovinen, T. (eds.) Mathematical Modeling and Optimization of Complex Structures, Springer Series: Computational Methods in Applied Sciences, vol. 40, pp. 61–91. Springer, Heidelberg (2016)
17. Wright, D.G., Feistel, R., Reissmann, J.H., Miyagawa, K., Jackett, D.R., Wagner, W., Overhoff, U., Guder, C., Feistel, A., Marion, G.: Numerical implementation and oceanographic application of the thermodynamic potentials of liquid water, water vapour, ice, seawater and humid air—Part 2: the library routines. Ocean Sci. **6**, 695–718 (2010)

18. Naifeh, A.H.: Introduction to Perturbation Techniques. Wiley, New York (2011)
19. Chashechkin, YuD: Singularly perturbed components of flows—linear precursors of shock waves. Math. Model. Nat. Phenom. **13**(2), 1–29 (2018)
20. Bardakov, R.N., Vasil'ev, A.Yu., Chashechkin, Yu.D.: Calculation and measurement of conical beams of three-dimensional periodic internal waves excited by a vertically oscillating piston. Fluid Dyn. **42**(4), 612–626 (2007)
21. Vasil'ev, AYu., Chashechkin, YuD: Three-dimensional periodic flows of an inhomogeneous fluid in the case of oscillations of part of an inclined plane. J. Appl. Math. Mech. **76**(3), 302–309 (2012)
22. Kistovich, A.V., Chashechkin, YuD: Fine structure of a conical beam of periodical internal waves in a stratified fluid. Izvestia. Atmos. Oceanic Phys. **50**(1), 103–110 (2014)
23. Kistovich, YuV, Chashechkin, YuD: Linear theory of the propagation of internal wave beams in an arbitrarily stratified liquid. J. Appl. Mech. Tech. Phys. **39**(5), 302–309 (1998)
24. Paoletti, M.S., Swinney, H.L.: Propagating and evanescent internal waves in a deep ocean model. J. Fluid Mech. **706**, 571–603 (2012)
25. Zagumennyi, Ia.V., Chashechkin, Yu.D.: Diffusion induced flow on a strip: theoretical, numerical and laboratory modeling. Proc IUTAM **8**, 256–266 (2013)
26. Chashechkin, Yu.D., Zagumennyi, Ia.V.: Hydrodynamics of horizontal stripe. Problems of evolution of open systems (The Republic of Kazakhstan) **18**(2), 25–49 (2015)
27. Chashechkin, YuD, Zagumennyi, IaV: Stratified flow fine structure around a sloping plate. In: Šimurda, D., Bodnár, T. (eds.) Topical Problems of Fluid Mechanics, pp. 87–94. Institute of Thermophysics, Prague (2017)
28. Chashechkin, YuD, Zagumennyi, I.V.: Formation of waves, vortices and ligaments in 2D stratified flows around obstacles. Phys. Scr. **94**(5), 1–17 (2019)
29. Hydrophysical Complex for Modeling Hydrodynamic Processes in the Environment and Their Impact on Underwater Technical Objects, as well as the Distribution of Impurities in the Ocean and Atmosphere, IPMech RAS, http://ipmnet.ru/uniqequip/gfk
30. Houcine, H., Chashechkin, YuD, Fraunie, Ph, Fernando, H., Gharbi, A., Lili, T.: Numerical modeling of the generation of internal waves by uniform stratified flow over a thin vertical barrier. Int. J. Numer. Meth. Fluids **68**, 451–466 (2012)
31. Chashechkin, YuD, Ilyinykh, AYu.: Capillary waves on the surface of the liquid droplets in submerging in a fluid drop. Dokl. Phys. **465**(4), 434–440 (2015)
32. Rogers, V.B.: On the formation of rotating rings by air and liquids under certain condition of discharge. Am. J. Sci. Arts. **26**(Second Series), 246–258 (1858)
33. Thomson, J.J., Newall, H.F.: On the formation of vortex rings by drops falling into liquids, and some allied phenomena. Proc. Roy. Soc. London **29**, 417–436 (1885)
34. Stepanova, E.V., Chashechkin, YuD: Marker transport in a composite vortex. Fluid Dyn. **45**(6), 843–858 (2010)

Dynamical System Theory of Flow Instability Using the Impulse and the Frequency Response Approaches

Tapan K. Sengupta, Soumyo Sengupta and Prasannabalaji Sundaram

Abstract We study the causal relation in a fluid dynamical system, for the impulse and frequency response approaches as instability theories and corresponding experiments. The zero-pressure-gradient (ZPG) boundary layer is analyzed to find complementary aspects of these approaches. The drawbacks of instability study are in formulating it as a homogeneous system. Another difficulty for the instability is in classifying it for either temporal or spatial growth. When viscous effects were included in the spatial theory, it predicted wave solution (known as Tollmien–Schlichting (TS) *waves*), which left many scientists unconvinced. Experimental verification remained difficult as instability does not require explicit excitation, and dependence on background noise makes experiment non-repeatable. The classic experiment of Schubauer and Skramstad for the boundary layer (J Aero Sci 14(2), 69–78, [24]) excited a monochromatic source inside to obtain spatially growing TS *waves*—considered as the frequency response of the boundary layer. In contrast, Gaster and Grant (Proc R Soc A 347(1649), 253–269, [13]) tried to create TS *waves* by a localized impulse excitation and ended up creating a wave-packet by the impulse response of the dynamical system. Here, we focus mainly on the impulse response of the ZPG boundary layer using Bromwich contour integral method (BCIM) developed by the authors for spatio-temporal growth of disturbance field in creating spatio-temporal wave-front (STWF). The main achievement of BCIM is in identifying the cause for the creation of STWF by both the approaches.

Keywords Impulse response · Frequency response · Bromwich contour integral method

T. K. Sengupta (✉) · P. Sundaram
High Performance Computing Laboratory, Department of Aerospace Engineering, Indian Institute of Technology Kanpur, Kanpur, Uttar Pradesh 208016, India
e-mail: tksen@iitk.ac.in

S. Sengupta
Graduate student, CERFACS, 31100 Toulouse, France

S. Bhattacharyya et al. (eds.), *Mathematical Modeling and Computational Tools*, Springer Proceedings in Mathematics & Statistics 320,
https://doi.org/10.1007/978-981-15-3615-1_11

1 Introduction

One of the principal tenets in developing dynamical system theory is to study the relationship between cause and effects. This is true for a fluid dynamical system characterized by large degrees of freedom, as compared to other dynamical systems in many fields of physics. While experimental verification of any theory is imperative, however, this is a difficult task for theories of instabilities. This is because instability theories rely on the omnipresent imperceptible ambient disturbances to produce the response which is difficult to quantify. Mathematically, the instability problem is posed as the output of a system governed by a homogeneous differential equation, for homogeneous boundary and initial conditions. Implicit in this scenario is the requirement of an equilibrium state, in which the imperceptible omnipresent disturbance resides and draws energy for its growth. For example, flow past a circular cylinder displays unsteadiness above a critical Reynolds number (based on oncoming flow speed and diameter of the cylinder), even when one is considering uniform flow over a perfectly smooth cylinder. While this can be rationalized for experimental investigation, where the prevalence of background disturbances cannot be ruled out, the situation is far from straightforward for computational efforts. Roles of various numerical sources of error triggering instability for uniform flow past a smooth circular cylinder are complicated. This issue has been dealt in [31]. Inability to compute the equilibrium flow past a circular cylinder is due to the presence of adverse pressure gradient experienced by the flow on the lee side of the cylinder.

The situation is equally difficult for the ZPG flow over a flat plate. As the equilibrium flow is obtained with significant precision, it is possible to study the ZPG flow past a flat plate as a receptivity problem, as has been done experimentally to study the existence of TS *waves* by Schubauer and Skramstad [24], where the disturbances were effectively created by a vibrating ribbon inside the boundary layer. The computations have been done with varying degrees of success in [12, 3, 6, 7, 20, 29, 39] for 2D and 3D instability routes, with results improving with advent of better computers and numerical methods. Early results obtained in small computational domain managed to show TS wave-packets (and not waves), but starting with the theoretical finding of STWF due to a linear mechanism [32] along with TS wave-packet has completely changed our perception of the field, both in terms of theoretical and computational approaches.

While the experiment in [24] virtually rescued the theoretical instability studies, it is necessary to understand the motivation of that experiment. Concomitant with the developed spatial instability studies by solving Orr–Sommerfeld equation (OSE) (as given in [10, 27]), the boundary layer was excited by a monochromatic localized source, and hence, this can be termed as the frequency response of the boundary layer. In the experiment, the authors could not create TS *waves* by acoustic excitation, and this drew the attention on the subject of receptivity of equilibrium flows to different types of input to the system. As the existence of TS wave-packet cannot be demonstrated outside the strict confines of the laboratory, Gaster and Grant [13] studied the ZPG boundary layer excited by a localized impulse. Mathematically, this is equivalent to using an input, which is a delta function in space and time, and the results provide the impulse response of the dynamical system. Interestingly, this experiment produced a wave-packet, which can be identified with the STWF found in [32]. It is noted that the search for STWF was sought in other branches of physics, with early efforts recounted in Brillouin [8] for electromagnetic wave propagation and by Bers [2] in plasma physics. Unfortunately, the authors in [13] thought that the impulse response was an ensemble of TS *waves*, which can be obtained by spatial instability theory for a parallel boundary layer, which was summed for the eigenfunctions with empirical weights. In a recent numerical study, Bhaumik and Sengupta [4] have shown the creation of the STWF by solving the complete Navier–Stokes equation (NSE) with an accurate numerical method. The authors identified the impulse response as the STWF, which is the building block that explains diverse physical and geophysical events, such as transition to turbulence, rogue waves and tsunamis. The role of STWF in creating transition to turbulence via frequency response route has been conclusively established in [3, 29, 30]. There are many efforts [19, 37] which have talked about transient growth, algebraic growth, as alternative routes of transition, without involving TS *waves*.

Thus, it is essential to bridge the theoretical gap between the impulse and the frequency response of a dynamical system, which are used in theoretical and experimental studies. Here, the results for ZPG boundary layer are used to theoretically explain the common elements of the impulse and frequency responses. In the context of flow instability, the difference between the two responses continues to baffle the research community. The primary goal of the present research is to theoretically explain from the solution of OSE, the existence of STWF and its ubiquitous role in manifesting unsteady effects, even when the excitation is imposed impulsively once, which continues to grow indefinitely. Such an exercise can show the presence of STWF even when the amplitude of the STWF is small at the onset. We note that the STWF was found due to a change of point of view when flow instability was solved for generic spatio-temporal growth.

In the beginning, Orr and Sommerfeld [21, 34] proposed OSE without any qualifier on the disturbance growth, whether it is in space or in time. When Rayleigh's theorem for temporal growth failed to explain the instability of ZPG boundary layer [10], it was assumed that the growth must be in space. Although Heisenberg, Tollmien and Schlichting [10, 17, 23, 27, 36] solved the temporal instability for OSE, the results were interpreted as growth in space, using the growth in time to growth in space, using the group velocity [8, 27]. With the advent of computers, OSE has been solved by few methods for stiff differential equations. Of all the methods, the most reliable one appears to be the compound matrix method (CMM) described in [10, 26, 27]. In Sengupta [25], CMM was used along with discrete fast Fourier transform (DFFT) to solve the problem corresponding to the experiment of [24] using the signal-problem assumption. This is the first numerical solution, while theoretical conjectures exist in [1, 14, 15].

Here, we explain how the STWF is created for different start-up conditions by BCIM in solving OSE for a 2D response field. The corresponding solution of NSE has been shown for impulsive and non-impulsive start-ups in [5]. The formulation of the problem is shown in Sect. 2. This is followed by a description of the utility of the signal problem in Sect. 3. Next, the impulse response for the ZPG boundary layer is shown in Sect. 4, for three different Reynolds numbers, based on displacement thickness. The frequency response cases are shown next in Sect. 5, for three streamwise exciter locations, with identical physical frequency of excitation, to confirm with the parallel flow approximation in solving OSE. In the following Sect. 6, we describe the receptivity of ZPG boundary layer, when the input has no specific time scale imposed, while the time variation of input corresponds to a Heaviside function, a ramp and a rapidly varying function, but with smooth variation at the onset and the final state. To emphasize the importance of boundary layer growth and the corresponding shortcoming of parallel flow approximation, the case of frequency response described in Sect. 5 by solving OSE is computed again by solving NSE in Sect. 7. The paper closes with a summary and conclusion.

2 Formulation of the Impulse and the Frequency Response

The schematic of the problem is shown in Fig. 1a in the physical plane, while it is solved in the spectral plane, involving streamwise wavenumber (α) and circular frequency (ω_0). For the 2D problem, the response is calculated for the linearized field following the governing OSE given by

$$D^4\phi = i\tilde{Re}\big[(\alpha U(\tilde{y}) - \omega_0)D^2\phi - \alpha U''(\tilde{y})\phi\big] \tag{1}$$

where $D^2 = \frac{d^2}{d\tilde{y}^2} - \alpha^2$, $\tilde{Re} = \frac{U_e\delta^*}{\nu}$. Here, the displacement thickness at the exciter location has been used as the length scale, while the free stream speed is used as the velocity scale. The time scale is derived with the help of these two scales. The disturbance stream function is given by its spectral transform as

$$\bar{\psi} = \int_{\alpha_{Br}} \int_{\omega_{Br}} \phi(\alpha, \tilde{y}, \omega_0) e^{i(\alpha\tilde{x} - \omega_0 t)} d\alpha d\omega_0 \tag{2}$$

which is solved for both the signal and spatio-temporal problems using BCIM. The difference between these two lies in choosing integration contours in the spectral plane, in the respective strip of convergence—known as the Bromwich contour [22, 27, 38]. Here, the response to wall excitation is studied for three types of excitation fields: (i) Case-I—where the input is simply a product of delta functions in space and time that represents the pure impulse response. The other cases are shown in Fig. 1b, with the impulsive start represented by the Heaviside function (Case-II) and the other represents a non-impulsive start (Case-III) given by

$$U_1(t - t_0) = 0.5\left[1 + \text{erf}\left(\frac{t - t_0}{2\sqrt{\pi\alpha_E}}\right)\right] \tag{3}$$

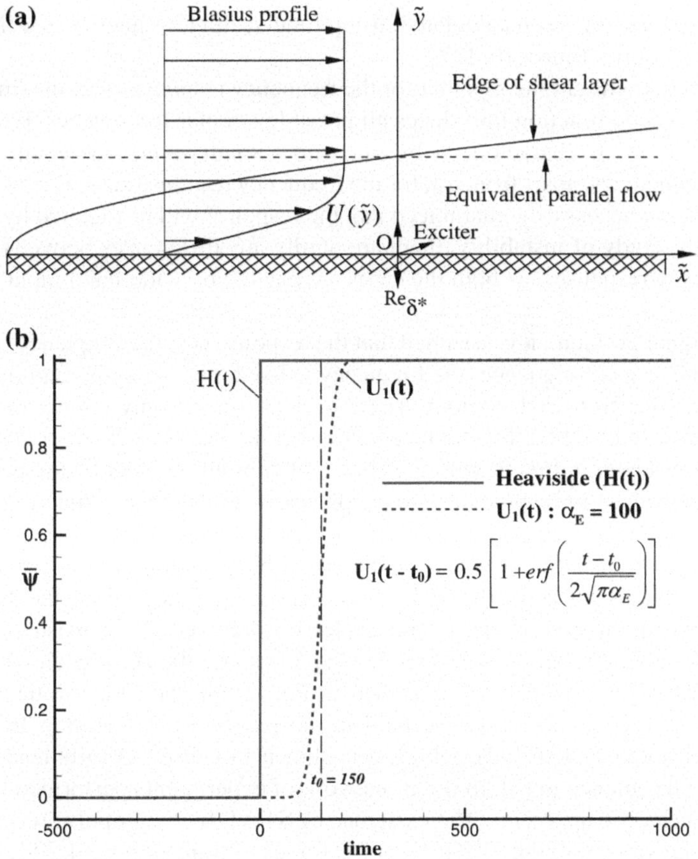

Fig. 1 **a** Schematic of the computation domains for the wall excitation of an equivalent parallel flow given by Blasius profile at a location indicated by the dashed line and **b** the envelope of the time-dependent excitations given by the Heaviside function ($H(t)$) and an error function ($U_1(t)$), triggered at the indicated times; $t = 0$ for $H(t)$ and $t = t_0$ for $U_1(t - t_0)$

which is related to the error function. One can study the impulse and frequency response cases, where $H(t)$ and $U_1(t)$ represent the envelope for the amplitude of input disturbance stream function, $\bar{\psi}$. If the excitation frequency is $\bar{\omega}_0$, then the excitation for the frequency response case is given by $\bar{\psi} e^{-i\bar{\omega}_0 t}$. Here, we have reported only one frequency response case, which is started impulsively using $H(t)$. We have also studied cases, where the dynamical system is excited by inputs, as shown in Fig. 1b without any imposed time scale, which will be termed as non-oscillatory transient cases. Additionally, a case of ramp start (Case-IV) is also studied which is non-oscillatory. Note that when α_E approaches zero in Eq. (3), one recovers the Heaviside function, $H(t)$. Also in Fig. 1b, the non-impulsive case $U_1(t - t_0)$ becomes nonzero from $t = 0$ onwards, while it is centered around t_0. For this reason, the

Fourier transform has been calculated, using time-scaling, frequency and time-shift theorems of Fourier transform [27].

We want to highlight the fact that for the frequency response case, the finite start-up with Heaviside function introduces all possible circular frequencies. Even in the case where $U_1(t)$ is characterized by α_E, with a small value, one excites a wide range of frequencies, apart from $\bar{\omega}_0$, for the frequency response case. For an unstable system, it is not necessarily guaranteed that the response will be dictated by $\bar{\omega}_0$ only. Thus, for the study of instability, there are hardly any differences between impulse and frequency responses, as both the cases are excited by wide-band input by finite start-up.

In the signal problem, it is assumed that the response is at the frequency of excitation, $\bar{\omega}_0$, and as a consequence, the frequency is fixed, i.e., $\omega_0 = \bar{\omega}_0$, and one solves Eq. (1) along the Bromwich contour in $\alpha(= \alpha_r + i\bar{\alpha}_i)$-plane only. Choice of constant $\bar{\alpha}_i$ facilitates use of DFFT for the inverse transform. The Bromwich contours used in BCIM are shown in Fig. 2, with the choice of contour dictated by the position of various eigenvalues in complex α and ω_0 planes, with details explained in [16, 27, 28].

As noted for unstable systems, the signal-problem assumption is incorrect. To solve the problems correctly, the BCIM was proposed [27, 28], where the dynamical system picks up the correct space-time scales for the fixed $\tilde{Re}$, consistent with the physical dispersion relation. After solving Eq. (1) along the Bromwich contours in the complex α- and ω_0-planes, as shown in Fig. 2, one performs double inverse transforms to recover the response field in the physical plane. Using BCIM, the STWF was noted first in [32], which was shown to cause 2D turbulence in [29, 30] and 3D turbulence in [3], in the framework of experiments performed using the frequency response approach. The existence of STWF by the impulse response has also been shown by solving 3D NSE for 3D routes of transition in [4, 35].

In the present work, the linearized problem is solved theoretically and computationally by considering different impulse and frequency response approaches. Only

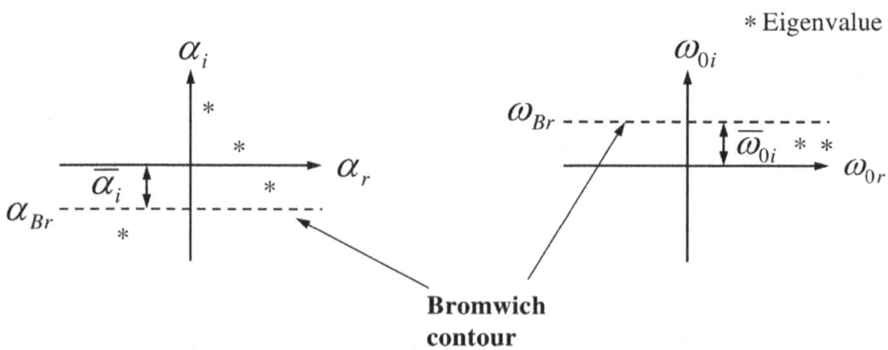

Fig. 2 Bromwich contours used here have been shown in complex α and ω_0-planes for the BCIM approach. For signal problems, only the contour in α-plane is used

one frequency response case is included here to demonstrate the difference between solution of OSE by BCIM and by direct simulation of NSE.

3 The Utility of the Signal Problem

Results of Eq. (1) have been obtained with the signal-problem assumption for the first time in [25] using CMM [27]. The same method has been used here, by considering the height of the domain in the wall-normal direction given by the similarity variable used in Blasius solution as $\eta_{\max} = 12$ with 3000 points. Along the Bromwich contour (α_{Br}), 8192 points are taken, for which Eq. (1) is solved, along with $\bar{\alpha}_i = -0.008$. While it has been reasoned above that the signal problem is inconsistent for instability studies, and instead, one should treat these as spatio-temporal growth problem, as in [27, 28, 32] to study frequency response cases. Thus, one should solve Eq. (1) for any type of excitation implied in Eq. (3), along the Bromwich contours shown in Fig. 2. Finally, double inverse Fourier transform is performed to obtain $\bar{\psi}$, as given in Eq. (2). This is the BCIM technique followed in [27, 28, 32], which led to the finding of the STWF. It is readily noted in BCIM that one needs to solve the signal problem, for every point along the Bromwich contour, ω_{Br} in the ω_0-plane.

In Fig. 3, $\bar{\psi}$ is plotted for three different cases with $\tilde{Re}$ and $\bar{\omega}_0$ combinations given by (1000, 0.1), (1500, 0.15) and (2000, 0.20), such that the physical frequency $F = \frac{\bar{\omega}_0}{\tilde{Re}}$ remains the same. The results are shown at a height which is close to the inner maximum of the disturbance field. The solution is determined by the instability

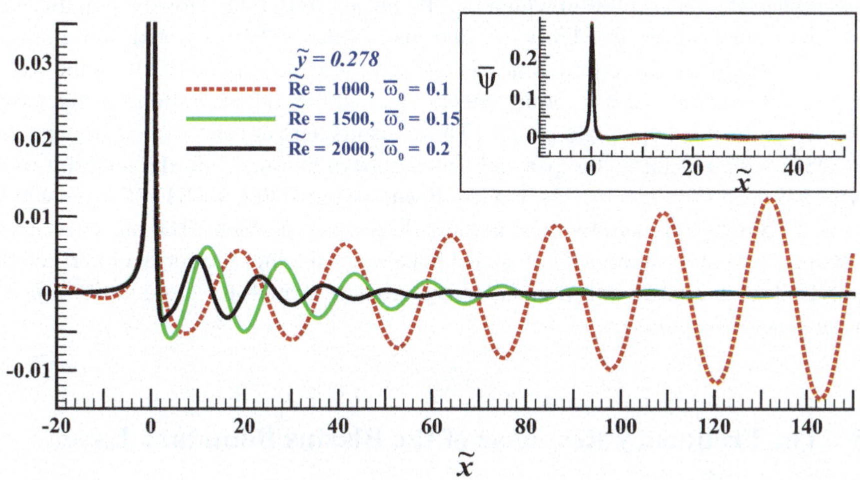

Fig. 3 Signal-problem solution for three representative $\tilde{Re}$ values, with results shown at the indicated height, $\tilde{y} = 0.278$. The non-dimensional frequencies are so chosen that one is tracking the same physical frequency. The Bromwich contour in α-plane is at $\bar{\alpha}_i = -0.008$, and α_r ranges from -4π to $+4\pi$, with 8192 points

property of the Blasius boundary layer, as given by the spatial analysis. Thus, the first combination shows growing TS wave. These results show the unique feature of receptivity analysis, in the form of a local solution in the vicinity of the exciter at $\tilde{x} = 0$, whose full view is shown in the inset, on the top right. These features of solution for the signal problem is noted in the solution using BCIM, except that the STWF is not seen, as one noted the STWF from the spatio-temporal solution of OSE and NSE in [28, 29, 32].

4 The Impulse Response of the Blasius Boundary Layer

In studying the spatio-temporal dynamics for the Blasius boundary layer, we first consider the case of pure impulse, with the wall excitation given by

$$\bar{\psi}(\tilde{x}, 0, t) = \delta(\tilde{x})\delta(t) \tag{4}$$

This is the type of wall excitation investigated in [13]. The results are obtained here by solving Eq. (1), for the input given by Eq. (4), using BCIM along the Bromwich contours, α_{Br} and ω_{Br}, using 8192 and 2048 points, respectively. The Bromwich contours are parallel to the real axis, located below at $\bar{\alpha}_i = -0.008$ in α-plane and above at $\bar{\omega}_{0i} = 0.01$ in the ω_0-plane. The height of the domain in the wall-normal direction is same, as that has been used in the signal problem. For each ω_0, one solves an equivalent signal problem, as described in the previous section. The results shown in Fig. 4 are for three $\tilde{Re}$ indicated in the frame. At the location of the exciter ($\tilde{x} = 0$), one notices the local solution which rapidly decays with time. However, in this case, one does not also see the TS wave, and instead the STWF is noted, that convects in the downstream direction, at nearly the same speed. For $\tilde{Re} = 1000$, the STWF appears at a downstream location, despite the fact that the excitation for this case is applied at the most upstream station. These results here are shown from the solution of OSE, which requires the parallel flow approximation, while the solution of 3D NSE has been shown in [4, 35]. In [13], it was assumed that the STWF is a weighted sum of TS *waves* created by the corresponding signal problem. The present solution not only shows the superiority of BCIM but also establishes the correct interpretation of STWF as the basic unit process of disturbance growth for the equilibrium flow arising as the impulse response.

5 The Frequency Response of the Blasius Boundary Layer

It has been noted already that the frequency response of a dynamical system is a misnomer for a physically unstable system, as the unstable modes are going to be

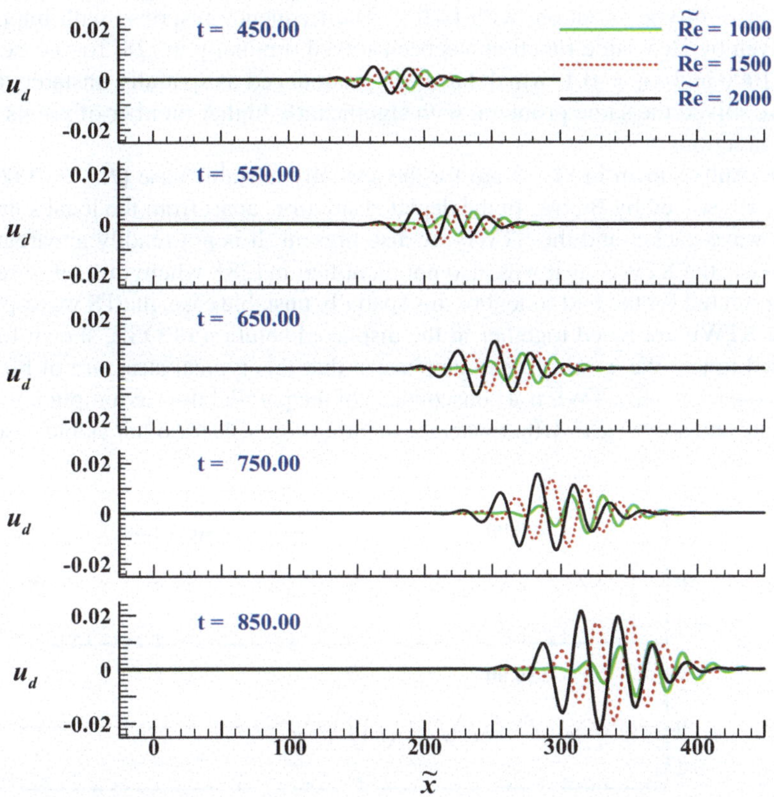

Fig. 4 Impulse response of the Blasius boundary layer to excitation as given by Eq. (4) for three representative $\tilde{Re}$ values, with results shown at the indicated height, $\tilde{y} = 0.278$. The Bromwich contour in α-plane is at $\bar{\alpha}_i = -0.008$, and α_r ranges from -4π to $+4\pi$ with 8192 points, and in the ω_0-plane the Bromwich contour is placed at $\bar{\omega}_i = 0.01$, and ω_{0r} varying from $-\pi/2$ to $+\pi/2$ with 2048 points

dominant, as compared to the forced response at the excitation frequency. Historically, this wrong perception arose due to adoption of spatial instability theory for fluid flow, in which one looks for spatial growth at the imposed frequency, associated with the signal-problem assumption. We have already noted in describing the various wall excitation cases that the finite-time start-up excites all possible circular frequencies, and the roles of various modes of transient variation have been noted in the previous section on impulse response. In this case the wall excitation is given by

$$\bar{\psi}(\tilde{x}, 0, t) = \delta(\tilde{x})\bar{\psi}_0 e^{-i\bar{\omega}_0 t} \tag{5}$$

where $\bar{\psi}_0 = H(t)$ or $U_1(t)$ with a chosen value of α_E, depending on whether the start-up is impulsive (as given by Heaviside function) or non-impulsive (as given by error function-type variation, with $U_1(t)$). The frequency response with impulsive start given by Heaviside function has been solved originally in [28] for a case with $\tilde{R}e = 1000$ and $\bar{\omega}_0 = 0.1$, which has been pronounced as spatially unstable. Here, we have solved the same problem, with significantly higher number of points in $\tilde{x}$- and $\tilde{y}$-directions.

The results shown in Fig. 5 are for the spatially unstable case ($\tilde{R}e = 1000$ and $\bar{\omega}_0 = 0.10$) solved by BCIM. In the depicted solution, apart from the local solution, the TS wave-packet and the STWF are also present. It is not readily apparent that there exists the STWF, as it was also not identified in [28], where this set of results were presented for the first time. For this spatially unstable case, the TS wave-packet and the STWF are fused together in the displayed solution of OSE, shown for the indicated times. We would like to emphasize that this typical structure of blended TS wave-packet and STWF is a consequence of the parallel flow assumption used to formulate and solve OSE. Otherwise, the solutions of OSE for other stable cases, as

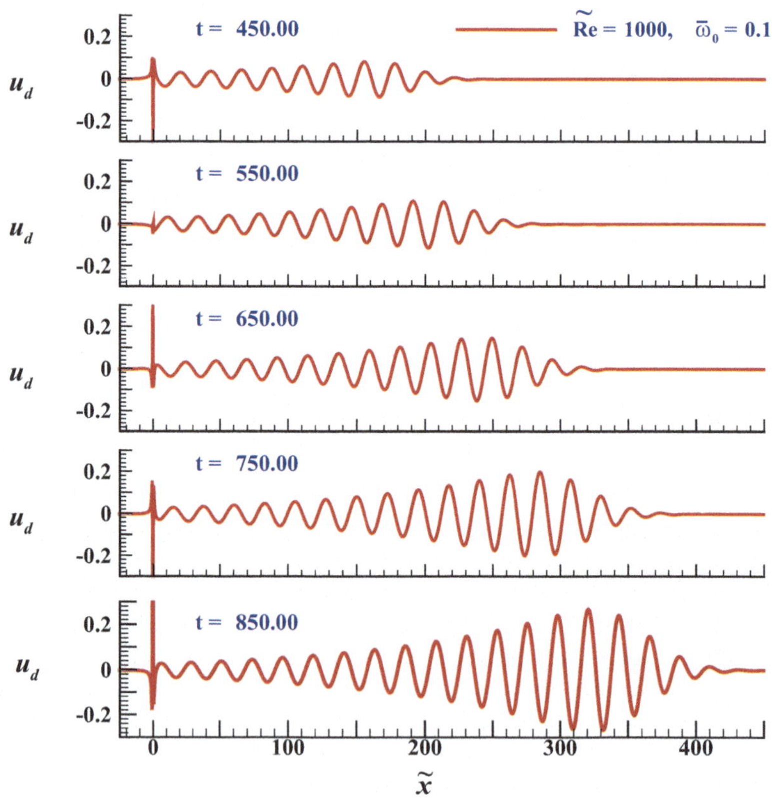

Fig. 5 Frequency response of the Blasius boundary layer to excitation as given by Eq. (5) for $\tilde{R}e = 1000$ and $\bar{\omega}_0 = 0.1$, with results shown at $\tilde{y} = 0.278$. The Bromwich contours are the same used in Fig. 4

will be shown later, display the separation of TS wave-packet and the STWF. Later, when BCIM was used to investigate spatially stable cases in [32, 33], the presence of STWF was easily discerned, with the TS wave-packet is seen to decay with space, while STWF grows and convects downstream. Two such stable cases are shown here in Fig. 6 for the indicated parameters.

The emergence of TS wave-packet is clearly visible from the local solution in all the frames. The property of the TS wave-packet is dictated primarily by the spatial stability property of the OSE at the location of the exciter, and it is easy to rationalize the decay of the TS wave-packet. However, the STWF has the property of growth in space and time and has little to do with spatial theory properties. The propagation properties are the same, as seen in Fig. 4. Consistent with the parallel flow assumption, the solutions shown in Figs. 5 and 6 are for the same constant physical frequency (f), for which $\frac{\bar{\omega}_0}{\tilde{Re}}$ remains constant, which in this case provides the non-dimensional physical frequency as $F = 2\pi f \nu / U_\infty^2$.

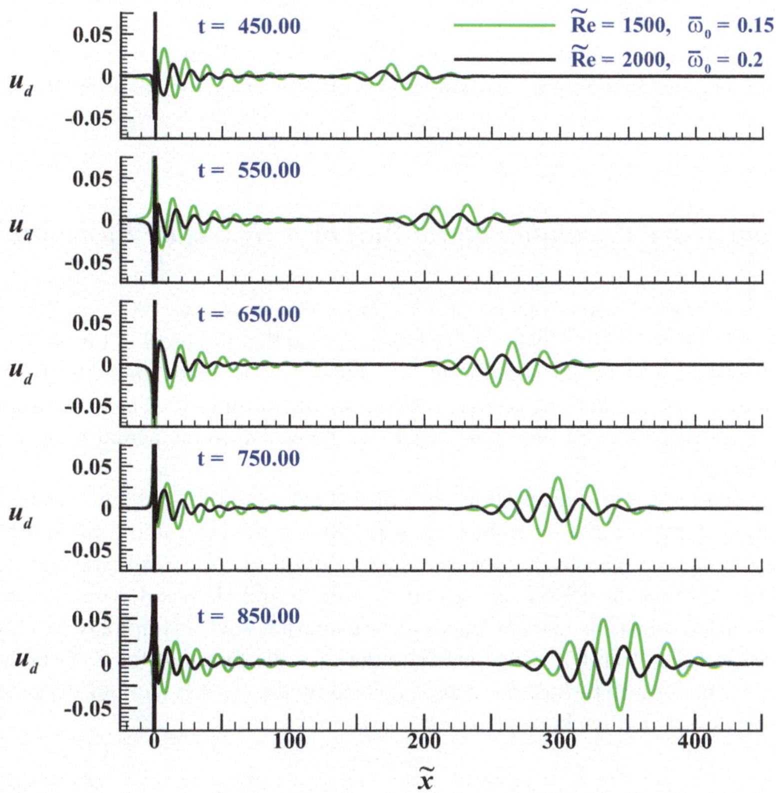

Fig. 6 Frequency response of the Blasius boundary layer to excitation as given by Eq. (5) for $\tilde{Re} = 1500$ and 2000, for $\bar{\omega}_0 = 0.15$ and 0.20, respectively. The results are shown at $\tilde{y} = 0.278$. The Bromwich contours are described in Fig. 4

6 Non-oscillatory Start-up Cases Solved by BCIM

Having noted the distinction between the impulse and the frequency response in the previous two sections, we note the absence of TS wave-packet for the former. At the same time, both cases have a local solution and STWF. However, the local solution for the impulse response is significantly smaller, and which furthermore rapidly decays with time. Thus, after some time, only the STWF will be the common link between the solutions of the impulse and the frequency response cases. It has been shown that the STWF is the precursor of transition to turbulence for 2D in [29] and 3D transition in [3, 4, 35]. It has also been shown that it is not necessary that STWF is created due to impulsive start for frequency response cases in [5]. The ever-growing STWF for both the impulse and frequency response cases shows that it is not necessary to impose any specific time scale to cause transition. However, imposition of time scale helps in creating TS wave-packets, which helps in transition for the frequencies which are closer to Branch-I of the neutral curve, where STWF is constantly fed by TS wave-packet and which does not remain stationary. These cases have been termed as interacting or I-type transition cases in [5]. Keeping this in view, next, we report response of Blasius boundary layer to wall excitations which are associated with a sudden jump used as the input, without any oscillation frequency associated with the input.

6.1 Impulsive Excitation at the Wall by a Heaviside Function

In this case, the exciter is placed at a location, where $\tilde{Re} = 1000$, and the input excitation is given by the Heaviside function. Given that the present investigation is for a linearized system, the amplitude of excitation is in non-dimensional form of unity value. Thus, the discussion here pertains to unit amplitude of excitation applied on the disturbance stream function, which can be scaled to the actual value of wall perturbation.

In Fig. 7, the streamwise component of disturbance velocity is shown as a function of streamwise distance at a height of $\tilde{y} = 0.278$, for the indicated time instants. In this case also, one can clearly observe the evolution of the STWF with space and time. The fact that the STWF is created by a delta and Heaviside function clearly establishes that transition to turbulence can be caused by such an impulsive excitation, as shown in Figs. 4 and 7. This clearly underlines the fact that for ZPG boundary layer, the transition to turbulence can be caused by the STWF without the presence of TS *waves* or wave-packets.

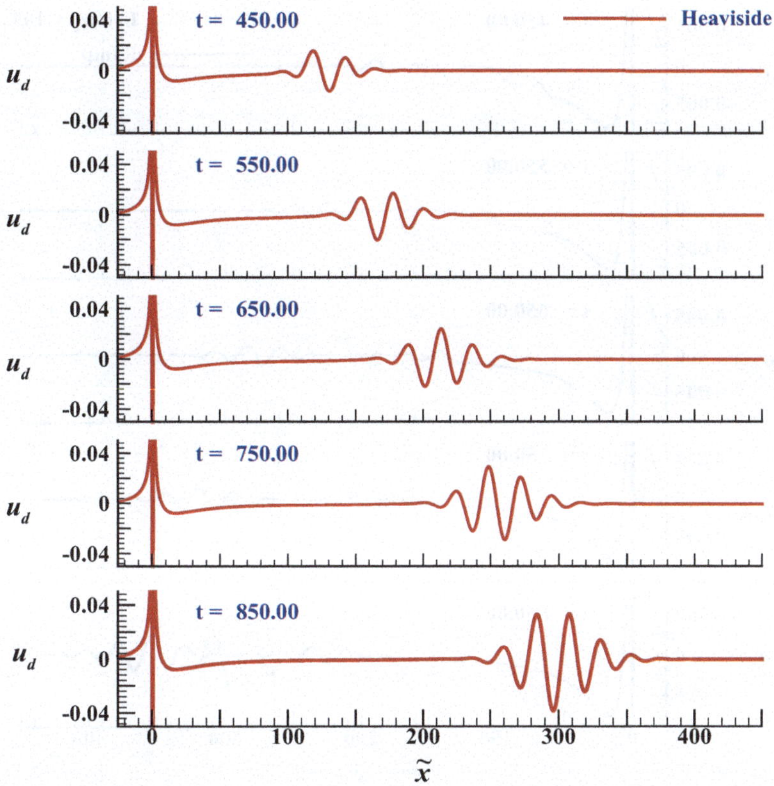

Fig. 7 Response of the Blasius boundary layer to excitation given by the Heaviside function for $\tilde{R}e = 1000$. Results are shown for $\tilde{y} = 0.278$. The Bromwich contours are as in Figs. 4, 5 and 6. The input is given in the form of unit disturbance stream function at the exciter location

6.2 Non-impulsive Excitation at the Wall Given by Ramp and Error Function

In these cases, we have used input disturbance stream function from Eq. (3) for the error function with $\alpha_E = 100$ and $t_0 = 150$, and the ramp function increases linearly from zero at $t = 0$ to unit value at $t = 300$. To solve OSE, the boundary conditions are obtained using DFFT of the time signal at the exciter. The results are obtained by solving OSE using BCIM, and Bromwich contours are chosen as before for the impulse and frequency response cases.

In Fig. 8, the streamwise component of disturbance velocity is shown as a function of streamwise distance for the two cases at the indicated times. We observe that these cases produce response fields which are one order of magnitude lower, as compared to the case shown in Fig. 7. Due to the faster growth rate of the error function excitation case, as compared to the ramp function case, the response field amplitude is higher

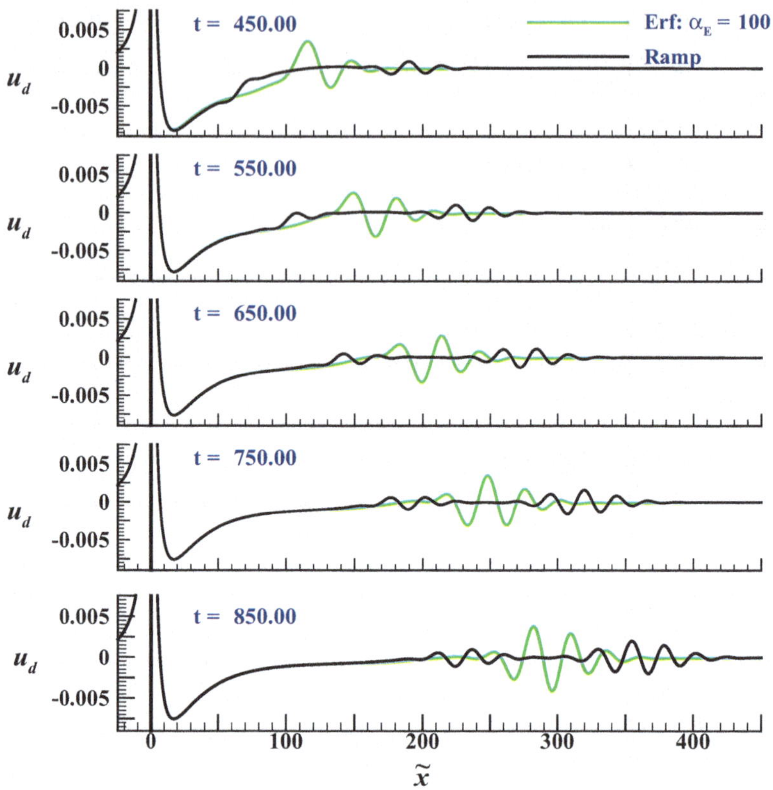

Fig. 8 Response of the Blasius boundary layer to excitation given by error function and ramp function for $\tilde{Re} = 1000$ during the time interval of $0 \leq t \leq 300$, with results shown for $\tilde{y} = 0.278$. The Bromwich contours are as in Figs. 4, 5 and 6. The input is given in the form of constant disturbance stream function at the exciter location

for the former. However, small is the approach of the input disturbance field to the same final value, one expects creation of the STWF, implying the ubiquitous nature of the STWF. Due to slope discontinuity during onset and terminal stage of the ramp start-up, one can see two distinct STWFs in the disturbance field as shown in Fig. 8. Given sufficient length and presence of wall shear, the STWF will grow eventually to cause transition to turbulence.

Although the response for the case of non-oscillatory Heaviside function is one order of magnitude higher than the other two cases, the spectrum of the response fields as shown in Fig. 9 indicates that the scales of the STWF for all the three cases are similar. One also notices that the STWF occurs not at a particular length scale but is a wide-band phenomenon centered around $\alpha_r \approx 0.3$ for the displayed time, $t = 450$. Subsequently, all the three cases amplify which is the universal feature of the STWF.

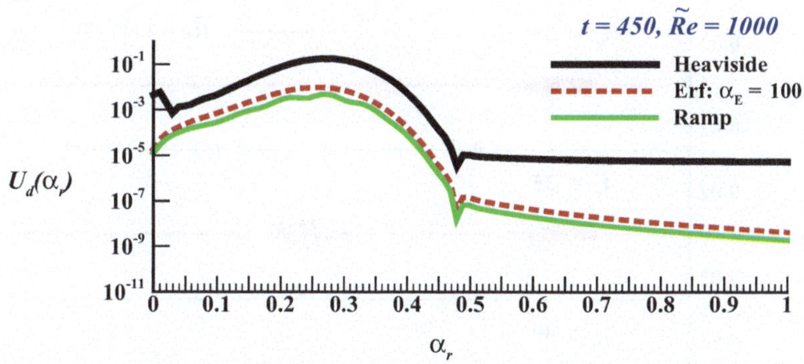

Fig. 9 Fourier transform of u_d for the three non-oscillatory input cases, whose responses are shown in Figs. 7 and 8 at the indicated time, $t = 450$

7 The Frequency Response Obtained from the Solution of the Navier–Stokes Equation

We have noted in Fig. 5 that the TS wave-packet and the STWF are together at all times. This led to confusion in [28], whereby the STWF was not recognized. Subsequently, when the spatial stable cases were solved by BCIM in [32, 33], one could distinguish between the TS wave-packet and the STWF, as also seen in Fig. 6. This particular feature for the spatially unstable cases is due to the parallel flow approximation, as was noted from the solution of NSE in [29].

The case considered in [29] was with a simultaneous blowing-suction strip extending from $\tilde{R}e = 656$–676, and such an excitation led to fully developed turbulence studied for different amplitude of excitation, displaying k^{-3} spectrum for u_d. For the case considered here in Fig. 5, we report the corresponding solution by solving NSE in Fig. 10.

We would like to point out that the scales used in representing the NSE are based on convection scales, while those used for OSE are viscous scales. For example, the viscous time scale is given by $T_{sc} = \frac{\delta^*}{U_\infty}$, whereas in solving the NSE, we have used a length scale (L), such that the corresponding Reynolds number is given by $\text{Re}_L = 10^5$ and the corresponding time scale is $T_c = \frac{L}{U_\infty}$. As a consequence, the ratio of the two time scales is given by $\frac{T_c}{T_{sc}} = \frac{\text{Re}_L}{\tilde{R}e}$. For the solution of NSE, the non-dimensional coordinates are given by x and y. From the top frame at $t_c = 25$, one can clearly observe that the STWF is distinctly different from the TS wave-packet. The solutions of OSE shown have extraordinarily high resolution as compared to the solution obtained by the NSE, because of the different time resolution of NSE and OSE. Thus, it is not possible to show solution of OSE corresponding to the top frame of Fig. 10 with the number of points taken in ω_0-plane. In Fig. 10, one notices continual growth and downstream propagation of the STWF, while the TS wave-packet appears to remain stationary, although this is a progressive wave, whose

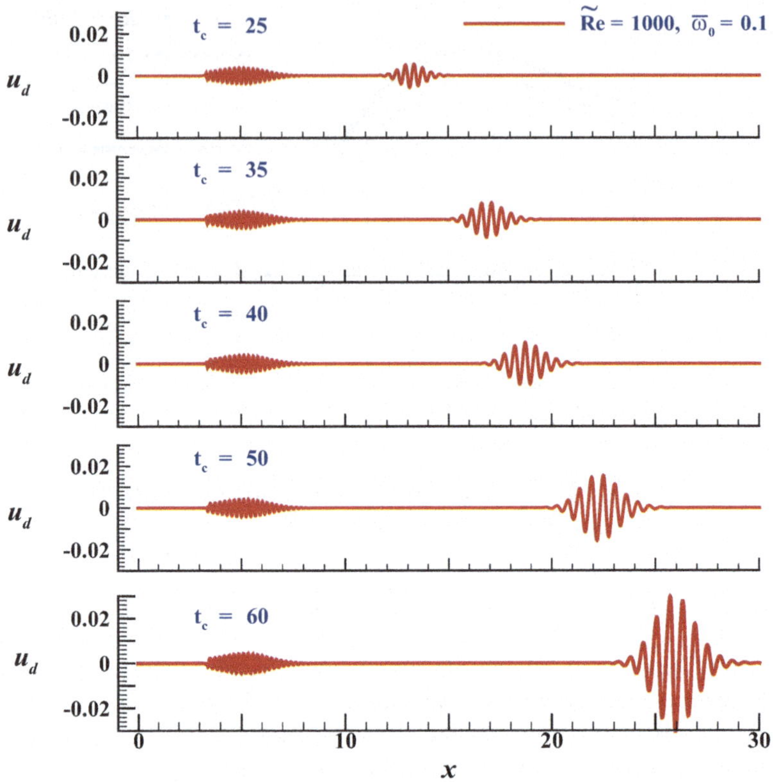

Fig. 10 Frequency response of the Blasius boundary layer to excitation as given by Eq. (5) with the exciter located where $\tilde{Re} = 1000$ for $\bar{\omega}_0 = 0.1$, and the results for u_d are shown at $y = 0.278$ for the indicated times

amplitude decays with downstream co-ordinate x. The observed stationary nature of the TS wave-packet is determined by the wave properties of the packet as determined by its growth and decay for the constant frequency wall excitation. The solution displayed in Fig. 10 is all during the linear growth stage of the STWF. The detailed 2D solution of similar cases has been reported in [29, 30].

8 Summary and Conclusion

Here, we have studied the impulse and frequency response cases to reconcile between the experiments reported in [24] (which has been termed as frequency response, as the input is provided at a fixed frequency consistent with the practice in spatial stability theory) and those in [13], where a wave-packet is created by a localized delta function excitation in space and time, as given in Eq. (4). The output of such an excitation can be termed indeed as the impulse response. Such an experimental approach is used in [13] to provide help with understanding natural transition. In contrast, the theoretical TS *waves* have been created only in a strict laboratory setting with a monochromatic excitation at a fixed frequency. In real flows, transition to turbulence is often noted as a turbulent spot or puff [11, 18]. We have reasoned that even the so-called frequency response starts at a finite time, and therefore, such an excitation is also similar to impulse excitation, and we have investigated three different start-ups: Impulsive (as given by Heaviside function), non-impulsive with varying acceleration [as given by Eq. (3)] and a linear ramp function. Only in the frequency response case, the input [as given by Eq. (5)] produces TS wave-packet as obtained from the solution of Navier–Stokes equation in Fig. 10, which have also been reported in [29, 30].

For both the cases of the impulse and frequency responses, one notices the common elements of the local solution and the spatio-temporal wave-front (STWF) here from the solution of linearized analysis of Orr–Sommerfeld equation (OSE). However, for impulse response, the local solution is insignificantly smaller for the impulse response, and furthermore, the amplitude of which decays with time. The presented results are from the solution of governing Navier–Stokes equation (NSE) in its full form or in its linearized version of OSE. This is distinctly different from various other approaches reported in the literature [9, 19]. It has been shown in [3, 29, 32] that frequency response cases create STWF, which is the precursor of transition to turbulence obtained from the solution of OSE and NSE. For the impulse response case, the existence of STWF has been shown from the solution of NSE in [4, 35]. It is shown here from the solution of OSE for the input excitation given by strictly delta function in space and time. Apart from this, existence of STWF is also shown, when the input is given by a Heaviside function, linearly varying ramp function and an error function. All of these excitations have varying degree of time variation of the input excitation for impulsive and non-impulsive start-ups. While all of these demonstrate the creation of STWF, none of these show TS wave-packets. The spectra of the various STWFs shown in Fig. 9 show the universality of the STWF. It is also explained that for the spatially unstable case shown in Fig. 5, one does not see the distinct STWF due to parallel flow assumption, as the same case solved using NSE in Fig. 10 display the STWF and the TS wave-packet. However, in Fig. 6, one can clearly see the demarcated STWF from the decaying TS wave-packet. All of these observations lead us to conclude that the STWF is the precursor of transition for both the impulse and frequency responses for the boundary layer and is created by the linear mechanism, governed by OSE. This point of view perfectly blends with experimentally observed transition to turbulence for not only wall-bounded flows but also for internal flows and free shear layers.

References

1. Ashpis, D.E., Reshotko, E.: The vibrating ribbon problem revisited. J. Fluid Mech. **213**, 531 (1990)

2. Bers, A.: Physique des Plasmas. Gordon and Breach, New York, USA (1975)
3. Bhaumik, S., Sengupta, T.K.: Precursor of transition to turbulence: Spatiotemporal wave front. Phys. Rev. E **89**(4), 043018 (2014)
4. Bhaumik, S., Sengupta, T.K.: Impulse response and spatio-temporal wave-packets: the common feature of rogue waves, tsunami and transition to turbulence. Phys. Fluids **29**, 124103 (2017)
5. Bhaumik, S., Sengupta, T.K., Shabab, Z.A.: Receptivity to harmonic excitation following non-impulsive start for boundary layer flows. AIAA J. **55**(10), 3233–3238 (2017)
6. Borrell, G., Sillero, J.A., Jiménez, J.: A code for direct numerical simulation of turbulent boundary layers at high Reynolds numbers in BG/P supercomputers. Comput. Fluids **80**, 37–43 (2013)
7. Breuer, K.S., Cohen, J., Haritonidis, J.H.: The late stages of transition induced by a low-amplitude wavepacket in a laminar boundary layer. J. Fluid Mech. **340**, 395–411 (1997)
8. Brillouin, L.: Wave Propagation and Group Velocity. Academic press, New York, USA (1960)
9. Chomaz, J.-M.: Global instabilities in spatially developing flows: non-normality and nonlinearity. Annu. Rev. Fluid Mech. **37**, 357–392 (2005)
10. Drazin, P.G., Reid, W.H.: Hydrodynamic Stability. Cambridge University Press, UK (1981)
11. Emmons, H.W.: The laminar-turbulent transition in a boundary layer-Part I. J. Aeronaut. Sci. **18**(7), 490–498 (1951)
12. Fasel, H., Konzelmann, U.: Non-parallel stability of a flat plate boundary layer using the complete Navier-Stokes equation. J. Fluid Mech. **221**, 331–347 (1990)
13. Gaster, M., Grant, I.: An experimental investigation of the formation and development of a wave packet in a laminar boundary layer. Proc. Royal Soc. A **347**(1649), 253–269 (1975)
14. Gaster, M.: On the generation of spatially growing waves in a boundary layer. J. Fluid Mech. **22**, 433 (1965)
15. Gaster, M.: Growth of disturbances in both space and time. Phys. Fluids **11**, 723–727 (1968)
16. Gaster, M., Sengupta, T.K.: The generation of disturbances in a boundary layer by wall perturbations: the vibrating ribbon revisited once more. In: Instabilities and Turbulence in Engineering Flows, Kluwer Academic Publisher, Dordrecht, The Netherlands (1993)
17. Heisenberg, W.: Über stabilität und turbulenz von flüssigkeitsströmen. Ann. Phys. Lpz. **379**, 577–627 (1924). (Translated as On stability and turbulence of fluid flows. NACA Tech. Memo. Wash. No 1291, 1951)
18. Hof, B., Doorne, C.W.H.V., Westerweel, J., Nieuwstadt, F.T.M., Faisst, H., Eckhardt, B., Wedin, H., Kerswell, R.R., Waleffe, F.: Experimental observation of nonlinear traveling waves in turbulent pipe flow. Science **305**(5690), 1594–1598 (2004)
19. Huerre, P., Monkewitz, P.A.: Absolute and convective instabilities in free shear layers. J. Fluid Mech. **159**, 151–168 (1985)
20. Kloker, M.J.: A robust high-resolution split-type compact FD scheme for spatial direct numerical simulation of boundary-layer transition. Appl. Sci. Res. **59**(4), 353–377 (1997)
21. Orr, McF.W.: The stability or instability of the steady motions of a perfect liquid and of a viscous liquid, Part I: A perfect liquid. Part II: A viscous liquid. Proc. Roy. Irish Acad., *A27*, 9–138 (1907)
22. Papoulis, A.: Fourier Integral and Its Applications. McGraw Hill, New York, USA (1962)
23. Schlichting, H.: Zur entstehung der turbulenz bei der plattenströmung. Nachr. Ges. Wiss. Goettingen, Math.-Phys. Kl., **42**, 181–208 (1933)
24. Schubauer, G.B., Skramstad, H.K.: Laminar boundary layer oscillations and the stability of laminar flow. J. Aero. Sci. **14**(2), 69–78 (1947)
25. Sengupta, T. K.: Impulse response of laminar boundary layer and receptivity. In: 7th International Conference on Numerical Methods In Laminar and Turbulent Flows. Pineridge Press (1991)
26. Sengupta, T.K.: Solution of the Orr-Sommerfeld equation for high wave numbers. Comput. Fluids **21**(2), 301–303 (1992)
27. Sengupta, T.K.: Instabilities of Flows and Transition to Turbulence. CRC Press, Taylor & Francis Group, Florida, USA (2012)

28. Sengupta, T.K., Ballav, M., Nijhawan, S.: Generation of Tollmien—Schlichting waves by harmonic excitation. Phys. Fluids **6**(3), 1213–1222 (1994)
29. Sengupta, T.K., Bhaumik, S.: Onset of turbulence from the receptivity stage of fluid flows. Phys. Rev. Lett. **154501**, 1–5 (2011)
30. Sengupta, T.K., Bhaumik, S., Bhumkar, Y.: Direct numerical simulation of two-dimensional wall-bounded turbulent flows from receptivity stage. Phys. Rev. E **85**(2), 026308 (2012)
31. Sengupta, T.K., Singh, N., Suman, V.K.: Dynamical system approach to instability of flow past a circular cylinder. J. Fluid Mech. **658**, 82–115 (2010)
32. Sengupta, T.K., Rao, A.K., Venkatasubbaiah, K.: Spatio-temporal growing wave fronts in spatially stable boundary layers. Phys. Rev. Lett. **96**(22), 224504–1–4
33. Sengupta, T.K., Rao, A.K., Venkatasubbaiah, K.: Spatio-temporal growth of disturbances in a boundary layer and energy based receptivity analysis. Phys. Fluids **18**, 094101 (2006)
34. Sommerfeld, A.: Ein Beitrag zur hydrodynamiscen Erklarung der turbulenten Flussigkeitsbewegung. In: Proceedings of 4th International Congress Mathematicians, Rome, pp. 116–124 (1908)
35. Sundaram, P., Sengupta, T.K., Bhaumik, S.: The three-dimensional impulse response of a boundary layer to different types of wall excitation. Phys. Fluids **30**, 124103 (2018)
36. Tollmien, W.: Über die enstehung der turbulenz. I. English translation: NACA TM 609 (1931)
37. Trefethen, L.N., Trefethen, A.E., Reddy, S.C., Driscoll, T.A.: Hydrodynamic stability without eigenvalues. Science **261**(5121), 578–584 (1993)
38. Van Der Pol, B., Bremmer, H.: Operational calculus based on two-sided Laplace integral. Cambridge University Press, Cambridge, UK (1959)
39. Yeo, K.S., Zhao, X., Wang, Z.Y., Ng, K.C.: DNS of wavepacket evolution in a Blasius boundary layer. J. Fluid Mech. **652**, 333–372 (2010)

Entropy Generation for a Mixed Convection Nanofluid Flow in an Inclined Channel Filled with Porous Medium with Thermal Radiation

Lalrinpuia Tlau and Surender Ontela

Abstract The current paper analyzes the generation of entropy in a sloped channel with a Cu–H_2O nanofluid-saturated porous media for the mixed convection of nanofluids under the influence of thermal radiation. The entropy characteristics and their dependence on flow parameters are studied and analyzed thoroughly, namely Darcy numbers, Brinkman numbers, Peclet numbers, radiation parameters, channel angle inclination, mixed convection parameters and volume fractions of nanoparticles. The results achieved are compared with the existing literature for limiting values and found to be excellent.

Keywords Nanofluid · Thermal radiation · Entropy generation · Inclined channel · Mixed convection

1 Introduction

Recent research niche has mainly focused on minimizing machines and maximizing their performances. Maximizing performances leads to the greater workload which leads to thermal energy generation. Optimizing performance requires machines to be at a stable temperature, hence requiring constant cooling. This has led to the development of nanofluid and its research, pioneered by Choi [1]. Nanofluids consist of nanoparticles, of the size of 1–100 nm in diameter, suspended in fluids. Applications are diverse and still under intense investigation, many of which can be found in [2–5].

Heat transfer for inclined channel problems has been studied by many researchers but lacks diversity as compared to other problems. In the investigation of an inclined parallel-walled channel with heat flux and impermeable walls, Barletta et al. [6] observed that there were a large number of flow solutions when viscous dissipation was neglected. The problem of the porous media-filled slope with a mixed-convective nanofluid flow was investigated by Cimpean and Pop [7]. They came to the conclusion that adding nanoparticles into the liquid significantly improves the heat transfer.

L. Tlau (✉) · S. Ontela
National Institute of Technology Mizoram, Aizawl, Mizoram 796012, India
e-mail: puiatlau0610@gmail.com

S. Bhattacharyya et al. (eds.), *Mathematical Modeling and Computational Tools*, Springer Proceedings in Mathematics & Statistics 320,
https://doi.org/10.1007/978-981-15-3615-1_12

Liu et al. [8] deliberated heat transfer on a sloping channel for the Poiseuille–Couette flow. They observed, with the Brinkman number increasing, that hydrodynamical and thermal profiles are increasing. In a tilt channel filled with porous medium with periodic conditions on the boundary, Jha et al. [9] investigated the hydrodynamic and thermal behavior for a mixed convection flow. It was perceived that for particular Darcy number values the flow reversal could be controlled. Reddy et al. [10] investigated a hydromagnetic peristaltic flow in an asymmetric porous medium-filled tilted channel of a radiating and reacting couple stress fluid. They observed that the temperature increased with the Prandtl number and decreased by radiation increase.

The generation of entropy and its related field is paramount to the exploration of heat transfer. Bejan [11] instigated the field of research. Baytas [12] was responsible for deliberation of entropy generation in a sloping porous cavity. He intimated that the irreversibility by heat transfer began to dominate entropy generation as the Rayleigh number declined. In an inclined channel, Cimpean and Pop [13] studied entropy generation reduction. They came to the conclusion that irreversibility by heat transfer dominated the mechanism of entropy generation. Dehsara et al. [14] have carried out a numerical study in the presence of radiation and magnetic field of entropy production in nanoflow on the transparent plate in a porous medium. The entropy generation surged with the hike in the Brinkman and Hartman numbers, respectively. Srinivasacharya and Hima Bindu [15] probed entropy production in flow of micropolar fluid in a tilted channel. The increasing angle of inclination increased the rate of entropy production. In a sloping channel filled with ferrofluids, Baskaya et al. [16] investigated the magnetic field effects on the generation of entropy. At a small angle, the magnetic field increase was shown to decrease the rate of entropy generation. Hussain et al. [17] conducted the investigation of the generation of entropy in an inclined channel with a nanofluid-filled cavity.

The present article investigates the generation of entropy in an inclined channel for a mixed convection flow with porous media and thermal radiation effects. By relevant substitution, non-dimensionalization of the governing equations is done. The equations are then analytically solved with the boundary conditions. Therefore, for the calculation of entropy and Bejan number, the temperature and velocity profiles are used. The ramifications of various relevant parameters on entropy and Bejan numbers are analyzed and displayed graphically.

2 Mathematical Formulation

Consider a fully developed mixed convection of a Cu–water nanofluid in a two-dimensional channel, bounded by impermeable walls at a D separation and full of a fluid-saturated porous medium as shown in the figure. The walls of the channel are heated with a q_w thermal flux, fluid has a uniform U_0 stream velocity and an approximation by Rossel and is utilized to define the thermal flux radiation in the energy equation. Darcy Law and Boussinesq approximation are used, and thermal and local equilibrium is considered in the porous medium. Thus, the governing equations in Cartesian coordinates can be described as follows (Fig. 1):

Fig. 1 Schematic diagram with coordinate axes

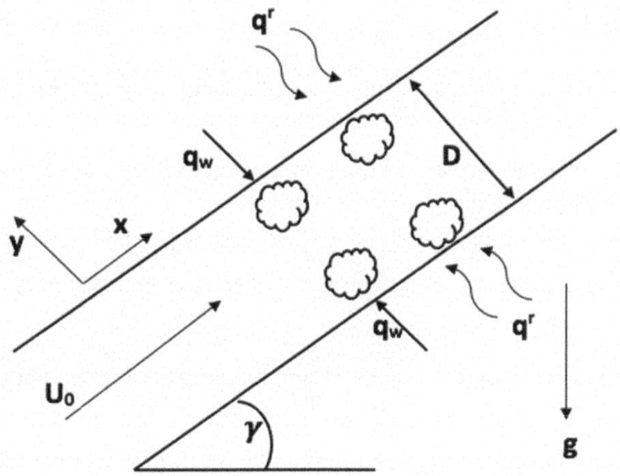

$$\frac{\partial v^{\bullet}}{\partial y}+\frac{\partial u^{\bullet}}{\partial x}=0 \tag{1}$$

$$\frac{\mu_{\rm nf}}{K}\left(\frac{\partial u^{\bullet}}{\partial y}-\frac{\partial v^{\bullet}}{\partial y}\right)=(\tau\beta)_{\rm nf}\left[\frac{\partial \Upsilon}{\partial y}{\rm Sin}\gamma-\frac{\partial \Upsilon}{\partial x}{\rm Cos}\gamma\right] \tag{2}$$

$$u^{\bullet}\frac{\partial \Upsilon}{\partial x}+v^{\bullet}\frac{\partial \Upsilon}{\partial y}=\alpha_{\rm nf}\left(\frac{\partial^2 \Upsilon}{\partial x^2}+\frac{\partial^2 \Upsilon}{\partial y^2}\right)-\frac{1}{\left(\tau\, C_{\rm p}\right)_{\rm nf}}\frac{\partial q^{r}}{\partial y} \tag{3}$$

under the boundary conditions:

$$v^{\bullet}(0)=0,\ \left.\frac{\partial Y}{\partial y}\right|_{y=0}=-\frac{q_{\rm w}}{\chi_{\rm nf}} \tag{4a}$$

$$v^{\bullet}(D)=0,\ \left.\frac{\partial Y}{\partial y}\right|_{y=D}=\frac{q_{\rm w}}{\chi_{\rm nf}} \tag{4b}$$

where $u^{\bullet}$ and $v^{\bullet}$ denote velocity along the Cartesian components, respectively,β is the thermal expansion, Y is the nanofluid temperature, τ is the density, K is the permeability of the porous medium, $\mu_{\rm nf}$ is the viscosity of the nanofluid, $\alpha_{\rm nf}$ is the thermal diffusivity of the nanofluid, γ is the inclination angle of the channel, and $\chi_{\rm nf}$ is the thermal conductivity of the nanofluid.

The forced flow condition is given by

$$\int_0^D u^{\bullet}{\rm d}y=\Lambda \tag{5}$$

where Λ is the constant nanofluid inflow prescribed at the entrance of the channel. The speed u depends on the transverse y coordinate as the flow is fully developed.

Hence,

$$\frac{\partial u^{\bullet}}{\partial x} = 0 \Rightarrow u^{\bullet} = u^{\bullet}(y)$$

Now, from Eq. 1 and the boundary conditions 4, we have $\upsilon = 0$. Hence, Eqs. 2 and 3 are reduced to

$$\frac{\mu_{\mathrm{nf}}}{K}\frac{\partial u^{\bullet}}{\partial y} = (\tau\beta)_{\mathrm{nf}}\left[\frac{\partial \Upsilon}{\partial y}\mathrm{Sin}\gamma - \frac{\partial \Upsilon}{\partial x}\mathrm{Cos}\gamma\right] \tag{6}$$

$$u\frac{\partial \Upsilon}{\partial x} + \frac{1}{\left(\tau\, C_{\mathrm{p}}\right)_{\mathrm{nf}}}\frac{\partial q^{r}}{\partial y} = \alpha_{\mathrm{nf}}\frac{\partial^2 \Upsilon}{\partial y^2} \tag{7}$$

For nanoparticles, nanofluid and base fluid, we consider the following terms for their physical characteristics:

$$(\tau\beta)_{\mathrm{nf}} = (1-\phi)(\tau\beta)_{\mathrm{f}} + \phi(\tau\beta)_{\mathrm{s}}$$

$$\frac{\chi_{\mathrm{nf}}}{\chi_{\mathrm{f}}} = \frac{(2\chi_{\mathrm{f}} + \chi_{\mathrm{s}}) + 2\phi(\chi_{\mathrm{s}} - \chi_{\mathrm{f}})}{(2\chi_{\mathrm{f}} + \chi_{\mathrm{s}}) - \phi(\chi_{\mathrm{s}} - \chi_{\mathrm{f}})}$$

$$\tau_{\mathrm{nf}} = (1-\phi)\tau_{\mathrm{f}} + \phi\tau_{\mathrm{s}}$$

$$\mu_{\mathrm{nf}} = \frac{\mu_{\mathrm{f}}}{(1-\phi)^{2.5}}$$

Implementing the following non-dimensional variables into Eqs. 6 and 7

$$Y = \frac{y}{D}, X = \frac{x}{D}, U = \frac{u^{\bullet}}{U_0}, \theta = \frac{\Upsilon - \Upsilon_0}{qD/\chi_{\mathrm{f}}} \tag{8}$$

such that $U_0 = \Lambda/D$ is the uniform velocity and Υ_0 is the uniform inflow fluid temperature, we have

$$\frac{\partial U}{\partial Y} = \lambda(1-\phi)^{2.5}\left[(1-\phi) + \phi\frac{(\tau\beta)_{\mathrm{s}}}{(\tau\beta)_{\mathrm{f}}}\right]\left[\frac{\partial \theta}{\partial Y}\mathrm{Sin}\gamma - \frac{\partial \theta}{\partial X}\mathrm{Cos}\gamma\right] \tag{9}$$

$$U\mathrm{Pe}\frac{\partial \theta}{\partial X} = \left[\frac{\chi_{\mathrm{nf}}}{\chi_{\mathrm{f}}} + \frac{4\mathrm{Rd}}{3}\right]\frac{1}{\left[(1-\phi) + \phi\frac{(\tau C_{\mathrm{p}})_{\mathrm{s}}}{(\tau C_{\mathrm{p}})_{\mathrm{f}}}\right]}\frac{\partial^2 \theta}{\partial Y^2} \tag{10}$$

with the associated non-dimensionalized conditions at the boundary

$$\left.\frac{\partial \theta}{\partial Y}\right|_{Y=0} = -1 \tag{11a}$$

$$\left.\frac{\partial \theta}{\partial Y}\right|_{Y=1} = 1 \tag{11b}$$

and the forced flow condition $\int_0^1 U(Y)\mathrm{d}Y = 1$.
The mixed convection parameter λ, radiation parameter Rd and Peclet number Pe are defined as

$$\lambda = \frac{g(\tau\beta)_f K q D}{U_0 \mu_f \chi_f}, \ \mathrm{Rd} = \frac{4\sigma \Upsilon_0^3}{\Xi \chi_f}, \ \mathrm{Pe} = \frac{U_0 D}{\alpha_f} \tag{12}$$

3 Solution of the Problem

We now solve Eqs. 9 and 10. Following the method used by Cimpean and Pop [7], the velocity and temperature are expressed as

$$U = U(Y), \ \theta(X, Y) = C_1 X + F(Y) \tag{13}$$

Substituting Eq. 14 into 10, we get

$$U \mathrm{Pe} C_1 = \left[\frac{\chi_{nf}}{\chi_f} + \frac{4\mathrm{Rd}}{3}\right] \frac{1}{\left[(1-\phi) + \phi \frac{(\tau C_p)_s}{(\tau C_p)_f}\right]} \frac{\partial^2 \theta}{\partial Y^2} \tag{14}$$

Integrating the above equation across the channel cross section, we get

$$\mathrm{Pe} C_1 \int_0^1 U \mathrm{d}Y = \left[\frac{\chi_{nf}}{\chi_f} + \frac{4\mathrm{Rd}}{3}\right] \frac{1}{\left[(1-\phi) + \phi \frac{(\tau C_p)_s}{(\tau C_p)_f}\right]} \int_0^1 \frac{\partial^2 \theta}{\partial Y^2} \mathrm{d}Y \tag{15}$$

$$\Rightarrow C_1 = \frac{2}{\mathrm{Pe}} \left[\frac{\chi_{nf}}{\chi_f} + \frac{4\mathrm{Rd}}{3}\right] \frac{1}{\left[(1-\phi) + \phi \frac{(\tau C_p)_s}{(\tau C_p)_f}\right]} \tag{16}$$

Using Eqs. 17 and 14 in 9 and 10, we obtain

$$\frac{\partial U}{\partial Y} = \lambda \left[(1-\phi) + \phi \frac{(\tau\beta)_s}{(\tau\beta)_f}\right] (1-\phi)^{2.5} \left[\frac{\partial F}{\partial Y} \mathrm{Sin}\gamma - \frac{2}{\mathrm{Pe}} \left[\frac{\chi_{nf}}{\chi_f} + \frac{4\mathrm{Rd}}{3}\right] \frac{\mathrm{Cos}\gamma}{\left[(1-\phi) + \phi \frac{(\tau C_p)_s}{(\tau C_p)_f}\right]}\right] \tag{17}$$

$$U = \frac{1}{2} \frac{\mathrm{d}^2 F}{\mathrm{d}Y^2} \tag{18}$$

Combining Eqs. 20 and 21, we get a third-order differential equation

$$\frac{\mathrm{d}^3 F}{\mathrm{d}Y^3} - 2A\mathrm{Sin}\gamma\frac{\mathrm{d}F}{\mathrm{d}Y} + \frac{4\lambda A A_1}{\mathrm{Pe}}\mathrm{Cos}\gamma = 0 \tag{19}$$

where

$$A = \left[(1-\phi) + \phi\frac{(\tau\beta)_\mathrm{s}}{(\tau\beta)_\mathrm{f}}\right](1-\phi)^{2.5},$$

$$A_1 = \left[\frac{\chi_\mathrm{nf}}{\chi_\mathrm{f}} + \frac{4\mathrm{Rd}}{3}\right]\frac{1}{\left[(1-\phi) + \phi\frac{(\tau C_\mathrm{p})_\mathrm{s}}{(\tau C_\mathrm{p})_\mathrm{f}}\right]}$$

and the boundary equations

$$\left.\frac{\mathrm{d}F}{\mathrm{d}Y}\right|_{Y=0} = -1 \tag{20a}$$

$$\left.\frac{\mathrm{d}F}{\mathrm{d}Y}\right|_{Y=1} = 1 \tag{20b}$$

As per the proposed solution form, $F(Y)$ has to be calculated so as to determine the temperature profile. A solution for $\frac{\mathrm{d}F}{\mathrm{d}Y}$ is obtained from Eq. 22. This expression is integrated but an arbitrary constant is introduced into the expression. This can be determined by integrating Eq. 10 and using Eqs. 14 and 19

$$\frac{\partial}{\partial X}\left(\int_0^1 \theta U \mathrm{d}Y\right) = \frac{2}{\mathrm{Pe}}\left[\frac{\chi_\mathrm{nf}}{\chi_\mathrm{f}} + \frac{4\mathrm{Rd}}{3}\right]\left[(1-\phi) + \phi\frac{(\tau\, C_\mathrm{p})_\mathrm{s}}{(\tau\, C_\mathrm{p})_\mathrm{f}}\right]^{-1} \tag{21}$$

$$\Rightarrow \int_0^1 \theta U \mathrm{d}Y = \frac{2X}{\mathrm{Pe}}\left[\frac{\chi_\mathrm{nf}}{\chi_\mathrm{f}} + \frac{4\mathrm{Rd}}{3}\right]\left[(1-\phi) + \phi\frac{(\tau\, C_\mathrm{p})_\mathrm{s}}{(\tau\, C_\mathrm{p})_\mathrm{f}}\right]^{-1} \tag{22}$$

Now, using Eq. 14 into 25 and using Eq. 12, the arbitrary constant can be determined using the obtained expression

$$\int_0^1 F(Y)U(Y)\mathrm{d}Y = 0 \tag{23}$$

4 Entropy Generation

The thermal gradient between the two media, i.e., fluid and channel wall, causing an unbalanced state, is the reason for the entropy generation in fluid transmission. In the present study under consideration, the commutation of energy and momentum within the saturated porous nanofluid media and the channel walls reinforces the setting of imbalance that generate entropy in the flow field. The local volumetric entropy generation rate for a viscous fluid, therefore, is specified under the influence of thermal radiation [18]:

$$S_G = \frac{\chi_{nf}}{Y_0}\left[\left(\frac{\partial \Upsilon}{\partial y}\right)^2 + \frac{16\sigma Y_0^3}{3\chi\chi_f}\left(\frac{\partial \Upsilon}{\partial y}\right)^2 + \left(\frac{\partial \Upsilon}{\partial x}\right)^2\right] + \frac{\mu_{nf}}{Y_0}\left(\frac{\partial u}{\partial y}\right)^2 + \frac{\mu_{nf}}{K Y_0}u^2 \tag{24}$$

Using the non-dimensional terms introduced in 8 and using the dimensionless entropy generation formula

$$N_s = \frac{D^2\Upsilon_0^2}{\chi_f(\Delta\Upsilon)^2}S_G \tag{25}$$

we get the expression for dimensionless entropy generation rate as

$$N_s = \frac{\chi_{nf}}{\chi_f}\left[\left(1+\frac{4}{3}\mathrm{Rd}\right)\left(\frac{\partial\theta}{\partial Y}\right)^2 + \left(\frac{\partial\theta}{\partial X}\right)^2\right] + \frac{1}{(1-\phi)^{2.5}}\frac{\mathrm{Br}}{\Omega}\left[\left(\frac{\partial U}{\partial Y}\right)^2 + \frac{U^2}{\mathrm{Da}}\right] \tag{26}$$

where $\mathrm{Br} = \mathrm{Ec}\cdot\mathrm{Pr} = \frac{\mu_f U_0^2}{\chi_f \Delta\Upsilon}$ is the Brinkman number and $\mathrm{Da} = \frac{K}{D^2}$ is the Darcy number.

The volumetric entropy is generated in a viscous, incompressible flow due to heat transfer and fluid friction. Therefore, we can write

$$N_s = N_h|_{\text{heat transfer}} + N_v|_{\text{fluid friction}} \tag{27}$$

such that

$$N_h = \frac{\chi_{nf}}{\chi_f}\left[\left(1+\frac{4}{3}\mathrm{Rd}\right)\left(\frac{\partial\theta}{\partial Y}\right)^2 + \left(\frac{\partial\theta}{\partial X}\right)^2\right] \tag{28}$$

$$N_v = \frac{1}{(1-\phi)^{2.5}}\frac{\mathrm{Br}}{\Omega}\left[\left(\frac{\partial U}{\partial Y}\right)^2 + \frac{U^2}{\mathrm{Da}}\right] \tag{29}$$

Bejan number, Be, is the ratio between the heat transfer entropy generation and the total entropy generation and takes values from 0 to 1. Thus, we have

$$\mathrm{Be} = \frac{N_\mathrm{h}}{N_\mathrm{h} + N_\mathrm{v}} \tag{30}$$

For Be = 1, irreversibility by heat transfer completely dominates the generation of entropy in fluid flow. With Be = 0, the entropy generation in the flow field is dominated completely by fluid friction. At Be = 0.5, heat transfer and fluid friction contribute equally to the entropy generation in the fluid flow.

5 Results and Discussion

The expression is acquired analytically for the velocity and temperature. Shown in Table 1 are the thermophysical properties of the nanoparticles and base fluid in question. Unless stated otherwise, we take the parameter values as $\lambda = 1$, $\gamma = \pi/4$, $\phi = 1\%$, Br = 0.01, Da = 10^{-3},Rd = 1 and Pe = 1 for all cases. The solution expression is compared to limiting cases. The graphs for U and F as functions of λ are obtained as shown in Figs. 2 and 3, respectively, for $\phi = 0$ and Rd = 0 and likened with the results procured by Cimpean and Pop [7]. As shown in Figs. 4 and 5, graphs for Bejan number are also obtained as a function of the mixed convection parameter and entropy generation rate as a function of Peclet number for $\phi = 0$ and Rd = 0 and compared with the results obtained by Cimpean and Pop [13]. All comparisons have been found to be well-conformed.

Figures 6 and 7 show the effects on the entropy generation rate and the Bejan number, respectively, of the varying Brinkman number (Br). An increase in Br results in a surge in the rate of entropy generation. An upsurge in Br shows a heat transfer increase due to viscous dissipation. Br has an inverse proportional impact on the Bejan number. Augmentation in Br shows that the Bejan number has declined. There is an increase in the Bejan number when one moves across the channel. This may therefore be due to a decrease in the heat transfer through viscous dissipation as you move through the channel from $Y = 0$ to $Y = 1$.

Darcy number's impact on the entropy and Bejan number is shown in Figs. 8 and 9, respectively. An increase in the number of Darcy leads to a fall in entropy.

Table 1 Base fluid (water) and nanoparticles' thermophysical properties

Property	Water	Copper
C_p ($\mathrm{Jkg^{-1}\,K^{-1}}$)	4079	385
K ($\mathrm{Wm^{-1}\,K^{-1}}$)	0.613	401
$\beta \times 10^{-5}$ ($\mathrm{K^{-1}}$)	21	1.67
τ ($\mathrm{kgm^{-3}}$)	997.1	8933

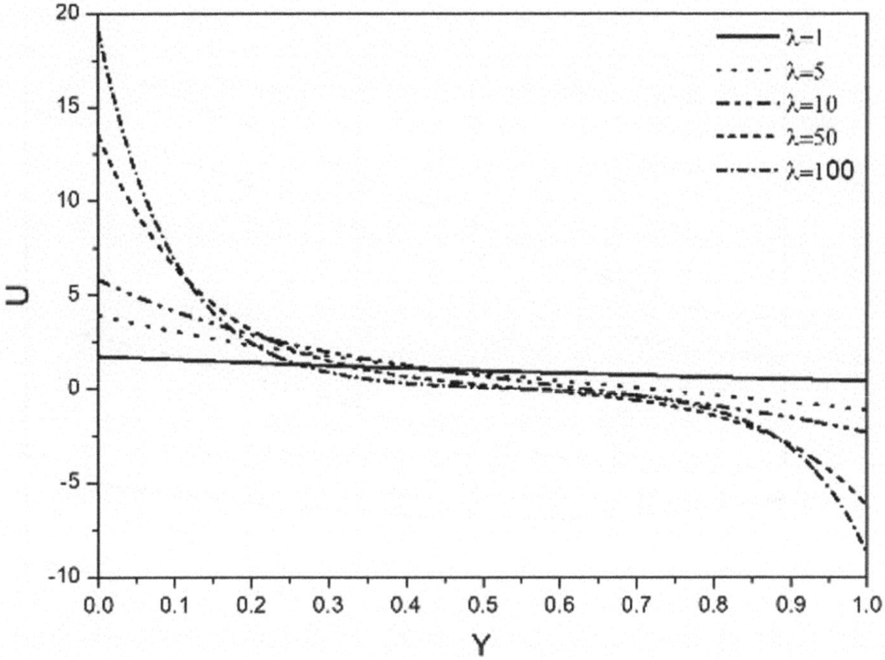

Fig. 2 Reaction of λ on velocity [7]

This is because of the inverse proportionality of the rate of entropy production and Darcy numbers. In addition, increasing the Darcy number results in escalating the permeability of the pore media which makes the flow of the fluid easier. In turn that reduces the rate of entropy production. The number of Bejan is growing with the number of Darcy. It can be seen that the irreversibility of heat transfer dominates the entropy generation of all Da values in the top half of the channel.

In Figs. 10 and 11, the effect of variation on the channel angle on the rate of generation of entropy and Bejan number is shown. Note that $\psi = 0$ represents the horizontal flow and $\psi = \pi/2$ depicts the vertical channel flow. The entropy generation at the base of the channel is at maximum for the horizontal channel flow and decreases slowly as we move upward. There is a minimum, and the entropy rate increases slightly at the top of the channel. The entropy generation rate for a vertical channel is similar near the channel wall but shows a little slump in the center of the channel. For an incline angle less than $\pi/2$, irreversibility by fluid friction dominates entropy generation close to the channel's lower wall, and irreversibility by heat transfer commands the entropy generation near the top of the channel. For a vertical channel, irreversibility by heat transfer is the prominent feature of entropy throughout the channel and is maximum at the center.

As shown in Fig. 12, the mixed convection parameter greatly affects the rate of entropy generation. Generation of entropy reduces near the center of the channel and

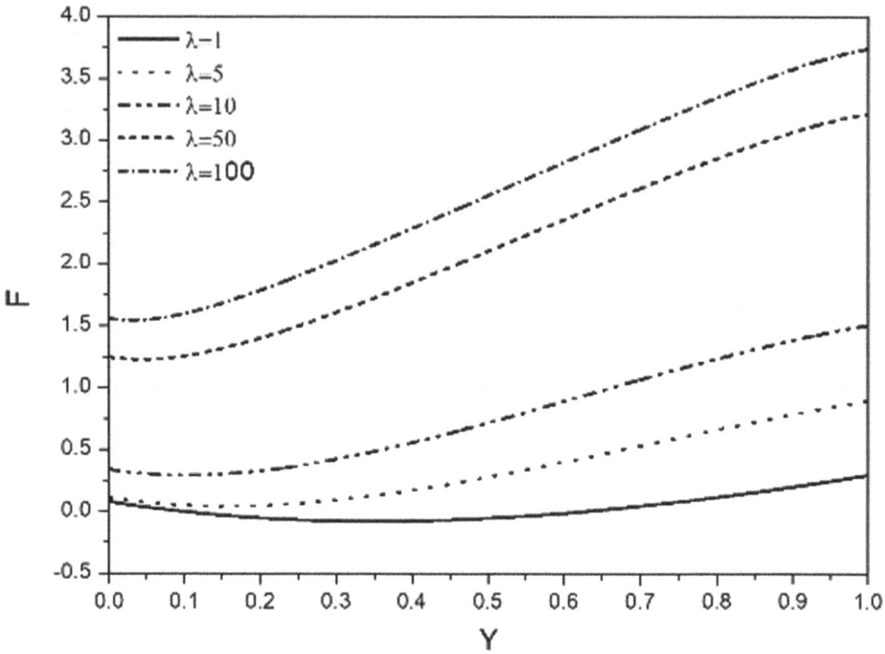

Fig. 3 Reaction of λ on F [7]

maximizes as you approach the walls of the channel. Variation of the mixed convection parameter leads to irreversibility by heat transfer, as seen in Fig. 13, dominating the entropy generation completely. The fluid friction dominates the entropy generation at the bottom wall of the channel at $\lambda = 1$ where buoyancy forces and velocity forces act equally on the flow. The irreversibility by heat transfer slowly takes precedence and reaches complete entropy generation domination near the channel's upper wall. The point where heat transfer completely dominates the rate of entropy generation occurs near the center of the channel as buoyancy forces dominate the flow. However, the irreversibility of fluid friction dominates the entropy generation close to the channel walls when the fluid flow is dominated by buoyancy forces.

Figures 14 and 15, respectively, show the influence of the Peclet numbers on entropy generation rates and Bejan numbers. The entropy generation rate, for high values of Peclet numbers, slightly decreases near the channel center and increases gradually as one moves in the direction of the channel walls. Irreversibility by fluid friction prevails in the entropy generation of high Peclet number flows. The irreversibility by the heat transfer totally dominates the rate of entropy generation in the center of the channel for higher Peclet number values.

From Figs. 16 and 17, the variation in the volume of nanoparticles and their impact on entropy generation rates and Bejan numbers can be noted. Along with the increase of nanoparticle volume fraction, the entropy rate is progressively increasing. This is because the rate of generation of entropy and the volume fraction of nanoparticles

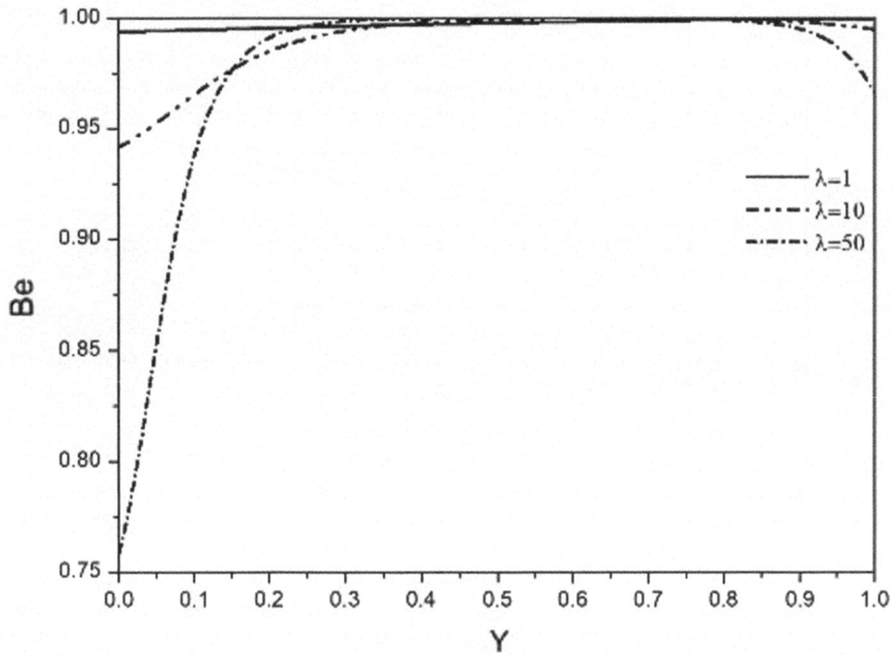

Fig. 4 Reaction of λ on Be [7]

are inversely proportional. For the subjected values of nanoparticle volume fraction, however, the entropy generation rate declines across the channel. Bejan number also shows an upsurge with the increase in the volume fraction of nanoparticles. The irreversibility by fluid friction dominates on the bottom while the irreversibility by heat transfer is domineering on the upper wall of the conduit.

Figures 18 and 19 show the radiation parameter influence on the entropy generation rates and Bejan number. Radiation increases lead to a surge in the rate of entropy generation. This is an expected phenomenon. The Bejan number shows growth with radiation parameter increase as well. It can be observed that the irreversibility by fluid friction prevails at the bottom of the canal, while heat transfer predominates at the top. There is a point near the channel top, where heat transfer dominates entropy generation completely.

6 Conclusion

This article explores the entropy generation analysis for a mixed nanofluid convection flow in a sloping conduit, with thermal radiation, filled with saturated porous medium. Analytically, the governing equations are solved. Inspection of the entropy generation is conducted for several relevant flow parameters. Graphs are plotted and studied meticulously. The following conclusions are made from our analysis:

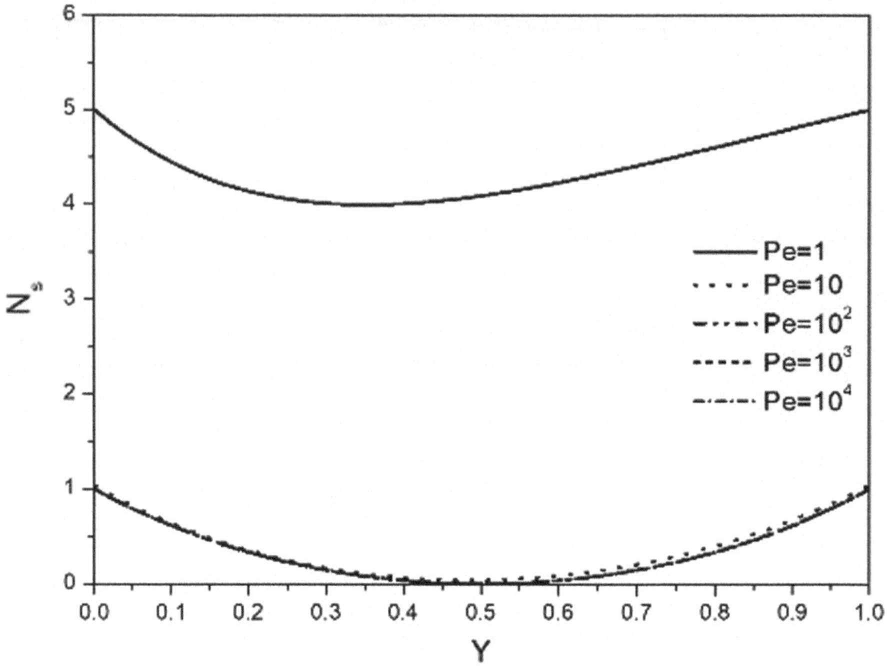

Fig. 5 Reaction of Pe on N_S [13]

- A radiation parameter increase stimulates flow entropy generation. The same is true of the Bejan number.
- In the entropy generation rate, a mixed convection parameter has a great influence. The entropy generation for the buoyancy-driven flows is commanded by fluid friction irreversibility.
- Brinkman number has a highly significant effect on the rate of entropy generation and Bejan number.
- The inclination angle of the channel and its effect on entropy and Bejan numbers are studied. For horizontal and vertical channel flows, there is a significant difference.

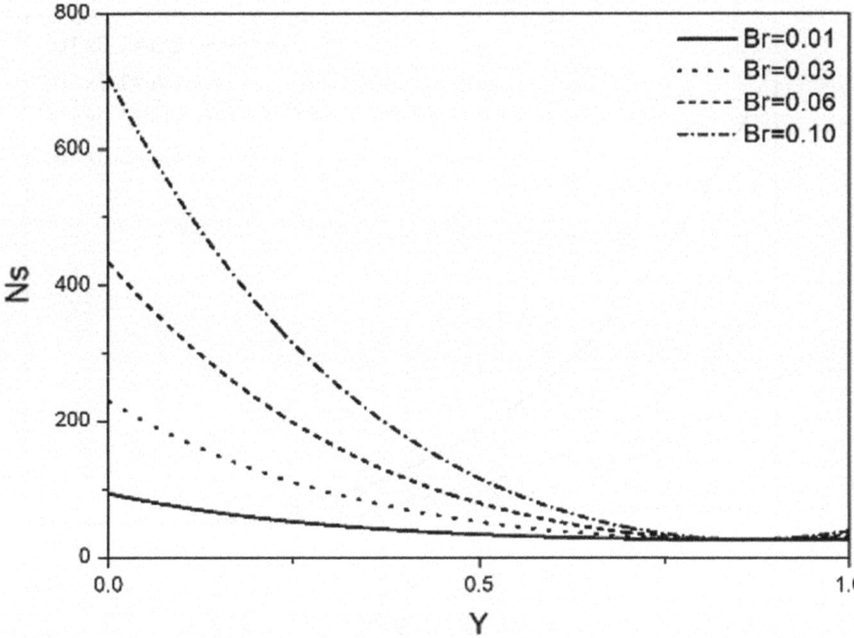

Fig. 6 Reaction of Br on entropy generation rate

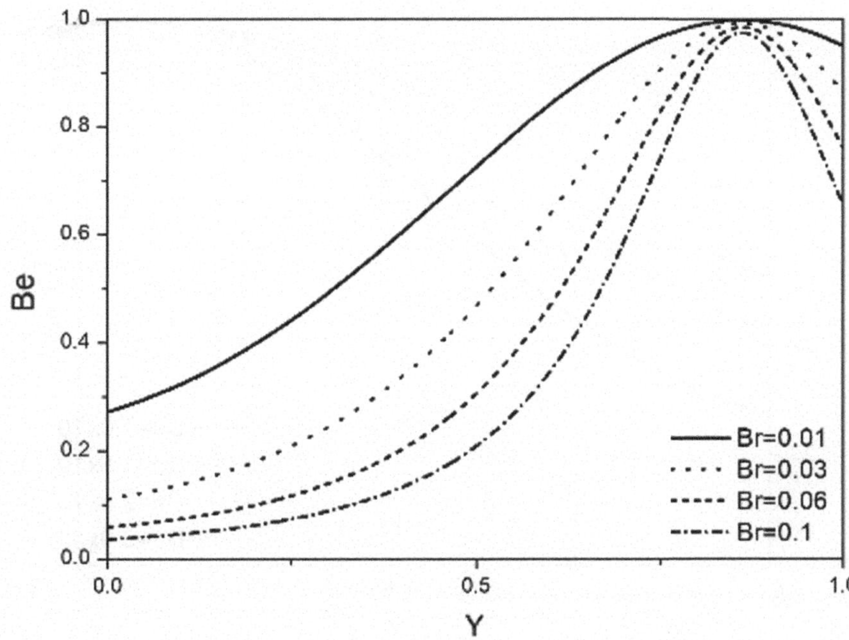

Fig. 7 Reaction of Br on Be

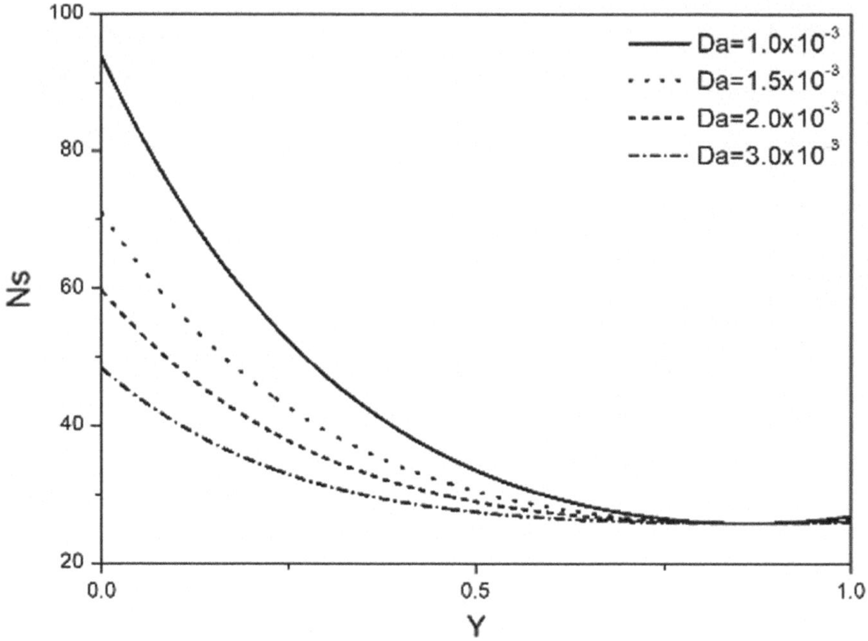

Fig. 8 Reaction of Da on N_S

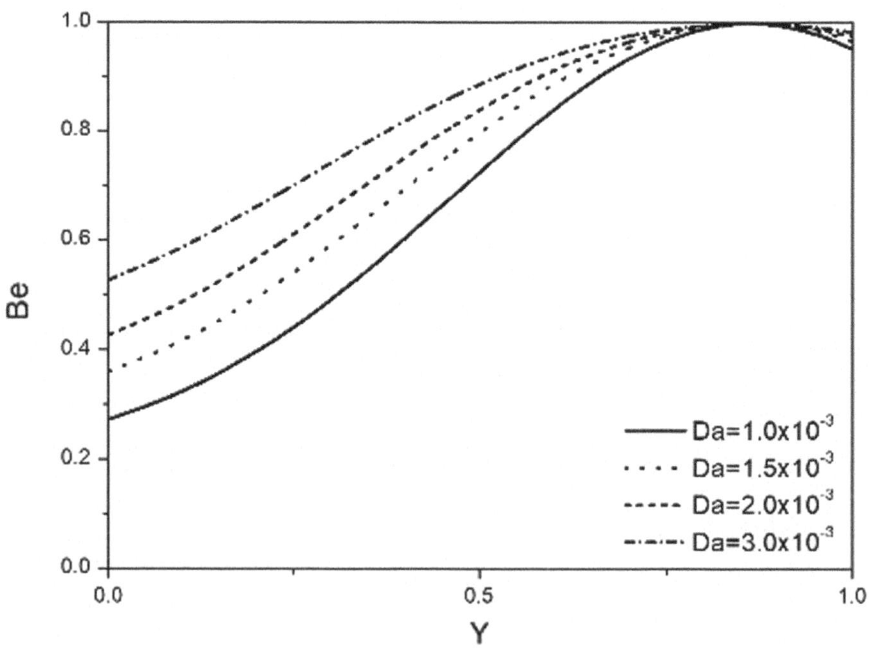

Fig. 9 Reaction of Da on Be

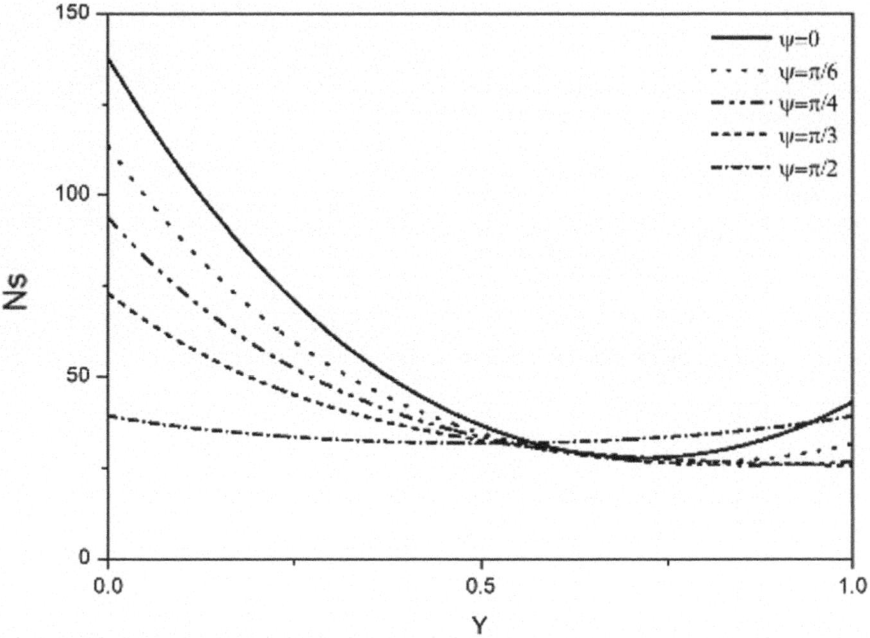

Fig. 10 Reaction of ψ on N_s

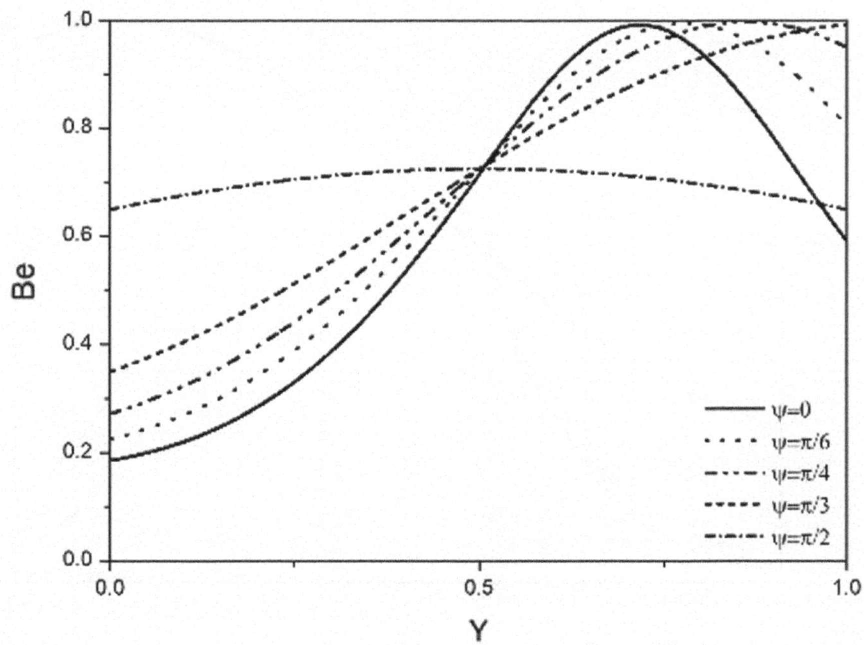

Fig. 11 Reaction of ψ on Be

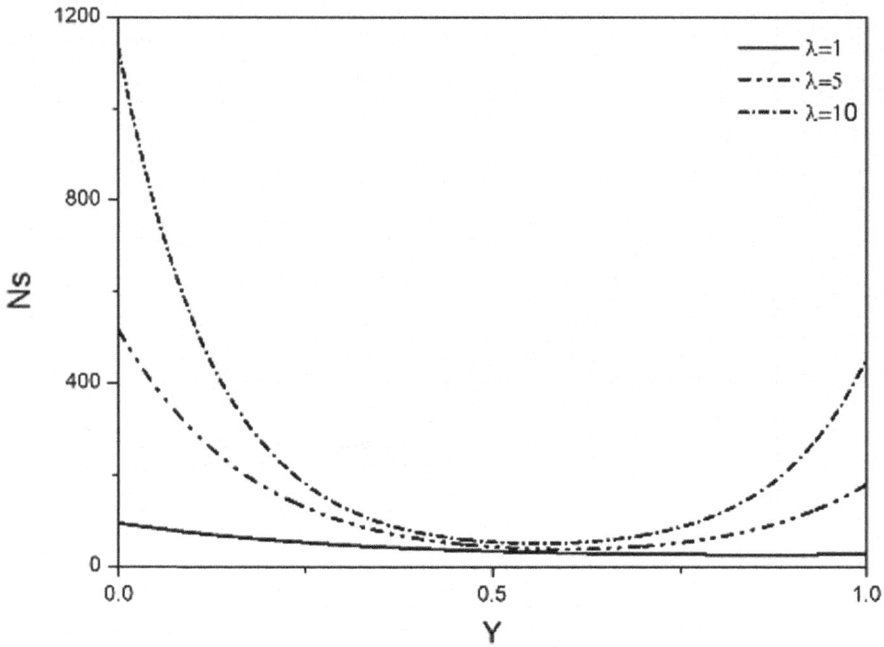

Fig. 12 Reaction of λ on N_s

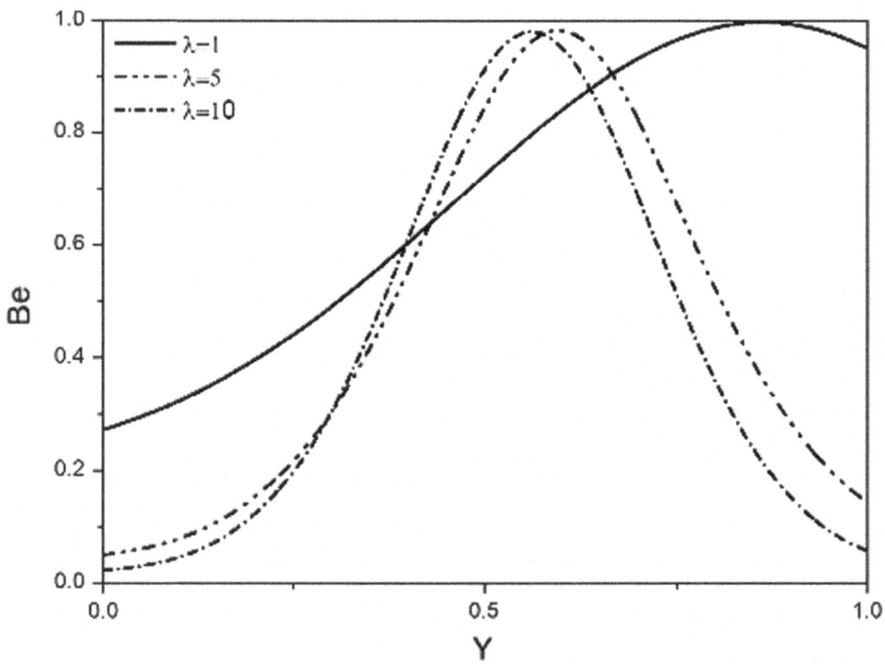

Fig. 13 Reaction of λ on Be

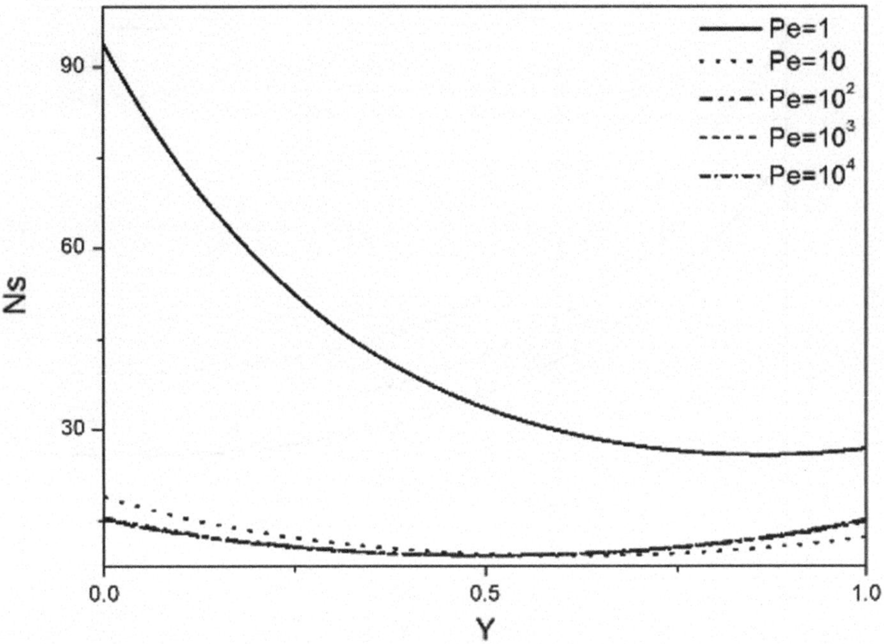

Fig. 14 Reaction of Pe on N_s

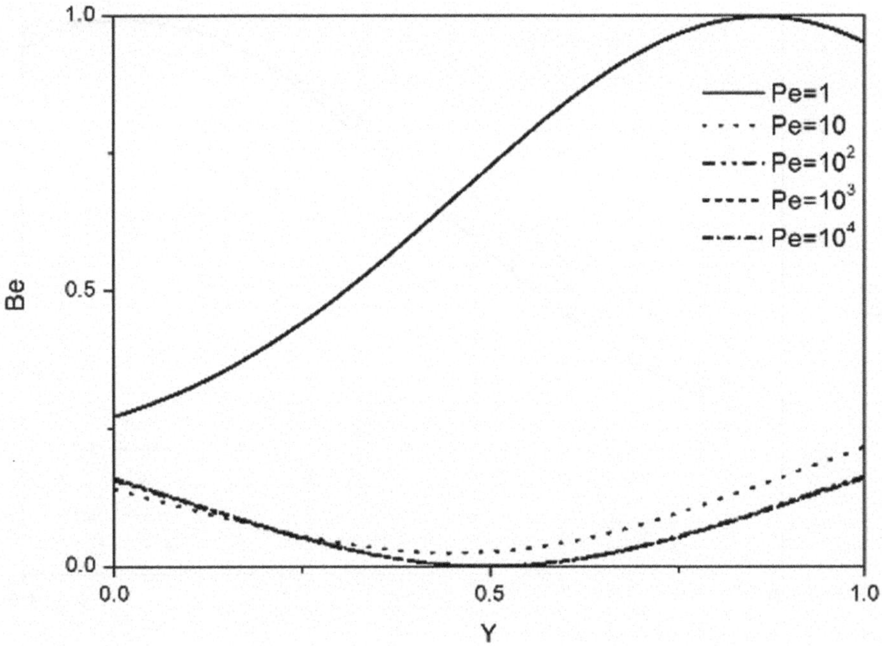

Fig. 15 Reaction of Pe on Be

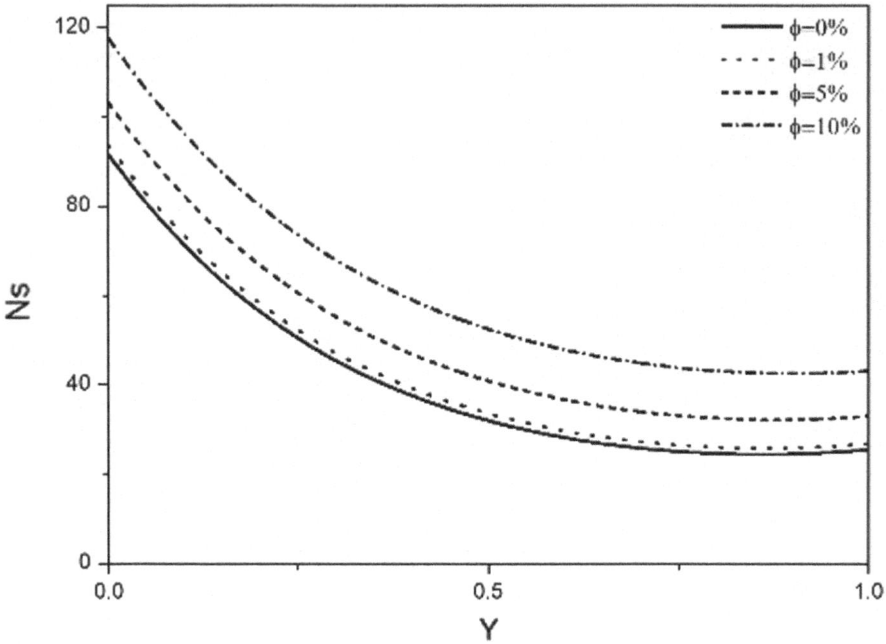

Fig. 16 Reaction of ϕ on N_s

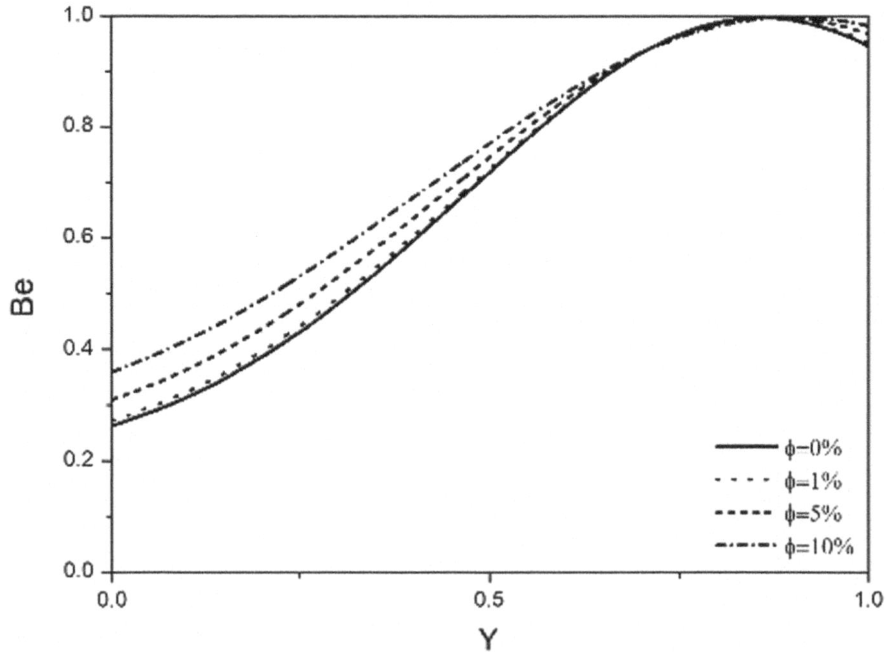

Fig. 17 Reaction of ϕ on Be

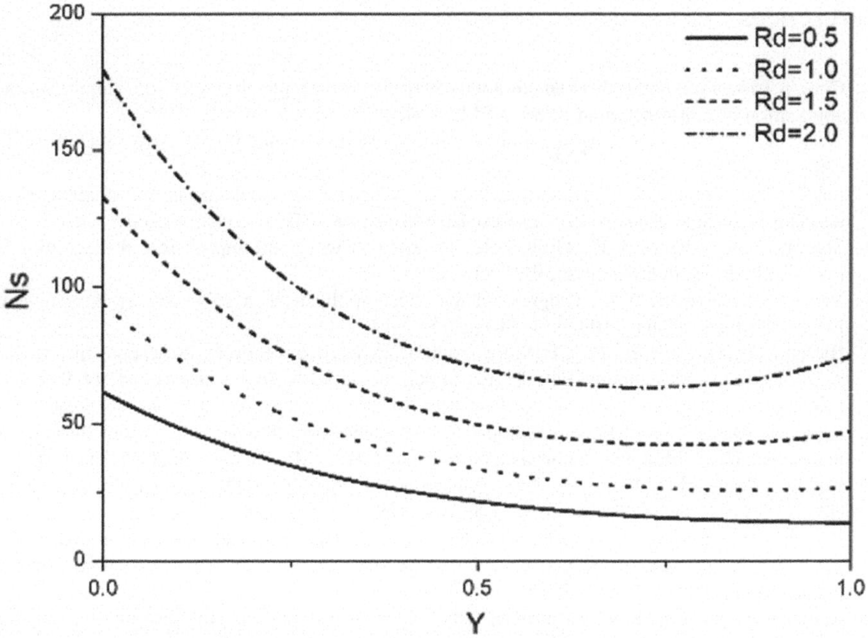

Fig. 18 Reaction of Rd on N_s

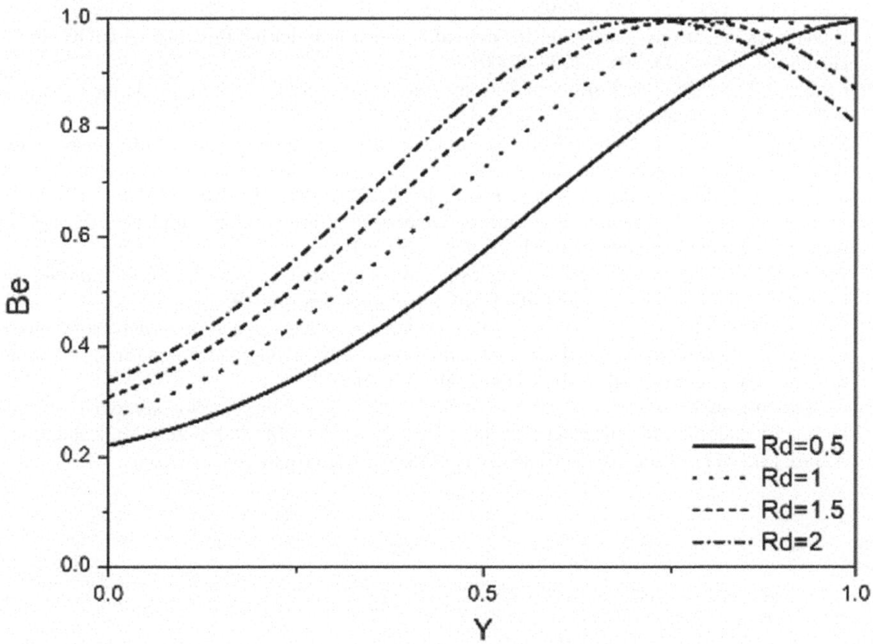

Fig. 19 Reaction of Rd on Be

References

1. Choi, S.U.S.: Enhancing thermal conductivity of fluids with nanoparticles, developments and application of non-newtonian flows. ASME J. Heat Transf. **66**, 99–105 (1995)
2. Wong, K.V., De Leon, O.: Applications of nanofluids: current and future. Adv. Mech. Eng. 11 (2010)
3. Saidura, R., Leong, K.Y., Mohammad, H.A.: A review on applications and challenges of nanofluids. Renew. Sustain. Energy Rev. **15**, 1646–1668 (2011)
4. Sharma, A.K., Tiwari, A.K., Dixit, A.R.: Progress of nanofluid application in machining: a review. Mater. Manuf. Process. **30**(7), 813–828 (2015)
5. Verma, S.K., Tiwari, A.K.: Progress of nanofluid application in solar collectors: a review. Energy Convers. Manag. **100**, 324–346 (2015)
6. Barletta, A., Magyari, E., Pop, I., Storesletten, L.: Mixed convection with viscous dissipation in an inclined porous channel with isoflux impermeable walls. Heat Mass Transf. **44**, 979–988 (2008)
7. Cimpean, D.S., Pop, I.: Fully developed mixed convection flow of a nanofluid through an inclined channel filled with a porous medium. Int. J. Heat Mass Transf. **55**, 907–914 (2012)
8. Liu, I.C., Wang, H.H., Umavathi, J.C..: Poiseuille-Couette flow and heat transfer in an inclined channel for composite porous medium. J. Mech. **28**, 171–178 (2012)
9. Jha, B.K., Daramola, D., Ajibade, A.O.: Mixed Convection in an inclined channel filled with porous material having time-periodic boundary conditions: steady-periodic regime. Transp. Porous Media **109**, 495–512 (2015)
10. Reddy, M.G., Reddy, K.V.I., Makinde, O.D.: Hydromagnetic peristaltic motion of a reacting and radiating couple stress fluid in an inclined asymmetric channel filled with a porous medium. Alexandria Eng. J. **55**, 1841–1853 (2016)
11. Bejan, A.: A study of entropy generation in fundamental convective heat transfer. ASME J. Heat Transf. **101**, 718–725 (1979)
12. Baytas, A.C.: Entropy generation for natural convection in an inclined porous cavity. Int. J. Heat Mass Transf. **43**, 2089–2099 (2000)
13. Cimpean, D.S., Pop, I.: A study of entropy generation minimization in an inclined channel. WSEAS Trans. Heat Mass Transf. **6**(2), 31–40 (2011)
14. Dehsara, M., Dalir, N., Nobari, M.R.H.: Numerical analysis of entropy generation in nanofluid flow over a transparent plate in porous medium in presence of solar radiation, viscous dissipation and variable magnetic field. J. Mech. Sci. Technol. **28**(5), 1819–1831 (2014)
15. Srinivasacharya, D., Bindu, K.H.: Entropy generation in a micropolar fluid flow through an inclined channel. Alexandria Eng. J. **55**, 973–982 (2016)
16. Baskaya, E., Komurgoz, G., Ozkol, I.: Investigation of oriented magnetic field effects on entropy generation in an inclined channel filled with ferrofluids. Entropy **19**, 377 (2017)
17. Hussain, S., Mehmood, K., Sagheer, M., Farooq, A.: Entropy generation analysis of mixed convective flow in an inclined channel with cavity with Al_2O_3-water nanofluid in porous medium. Int. Commun. Heat Mass Transf. **89**, 198–210 (2017)
18. Freidoonimehr, N., Rahimi, A.B.: Comment on "Effects of thermophoresis and Brownian motion on nanofluid heat transfer and entropy generation" by M. Mahmoodi, Sh. Kandelousi. J. Mol. Liq. **211**, 15–24 (2015), J. Mol. Liq. **216**, 99–102 (2016)

Numerical Techniques to Physical Problems

Mixed Convection in a Lid-Driven Inclined Cavity with Discrete Heater on the Lower Wall

Subhasree Dutta and Somnath Bhattacharyya

Abstract The analysis of fluid flow and heat transfer enhancement in a lid-driven square enclosure inclined at an angle ψ and partially heated from below is developed numerically. A heater is placed at the middle of the bottom wall whereas the upper wall, moving horizontally at a constant speed, is maintained at a lessened temperature. Governing discretized equations are solved by applying the finite volume method with a pressure correction-based SIMPLE algorithm. Results are obtained for various parameters such as Richardson number ($0.1 \leq \mathrm{Ri} \leq 3$), solid volume fraction ($0 \leq \phi \leq 0.1$) with the inclination angle varying from $-60°$ to $60°$. The change in the rate of heat transfer due to inclusion of the nanoparticles is investigated. Flow field as well as the heat transfer has dependency on the inclination angle of the enclosure. The augmentation in heat transfer is obtained at a comparatively higher rate than that of the entropy generation in our proposed model.

Keywords Mixed convection · Inclination angle · Entropy generation · Nanofluid

1 Introduction

Convective heat transfer is widely used because of its utilization in engineering, technological and natural processes [1–3]. Many analysis on heat transfer and cavity flow have been conducted using experimental or numerical methods during the last three decades using fluids such as clear fluid and nanofluid. Nanofluid is considered to be a mixture of solid and liquid in where the metallic nanoparticles of approximate size 1–100 nm are suspended within the clear fluid, is considered due to its high heat transfer performance than that of the base fluid. Thermal conductivity as well as the heat transfer rate increases due to the consideration of nanoparticles [4] within the base fluid. The heat transfer characteristics of the nanofluid have a dependency on the volume fraction, shape, size and the thermophysical properties of the base fluid as well as the nanoparticles. Many studies have been done on convection in

S. Dutta (✉) · S. Bhattacharyya
Department of Mathematics, Indian Institute of Technology Kharagpur, Kharagpur 721302, India
e-mail: subhdutt050293@gmail.com

S. Bhattacharyya et al. (eds.), *Mathematical Modeling and Computational Tools*, Springer Proceedings in Mathematics & Statistics 320,
https://doi.org/10.1007/978-981-15-3615-1_13

an enclosure using nanofluid and their heat transfer performance. The experimental study of Xuan and Li [5] shows that the enhancement in heat transfer in the presence of nanofluid is due to the random movement of nanoparticles, which raises the thermal conductivity of the fluid. The experimental results of Ho et al. [6] on Al_2O_3-water nanofluid in the vertically placed enclosures represent that low nanoparticle volume fraction ($\phi \ll 1\%$) attains higher heat transfer rate in comparison with the higher solid volume fraction ($\phi \gg 2\%$). Several numerical studies on the utilization of nanofluid in the convective heat transfer have been reported by researchers [7–11]. Mohammad [12] studied numerically the effect of heat transfer as well as the drop in pressure due to different composition of nanoparticles and clear fluid and concluded that for the water-based nanofluids the pressure drop is minimum, whereas the heat transfer coefficient is maximum in comparison with the others. Convective flow using nanofluid based on different viscosity models on single as well as double lid-driven square enclosures is studied by Chamkha and Abu-Nada [13]. A notable increment is observed in heat transfer for higher values of Ri on the presence of the nanoparticles. The analysis of heat transfer using nanofluid is numerically made by Tiwari and Das [14] considering the variation of solid volume fraction and observed that the increment in heat transfer varies with the solid volume fraction. The flow pattern differs for natural and forced convection-dominated regime due to the presence of nanoparticles.

There are mainly two different approaches for modeling the heat transfer and fluid flow properties of the nanofluid, one of which is homogeneous model. In single-phase model, a thermal equilibrium is maintained between the base fluid and the nanoparticles, moving with the same velocity. On the contrary, in the two-phase model, a velocity is considered between the nanoparticles and the base fluid, and the nanofluid is assumed as nonhomogeneous composition of base fluid along with the nanoparticles. There are several slip mechanisms to generate the relative velocity of which Brownian diffusion and thermophoresis are considered to be the most effective slip mechanisms [15, 16]. For the evaluation of the thermophysical properties of nanofluid, several models are proposed in the literature [17–21]. For the estimation of the thermal conductivity of the nanofluid, Maxwell-Garnett's model [20] is highly used, whereas the Brinkman model [21] is used to estimate the effective viscosity.

Convective heat transfer in rectangular enclosure for natural and mixed convection is studied by several researchers [22–30]. The inclined enclosure is studied by many researchers nowadays because of its importance on the heat and fluid flow [3, 31–33]. Consideration of the inclination angle of the enclosure is also taken into account to study the effect of heat transfer as the inclination angle has a major role on temperature and velocity field. Abu-Nada and Chamkha [34] analyzed numerically the convective heat transfer in an inclined lid-driven square enclosure in presence of nanofluid. They found that the heat transfer varies linearly with the increment of inclination angle for natural and mixed convection-dominated regime whereas remain almost invariable in forced convection-dominated case. Effect of inclination angle and nanoparticles on natural convection is studied by Abu-Nada and Ozotop [35]. They observed that the effect of inclination angle on heat transfer has a strong dependency on Rayleigh number and the heat transfer becomes almost negligible at low Rayleigh number.

Ghasemi and Aminossadati [36] considered a suitable range of inclination angle to analyze the effect of heat transfer and found an optimal value of the inclination angle to achieve the maximum rate of heat transfer.

The effect fluid flow and heat transfer due to the convective heat transfer within an enclosure with localized heat source has importance in nowadays research because of its various technological and industrial applications such as in solar energy collectors, air-cooled electronic devices, nuclear reactors and many others. The study of Sivakumar et al. [37] concluded that the effect of size and location of the heat source has an important impact in the heat transfer augmentation as it has dependency on both the position and length of the heater. Studies on buoyancy-dominated heat transfer in the presence of heat sources in the wall of the enclosures were studied by several researchers [38–42]. Mansour and Habib [43] represented the importance of nanofluid for cooling in the presence of three symmetrically spaced heaters. Elif et al. [41] studied the effect of natural convection in inclined cavity, differentially heated, in the presence of different water-based nanofluids. Guo and Muhammad [44] analyzed the effect of partial heat source of constant heat flux on the mixed convection of a square enclosure at different aspect ratios and found an optimal aspect ratio for which the heat transfer rate is maximum.

In our study, we consider the mixed convection using Al_2O_3-water nanofluid in an inclined enclosure. A localized heat source of uniform temperature is kept on the lower wall of the enclosure, whereas the top wall of the enclosure, sliding in horizontally is kept at a lower temperature. The viscosity and thermal conductivity are determined by using MG-Brinkman model. The single-phase model, which ignores the slip velocity of the nanofluid, having the capability of the evaluation of the heat transfer characteristics of the nanofluid, is considered. Consequently, flow pattern, thermal field and heat transfer due to the variation of bulk volume fraction ($0 \leq \phi \leq 0.05$), inclination angle ($-60° \leq \psi \leq 60°$) and Richardson number ($0.1 \leq \mathrm{Ri} \leq 3$) are discussed.

2 Mathematical Model

The physical model of our computation consists of a square enclosure of dimension H, filled with water-Al_2O_3 nanofluid, inclined at an angle ψ with the horizontal (Fig. 1). A heat source of length l is assumed at the center of the bottom wall having an uniform temperature T_{h}. The top wall, moving with constant speed U_0, is considered to be cold (T_{c}). The left and right vertical wall and the rest portion of the lower wall are kept thermally insulated. The nanofluid is assumed to be sufficiently dilute with volume fraction $\phi \leq 0.1$.

The flow is assumed to be two dimensional, Newtonian, laminar and incompressible. The base fluid and the nanoparticles are presumed to be in thermal equilibrium having no slip velocity between them. All the thermophysical properties are assumed

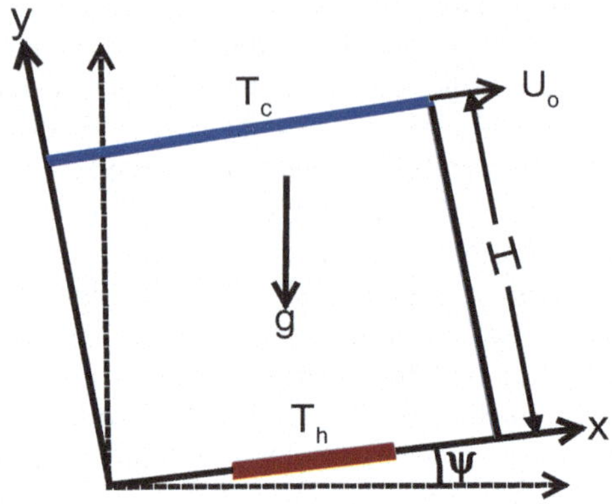

Fig. 1 Geometry of the present model

to be constant, where the density follows the Boussinesq approximation. The chemical reaction between the nanoparticles and the base fluid is assumed to have a negligible effect.

The governing equations in non-dimensional can be expressed as

$$\frac{\partial u}{\partial x}+\frac{\partial v}{\partial y}=0 \tag{1}$$

$$\begin{aligned}\frac{\partial u}{\partial t}+u\frac{\partial u}{\partial x}+v\frac{\partial u}{\partial y}&=-\frac{\partial p}{\partial x}+\frac{1}{\mathrm{Re}}\frac{\rho_{\mathrm{f}}}{\rho_{\mathrm{nf}}}\frac{1}{(1-\phi)^{2.5}}\left(\frac{\partial^2 u}{\partial x^2}+\frac{\partial^2 u}{\partial y^2}\right)\\&+\frac{\mathrm{Gr}}{\mathrm{Re}^2}\frac{\rho_{\mathrm{f}}}{\rho_{\mathrm{nf}}}\left(1-\phi+\phi\frac{\rho_{\mathrm{p}}\beta_{\mathrm{p}}}{\rho_{\mathrm{f}}\beta_{\mathrm{f}}}\right)\theta\sin\psi\end{aligned} \tag{2}$$

$$\begin{aligned}\frac{\partial v}{\partial t}+u\frac{\partial v}{\partial x}+v\frac{\partial v}{\partial y}&=-\frac{\partial p}{\partial y}+\frac{1}{\mathrm{Re}}\frac{\rho_{\mathrm{f}}}{\rho_{\mathrm{nf}}}\frac{1}{(1-\phi)^{2.5}}\left(\frac{\partial^2 v}{\partial x^2}+\frac{\partial^2 v}{\partial y^2}\right)\\&+\frac{\mathrm{Gr}}{\mathrm{Re}^2}\frac{\rho_{\mathrm{f}}}{\rho_{\mathrm{nf}}}\left(1-\phi+\phi\frac{\rho_{\mathrm{p}}\beta_{\mathrm{p}}}{\rho_{\mathrm{f}}\beta_{\mathrm{f}}}\right)\theta\cos\psi\end{aligned} \tag{3}$$

$$\frac{\partial \theta}{\partial t}+u\frac{\partial \theta}{\partial x}+v\frac{\partial \theta}{\partial y}=\frac{k_{\mathrm{nf}}}{k_{\mathrm{f}}}\frac{(\rho C_{\mathrm{p}})_{\mathrm{f}}}{(\rho C_{\mathrm{p}})_{\mathrm{nf}}}\frac{1}{\mathrm{Re\,Pr}}\left(\frac{\partial^2 \theta}{\partial x^2}+\frac{\partial^2 \theta}{\partial y^2}\right) \tag{4}$$

The applied boundary conditions for the defined computational domain are as follows:

$u=1,\ v=0,\ \theta=0$ at $y=1$ and $0\le x\le 1$.
$u=v=0,\ \frac{\partial\theta}{\partial x}=0$ at $x=0,1$ and $0\le y\le 1$.
$u=v=0,\ \theta=1$ at $y=0$ and $l\le x\le l+\varepsilon$.
$u=v=0,\ \frac{\partial\theta}{\partial \mathrm{x}}=0$ at $y=0$ and $0\le x\le l,\ l+\varepsilon\le x\le 1$.

Table 1 Thermophysical properties of clear fluid and Al_2O_3 nanoparticles

Parameter	Water	Al_2O_3
ρ (kg/m^3)	993	3970
k (W/mK)	0.628	40
cp (J/kgK)	4179	765
β (K^{-1})	3.6×10^{-4}	0.85×10^{-5}

l and ε being the dimensionless length of the heater and the distance of the heat source from origin, respectively, i.e. $\varepsilon = l = 1/3$.

The defined non-dimensional variables are characterized by $x = x^*/H, y = y^*/H, t = t^*U_0/H, h = h*/H, u = u^*/U_0, v = v^*/U_0, \theta = (T - T_c)/(T_h - T_c), p = p^*/\rho_{nf}U_0^2$. The dimensionless parameters are defined as Richardson number $Ri = Gr/Re^2$, Grashof number $Gr = \frac{\beta_f g(T_h - T_c)H^3}{\nu_f^2}$, Prandtl number $Pr = \frac{\nu_f}{\alpha_f}$ and Reynolds number $Re = \frac{\rho_f U_0 H}{\mu_f}$.

The heat capacitance for nanofluid is $(\rho_{cp})_{nf} = (1-\phi)(\rho_{cp})_f + \phi(\rho_{cp})_p$. The effective density of nanofluid is given by $(\rho)_{nf} = (1-\phi)\rho_f + \phi\,\rho_p$. The thermal diffusivity is given by $\alpha_{nf} = \frac{k_{nf}}{(\rho_{cp})_{nf}}$. The thermal conductivity of the nanofluid is determined using Maxwell-Garnett's model as $\frac{k_{nf}}{k_f} = \frac{k_p + 2k_f - 2\phi(k_f - k_p)}{k_p + 2k_f + \phi(k_f - k_p)}$ [20]. The effective viscosity is obtained as $\mu_{nf} = \frac{\mu_f}{(1-\phi)^{2.5}}$ using Brinkman model [21].

The thermophysical properties for clear fluid and Al_2O_3 used in our computation are in Table 1.

2.1 Nusselt Number and Entropy Generation

The expression for the local Nusselt number in non-dimensional form is given by $Nu = -\frac{k_{nf}}{k_f}\frac{\partial\theta}{\partial n}$, n being the unit normal to the bottom wall. Averaged value of Nusselt number (Nu_{av}) can be obtained by integrating the local Nu along the heater.

The non-dimensional entropy generation can be defined as

$$S_{gen} = \frac{k_{nf}}{k_f}\left[\left(\frac{\partial\theta}{\partial x}\right)^2 + \left(\frac{\partial\theta}{\partial y}\right)^2\right] + \chi\frac{\mu_{nf}}{\mu_f}\left[2\left(\frac{\partial u}{\partial x}\right)^2 + \left(\frac{\partial v}{\partial y}\right)^2 + \left(\frac{\partial u}{\partial y} + \frac{\partial v}{\partial x}\right)^2\right]$$
$$= S_h + S_f$$

S_h and S_f being the entropy generated by the heat transfer and fluid friction irreversibility and χ is the irreversibility factor, can be defined as $\chi = (\mu_f T_0 U_0^2)/k_f(\Delta T)$, where $T_0 = (T_h + T_c)/2$ is the reference temperature. The average entropy generation S_{av} is defined as

$$S_{\text{av}} = \frac{1}{A} \int_A S_{\text{gen}}\, \mathrm{d}x\, \mathrm{d}y.$$

3 Numerical Procedure

The governing equations in non-dimensional form are solved numerically using finite volume method. The nonlinear governing equations are integrated over each cell of the control volume. A pressure correction-based Semi-Implicit Method for Pressure Linked Equations (SIMPLE) [45] algorithm is used for computation. In the staggered grid arrangement, each of the velocity components (u, v) is stored at the midpoint of the sides on which they are normal whereas the pressure and temperature are stored at the center of each cell. The algebraic equation is solved iteratively by a cyclic series of guess and correct operations using block elimination algorithm. The convergence criterion of this iteration is expressed as $\max_{ij} |\xi_{ij}^{k+1} - \xi_{ij}^{k}| \leq 10^{-5}$ where the symbol ξ denotes for the nondimensional velocities and temperature and the subscripts i, j indicates the index of cell, and superscript k is the index of the computed iteration.

4 Grid Independence Test and Validation of Code

The grid independence test to evaluate the proper grid size for the present model is performed. For this, we compute the local Nusselt number for grid size 150 × 150, 180 × 180, 270 × 270 at Re = 100, $\phi = 0.05$, Ri = 1, and $\psi = 0°$ along the heated portion of the bottom wall (Fig. 2a). It is evident from the result that further improvement from 180 × 180 does not make any noticeable change in the result (Fig. 2a). The 180 × 180 grid system is considered to be optimal. To validate

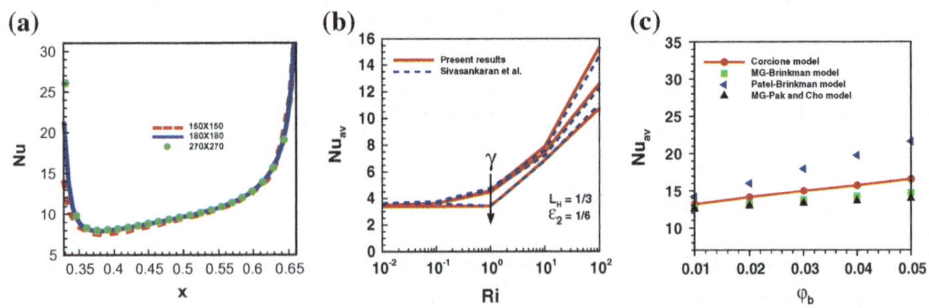

Fig. 2 Grid independence test and code validation with existing result; (**a**) effect of mesh sizes for computing local Nu with different grid sizes, (**b**) comparative result for $\mathrm{Nu_{av}}$ with the numerical result by Sivasankaran et al. [42] at $\phi = 0$, (**c**) comparative study for $\mathrm{Nu_{av}}$ with several models for viscosity and thermal conductivity Ri = 1 and Re = 100.

our present code, the result for the Nu_{av} is compared with the numerically obtained results by Sivasankaran et al. [42] in a lid-driven square enclosure considering the pure fluid ($\phi = 0$) and Re = 100, with the heater at the bottom of the left wall. Analysis indicates a good agreement between the existing result and the present one. Figure 2c presents a comparative study of several models to compute the thermal conductivity and viscosity for obtaining the Nu_{av} for the mixed convection in a square cavity filled with Al_2O_3-water nanofluid with Re = 100 and Ri = 1. It is observed from the result (Fig. 2c) that the heat transfer due to Corcione model [17], MG-Pak and Cho [18] model and MG-Brinkman model [20, 21] is almost same compared to the model suggested by Patel [19]. In the present study, to determine the viscosity and the thermal conductivity, we use MG-Brinkman model in our computation.

5 Results and Discussions

Mixed convection of Al_2O_3-water nanofluid in a square cavity with discrete heat source has been studied for different inclination angles ($-60° \leq \psi \leq 60°$), bulk volume fraction ($0 \leq \phi \leq 0.1$). In our present study, we kept fixed the value of the Reynolds number at Re = 100 and varied the value of the Grashof number (Gr) from 10^3 to 3×10^4 to study the relative effect of buoyancy-dominated natural convection and lid-driven forced convection. Streamlines and isotherms are studied to describe the effect of nanofluid on flow and thermal field. Enhancement in heat transfer and the analysis of energy variation of the system are discussed through the variation of Nu_{av} and S_{av}.

5.1 Fluid Flow and Thermal Fields

Figure 3 illustrates the variation of the flow field with the deviation of inclination angle (ψ) at different Ri. Streamlines are studied in the presence of nanoparticles in all modes of convection. Due to the existence of temperature gradient between the hot and cold walls and movement of the top lid, the cold fluid goes downward whereas the heated fluid rises from the bottom wall in upward direction forming a clockwise flow pattern inside the cavity. The flow strength rises, and the streamlines become denser for increased value of Ri. The effect of buoyancy force is negligible in comparison with the shear effect for lower values of Ri. Figure 3 shows that in forced convection-dominated regime (Ri < 1) (at $\psi = -30°$, 0° and 30°), the dominating primary eddy occupies most of the cavity generated by the moving lid and two negligible secondary eddies are formed near the bottom wall of the cavity. For higher values of Ri (Ri = 1 and 3), where the buoyancy effect becomes stronger, the primary eddy becomes stronger as compared with the shear-dominated case. In fact, the buoyancy effect grows up when the inclination angle becomes positive ($\psi > 0$). It is found that for a positive inclination angle ($\psi = 30°$) increment in Ri causes

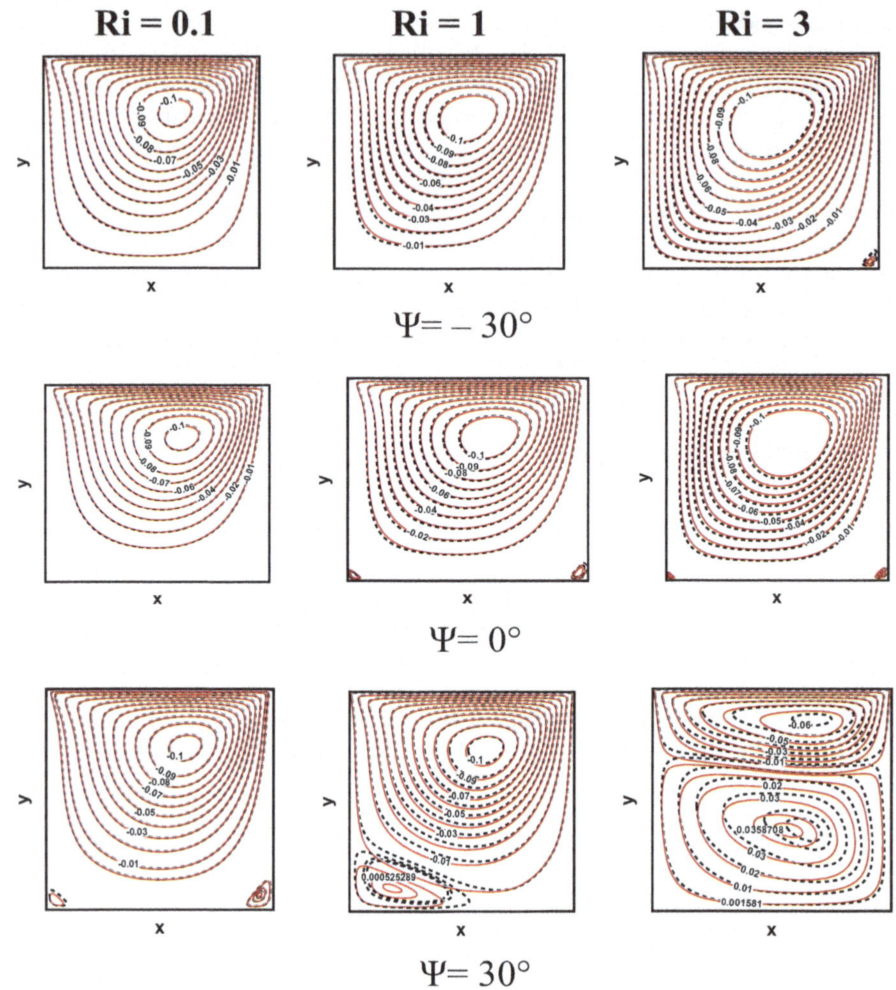

Fig. 3 Variation of flow field with inclination angle (ψ) and bulk volume fraction (ϕ) at different Ri = 0.1, 1 and 3. Dotted and solid lines represent clear fluid ($\phi = 0$) and nanofluid ($\phi = 0.1$), respectively

the formation of strong secondary eddy due to the fact that the primary vortex is created for the presence of shear effect whereas the secondary one for the thermal buoyancy. In fact, recirculation flow size becomes increasing near the bottom wall with the development of buoyancy force. It also should be noted that the inclusion of nanoparticles increases the strength of the flow within the cavity. The primary vortex expands, whereas the secondary eddy reduces with the increase of solid volume fraction.

Figure 4 shows the effect of inclination angle (ψ) and Ri on the thermal field for nanofluid as well as the clear fluid. From the figure, it is seen that the isotherms, heavily clustered near the heated bottom wall, are almost parallel to each other due to the formation of a steep temperature gradient in this region. They are also clustered near the left vertical walls due to the movement of the top wall to the right side. The temperature gradients are weak in the remaining area of the cavity, indicating lower temperature difference in the interior of the enclosure. Due to the increment of Ri, the isotherms move in an upward direction indicating a moderate temperature gradient along the vertical direction of the enclosure. For $\psi = 0°$ i.e. when the enclosure is parallel to the horizontal, the isotherms are nearly parallel to the adiabatic wall

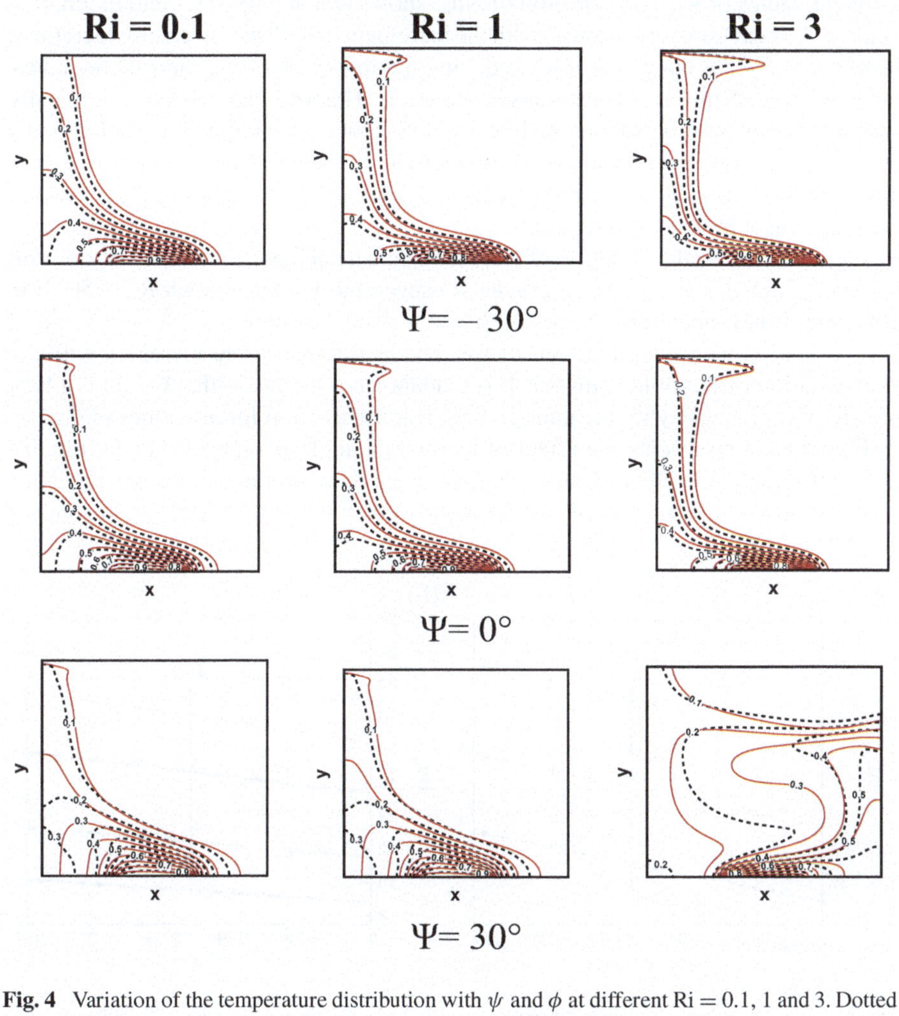

Fig. 4 Variation of the temperature distribution with ψ and ϕ at different Ri = 0.1, 1 and 3. Dotted and solid lines represent clear fluid ($\phi = 0$) and nanofluid ($\phi = 0.1$), respectively.

on the left portion of the cavity, indicating a stratification. The thermal distortion occurs when the inclination angle $\psi > 0°$, indicating a well mixing. The inclusion of nanoparticle enhances the thermal conductivity of the nanofluid as well as thermal gradient near the heated wall. This shows that the inclusion of nanoparticles has a significant effect in the enhancement of heat transfer throughout the enclosure.

5.2 *Effect of Different Parameters on Nu_{av}*

Figure 5a presents the influence of solid volume fraction on heat transfer rate at different values of Ri. The variation of Nu_{av} shows that at a fixed Gr and inclination angle ψ the heat transfer enhances with the increment in Ri. This is because increment in Ri enhances the buoyancy force reducing the thickness of the thermal boundary layer. As a result, the rate of heat transfer increases. The Nu_{av} enhances monotonically with the increment of solid volume fraction ϕ [30]. Increment of nanoparticles inside the enclosure augmented the thermal conductivity of the nanofluid, resulting a higher amount of heat absorption and removal from the hot wall by the nanofluid. As a result, the rate of heat transfer is increased.

Figure 5b shows the variation of Nu_{av} along the heated portion of the bottom wall because of the presence of nanoparticles for several Reynolds number Re = 50, 100, 200, 300. It is found from the result that at a fixed inclination angle, the value of Nu_{av} enhances with the increment of Re. The heat transfer rate increases with the augmentation of Reynolds number. It is evident from the result that the rate of heat transfer rises linearly with the nanoparticle volume fraction for all values of Re.

Figure 6a–c represents the effect of inclination angle ψ on heat transfer rate for different values of Ri. Increment of inclination angle ψ produces a decrease in Nu_{av} for different volume fractions ϕ. As the angle of inclination increases, the secondary

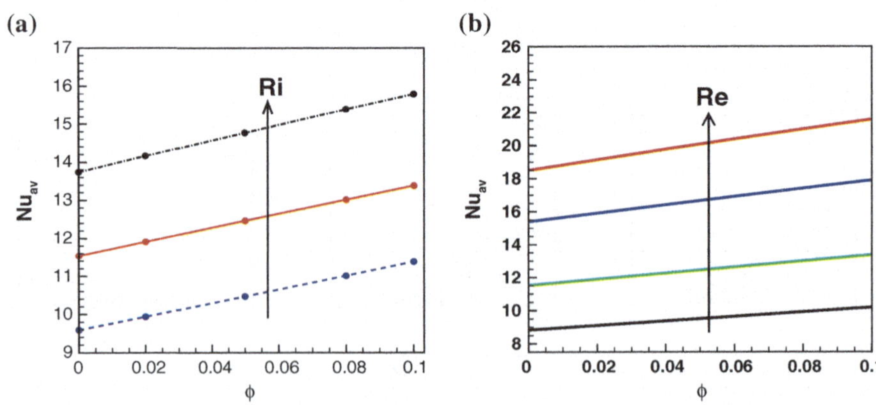

Fig. 5 Variation of Nu_{av} for different (**a**) Ri (= 0.1, 1, 3), (**b**) Re (= 50, 100, 200, 300) with the variation of ϕ at $\psi = 0°$

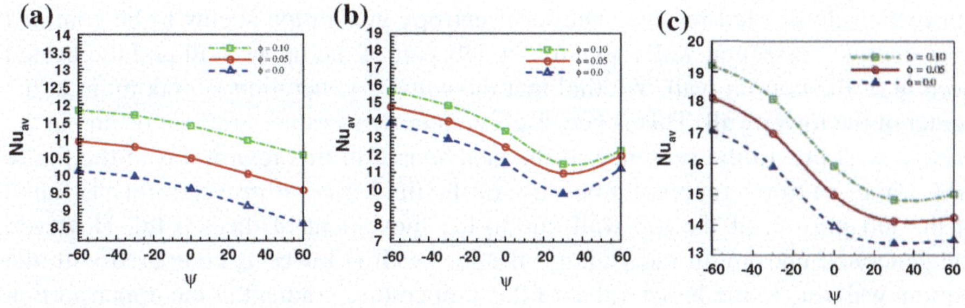

Fig. 6 Variation of Nu_{av} with inclination angle for different ϕ ($\phi = 0, 0.05, 0.1$) at (**a**) Ri = 0.1, (**b**) Ri = 1 and (**c**) Ri = 3

vortex appears within the enclosure. So the flow being trapped, the intensity reduces. At Ri = 0.1, the pattern reduces monotonically with the increment of inclination angle. In mixed convection-dominated regime, where the buoyancy force and the shear force are relatable in the flow field, the heat transfer rate reduces with the increase of ψ. It again increases after $\psi = 30°$ due to the enhancement in buoyancy force with the increment of inclination angle. Similar pattern occurs for higher inclination angle where the natural convection dominates. The maximum Nu_{av} is obtained at $\psi = -60°$ in all modes of convection. It is also found that the Nu_{av} increases significantly due to the rise of bulk volume fraction, for considered values of the inclination angle ψ and Ri.

5.3 Effect of Different Parameters on S_{av}

The impact of fluid friction and heat transfer irreversibility on the generation of entropy is shown in Fig. 7a–c. Results represent the distribution of local entropy generation for clear fluid ($\phi = 0$) as well at $\psi = -30°$, $\psi = 0°$, $\psi = 30°$ in mixed

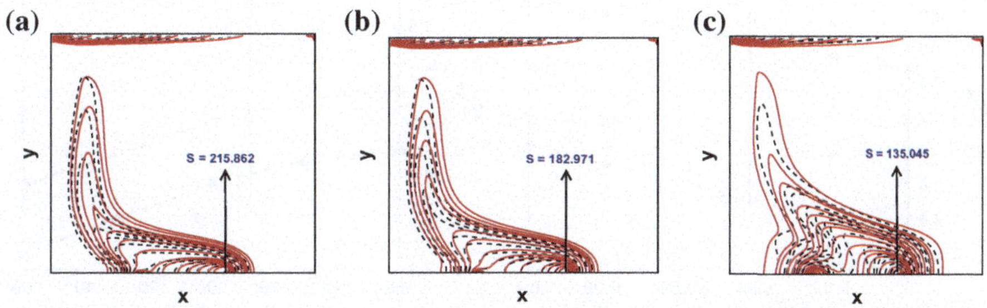

Fig. 7 Variation of local entropy generation as a function of ψ at Ri = 1; inclination angle (**a**) $\psi = -30°$, (**b**) $\psi = 0°$, and (**c**) $\psi = 30°$ for clear fluid ($\phi = 0$ by dotted lines) and nanofluid ($\phi = 0.1$ by solid lines)

convection-dominated regime. The local entropy generation seems to be confined near the two horizontal walls, mainly the left part of the upper wall and the heated portion of the bottom wall. We find that the entropy generation is maximum at the center of the lower wall. This is because a greater temperature gradient occurs in the bottom wall due to the presence of the heat source in this region. From the figure (Fig. 7a–c), entropy generation because of the fluid friction irreversibility is found at the left portion of the top wall due to the movement of the top lid. However, the generated entropy in the vicinity of upper wall is lower as compared with the bottom wall due to the lesser value of the temperature gradient at the upper portion of the enclosure. Inside the core of the cavity, the entropy generation is almost diminished due to negligible temperature gradient compared to the other segment of the enclosure. Results show that the entropy generation is highly dependent on the inclination angle. The maximum entropy generation decreases with the increment of the inclination angle. It is noted that the inclusion of the nanoparticles inside the enclosure enhances the entropy generation. Thermal gradient plays the leading role in the enhancement of entropy generation due to the addition of nanoparticles. This is because the presence of nanoparticle creates an increment in the fluid viscosity and the fluid friction irreversibility rises, although it has negligible contribution in entropy generation in comparison with the entropy due to the heat transfer.

Figure 8a presents the influence of the inclusion of nanoparticles on the entropy generation for different inclination angles (ψ). From the result, it is seen that the entropy generation rises with the increasing Ri at Re = 100. This is because the buoyancy force enhances the heat transfer rate, with the increasing Ri. This creates an enhancement in the velocity gradient, consequently the entropy generation due to heat transfer irreversibility [46]. It is evident from the result that S_{av} obtained a linear increment with the inclusion of nanoparticles as described earlier (Fig. 7a–c) in all modes of convection. Figure 8b indicates the effect of the inclination angle on the S_{av} at a fixed Ri = 0.1 for different bulk volume fractions (ϕ). Likewise

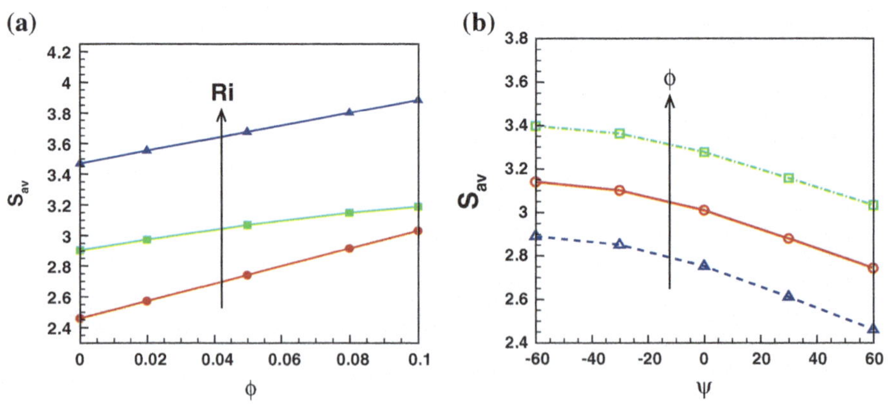

Fig. 8 Variation of S_{av} as a function of (**a**) ϕ for different Ri (0.1, 1, 3) at $\psi = 60°$, (**b**) inclination angle for different ϕ (0, 0.05, 0.1) at Re = 100

the heat transfer, S_{av} also decreases monotonically with the increase of inclination angle (ψ) in forced convection-dominated regime (Ri < 1). For small value of Ri, the effect of fluid friction on entropy generation is negligible. Hence, the viscous effect dominates the energy loss of the system. Also, the value of S_{av} is large for higher ϕ. Inclusion of nanoparticle enhances the thermal conductivity and hence the heat transfer irreversibility, resulting a higher entropy generation for the nanofluid in comparison with the clear fluid ($\phi = 0$). For the sake of brevity, other cases are not shown here.

5.4 Enhancement Factor

We define enhancement factor of Nu_{av} and S_{av} of nanofluid with respect to the clear fluid ($\phi = 0$) as Nu^*_{av} and S^*_{av} given by $\mathrm{Nu}^*_{av} = \mathrm{Nu}_{av}/\mathrm{Nu}_{av}(\phi = 0)$ and $S^*_{av} = S_{av}/S_{av}(\phi = 0)$, respectively. The ratios represent the enhancement of heat transfer and entropy generation of the nanofluid in comparison with the clear fluid ($\phi = 0$). Figure 9 represents the effect of inclination angle on Nu^*_{av} and S^*_{av} for different ϕ. Result shows that the ratios for heat transfer and the entropy generation are greater than 1 indicating a strong influence in heat transfer and entropy generation due to inclusion of nanoparticles inside the enclosure. The rate of enhancement in both the cases increases with the rise of nanoparticle volume fraction as the addition of nanoparticles enhances the thermal conductivity of the nanofluid, and hence, the increment in heat transfer and entropy generation occurs. Figure 9 shows that the heat transfer is enhanced at a higher rate than that of the entropy generation for each nanoparticle volume fraction. In forced convection-dominated regime (Ri < 1), both the ratios increase with the increment of the inclination angle as the buoyancy force

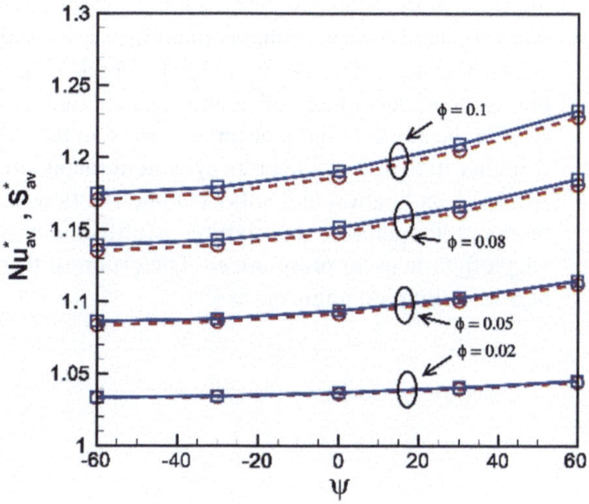

Fig. 9 Variation of Nu^*_{av} (solid lines) and S^*_{av} (dotted lines) with inclination angle for different ϕ at Re = 100 and Ri = 0.1

increases with the increment of inclination angle, creating an enhancement in both the Nu_{av} and S_{av}.

6 Conclusion

The analysis of the flow and thermal field for Al_2O_3-water nanofluid in the presence of discrete heat source is made for a range of inclination angles, bulk volume fractions and the effects of the non-dimensional parameters are discussed in the mixed convective heat transfer. The Nu_{av} and S_{av} are plotted with respect to various parameters to find the influence of nanoparticles on heat transfer and energy loss. Our computation is based upon Maxwell-Garnett's Model and Brinkman model, respectively, for the computation of thermal conductivity and effective viscosity. The observations we get from the analysis of the present study are as follows:

1. The rate of heat transfer as well as the entropy generation augmented with the increment of solid volume fraction at a fixed inclination angle. Inclusion of nanoparticles enhances the heat transfer due to the increment of thermal conductivity of the fluid. It is found that the Nu_{av} is a strictly increasing function of Ri for the reason that buoyancy force dominates the shear-dominated force. Increment in inclination angle decreases the Nu_{av}, and it occurs for higher Ri, when the shear effect is dominated by the buoyancy force, maximum being obtained at $\psi = -60°$ in all modes of convection.
2. Likewise the heat transfer, entropy generation rate is also dependent on solid volume fraction as well as Ri. Increment in S_{av} is due to the large influence of buoyancy effect. It also increases with the increment of nanoparticle volume fraction as the fluid friction irreversibility dominates.
3. The intensification in the rate of heat transfer due to nanofluid in comparison with the clear fluid reduces with the enhancement in Ri, at a fixed inclination angle. Also, the heat transfer enhancement increases with the increment of inclination angle as well as with the increment of bulk volume fraction. The enhancement rate for heat transfer as well as entropy generation due to the presence of nanofluid rises as the angle of inclination increases. In fact, the heat transfer increment rate is higher than that of the entropy generation at a fixed Re.
4. Angle of inclination and solid volume fraction have a strong influence on flow field and temperature distribution. Multicellular vortex appears when the buoyancy effect is more pronounced. Distortion in thermal distribution develops for higher inclination angle ($\psi > 0°$).

References

1. Mehmood, K., Hussain, S., Sagheer, M.: Mixed convection in alumina-water nanofluid filled lid-driven square cavity with an isothermally heated square blockage inside with magnetic field effect, Introduction. Int. J. Heat Mass Transf. **109**, 397–409 (2017)
2. Sheremet, A.M., Pop, I.: Mixed convection in a lid-driven square cavity filled by a nanofluid: Buongiorno's mathematical model. Appl. Math. Comput. **266**, 792–808 (2015)
3. Teamah, M.A., Sorour, M.M., El-Maghlany, W.M., Afifi, A.: Numerical simulation of double diffusive laminar mixed convection in shallow inclined cavities with moving lid. Alexandria Eng. J. **52**(3), 227–239 (2013)
4. Wang, X., Xu, X., Choi, S.U.S.: Thermal conductivity of nanoparticle-fluid mixture. J. Thermophys. Heat Transfer **13**(4), 474–480 (1999)
5. Xuan, Y., Li, Q.: Investigation on convective heat transfer and flow features of nanofluids. J. Heat Transf. **125**(1), 151–155 (2003)
6. Ho, C.J., Liu, W.K., Chang, Y.S., Lin, C.C.: Natural convection heat transfer of alumina-water nanofluid in vertical square enclosures: an experimental study. Int. J. Therm. Sci. **49**(8), 1345–1353 (2010)
7. Abu-Nada, E., Masoud, Z., Oztop, H.F., Campo, A.: Effect of nanofluid variable properties on natural convection in enclosures. Int. J. Therm. Sci. **49**(3), 479–491 (2010)
8. Khanafer, K., Vafai, K., Lightstone, M.: Buoyancy-driven heat transfer enhancement in a two-dimensional enclosure utilizing nanofluids. Int. J. Heat Mass Transf. **46**(19), 3639–3653 (2003)
9. Maga, S.E.B., Nguyen, C.T., Galanis, N., Roy, G.: Heat transfer behaviors of nanofluids in a uniformly heated tube. Superlattices Microstruct. **35**(3), 543–557 (2004)
10. Roy, G., Nguyen, C.T., Lajoie, P.-R.: Numerical investigation of laminar flow and heat transfer in a radial flow cooling system with the use of nanofluids. Superlattices Microstruct. **35**(3–6), 497–511 (2004)
11. Cho, C.C., Chen, C.L.: Mixed convection heat transfer performance of water-based nanofluids in lid-driven cavity with wavy surfaces. Int. J. Therm. Sci. **68**, 181–190 (2013)
12. Kalteh, M.: Investigating the effect of various nanoparticle and base liquid types on the nanofluids heat and fluid flow in a microchannel. Appl. Math. Model. **37**(18-19), 8600–8609 (2013)
13. Chamkha, A.J., Abu-Nada, E.: Mixed convection flow in single-and double-lid driven square cavities filled with water-Al_2O_3 nanofluid: effect of viscosity models. Eur. J. Mech. B/Fluids **36**, 82–96 (2012)
14. Tiwari, R.K., Das, M.K.: Heat transfer augmentation in a two-sided lid-driven differentially heated square cavity utilizing nanofluids. Int. J. Heat Mass Transf. **50**(9-10), 2002–2018 (2007)
15. Buongiorno, J.: Convective transport in nanofluids. J. Heat Transf. **128**(3), 240–250 (2006)
16. Alsabery, A.I., Ismael, M.A., Chamkha, A.J., Hashim, I.: Mixed convection of Al_2O_3-water nanofluid in a double lid-driven square cavity with a solid inner insert using Buongiorno's two-phase model. Int. J. Heat Mass Transf. **119**, 939–961 (2018)
17. Corcione, M.: Empirical correlating equations for predicting the effective thermal conductivity and dynamic viscosity of nanofluids. Energy Convers. Manag. **52**(1), 789–793 (2011)
18. Pak, B.C., Cho, Y.I.: Hydrodynamic and heat transfer study of dispersed fluids with submicron metallic oxide particles. Exp. Heat Transf. Int. J. **11**(2), 151–170 (1998)
19. Patel, H.E., Anoop, K.B., Sundararajan, T., Das, S.K.: A micro-convection model for thermal conductivity of nanofluids. In: International Heat Transfer Conference 13. Begel House Inc. (2006)
20. Maxwell, J.: A Treatise on Electricity and Magnetism, vol. 1. Clarendon press (1881)
21. Brinkman, H.C.: The viscosity of concentrated suspensions and solutions. J. Chem. Phys. **20**(4), 571 (1952)
22. Basak, T., Chamkha, A.J.: Heatline analysis on natural convection for nanofluids confined within square cavities with various thermal boundary conditions. Int. J. Heat Mass Transf. **55**(21–22), 5526–5543 (2012)

23. Kuznetsov, G.V., Sheremet, M.A.: Conjugate natural convection in an enclosure with a heat source of constant heat transfer rate. Int. J. Heat Mass Transf. **54**(1–3), 260–268 (2011)
24. Choi, S.K., Kim, S.O., Lee, T.H., Dohee-Hahn, : Computation of the natural convection of nanofluid in a square cavity with homogeneous and nonhomogeneous models. Numer. Heat Transf., Part A: Appl. **65**(4), 287–301 (2014)
25. Rahman, M.M., Billah, M.M., Hasanuzzaman, M., Saidur, R., Rahim, N.A.: Heat transfer enhancement of nanofluids in a lid-driven square enclosure. Numer. Heat Transf., Part A: Appl. **62**(12), 973–991 (2012)
26. Talebi, F., Mahmoudi, A.H., Shahi, M.: Numerical study of mixed convection flows in a square lid-driven cavity utilizing nanofluid. Int. Commun. Heat Mass Transf. **37**(1), 79–90 (2010)
27. Sebdani, S.M., Mahmoodi, M., Hashemi, S.M.: Effect of nanofluid variable properties on mixed convection in a square cavity. Int. J. Therm. Sci. **52**, 112–126 (2012)
28. Sheikhzadeh, G.A., Qomi, M.E., Hajialigol, N., Fattahi, A.: Numerical study of mixed convection flows in a lid-driven enclosure filled with nanofluid using variable properties. Results Phys. **2**, 5–13 (2012)
29. Mahmoodi, M.: Mixed convection inside nanofluid filled rectangular enclosures with moving bottom wall. Therm. Sci. **15**(3), 889–903 (2011)
30. Nayak, R.K., Bhattacharyya, S., Pop, I.: Numerical study on mixed convection and entropy generation of a nanofluid in a lid-driven square enclosure. J. Heat Transf. **138**(1), 012503 (2016)
31. Ben-Nakhi, A., Chamkha, A.J.: Natural convection in inclined partitioned enclosures. Heat mass Transf. **42**(4), 311–321 (2006)
32. Cheong, H.T., Siri, Z., Sivasankaran, S.: Effect of aspect ratio on natural convection in an inclined rectangular enclosure with sinusoidal boundary condition. Int. Commun. Heat Mass Transf. **45**, 75–85 (2013)
33. Nayak, R.K., Bhattacharyya, S., Pop, I.: Heat transfer and entropy generation in mixed convection of a nanofluid within an inclined skewed cavity. Int. J. Heat Mass Transf. **102**, 596–609 (2016)
34. Abu-Nada, E., Chamkha, A.J.: Mixed convection flow in a lid-driven inclined square enclosure filled with a nanofluid. Eur. J. Mech.-B/Fluids **29**(6), 472–482 (2010)
35. Abu-Nada, E., Oztop, H.F.: Effects of inclination angle on natural convection in enclosures filled with Cu-water nanofluid. Int. J. Heat Fluid Flow **30**(4), 669–678 (2009)
36. Ghasemi, B., Aminossadati, S.M.: Natural convection heat transfer in an inclined enclosure filled with a water-CuO nanofluid. Numer. Heat Transf., Part A: Appl. **55**(8), 807–823 (2009)
37. Sivakumar, V., Sivasankaran, S., Prakash, P., Lee, J.: Effect of heating location and size on mixed convection in lid-driven cavities. Comput. Math Appl. **59**(9), 3053–3065 (2010)
38. Nithyadevi, N., Kandaswamy, P., Lee, J.: Natural convection in a rectangular cavity with partially active side walls. Int. J. Heat Mass Transf. **50**(23-24), 4688–4697 (2007)
39. Cheikh, N.B., Beya, B.B., Lili, T.: Influence of thermal boundary conditions on natural convection in a square enclosure partially heated from below. Int. Commun. Heat Mass Transf. **34**(3), 369–379 (2007)
40. Alam, P., Kumar, A., Kapoor, S., Ansari, S.R.: Numerical investigation of natural convection in a rectangular enclosure due to partial heating and cooling at vertical walls. Commun. Nonlinear Sci. Numer. Simul. **17**(6), 2403–2414 (2012)
41. Elif, B.O.: Natural convection of water-based nanofluids in an inclined enclosure with a heat source. Int. J. Therm. Sci. **48**(11), 2063–2073 (2009)
42. Sivasankaran, S., Sivakumar, V., Hussein, A.K.: Numerical study on mixed convection in an inclined lid-driven cavity with discrete heating. Int. Commun. Heat Mass Transf. **46**, 112–125 (2013)
43. Ben-Mansour, R., Habib, M.A.: Use of nanofluids for improved natural cooling of discretely heated cavities. Adv. Mech. Eng. **5**, 383267 (2013 2013
44. Guo, G., Sharif, M.A.: Mixed convection in rectangular cavities at various aspect ratios with moving isothermal sidewalls and constant flux heat source on the bottom wall. Int. J. Therm. Sci. **43**(5), 465–475 (2004)

45. Patankar, S.: Numerical Heat Transfer and Fluid Flow. CRC press (1980)
46. Wang, T., Huang, Z., Xi, G.: Entropy generation for mixed convection in a square cavity containing a rotating circular cylinder using a local radial basis function method. Int. J. Heat Mass Transf. **106**, 1063–1073 (2017)

Discrete Prey–Predator Model with Square Root Functional Response Under Imprecise Biological Parameters

P. Santra and G. S. Mahapatra

Abstract This paper presents a discrete-time prey–predator model in which the prey exhibits herd behavior, and hence, the predator interacts along the outer corridor of the herd of the prey. Due to the unavailability of numerical information of the biological parameters, we consider the model with interval parameters in the parametric functional form. The existence and stability of the proposed model are analyzed. We give a flip bifurcation analysis and chaos control procedure. The bifurcation diagrams, phase portraits and time graphs are presented for different model parameters. Here, we introduce a new concept in bifurcation analysis. The codimension of a bifurcation is the number of parameters which must be varied for the bifurcation to occur. When we consider p as bifurcation parameter, ultimately, we consider here 4 bifurcation parameter in a certain range, but interesting fact is that using our technic, we convert this 4 codim bifurcation in 1 codim. Numerical simulations exhibit that the present model is a chaotic with rich dynamics.

Keywords Discrete prey–predator model · Stability · Bifurcation · Chaos · Interval parameters

1 Introduction

One of the important interactions among species is the predator-prey relationship. The words "predator" and "prey" are almost always used to mean only animals that eat animals, but this idea also applies to plants. The dynamics of prey–predator has been extensively studied because of its universal existence. Several factors affecting the

P. Santra
Maulana Abul Kalam Azad University of Technology, Kolkata 700064, India
e-mail: prasunsantra5@gmail.com

G. S. Mahapatra (✉)
Department of Mathematics, National Institute of Technology Puducherry, Karaikal 609609, India
e-mail: gs.mahapatra@nitpy.ac.in

S. Bhattacharyya et al. (eds.), *Mathematical Modeling and Computational Tools*, Springer Proceedings in Mathematics & Statistics 320,
https://doi.org/10.1007/978-981-15-3615-1_14

dynamics of predator-prey models, such a familiar factors is the functional response. The functional response is linear in the Lotka–Volterra model, which is valid first-order approximations of more general interaction.

In general, researchers [1–20] always developed the prey–predator system with the assumption that the biological parameters are exactly known; however, the scenario is different in practical world. In reality, each of the biological parameters may not be fixed rather varying due to several reasons. Therefore, the biological parameters are very sensible and treated as nonnegative imprecise number instead of fixed real number. Peixoto et al. [21] studied predator-prey fuzzy model. Pal et al. [22] proposed optimal harvesting prey–predator bio-economic model with interval biological parameters. Pal et al. [23] presented quota harvesting model under fuzziness. In our work, we use interval approach.

This paper considers one-prey one-predator discrete system and calculates equilibrium points, stability and bifurcation of the prey–predator system, where at least one biological parameters of the model is an interval number. We present the interval parameters in the parametric function form and then study the parametric prey–predator discrete model. A parametric mathematical program is formulated to find the different behavior of the system for different value of parameter. The proposed procedure is more effective and interesting since we get different behavior of the model using functional form of an interval parameter based on interval-valued technique. The proposed procedure can present different characteristics of the model in a single framework.

The rest of the paper is organized as follows: The second section introduces mathematics for this paper. In section 3, a discrete-time prey– predator model under non-overlapping generation with refuge is formulated. Section 4 expands this model under imprecise biological parameters. Section 5 presents the local stability analysis around the interior fixed point of the proposed model. Discussion on flip bifurcation is on Sect. 6 Chaos Control procedure is given in Sect. 7. Section 8 gives a numerical simulations to support of the proposed model. Finally, this paper ends with a conclusion in Sect. 9.

2 Prerequisite Mathematics

An interval number A is represented by closed interval $[a_l, a_r]$ and defined by $A = [a_l, a_r] = \{x : a_l \leq x \leq a_r, x \in R\}$, where R is the set of real numbers and a_l, a_r are the left and right limit of the interval number, respectively.

Interval-valued function: Let $a, b > 0$ and the interval $[a, b]$ can represent by the interval-valued function as $h(p) = a^{1-p}b^p$ for $p \in [0, 1]$.

Here, we present some arithmetic operations as follows:

Let $A = [a_l, a_u]$ and $B = [b_l, b_u]$ be two interval numbers.

Addition: The interval-valued function for the interval $A + B = [a_l + b_l, a_u + b_u]$, provided $a_l + b_l > 0$, is given by $h(p) = a_L^{1-p} a_U^p$ where $a_L = a_l + b_l$ and $a_U = a_u + b_u$.

Subtraction: The interval-valued function for the interval $A - B = [a_l - b_u, a_u - b_l]$, provided $a_l - b_u > 0$, is given by $h(p) = b_L^{1-p} b_U^p$ where $b_L = a_l - b_u$ and $a_L = a_u - b_l$.

Scalar Multiplication: $\eta A = \eta [a_l, a_u] = \begin{cases} [\eta a_l, \eta a_u]\,;\, if\, \eta \geq 0 \\ [\eta a_u, \eta a_l]\,;\, if\, \eta < 0 \end{cases}$
provided $a_l > 0$ and $b_l > 0$. The interval-valued function ηA is given by $h(p) = c_L^{1-p} c_U^p$ if $\alpha \geq 0$ and $h(p) = -d_U^{1-p} d_L^p$ if $\eta < 0$, where $c_L = \eta a_l$, $c_U = \eta a_u$, $d_U = |\eta| a_u$ and $d_L = |\eta| a_l$.

3 Description of Prey–Predator Model

We consider populations with non-overlapping generation, where all the adults die after they have given birth. General form of prey–predator system in discrete time is as follows:

$$
\begin{aligned}
x_{n+1} &= x_n f(x_n, y_n) = a x_n (1 - x_n) - b\sqrt{x_n} y_n \\
y_{n+1} &= y_n g(x_n, y_n) = c\sqrt{x_n} y_n - d y_n
\end{aligned}
\tag{1}
$$

where $\frac{df}{dy_n} \leq 0$ and $\frac{dg}{dx_n} \geqslant 0$. Here, a, b, c and d are the nonnegative model parameters. The dynamical properties of the above system allow us to get information about the long-run behavior of prey–predator populations. Starting from given initial condition (x_0, y_0), the iteration of Eq. (1) uniquely determines a trajectory of the states of population output in the form of $(x_n, y_n) = T^n(x_0, y_0)$, where $n = 0, 1, 2, ...$

4 Proposed Model Under Impreciseness

So far, most of the prey–predator model are considered in precise environment, but data can not be recorded or collected precisely due to several reasons in reality. Hence, analysis of the model with imprecise parameters gives better results in modeling respect. Uncertain growth rate of prey populations, interspecific competition rates of prey species, predation coefficient and reduction rates of predator species are usually considered as an effect of environmental fluctuations. Reproduction of species depends on various factors, such as temperature, parasites, pathogens, humidity and environmental pollution. Since biological environments of populations are not entirely predictable, the biological parameters of modeling of prey–predator system should be considered as imprecise in nature.

The proposed discrete-time prey–predator model is presented here with the interval coefficient due to the uncertainty of parameter of practical problem in nature.

4.1 Model with Interval Coefficient

Let $\widehat{a}$, $\widehat{b}$, $\widehat{c}$ and $\widehat{d}$ be the interval counterparts of a, b, c and d, respectively. Then, the modified model is

$$\begin{aligned} x_{n+1} &= \widehat{a}x_n(1-x_n) - \widehat{b}\sqrt{x_n}y_n \\ y_{n+1} &= \widehat{c}\sqrt{x_n}y_n - \widehat{d}y_n \end{aligned} \tag{2}$$

where $\widehat{a} \in [a_l, a_u]$, $\widehat{b} \in [b_l, b_u]$, $\widehat{c} \in [c_l, c_u]$ and $\widehat{d} \in [d_l, d_u]$. Also, $a_l > 0, b_l > 0$, $c_l > 0$, and $d_l > 0$.

4.2 Model with Parametric Interval Coefficient

The Eq. (2) can be written in the parametric form as follows

$$\begin{aligned} x_{n+1} &= (a_l)^{1-p}(a_u)^p x_n(1-x_n) - (b_l)^{1-p}(b_u)^p\sqrt{x_n}y_n \\ y_{n+1} &= (c_l)^{1-p}(c_u)^p\sqrt{x_n}y_n - (d_l)^{1-p}(d_u)^p y_n \end{aligned} \tag{3}$$

for $p \in [0, 1]$.

5 Fixed Points and Stability Analysis of Prey–Predator System

To find the fixed points of the system, we have to solve the following nonlinear system of equations:

$x = (a_l)^{1-p}(a_u)^p x(1-x) - (b_l)^{1-p}(b_u)^p\sqrt{x}y$

$y = (c_l)^{1-p}(c_u)^p\sqrt{x}y - (d_l)^{1-p}(d_u)^p y$

From the above nonlinear system of equations, we get these nonnegative fixed points as follows:

$(i)\, P_0 = (0, 0)$, $(ii)\, P_1 = \left(\frac{(a_l)^{1-p}(a_u)^p - 1}{(a_l)^{1-p}(a_u)^p}, 0\right)$, $(a_l)^{1-p}(a_u)^p > 1$, $(iii)\, P_2 = (x^*, y^*)$

where $x^* = \left(\frac{(d_l)^{1-p}(d_u)^p + 1}{(c_l)^{1-p}(c_u)^p}\right)^2$

and $y^* = \frac{(a_l)^{1-p}(a_u)^p((d_l)^{1-p}(d_u)^p+1)}{(b_l)^{1-p}(b_u)^p(c_l)^{1-p}(c_u)^p}\left[1 - \frac{1}{(a_l)^{1-p}(a_u)^p} - \left(\frac{(d_l)^{1-p}(d_u)^p+1}{(c_l)^{1-p}(c_u)^p}\right)^2\right]$,

$\left[\frac{1}{(a_l)^{1-p}(a_u)^p} + \left(\frac{(d_l)^{1-p}(d_u)^p+1}{(c_l)^{1-p}(c_u)^p}\right)^2\right] < 1$

5.1 Dynamic Behavior of the Model

This section presents the local behavior of the model (3) for each equilibrium points of the prey–predator system. The stability of the system (3) is carried out by computing the Jacobian matrix corresponding to each equilibrium point. The Jacobian matrix J for the system (3) is

$$J = \begin{bmatrix} (a_l)^{1-p}(a_u)^p(1-2x) - \frac{(b_l)^{1-p}(b_u)^p y}{2\sqrt{x}} & -(b_l)^{1-p}(b_u)^p\sqrt{x} \\ \frac{(c_l)^{1-p}(c_u)^p y}{2\sqrt{x}} & (c_l)^{1-p}(c_u)^p\sqrt{x} - (d_l)^{1-p}(d_u)^p \end{bmatrix}$$

Characteristic equation of matrix J is $\lambda^2 - \text{Tr}(J)\,\lambda + \text{Det}(J) = 0$ where

$$\begin{aligned}\text{Tr}(J) &= \text{Trace of matrix } J \\ &= \left[(a_l)^{1-p}(a_u)^p(1-2x) - \frac{(b_l)^{1-p}(b_u)^p y}{2\sqrt{x}}\right] + \left[(c_l)^{1-p}(c_u)^p\sqrt{x} - (d_l)^{1-p}(d_u)^p\right]\end{aligned}$$

$$\begin{aligned}\text{Det}(J) &= \text{Determinant of matrix } J \\ &= (a_l)^{1-p}(a_u)^p(1-2x)\left((c_l)^{1-p}(c_u)^p\sqrt{x} - (d_l)^{1-p}(d_u)^p\right) \\ &\quad + \frac{(b_l)^{1-p}(b_u)^p(d_l)^{1-p}(d_u)^p y}{2\sqrt{x}}\end{aligned}$$

Hence, the model (3) is a dissipative dynamical system if

$$\left|(a_l)^{1-p}(a_u)^p(1-2x)\left((c_l)^{1-p}(c_u)^p\sqrt{x} - (d_l)^{1-p}(d_u)^p\right) + \frac{(b_l)^{1-p}(b_u)^p(d_l)^{1-p}(d_u)^p y}{2\sqrt{x}}\right| < 1$$

conservative dynamical one, if and only if

$$\left|(a_l)^{1-p}(a_u)^p(1-2x)\left((c_l)^{1-p}(c_u)^p\sqrt{x} - (d_l)^{1-p}(d_u)^p\right) + \frac{(b_l)^{1-p}(b_u)^p(d_l)^{1-p}(d_u)^p y}{2\sqrt{x}}\right| = 1$$

and is an un-dissipated dynamical system otherwise.

In order to study the stability of the fixed points of the model, we first give the following lemma

Lemma 1 *Let $F(\lambda) = \lambda^2 - B\lambda + C$. Suppose that $F(1) > 0$, λ_1 and λ_2 are the two roots of $F(\lambda) = 0$. Then*

(i) $|\lambda_1| < 1$ and $|\lambda_2| < 1$ if and only if $F(-1) > 0$ and $C < 1$;
(ii) $|\lambda_1| < 1$ and $|\lambda_2| > 1$ (or $|\lambda_1| > 1$ and $|\lambda_2| < 1$) if and only if $F(-1) < 0$;
(iii) $|\lambda_1| > 1$ and $|\lambda_2| > 1$ if and only if $F(-1) > 0$ and $C > 1$;
(iv) $\lambda_1 = -1$ and $|\lambda_2| \neq 1$ if and only if $F(-1) = 0$ and $B \neq 0, 2$;
(v) λ_1 and λ_2 are complex and $|\lambda_1| = |\lambda_2| = 1$ if and only if $B^2 - 4C < 0$ and $C = 1$.

Let λ_1 and λ_2 be the two eigenvalues of the fixed point (x, y). We recall some definitions of topological types for a fixed point (x, y).

A fixed point (x, y) is called
(i) a sink if $|\lambda_1| < 1$ and $|\lambda_2| < 1$, so the sink is locally asymptotically stable.
(ii) a source if $|\lambda_1| > 1$ and $|\lambda_2| > 1$, so the source is locally unstable.
(iii) a saddle if $|\lambda_1| > 1$ and $|\lambda_2| < 1$ or ($|\lambda_1| < 1$ and $|\lambda_2| > 1$).
(iv) non-hyperbolic if either $|\lambda_1| = 1$ or $|\lambda_2| = 1$.

5.2 Stability and Dynamic Behavior of P_1

At $P_1 = \left(\frac{(a_l)^{1-p}(a_u)^p - 1}{(a_l)^{1-p}(a_u)^p}, 0\right)$, the Jacobian matrix J for the system is

$$J = \begin{bmatrix} 2-(a_l)^{1-p}(a_u)^p & -(b_l)^{1-p}(b_u)^p\sqrt{\left[\frac{(a_l)^{1-p}(a_u)^p-1}{(a_l)^{1-p}(a_u)^p}\right]} \\ 0 & (c_l)^{1-p}(c_u)^p\sqrt{\left[\frac{(a_l)^{1-p}(a_u)^p-1}{(a_l)^{1-p}(a_u)^p}\right]} - (d_l)^{1-p}(d_u)^p \end{bmatrix}$$

Equilibrium point is

Sink if $\left|2-(a_l)^{1-p}(a_u)^p\right| < 1$ and $\left|(c_l)^{1-p}(c_u)^p\sqrt{\left[\frac{(a_l)^{1-p}(a_u)^p-1}{(a_l)^{1-p}(a_u)^p}\right]} - (d_l)^{1-p}(d_u)^p\right| < 1$

Source if $\left|2-(a_l)^{1-p}(a_u)^p\right| > 1$ and $\left|(c_l)^{1-p}(c_u)^p\sqrt{\left[\frac{(a_l)^{1-p}(a_u)^p-1}{(a_l)^{1-p}(a_u)^p}\right]} - (d_l)^{1-p}(d_u)^p\right| > 1$

Saddle if $\left|2-(a_l)^{1-p}(a_u)^p\right| > 1$ and $\left|(c_l)^{1-p}(c_u)^p\sqrt{\left[\frac{(a_l)^{1-p}(a_u)^p-1}{(a_l)^{1-p}(a_u)^p}\right]} - (d_l)^{1-p}(d_u)^p\right| < 1$ or

$\left|2-(a_l)^{1-p}(a_u)^p\right| < 1$ and $\left|(c_l)^{1-p}(c_u)^p\sqrt{\left[\frac{(a_l)^{1-p}(a_u)^p-1}{(a_l)^{1-p}(a_u)^p}\right]} - (d_l)^{1-p}(d_u)^p\right| > 1$

Non-hyperbolic if $\left|2-(a_l)^{1-p}(a_u)^p\right| = 1$ or $\left|(c_l)^{1-p}(c_u)^p\sqrt{\left[\frac{(a_l)^{1-p}(a_u)^p-1}{(a_l)^{1-p}(a_u)^p}\right]} - (d_l)^{1-p}(d_u)^p\right| = 1$

If $(a_l)^{1-p}(a_u)^p = 3$ and $\left|(c_l)^{1-p}(c_u)^p\sqrt{\left[\frac{(a_l)^{1-p}(a_u)^p-1}{(a_l)^{1-p}(a_u)^p}\right]} - (d_l)^{1-p}(d_u)^p\right| \neq 1$, then $P_1 = \left(\frac{(a_l)^{1-p}(a_u)^p-1}{(a_l)^{1-p}(a_u)^p}, 0\right)$ can undergo flip bifurcation when the parameters vary in the neighborhood of $(a_l)^{1-p}(a_u)^p = 3$.

5.3 Local Stability and Dynamic Behavior Around Interior Fixed Point

The dynamic behavior for the interior equilibrium point of the system is presented here:

$$\begin{aligned}
&1 - \mathrm{Tr}(J) + \mathrm{Det}(J) \\
&= 1 - \left[(a_l)^{1-p}(a_u)^p(1-2x) - \frac{(b_l)^{1-p}(b_u)^p y}{2\sqrt{x}}\right] \\
&\quad - \left[(c_l)^{1-p}(c_u)^p\sqrt{x} - (d_l)^{1-p}(d_u)^p\right] \\
&\quad + (a_l)^{1-p}(a_u)^p(1-2x)\left((c_l)^{1-p}(c_u)^p\sqrt{x} - (d_l)^{1-p}(d_u)^p\right) \\
&\quad + \frac{(b_l)^{1-p}(b_u)^p(d_l)^{1-p}(d_u)^p y}{2\sqrt{x}}
\end{aligned}$$

$$
\begin{aligned}
&1+\mathrm{Tr}\,(J)+\mathrm{Det}\,(J)\\
&=1+\left[(a_l)^{1-p}(a_u)^p(1-2x)-\frac{(b_l)^{1-p}(b_u)^p y}{2\sqrt{x}}\right]\\
&\quad+\left[(c_l)^{1-p}(c_u)^p\sqrt{x}-(d_l)^{1-p}(d_u)^p\right]+(a_l)^{1-p}(a_u)^p(1-2x)\\
&\left((c_l)^{1-p}(c_u)^p\sqrt{x}-(d_l)^{1-p}(d_u)^p\right)+\frac{(b_l)^{1-p}(b_u)^p(d_l)^{1-p}(d_u)^p y}{2\sqrt{x}}
\end{aligned}
$$

$$
\begin{aligned}
\mathrm{Det}\,(J)=&\,(a_l)^{1-p}(a_u)^p(1-2x)\left((c_l)^{1-p}(c_u)^p\sqrt{x}\right.\\
&\left.-(d_l)^{1-p}(d_u)^p\right)+\frac{(b_l)^{1-p}(b_u)^p(d_l)^{1-p}(d_u)^p y}{2\sqrt{x}}
\end{aligned}
$$

At $P_2=(x^*,y^*)$, if $1-\mathrm{Tr}\,(J)+\mathrm{Det}\,(J)>0$, then interior equilibrium point is
Sink if $1+\mathrm{Tr}\,(J)+\mathrm{Det}\,(J)>0$ and $\mathrm{Det}\,(J)<1$
Source if $1+\mathrm{Tr}\,(J)+\mathrm{Det}\,(J)>0$ and $\mathrm{Det}\,(J)>1$
Saddle if $1+\mathrm{Tr}\,(J)+\mathrm{Det}\,(J)<0$
Non-hyperbolic if $1+\mathrm{Tr}\,(J)+\mathrm{Det}\,(J)=0$ and $\mathrm{Tr}\,(J)\neq 0,2.$ or $[\mathrm{Tr}\,(J)]^2-4\mathrm{Det}\,(J)<0$ and $\mathrm{Det}\,(J)=1$.

At $P_2=(x^*,y^*)$, if $1-\mathrm{Tr}\,(J)+\mathrm{Det}\,(J)>0$, $1+\mathrm{Tr}\,(J)+\mathrm{Det}\,(J)=0$, and $\mathrm{Tr}\,(J)\neq 0 and 2$, then (x^*,y^*) can undergo flip bifurcation.

At $P_2=(x^*,y^*)$, if $1-\mathrm{Tr}\,(J)+\mathrm{Det}\,(J)>0$, $(\mathrm{Tr}\,(J))^2-4\mathrm{Det}\,(J)<0$ and $\mathrm{Det}\,(J)=1$, then (x^*,y^*) can undergo Hopf bifurcation.

6 Flip Bifurcation

From Lemma 1, one of the eigenvalues of the positive fixed point $P_2=(x^*,y^*)$ is $\lambda_1=-1$ and the other (λ_2) is neither 1 nor -1 if parameters of the model are located in the following set $A=\{(a_l,a_u,b_l,b_u,c_l,c_u,d_l,d_u,p)$: $1-\mathrm{Tr}\,(J)+\mathrm{Det}\,(J)>0$, $1+\mathrm{Tr}\,(J)+\mathrm{Det}\,(J)=0$, $\mathrm{Tr}\,(J)\neq 0,2$ and $p\in[0,1]\}$.

Here, we discuss flip bifurcation of the model (3) at $P_2=(x^*,y^*)$ when parameters vary in a small neighborhood of A. In analyzing the flip bifurcation, p is used as the bifurcation parameter. Further, p^* is the perturbation of p, we consider a perturbation of the system as follows:

$$
\begin{aligned}
x_{n+1}&=(a_l)^{1-(p+p^*)}(a_u)^{(p+p^*)}x_n(1-x_n)-(b_l)^{1-(p+p^*)}(b_u)^{(p+p^*)}\sqrt{x_n}y_n\equiv f(x_n,y_n,p^*)\\
y_{n+1}&=(c_l)^{1-(p+p^*)}(c_u)^{(p+p^*)}\sqrt{x_n}y_n-(d_l)^{1-(p+p^*)}(d_u)^{(p+p^*)}y_n\equiv g(x_n,y_n,p^*)
\end{aligned}
\tag{4}
$$

where $|p^*|\lll 1$

Let $u_n=x_n-x^*$, $v_n=y_n-y^*$, then equilibrium $P_2=(x^*,y^*)$ is transformed into the origin, and further expanding f and g as a Taylor series at $(u_n,v_n,p^*)=(0,0,0)$ to the third order, the model (4) becomes

$$\begin{aligned} u_{n+1} &= \alpha_1 u_n + \alpha_2 v_n + \alpha_{11} u_n^2 + \alpha_{12} u_n v_n + \alpha_{13} u_n p^* + \alpha_{23} v_n p^* + \\ &\quad \alpha_{111} u_n^3 + \alpha_{112} u_n^2 v_n + \alpha_{113} u_n^2 p^* + \alpha_{123} u_n v_n p^* + O((|u_n| + |v_n| + |p^*|)^4) \\ v_{n+1} &= \beta_1 u_n + \beta_2 v_n + \beta_{11} u_n^2 + \beta_{12} u_n v_n + \beta_{22} v_n^2 + \beta_{13} u_n p^* + \beta_{23} v_n p^* + \beta_{111} u_n^3 + \\ &\quad \beta_{112} u_n^2 v_n + \beta_{113} u_n^2 p^* + \beta_{123} u_n v_n p^* + \beta_{223} v_n^2 p^* + O((|u_n| + |v_n| + |p^*|)^4) \end{aligned} \tag{5}$$

where $\alpha_1 = f_x(x^*, y^*, 0)$, $\alpha_2 = f_y(x^*, y^*, 0)$, $\alpha_{11} = f_{xx}(x^*, y^*, 0)$, $\alpha_{12} = f_{xy}(x^*, y^*, 0)$, $\alpha_{13} = f_{xp^*}(x^*, y^*, 0)$, $\alpha_{23} = f_{yp^*}(x^*, y^*, 0)$, $\alpha_{111} = f_{xxx}(x^*, y^*, 0)$, $\alpha_{112} = f_{xxy}(x^*, y^*, 0)$, $\alpha_{113} = f_{xxp^*}(x^*, y^*, 0)$, $\alpha_{123} = f_{xyp^*}(x^*, y^*, 0)$

$\beta_1 = g_x(x^*, y^*, 0)$, $\beta_2 = g_y(x^*, y^*, 0)$, $\beta_{11} = g_{xx}(x^*, y^*, 0)$, $\beta_{12} = g_{xy}(x^*, y^*, 0)$, $\beta_{22} = g_{yy}(x^*, y^*, 0)$, $\beta_{13} = g_{xp^*}(x^*, y^*, 0)$, $\beta_{23} = g_{yp^*}(x^*, y^*, 0)$, $\beta_{111} = g_{xxx}(x^*, y^*, 0)$, $\beta_{112} = g_{xxy}(x^*, y^*, 0)$, $\beta_{113} = g_{xxp^*}(x^*, y^*, 0)$, $\beta_{123} = g_{xyp^*}(x^*, y^*, 0)$, $\beta_{223} = g_{yyp^*}(x^*, y^*, 0)$

We define $T = \begin{bmatrix} \alpha_2 & \alpha_2 \\ -1-\alpha_1 & \lambda_2 - \alpha_1 \end{bmatrix}$, where T is invertible, and using the transformation $\begin{bmatrix} u_n \\ v_n \end{bmatrix} = T \begin{bmatrix} \overline{x}_n \\ \overline{y}_n \end{bmatrix}$, the model (5) becomes

$$\begin{aligned} \overline{x}_{n+1} &= -\overline{x}_n + f_1(u_n, v_n, p^*) \\ \overline{y}_{n+1} &= \lambda_2 \overline{y}_n + g_1(u_n, v_n, p^*) \end{aligned} \tag{6}$$

where the functions f_1 and g_1 denote the terms in the model (6) in variables (u_n, v_n, p^*) with the order at least two.

From the theorem of center manifold, there exists a center manifold $W^c(0, 0, 0)$ of the model (6) at (0, 0) in a small neighborhood of $p^* = 0$, which can be approximately described as follows:

$W^c(0, 0, 0) = \left\{ \left(\overline{x}_n, \overline{y}_n, p^* \right) \epsilon R^3 : \overline{y}_{n+1} = \overline{\alpha}_1 \overline{x}_n^2 + \overline{\alpha}_2 \overline{x}_n p^* + O((|\overline{x}_n| + |p^*|)^3) \right\}$

where $\overline{\alpha}_1 = \dfrac{\alpha_2[(1+\alpha_1)\alpha_{11} + \alpha_2 \beta_{11}]}{1-\lambda_2^2} + \dfrac{\beta_{22}(1+\alpha_1)^2}{1-\lambda_2^2} - \dfrac{(1+\alpha_1)[\alpha_{12}(1+\alpha_1) + \alpha_2 \beta_{12}]}{1-\lambda_2^2}$,
$\overline{\alpha}_2 = \dfrac{(1+\alpha_1)[\alpha_{23}(1+\alpha_1) + \alpha_2 \beta_{23}]}{\alpha_2(1+\lambda_2)^2} - \dfrac{(1+\alpha_1)\alpha_{13} + \alpha_2 \beta_{13}]}{(1+\lambda_2)^2}$.

We obtain the system (6) restricted to center manifold $W^c(0, 0, 0)$, which has the following form

$$\overline{x}_{n+1} = -\overline{x}_n + h_1 \overline{x}_n^2 + h_2 \overline{x}_n p^* + h_3 \overline{x}_n^2 p^* + h_4 \overline{x}_n p^{*2} + h_5 \overline{x}_n^3 + O((|\overline{x}_n| + |p^*|)^3) \equiv F(\overline{x}_n, p^*)$$

$$\begin{aligned} h_1 &= \frac{\overline{\alpha}_2[(\lambda_2 - \overline{\alpha}_1)\alpha_{11} - \overline{\alpha}_2 \beta_{11}]}{1+\lambda_2} - \frac{\beta_{22}(1+\overline{\alpha}_1)^2}{1+\lambda_2} - \frac{(1+\overline{\alpha}_1)[(\lambda_2 - \overline{\alpha}_1)\alpha_{12} - \overline{\alpha}_2 \beta_{12}]}{1+\lambda_2}, \\ h_2 &= \frac{(\lambda_2 - \overline{\alpha}_1)\alpha_{13} - \overline{\alpha}_2 \beta_{13}}{1+\lambda_2} - \frac{(1+\overline{\alpha}_1)[(\lambda_2 - \overline{\alpha}_1)\alpha_{23} - \overline{\alpha}_2 \beta_{23}]}{\overline{\alpha}_2 (1+\lambda_2)}, \\ h_3 &= \frac{(\lambda_2 - \alpha_1)\overline{\alpha}_1 \alpha_{13} - \alpha_2 \beta_{13}}{1+\lambda_2} + \frac{[(\lambda_2 - \alpha_1)\alpha_{23} - \alpha_2 \beta_{23}](\lambda_2 - \alpha_1)\overline{\alpha}_1}{\alpha_2 (1+\lambda_2)} \\ &\quad - \frac{(1+\alpha_1)[(\lambda_2 - \alpha_1)\alpha_{123} - \alpha_2 \beta_{123}]}{1+\lambda_2} + \frac{\alpha_2[(\lambda_2 - \alpha_1)\alpha_{113} - \alpha_2 \beta_{113}]}{1+\lambda_2} \end{aligned}$$

$$
\begin{aligned}
&-\frac{\beta_{223}(1+\alpha_1)^2}{1+\lambda_2}+\frac{2\alpha_2\overline{\alpha}_2[(\lambda_2-\alpha_1)\alpha_{11}-\alpha_2\beta_{11}]}{1+\lambda_2}-\frac{2\beta_{22}\overline{\alpha}_2(1+\alpha_1)(\lambda_2-\alpha_1)}{1+\lambda_2}\\
&+\frac{\overline{\alpha}_2[(\lambda_2-\alpha_1)\alpha_{12}-\alpha_2\beta_{12}](\lambda_2-1-2\alpha_1)}{1+\lambda_2},\\
h_4=&\frac{\overline{\alpha}_2[(\lambda_2-\alpha_1)\alpha_{13}-\alpha_2\beta_{13}]}{1+\lambda_2}+\frac{[(\lambda_2-\alpha_1)\alpha_{23}-\alpha_2\beta_{23}](\lambda_2-\alpha_1)\overline{\alpha}_2}{\alpha_2(1+\lambda_2)}\\
&+\frac{2\alpha_2\overline{\alpha}_2[(\lambda_2-\alpha_1)\alpha_{11}-\alpha_2\beta_{11}]}{1+\lambda_2}\\
&+\frac{2\beta_{22}\overline{\alpha}_2(1+\alpha_1)(\lambda_2-\alpha_1)}{1+\lambda_2}+\frac{\overline{\alpha}_2[(\lambda_2-\alpha_1)\alpha_{12}-\alpha_2\beta_{12}](\lambda_2-1-2\alpha_1)}{1+\lambda_2},\\
h_5=&\frac{2\alpha_2\overline{\alpha}_1[(\lambda_2-\alpha_1)\alpha_{11}-\alpha_2\beta_{11}]}{1+\lambda_2}+\frac{2\beta_{22}\overline{\alpha}_1(\lambda_2-\alpha_1)(1+\alpha_1)}{1+\lambda_2}\\
&+\frac{[(\lambda_2-\alpha_1)\alpha_{11}-\alpha_2\beta_{11}](\lambda_2-1-2\alpha_1)\overline{\alpha}_1}{1+\lambda_2}\\
&+\frac{\overline{\alpha}_2^2[(\lambda_2-\alpha_1)\alpha_{111}-\alpha_2\beta_{111}]}{1+\lambda_2}-\frac{\overline{\alpha}_2(1+\alpha_1)[(\lambda_2-\alpha_1)\alpha_{112}-\alpha_2\beta_{112}]}{1+\lambda_2}.
\end{aligned}
$$

For flip bifurcation, we require the two discriminatory quantities ξ_1 and ξ_2 to be nonzero,

$$\xi_1=\left(\frac{\partial^2 F}{\partial\overline{x}\partial p^*}+\frac{1}{2}\frac{\partial F}{\partial p^*}\frac{\partial^2 F}{\partial\overline{x}^2}\right)|_{(0,0)}$$

$$\xi_2=\left(\frac{1}{6}\frac{\partial^3 F}{\partial\overline{x}^3}+\left(\frac{1}{2}\frac{\partial^2 F}{\partial\overline{x}^2}\right)^2\right)|_{(0,0)}$$

Finally, from the above analysis , we have the following result.

Theorem 2 *If $\xi_1 \neq 0$ and $\xi_2 \neq 0$ then the model (3) undergoes flip bifurcation at $P_2 = (x^*, y^*)$, if $\xi_2 > 0$ (resp. $\xi_2 < 0$), then the period-2 points that bifurcation from $P_2 = (x^*, y^*)$ are stable.*

7 Chaos Control

This section presents a feedback control method to stabilize chaotic orbits at an unstable positive fixed point of system (3).

Consider the following controlled form of model (3):

$$
\begin{aligned}
x_{n+1}&=(a_l)^{1-p}(a_u)^p x_n(1-x_n)-(b_l)^{1-p}(b_u)^p\sqrt{x_n}y_n+S\\
y_{n+1}&=(c_l)^{1-p}(c_u)^p\sqrt{x_n}y_n-(d_l)^{1-p}(d_u)^p y_n
\end{aligned}
\tag{7}
$$

with the following feedback control law as the control force:

$$S=-q_1\left(x_n-x^*\right)-q_2\left(y_n-y^*\right)$$

where q_1 and q_2 are the feedback gain and (x^*, y^*) is a positive fixed point of model.

The Jacobian matrix J for the system (7) at (x^*, y^*) is
$J = \begin{bmatrix} a_{11} - q_1 & a_{12} - q_2 \\ a_{21} & a_{22} \end{bmatrix}$
where $a_{11} = {a_l}^{1-p}{a_u}^p(1-2x^*) - \frac{{b_l}^{1-p}{b_u}^p y^*}{2\sqrt{x^*}}$, $a_{12} = -{b_l}^{1-p}{b_u}^p\sqrt{x^*}$, $a_{21} = \frac{{c_l}^{1-p}{c_u}^p y^*}{2\sqrt{x^*}}$, $a_{22} = {c_l}^{1-p}{c_u}^p\sqrt{x^*} - {d_l}^{1-p}{d_u}^p$. The corresponding characteristic equation of matrix J is
$\lambda^2 - (a_{11} + a_{22} - q_1)\lambda + a_{22}(a_{11} - q_1) - a_{21}(a_{12} - q_2)$
Let λ_1 and λ_2 are the eigenvalues

$$\lambda_1 + \lambda_2 = a_{11} + a_{22} - q_1 \tag{8}$$

and

$$\lambda_1\lambda_2 = a_{22}(a_{11} - q_1) - a_{21}(a_{12} - q_2) \tag{9}$$

The lines of marginal stability are determined by solving the equation $\lambda_1 = \pm 1$ and $\lambda_1\lambda_2 = 1$. These conditions guarantee that the eigenvalues λ_1 and λ_2 have modulus less than 1.

Suppose $\lambda_1\lambda_2 = 1$; from (9) we have line l_1 as follows:
$a_{22}q_1 - a_{21}q_2 = a_{22}a_{11} - a_{21}a_{12} - 1$
Suppose $\lambda_1 = \pm 1$; from (8, 9), we have line l_2 and l_3 as follows:
$(1 - a_{22})q_1 + a_{21}q_2 = a_{11} + a_{22} - 1 - a_{22}a_{11} + a_{21}a_{12}$
and
$(1 + a_{22})q_1 - a_{21}q_2 = a_{11} + a_{22} + 1 + a_{22}a_{11} - a_{21}a_{12}$
The stable eigenvalues lie within a triangular region by line l_1, l_2 and l_3.

8 Numerical Simulation

Here, we consider a numerical example of the above model and carried out mathematical calculation that depends on some artificial data. We calculated the equilibrium points and analyzed their stability. For the model (3) given in the paper, we consider the parameter values $\widehat{a} \in [a_l, a_u] = [4.0, 4.2]$, $\widehat{b} \in [b_l, b_u] = [1.8, 2.0]$, $\widehat{c} \in [c_l, c_u] = [1.7, 1.9]$, $\widehat{d} \in [d_l, d_u] = [0.1, 0.2]$. Performing computer simulation on that chosen data, we calculate the equilibria points, eigenvalues and stability of every equilibrium points for different values of p. The obtained results are given in Table 1.

Figures 1 and 2 are drawn in the basis of the parameter values $\widehat{a} \in [a_l, a_u] = [4.0, 4.2]$, $\widehat{b} \in [b_l, b_u] = [1.8, 2.0]$, $\widehat{c} \in [c_l, c_u] = [1.7, 1.9]$, $\widehat{d} \in [d_l, d_u] = [0.1, 0.2]$. Here, we observe damped oscillation for time plot in Fig. 1 for $p = 0.0, 0.2, 0.4, 0.6, 0.8$. In Fig. 2, all trajectories spiral into the stable fixed point for $p = 0.0, 0.2, 0.4, 0.6, 0.8$. Here, we found constant oscillation about interior equilibrium points for time plot in Fig. 1 for $p = 1.0$. In Fig. 2, trajectories are attracted to a limit cycle about interior equilibrium points for $p = 1.0$. Hence, there exist a bi-

Table 1 Equilibrium points, Eigenvalues and stability of equilibrium points

Value of p	Equilibrium points	Eigenvalues	Stability
$p = 0.0$	(0.7500, 0)	−2.0000, 1.3722	Unstable point
$p = 0.0$	(0.4187, 0.4764)	$0.4939 - 0.6876i, 0.4939 + 0.6876i$	Stable point
$p = 0.2$	(0.7524, 0)	−2.0390, 1.3929	Unstable point
$p = 0.2$	(0.4114, 0.4806)	$0.5135 - 0.7288i, 0.5135 + 0.7288i$	Stable point
$p = 0.4$	(0.7548, 0)	−2.0786, 1.4122	Unstable point
$p = 0.4$	(0.4056, 0.4832)	$0.5289 - 0.7644i, 0.5289 + 0.7644i$	Stable point
$p = 0.6$	(0.7572, 0)	−2.1187, 1.4298	Unstable point
$p = 0.6$	(0.4015, 0.4841)	$0.5394 - 0.7946i, 0.5394 + 0.7946i$	Stable point
$p = 0.8$	(0.7596, 0)	−2.1595, 1.4454	Unstable point
$p = 0.8$	(0.3992, 0.4836)	$0.5445 - 0.8200i, 0.5445 + 0.8200i$	Stable point
$p = 1.0$	(0.7619, 0)	−2.2000, 1.4585	Unstable point
$p = 1.0$	(0.3989, 0.4815)	$0.5434 - 0.8405i, 0.5434 + 0.8405i$	Unstable point

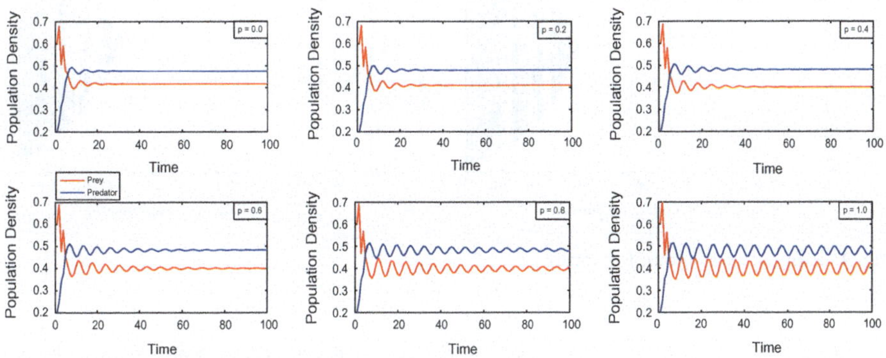

Fig. 1 Time graph for different p

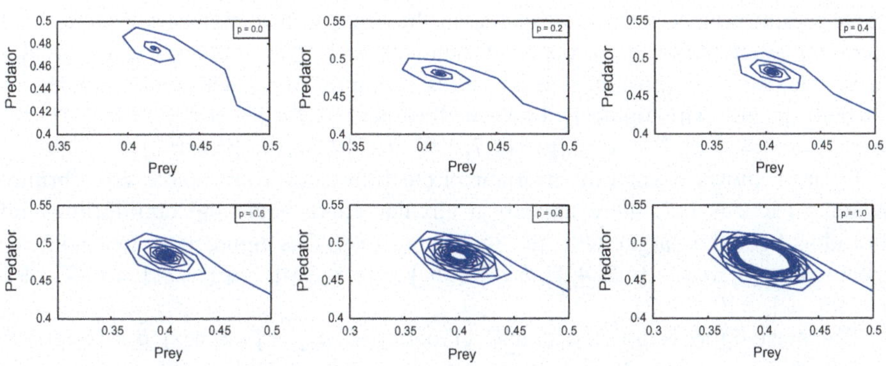

Fig. 2 Phase portrate for different p

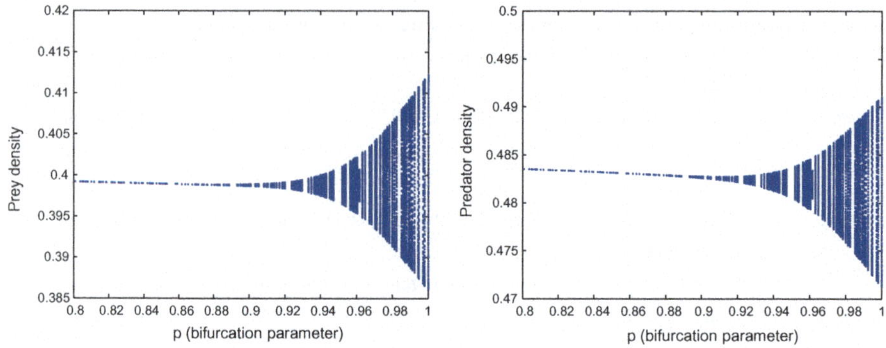

Fig. 3 Bifurcation diagram for varying p

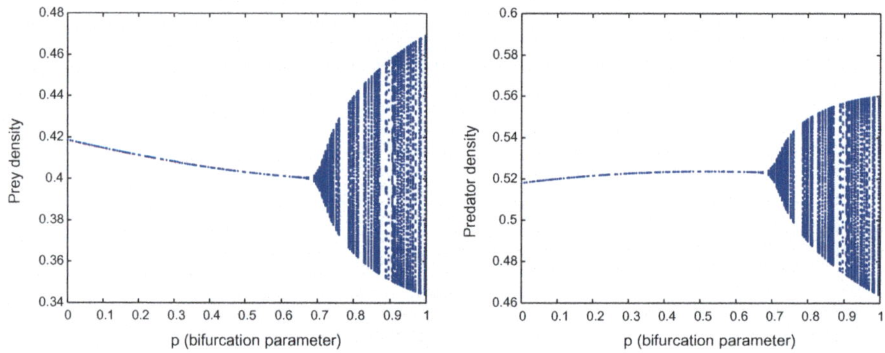

Fig. 4 Bifurcation diagram for varying p

furcation for p. This bifurcation is supercritical—after the fixed point loses stability, it is surrounded by a stable limit cycle.

Figure 3 depicts smooth invariant circle bifurcates for both prey and predator from stable equilibrium. As the p value increases, the behavior becomes more complex and more unpredictable for both species. When p exceeds 0.91, there appears a circular curve enclosing equilibrium and its radius becomes larger with chaotic behavior for both species. This figure is drawn with respect to $\widehat{a} \in [a_l, a_u] = [4.0, 4.2]$, $\widehat{b} \in [b_l, b_u] = [1.8, 2.0]$, $\widehat{c} \in [c_l, c_u] = [1.7, 1.9]$, $\widehat{d} \in [d_l, d_u] = [0.1, 0.2]$.

Figure 4 shows a smooth invariant circle bifurcates from stable equilibrium. When p exceeds 0.7, there appears a circular curve enclosing equilibrium and its radius becomes larger with the increasing of p.This figure is drawn with respect to $\widehat{a} \in [a_l, a_u] = [4.2, 4.4]$, $\widehat{b} \in [b_l, b_u] = [1.8, 2.0]$, $\widehat{c} \in [c_l, c_u] = [1.7, 1.9]$, $\widehat{d} \in [d_l, d_u] = [0.1, 0.2]$.

The above figure is drawn with respect to $\widehat{a} \in [a_l, a_u] = [4.5, 4.7]$, $\widehat{b} \in [b_l, b_u] = [1.8, 2.0]$, $\widehat{c} \in [c_l, c_u] = [1.7, 1.9]$, $\widehat{d} \in [d_l, d_u] = [0.1, 0.2]$. Figure 5 shows smooth invariant circle bifurcates for both species from stable equilibrium. Furthermore, if p exceeds 0.45, there appears a circular curve enclosing equilibrium and its radius

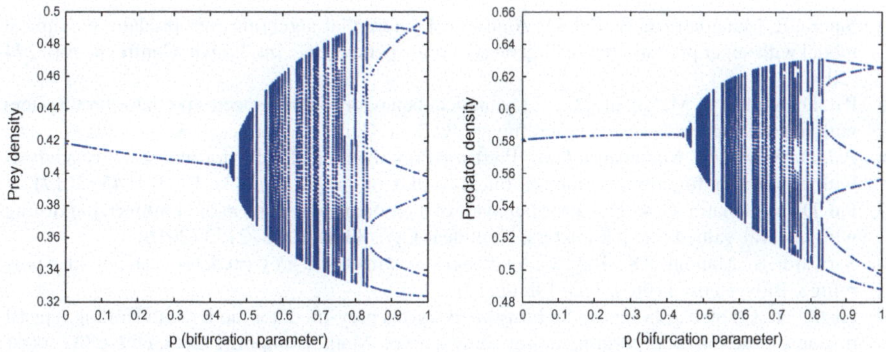

Fig. 5 Bifurcation diagram for varing p

becomes larger with the growth of p. At p values above 0.83, the systems behave as a limit cycle for both species.

9 Conclusion

This work is related to the qualitative behavior of a discrete-time predator-prey model under imprecise biological parameters. We have found the fixed points of the system and discussed their stability analytically. We give a flip bifurcation analysis and chaos control procedure. The phase portraits, bifurcation and time graphs are obtained for different parameters of the model. Here, we introduce a new concept in bifurcation analysis. The codimension of a bifurcation is the number of parameters which must be varied for the bifurcation to occur. When we consider p as bifurcation parameter, ultimately, we consider here 4 bifurcation parameter in a certain range, but interesting fact is that using our technic we convert this 4 codim bifurcation in 1 codim. The proposed study will be very useful for the mathematical modeling and analysis of a wide range of predator–prey interactions. Our study suggests that herd behavior has stabilizing effect on population dynamics.

References

1. Kar, T.K.: Stability analysis of a prey-predator model incorporating a prey refuge. Commun. Nonlinear Sci. Numer. Simul. **10**, 681–691 (2005)
2. Pal, D., Mahapatra, G.S., Samanta, G.P.: A proportional harvesting dynamical model with fuzzy intrinsic growth rate and harvesting quantity. Pac.-Asian J. Math. **6**, 199–213 (2012)
3. Santra, P., Mahapatra, G.S.: Prey-predator model for optimal harvesting with functional response incorporating prey refuge. Int. J. Biomath. **09**, ID1650014 (2016)

4. Santra, P., Mahapatra, G.S., Pal, D.: Analysis of deferential-algebraic prey-predator dynamical model with super predator harvesting on economic perspective. Int. J. Dyn. Control **4**, 266–274 (2016)
5. Pal, D., Santra, P., Mahapatra, G.S.: Dynamical behavior of three species predator prey system with mutual support between non refuge prey. Ecol. Genet. Genomics **3–5**, 1–6 (2017)
6. Pal, D., Santra, P., Mahapatra, G.S.: Predator-Prey dynamical behavior and stability analysis with square root functional response. Int. J. Appl. Comput. Math. **3**(3), 1833–1845 (2017)
7. Pal, D., Mahapatra, G.S.: Dynamic behavior of a predator-prey system of combined harvesting with interval-valued rate parameters. Nonlinear Dyn. **83**(4), 2113–2123 (2016)
8. Sarwardi, S., Mandal, P.K., Ray, S.: Analysis of a competitive prey-predator system with a prey refuge. Biosystems **110**(3), 133–148 (2012)
9. Huang, Y., Chen, F., Zhong, L.: Stability analysis of a prey-predator model with Holling type III response function incorporating a prey refuge. Appl. Math. Comput. **182**(1), 672–683 (2006)
10. Devi, Sapna: Nonconstant prey harvesting in ratio-dependent predator-prey system incorporating a constant prey refuge. Int. J. Biomathem. **5**(2), 1250021 (2012)
11. Mukhopadhyay, B., Bhattacharyya, R.: Effects of deterministic and random refuge in a prey-predator model with parasite infection. Math. Biosci. **239**(1), 124–130 (2012)
12. Jing, Z.J., Yang, J.: Bifurcation and chaos discrete-time predator-prey system. Chaos, Solitons Fractals **27**, 259–277 (2006)
13. Liu, X., Xiao, D.: Complex dynamic behaviors of a discrete-time predator-prey system. Chaos, Solitons Fractals **32**, 80–94 (2006)
14. Liu, X.: A note on the existence of periodic solution in discrete predator-prey models. Appl. Math. Model. **34**, 2477–2483 (2006)
15. Wang, W.X., Zhang, B.Y., Liu, C.Z.: Analysis of a discrete-time predator–prey system with Allee effect. Ecol. Complex. **8**, 81–85 (2011)
16. Elsadany, A.E.A.: Dynamical complexities in a discrete-time food chain. Comput. Ecol. Softw. **2**(2), 124–139 (2012)
17. Wu, T.: Dynamic behaviors of a discrete two species predator-prey system incorporating harvesting. Discrete Dyn. Nat. Soc. Article ID **429076** (2012)
18. Jana, D.: Chaotic dynamics of a discrete predator-prey system with prey refuge. Appl. Math. Comput. **224**, 848–865 (2013)
19. Din, Q., Elsayed, E.M.: Stability analysis of a discrete ecological model. Comput. Ecol. Softw. **4**(2), 89–103 (2014)
20. Tripathi, J.P., Abbas, S., Thakur, M.:. Dynamical analysis of a prey–predator model with Beddington–DeAngelis type function response incorporating a prey refuge. Nonlinear Dyn. **80**, 177–196 (2015)
21. Peixoto, M., Barros, L.C., Bassanezi, R.C.: Predator-prey fuzzy model. Ecol. Model. **214**, 39–44 (2008)
22. Pal, D., Mahapatra, G.S., Samanta, G.P.: Optimal harvesting of prey-predator system with interval biological parameters: a bioeconomic model. Math. Biosci. **24**, 181–187 (2013)
23. Pal, D., Mahapatra, G.S., Samanta, G.P.: Quota harvesting model for a single species population under fuzziness. Int. J. Mathe. Sci. **12**, 33–46 (2013)
24. Malthus, T.R.: An Essay on the Principle of Population, and a Summary View of the Principle of Populations. Penguin, Harmondsworth, England (1798)
25. Lotka, A.J.: Elements of Physical Biology. Williams and Wilkins, Baltimore (1925)
26. Volterra, V.: Leconssen la theorie mathematique de la leitte pou lavie. Gauthier-Villars, Paris (1931)
27. Zhao, M., Du, Y.: Stability of a discrete-time predator-prey system with Allee effect. Nonlinear Anal. Diff. Equ. **4**(5), 225–233 (2016)
28. Santra, P., Mahapatra, G.S., Pal, D.: Prey-predator nonlinear harvesting model with functional response incorporating prey refuge. Int. J. Dyn. Control **4**, 293–302 (2016)
29. Mahapatra, G.S., Mandal, T.K.: Posynomial parametric geometric programming with interval valued coefficient. J. Optim. Theory Appl. **154**, 120–132 (2012)

30. Bassanezi, R.C., Barros, L.C., Tonelli, A.: Attractors and asymptotic stability for fuzzy dynamical systems. Fuzzy Sets Syst. **113**, 473–483 (2000)
31. Barros, L.C., Bassanezi, R.C., Tonelli, P.A.: Fuzzy modelling in population dynamics. Ecol. Model. **128**, 27–33 (2000)
32. Tuyako, M.M., Barros, L.C., Bassanezi, R.C.: Stability of fuzzy dynamic systems. Int. J. Uncertainty Fuzziness Knowl.-Based Syst. **17**, 69–83 (2009)
33. Pereira, C.M., Cecconello, M.S., Bassanezi, R.C.: Prey-predator model under fuzzy uncertanties. In: Barreto, G., Coelho, R. (eds) Fuzzy Information Processing, NAFIPS 2018. Communications in Computer and Information Science, vol. 831, Springer, Cham (2018)
34. Barros, L.C., Oliveira, R.Z.G., Leite, M.B.F., Bassanezi, R.C.: Epidemiological models of directly transmitted diseases: an approach via fuzzy sets theory. Int. J. Uncertainty Fuzziness Knowl.-Based Syst. **22**(5), 769–781 (2014)
35. Gámeza, M., Lópeza, I., Rodrígueza, C., Vargab, Z., Garayc, J.: Ecological monitoring in a discrete-time prey-predator model. J. Theor. Biol. **429**, 52–60 (2017)
36. Huang, J., Liu, S., Ruan, S., Xiao, D.: Bifurcations in a discrete predator-prey model with nonmonotonic functional response. J. Math. Anal. Appl. **464**, 201–230 (2018)

Comparison of Explicit and Implicit Finite Difference Schemes on Diffusion Equation

Malabika Adak

Abstract In physics and mathematics, heat equation is a special case of diffusion equation and is a partial differential equation (PDE). Partial differential equations are useful tools for mathematical modeling. A few problems can be solved analytically, whereas difficult boundary value problem can be solved by numerical methods easily. A very popular numerical method known as finite difference methods (explicit and implicit schemes) is applied expansively for solving heat equations successfully. Explicit schemes are Forward Time and Centre Space (FTCS), Dufort and Frankel methods, whereas implicit schemes are Laasonen and Crank-Nicolson methods. In this study, explicit and implicit finite difference schemes are applied for simple one-dimensional transient heat conduction equation with Dirichlet's initial-boundary conditions. MATLAB code is used to solve the problem for each scheme in fine mesh grids. Comparing results with analytical results, Crank-Nicolson method gives the best approximate solution. FTCS scheme is conditionally stable, whereas other schemes are unconditionally stable. Convergence, stability and truncation error analysis are investigated. Transient temperature distribution plot and surface temperature plots for different time are presented. Also, unstable plot for FTCS method is represented.

Keywords Dirichlet boundary condition · Finite difference scheme · Truncation error · Convergence · Stability

1 Introduction

In most of the research work in the fields like applied elasticity, theory of plates and shells hydrodynamics, quantum mechanics, the problem reduces to partial differential equations. The heat equation is fundamental in diverse scientific fields, which describe the distribution of heat (or variation of temperature) in a given region over

M. Adak (✉)
Department of Applied Mathematics and Humanities, Yeshwantrao Chavan College of Engineering, Nagpur, Maharashtra 440010, India
e-mail: malabikaadak@yahoo.co.in

S. Bhattacharyya et al. (eds.), *Mathematical Modeling and Computational Tools*, Springer Proceedings in Mathematics & Statistics 320,
https://doi.org/10.1007/978-981-15-3615-1_15

time. In the heat equation, there are derivatives with respect to time and derivatives with respect to space. Different combinations of mesh points in the different formulas result in different schemes as used. As the mesh spacing (Δx and Δt) goes to zero, the numerical solution obtained with any useful scheme will approach to the true solution of the original differential equation. However, the rate at which the numerical solution approaches the true solution varies with the scheme. In addition, some practically useful schemes can fail to yield a solution for bad combinations of Δx and Δt. Four different schemes for the solution to heat equation are developed. Ames [1], Morton and Mayers [2], Cooper [3], Clive [4], Golub and Ortega [5], Burden and Faires [6], Thomas [7], Strikwerda [8], Arnold [9], Trefethen [10], Olsen-Kettle [11] and Ames [1] provide a development of finite difference methods and modern introduction to the theory of partial differential equation along with a brief coverage of numerical methods. The explicit and implicit Euler schemes are constructed and investigated for hyperbolic heat conduction equation by Ciegis [12].

Recktenwald [13] discussed the three finite difference methods (FTCS, BTCS and Crank-Nicolson) to solve one-dimensional boundary problem. Gerald used the MATLAB code for numerical solution. Karatay et al. [14] obtained the solution of time fractional heat equation using Crank-Nicolson method. Aswin et al. [15] described three different numerical schemes to approximate the solution of the convection–diffusion equation. Azad and Andallah [16] studied stability analysis for two standard finite difference schemes forward time backward space and centered space (FTBSCS) and forward time and centered space (FTCS) for convection–diffusion equation. Mebrate [17] presented the comparative result of finite difference and finite element method for one-dimensional heat equation. Finite element method gave better result than the finite difference method. Olusegun [18] solved the one-dimensional heat equation using explicit scheme. Adak [18–20] solved the transient heat equation with convection boundary condition using explicit finite difference scheme.

The main objective of this paper is to study the effect of explicit and implicit schemes on one-dimensional diffusion equation with Dirichlet boundary condition. The paper is organized in the following ways: First, the second time level scheme to solve parabolic PDEs followed by the third time level scheme to solve parabolic PDEs is discussed. Subsequently, convergence, stability and truncation error analysis are presented for different schemes. Then, the numerical results are compared with the exact solution.

2 Finite Difference Schemes

Consider one-dimensional diffusion equation in a L m length rod without any sources or sinks

$$\frac{\partial T}{\partial t} = \alpha \frac{\partial^2 T}{\partial x^2} \quad 0 \le x \le L,\ t \ge 0 \tag{1}$$

Fig. 1 Mesh grids along distance and time direction

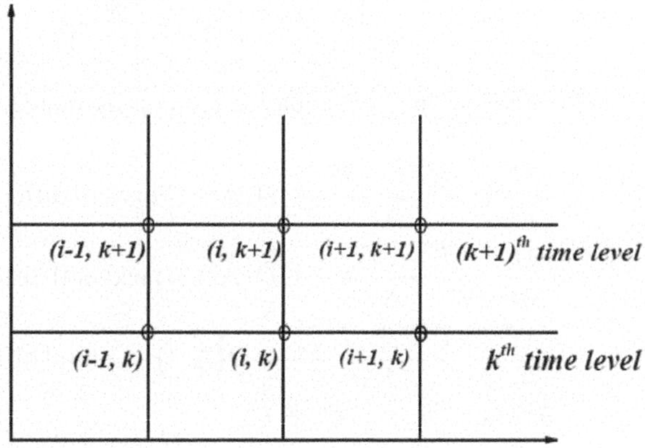

with initial condition $T(x, 0) = f(x)$, and Dirichlet's boundary conditions are

$$T(0, t) = T_0, \quad T(L, t) = T_L$$

where T = temperature (°C), t = time (s), x = length (m). $T_0 = T_L$ = constant temperature.
$\alpha = \frac{k}{\rho c}$ = thermal diffusivity of material depends on k = thermal conductivity (W/m °C) and c = heat capacity of material (J/m^3 °C) and ρ = density (kg/m^3).

This section represents the formulation of various numerical schemes with two time level and three time level. An approximate solution for $T(x, t)$ at a finite set of x and t is obtained by using finite difference schemes. Divide the (x, t) plane into smaller rectangular as shown in Fig. 1 by

$$x = i\Delta x, \quad i = 0, 1, 2 \ldots \quad t = k\Delta t, \quad i = 0, 1, 2 \ldots$$

For the code developed in this article, the discrete x is uniformly spaced in the interval such that

$$T(x, t) = T(i\Delta x, k\Delta t) = T_i^k \quad 0 \le x \le L$$
$$x_i = (i - 1)\Delta x, \quad i = 1, 2, \ldots N$$

where N is the total number of special nodes, including those on the boundary. Given L and N, the spacing between the x_i is computed with $\Delta x = \frac{L}{N-1}$.

Similarly, the discrete t is uniformly spaced in $0 \le t \le t_{\max}$

$$t_k = (k - 1)\Delta t, \quad k = 1, 2, 3 \ldots M$$

where M is the number of time steps and Δt is the size of a time step

$$\Delta t = \frac{t_{\max}}{M-1}$$

Derivatives in the heat equation are approximated by Taylor's series expansion

$$\frac{\partial T}{\partial t} = \frac{T_i^{n+1} - T_i^n}{\Delta t} + O(\Delta t) \text{ (Forward difference in time)}$$
$$\frac{\partial T}{\partial t} = \frac{T_i^n - T_i^{n-1}}{\Delta t} + O(\Delta t) \text{ (Backward difference in time)}$$
$$\frac{\partial T}{\partial t} = \frac{T_i^{n+1} - T_i^{n-1}}{2\Delta t} + O\left(\Delta t^2\right) \text{ (Central difference in time)}$$
$$\frac{\partial^2 T}{\partial x^2} = \frac{T_{i-1}^n - 2T_i^n + T_{i+1}^n}{(\Delta x)^2} + O\left(\Delta x^2\right) \text{ (Central difference in space)}$$

The terms $O\left(\Delta t + \Delta x^2\right)$ and $O\left(\Delta t^2 + \Delta x^2\right)$ denote the order of local truncation error and is also known as the order of method. After neglecting the truncation, error and simplifying, obtain the following difference schemes.

2.1 *Explicit Scheme*

Forward Time and Centre Space (FTCS) Method. In Eq. (1), first-order derivative is replaced by forward difference in time as well as second order is replaced by central difference in space. We get

$$\frac{T_i^{n+1} - T_i^n}{\Delta t} = \alpha \frac{T_{i-1}^n - 2T_i^n + T_{i+1}^n}{(\Delta x)^2}$$

which can be written as

$$T_i^{n+1} = (1 - 2\lambda)T_i^n + \lambda\left(T_{i+1}^n + T_{i-1}^n\right) \tag{2}$$

where $\lambda = \frac{\alpha \Delta t}{\Delta x^2}$ is called mesh ratio parameter.

In Eq. (2), T_i^{n+1} is expressed explicitly in terms of T_{i-1}^n, T_i^n and T_{i+1}^n.

Hence, it is called the explicit formula for the solution of one-dimensional heat equation. It can be shown that Eq. (2) is valid only for $0 \le \lambda \le \frac{1}{2}$, which is called the stability condition for explicit formula. Using Dirichlet initial and boundary condition in Eq. (2), we get system of linear equations for $n = 0, 1, 2\ldots$ These linear equations are solved to get the solution for new time step.

If we set $\lambda = \frac{1}{2}$ in Eq. (2), we obtain the simple formula

$$T_i^{n+1} = \frac{1}{2}\left(T_{i+1}^n + T_{i-1}^n\right) \tag{3}$$

which is called **Bender-Schmidt scheme**. It is clear that Eqs. (2) and (3) have limited application because of the restriction on the values of λ.

Dufort and Frankel Scheme. In Eq. (1), first-order derivative is replaced by central difference in time as well as second order is replaced by central difference in space. We get

$$\frac{T_i^{n+1} - T_i^{n-1}}{2\Delta t} = \alpha \frac{T_{i-1}^n - 2T_i^n + T_{i+1}^n}{(\Delta x)^2}$$

Also, replace T_i^n by the mean of the values T_i^{n+1} and T_i^{n-1} that means $T_i^n \approx \frac{1}{2}\left(T_i^{n+1} + T_i^{n-1}\right)$ and simplifying, Eq. (1) is converted to

$$T_i^{n+1} = \frac{1 - 2\lambda}{1 + 2\lambda} T_i^{n-1} + \frac{2\lambda}{1 + 2\lambda}\left(T_{i-1}^n + T_{i+1}^n\right) \tag{4}$$

where $\lambda = \frac{\alpha \Delta t}{\Delta x^2}$ is called mesh ratio parameter.

Equation (4) is explicit scheme. In this method, to calculate nth level approximate solution $(n-1)$th time level value is used that for calculating first time level (when $n =$ 0), (-1)th time level value is required. It is not possible physically. To overcome the critical situation FCTS scheme is used at $n = 0$; remaining time level approximation is calculated using Dufort-Frankel method. Therefore, FTCS scheme is very simple and straightforward.

2.2 Implicit Scheme

Laasonen Scheme. In Eq. (1), first-order derivative is replaced by backward difference in time as well as second order is replaced by central difference in space. We get

$$\frac{T_i^n - T_i^{n-1}}{\Delta t} = \alpha \frac{T_{i-1}^n - 2T_i^n + T_{i+1}^n}{(\Delta x)^2}$$

After rearranging equation and at $(n+1)$th level equation is given by

$$-\lambda T_{i-1}^{n+1} + (1 + 2\lambda) T_i^{n+1} + \lambda T_{i+1}^{n+1} = T_i^n \tag{5}$$

where $\lambda = \frac{\alpha \Delta t}{(\Delta x)^2}$ is called mesh ratio parameter.

Equation (5) is called Laasonen method, also called two level scheme since nth and $(n+1)$th levels are involved in equation. It is also known as the implicit scheme.

Using boundary and initial conditions in Eq. (5), represent system of linear equations

$$\begin{bmatrix} 1+2\lambda & -\lambda & 0 & 0 & 0 & 0 \\ -\lambda & 1+2\lambda & -\lambda & 0 & 0 & 0 \\ 0 & -\lambda & 1+2\lambda & -\lambda & 0 & 0 \\ 0 & 0 & -\lambda & 1+2\lambda & -\lambda & 0 \\ 0 & 0 & 0 & -\lambda & 1+2\lambda & -\lambda \\ 0 & 0 & 0 & 0 & -\lambda & 1+2\lambda \end{bmatrix} \begin{bmatrix} T_1^1 \\ T_2^1 \\ T_3^1 \\ T_4^1 \\ T_5^1 \\ T_6^1 \end{bmatrix} = \begin{bmatrix} T_1^0 \\ T_2^0 \\ T_3^0 \\ T_4^0 \\ T_5^0 \\ T_6^0 \end{bmatrix}$$

which is solved to determine the solution. Since it is implicit scheme, it is unconditionally stable method.

Crank-Nicolson Scheme. If we replace $\frac{\partial T}{\partial t}$ by forward difference approximation and $\frac{\partial^2 T}{\partial x^2}$ by average of central difference in space at n and $n+1$ level, after simplifying Eq. (1) becomes as

$$\frac{T_i^{n+1} - T_i^n}{\Delta t} = \alpha \frac{1}{2} \left(\frac{T_{i-1}^n - 2T_i^n + T_{i+1}^n}{(\Delta x)^2} + \frac{T_{i-1}^{n+1} - 2T_i^{n+1} + T_{i+1}^{n+1}}{(\Delta x)^2} \right)$$

It can be written as

$$-\lambda T_{i-1}^{n+1} + (2+2\lambda) T_i^{n+1} - \lambda T_{i+1}^{n+1} = \lambda T_{i-1}^n + (2-2\lambda) T_i^n + \lambda T_{i+1}^n \tag{6}$$

where $\lambda = \frac{\alpha \Delta t}{\Delta x^2}$ is called mesh ratio parameter.

This method is also implicit scheme and two level schemes.

The solution of Crank-Nicolson scheme represents the tri-diagonal matrix form as

$$\begin{bmatrix} 2+2\lambda & -\lambda & 0 & 0 & 0 & 0 \\ -\lambda & 2+2\lambda & -\lambda & 0 & 0 & 0 \\ 0 & -\lambda & 2+2\lambda & -\lambda & 0 & 0 \\ 0 & 0 & -\lambda & 2+2\lambda & -\lambda & 0 \\ 0 & 0 & 0 & -\lambda & 2+2\lambda & -\lambda \\ 0 & 0 & 0 & 0 & -\lambda & 2+2\lambda \end{bmatrix} \begin{bmatrix} T_1^1 \\ T_2^1 \\ T_3^1 \\ T_4^1 \\ T_5^1 \\ T_6^1 \end{bmatrix} = \begin{bmatrix} T_1^0 \\ T_2^0 \\ T_3^0 \\ T_4^0 \\ T_5^0 \\ T_6^0 \end{bmatrix}$$

Convergence. If T_i^n is the approximate solution of PDE and T is the true solution, then the convergence is the requirement that $\lim_{\Delta t,\, \Delta x \to 0} ||T_i^n - T|| = 0$ that means that for very smaller value of $\Delta x,\ \Delta t$, approximate solution becomes very closer to true value. At each level, convergence condition $\left|T^{n+1} - T^n\right| < \varepsilon$.
Truncation Error. It is seen that the truncation errors for forward and backward differences are of first order, whereas centered differences are of second order in time and space (using by Taylor series expansions). So, the terms $O\left(k + h^2\right)$ denote the order of local truncation error of FTCS, Bender-Schmidt, Laasonen, Crank-Nicolson and $O\left(k^2 + h^2\right)$ denote the order of local truncation error of Dufort-Frankel scheme.

Consistency. If FD scheme is presented without any error terms, then we can show consistency by Taylor expansion in the spatial approximation and temporal approximation separately; thus, the total truncation error goes to zero. Then, finite difference must be consistent at least for first-order truncation error $(O(\Delta t) + O(\Delta x))$.
Stability Criteria. For stability, error at $(n + 1)$th time level is less than equal to the error at nth time level. So, $\|e^{n+1}\| \leq \|e^{n}\| \rightarrow \|T_i^{n+1}\| \leq \|T_i^{n}\|$. Stability condition for FTCS scheme is $0 < \lambda \leq 1/2$. λ depends on mesh size in time and space. If $\lambda > 1/2$, scheme would be unstable, whereas Laasonen, Crank-Nicolson, Dufort-Frankel methods are unconditionally stable.

3 Test Problem and Verification

Various level finite difference schemes are used to approximate solution of parabolic Eq. (1). It is required to experiment with these numerical techniques. It is hoped that by writing computer codes and analyzing the results, numerical techniques show the gainful result. Therefore, this section proposes a simple example and presents solutions by described schemes.

In this study, consider a 1-m-long thin metal rod at temperature of wave equation. At $t = 0$, both of its ends are placed on ice 0 °C. Assume that the heat can only flow between rod and ice.

Governing equation of the above problem is given by Eq. (1) with initial condition $T(x, 0) = \sin \pi x$, $0 \leq x \leq 1$, and Dirichlet's boundary conditions are $T(0, t) = T(1, t) = 0$.

The exact solution of the problem is $T(x, t) = e^{-\pi^2 t} \sin \pi x$.

As the mesh spacing (Δx and Δt) goes to zero, truncation error tends to zero, so approximate solution will be very nearer to the exact solution.

Case I Consider $\Delta x = 0.1429\,\text{m}, \ \Delta t = 0.01\,\text{s}$.

So, $\lambda = \frac{\alpha \Delta t}{(\Delta x)^2} = 0.49 < 0.5$.

Therefore, stability condition of explicit (FTCS) finite scheme is satisfied and a stable condition is expected.

Other schemes that means Laasonen, Crank-Nicolson and Dufort-Frankle methods are unconditionally stable. The temperature profile for two-three level schemes is presented for three iterations as shown in Fig. 2.

Figure 3 shows that the comparison result of explicit (FTCS) and exact solution for 1st–25th iteration that means $t = 0$–0.25 s at point $x = 0.1429$ m. The graph indicates that temperature was high initially and then gradually was decreased due to ends kept at ice 0 °C. FTCS scheme is stable for $\lambda < 0.5$, so scheme is stable for $\lambda = 0.49$ from convergence plot which is shown in Fig. 4.

Figure 5 shows temperature at each point of x domain from initial to 25th time level for $\lambda = 0.49$ of FTCS scheme. It follows from the presented results that the temperature at middle of the x-axis is higher due to sine curve than ends of rod due

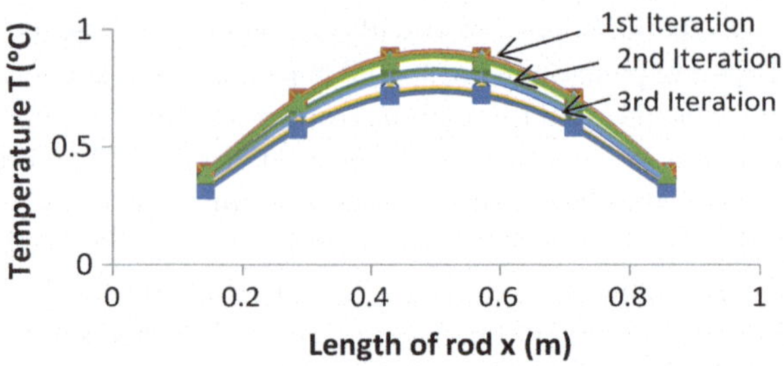

Fig. 2 Temperature profile with $\Delta x = 0.1429\,\text{m}$, $\Delta t = 0.01$ of various schemes

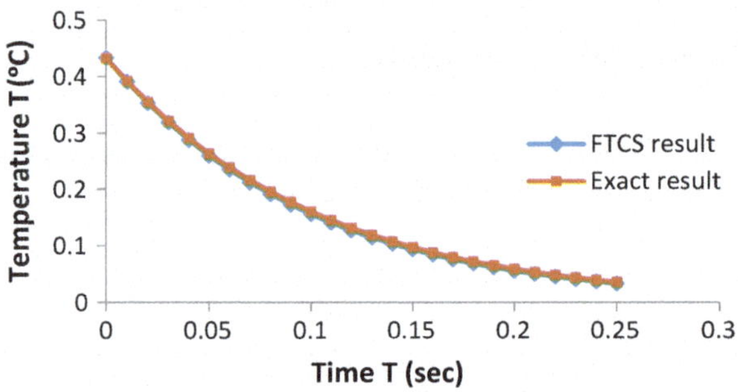

Fig. 3 Comparison temperature profile for FTCS scheme and exact solution

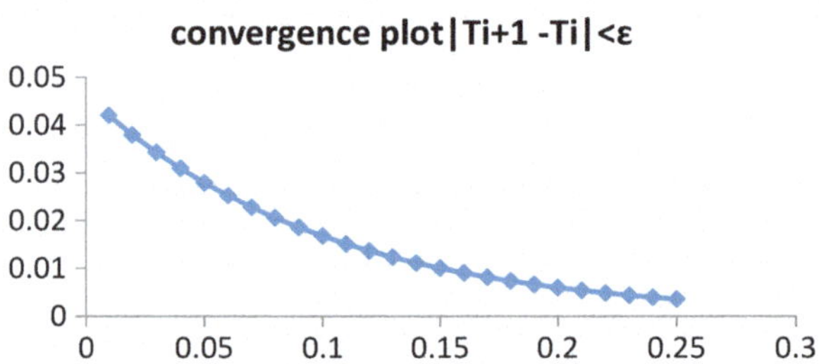

Fig. 4 Convergence plot of FTCS scheme for $\Delta x = 0.1429,\ \Delta t = 0.01$

to boundary values 0 °C. Temperature distributions are calculated for FTCS scheme at different time levels $t = 0,\ 0.05,\ 0.1,\ 0.15,\ 0.2,\ 0.25\,\text{s}$ as shown in Fig. 6.

Case II When time step is increased to 0.02 s with same space size. Therefore, $\Delta x = 0.1429,\ \Delta t = 0.02$.

$\lambda = \frac{\alpha \Delta t}{(\Delta x)^2} = 0.98 > 0.5$ which exceeds the stability requirement.

Therefore, FTCS scheme is unstable. So, unstable solution is appeared in Fig. 7.

In Case II, time step is increased with the same space size, so the λ is greater than 0.5.

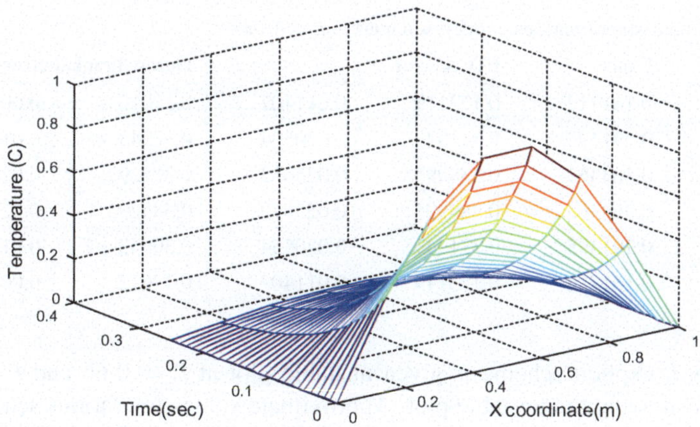

Fig. 5 Temperature profile of FTCS in x domain from time $t = 0$–0.25 s with $\Delta x = 0.1429,\ \Delta t = 0.01,\ \lambda = 0.49$

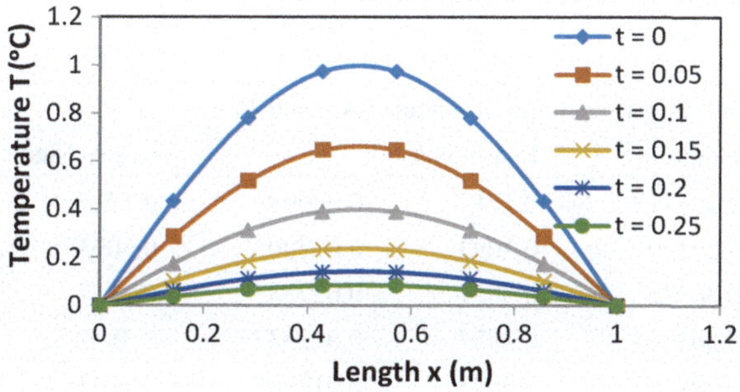

Fig. 6 Temperature profile for FTCS scheme at different time in x domain for $\Delta x = 0.1429\,\text{m},\ \Delta t = 0.01$

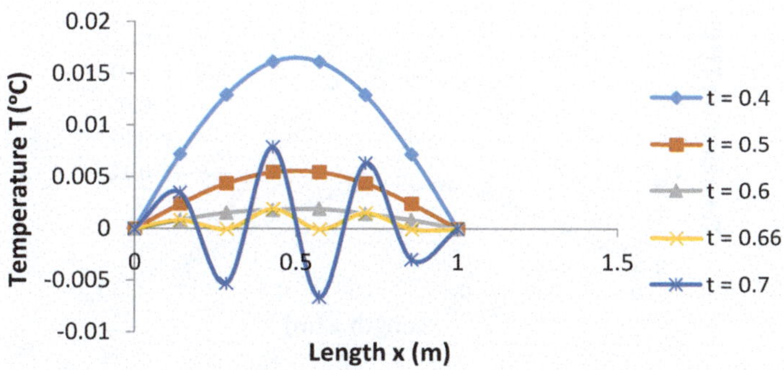

Fig. 7 Temperature profile of FTCS scheme for $\Delta x = 0.1429,\ \Delta t = 0.02$

Table 1 Comparison of various explicit schemes at $t = 0.1$ s

X	Exact	FTCS/error		Dufort-Frankel/error	
0.142857	0.161712	0.173119	0.011407	0.17012	0.008408
0.285714	0.291395	0.311949	0.020554	0.30943	0.018035
0.428571	0.363363	0.388995	0.025632	0.385292	0.021929
0.571429	0.363363	0.388995	0.025632	0.385292	0.021929
0.714286	0.291395	0.311949	0.020554	0.30943	0.018035
0.857143	0.161712	0.173119	0.011407	0.17012	0.008408

Therefore, explicit scheme is given unstable plot at $t = 0.66$ and $t = 0.7$ s. Figure 6 is showing the unstable plot. Approximate values for various schemes are compared with exact values at 10th time level ($t = 0.1$ s) at all x points. Absolute errors for explicit and implicit schemes are calculated as shown in Tables 1 and 2. From the table, it is clear that the Crank-Nicolson method gave the more accurate solution for transient heat conduction problem (Fig. 8).

Table 2 Comparison of various implicit schemes at $t = 0.1$ s

X	Exact	Laasonen/error		Crank-Nicolson/error	
0.142857	0.161712	0.1717	0.009988	0.1717	0.009988
0.285714	0.291395	0.3093	0.017905	0.3093	0.017905
0.428571	0.363363	0.3857	0.022337	0.3857	0.022337
0.571429	0.363363	0.3857	0.022337	0.3857	0.022337
0.714286	0.291395	0.3093	0.017905	0.3093	0.017905
0.857143	0.161712	0.1717	0.009988	0.1717	0.009988

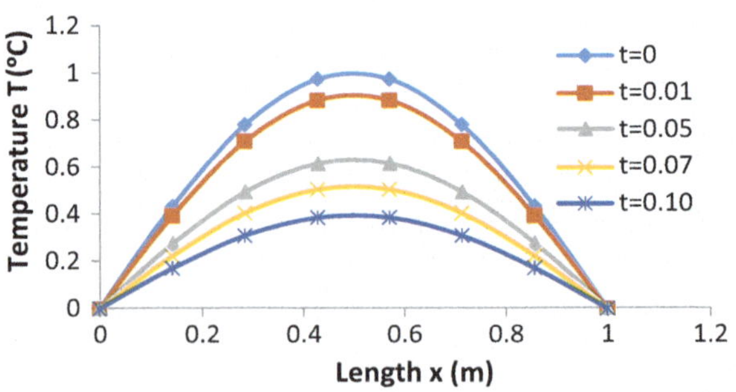

Fig. 8 Temperature profile for Laasonen scheme at various time levels for $\lambda = 0.49$

Table 3 Percentile errors for various level schemes at $t = 0.1$ s

x	FTCS % error	Laasonen % error	Crank-Nicolson % error	Dufort-Frankel % error
0.142857	7.053898	6.176412	0.425448	5.199367
0.285714	7.053656	6.14458	0.482163	6.189193
0.428571	7.054103	6.147296	0.533076	6.035012
0.571429	7.054103	6.147296	0.615638	6.035012
0.714286	7.053656	6.14458	0.688069	6.189193

4 Conclusion

Explicit and implicit finite difference schemes are described for approximate solution of unsteady state one-dimensional heat problem. From Fig. 2 and Tables 1, 2 and 3, one can say that Crank-Nicolson method gives the best numerical approximation to analytical solution. Laasonen, Crank-Nicolson, Dufort-Frankel schemes are unconditionally stable, whereas explicit (FTCS) scheme is conditionally stable. Therefore, explicit scheme is tested for stable and unstable conditions. Unstable solution is appeared in Fig. 7 for increased time step $\Delta t = 0.02$ for FTCS scheme. Also, convergence plot is presented for stability. The aim of this paper is comparative study for various time level finite difference schemes. These numerical techniques can be implemented for more dimensional heat problems, advection–diffusion and Burger equations.

References

1. Ames, W.F.: Numerical Methods for Partial Differential Equations, 3rd edn. Academic Press Inc., Boston (1992)
2. Morton, K.W., Mayers, D.F.: Numerical Solution of Partial Differential Equations: An Introduction. Cambridge University Press, Cambridge, England (1994)
3. Cooper, J.: Introduction to Partial Differential Equations with Matlab. Birkhauser, Boston (1998)
4. Clive, A.J.F.: Computational Techniques for Fluid Dynamics. Springer-Verlag, Berlin (1988)
5. Golub, G., Ortega, J.M.: Scientific Computing: An Introduction with Parallel Computing. Academic Press, Inc., Boston (1993)
6. Burden, R.L., Faires, J.D.: Numerical Analysis, 6th edn. Brooks/Cole Publishing Co., New York (1997)
7. Thomas, J.W.: Numerical Partial Differential Equations: Finite Difference Methods, vol. 22. Springer Science & Business Media (2013)
8. Strikwerda, J.C.: Finite difference schemes and partial differential equations. SIAM J. Appl. Sci. Environ. Sustain. **3**(7), 188–200 (2004). e-ISSN 2360-8013 200 | P a g e
9. Arnold, D.N.: Lecture Notes on Numerical Analysis of Partial Differential Equations. Available at http://www.math.umn.edu/~arnold/8445/notes.pdf (2015)
10. Trefethen, L.N.: Finite Difference and Spectral Methods for Ordinary and Partial Differential Equations. Unpublished Text. Available at https://people.maths.ox.ac.uk/trefethen/pdetext.html (1996)

11. Olsen-Kettle, L.: Numerical Solution of Partial Differential Equations. Retrieved from http://espace.library.uq.edu.au/view/UQ:239427 (2015)
12. Ciegis, R.: Numerical solution of hyperbolic heat conduction equation. Math. Model. Anal. **14**(1), 11–24 (2009)
13. Recktenwald, G.W.: Finite-Difference Approximations to the Heat Equation. http://www.nada.kth.se/~jjalap/numme/FDheat.pdf (2011)
14. Karatay, I., Kale, N., Bayramoglu, S.: A new difference scheme for time fractional heat equations based on the Crank-Nicholson method. Fract. Calc. Appl. Anal. **16**(4), 892–910 (2013)
15. Aswin, V.S., Awasthi, A., Anu, C.: A comparative study of numerical schemes for convection-diffusion equation. Procedia Eng. **127**, 621–627 (2015)
16. Azad, T.M.A.K., Andallah, L.S.: Stability analysis of finite difference schemes for an advection diffusion equation. Bangladesh J. Sci. Res. **29**(2), 143–151 (2016)
17. Mebrate, B.: Numerical solution of one dimensional heat equation with Dirichlet boundary condition. Am. J. Appl. Math. **3**(6), 305–311 (2015)
18. Adak, M., Mandal, N.R.: Numerical and experimental study of mitigation of welding distortion. Appl. Math. Model. **34**, 146–158 (2010)
19. Adak, M., Soares, C.G.: Effects of different restraints on the weld-induced residual deformations and stresses in a steel plate. Int. J. Adv. Manuf. Technol. **71**, 699–710 (2014)
20. Adak, M., Soares, C.G.: Residual deflections and stresses in a thick T joint plate structure. J. Appl. Mech. Eng. **5**, 6 (2016)

Numerical Solution of Space and Time Fractional Advection–Diffusion Equation by Meshless Approach

Hitesh Bansu and Sushil Kumar

Abstract In this paper, fractional version of advection–diffusion equation (FADE) has been considered for the numerical solution. It is acquired from the classical advection–diffusion equation (ADE) by substituting the space and time derivatives with a generalized Caputo fractional derivative. Moreover, we have proposed novel discretization for space and time using radial basis functions and Chebyshev polynomials, respectively. The proposed scheme is truly meshless thereby able to manage both space and time fractional derivatives simultaneously with appropriate boundary conditions. Lastly, we have discussed numerical example to affirm this proposed scheme whilst revealing the accuracy and performance of the same.

Keywords Radial basis function · Chebyshev polynomials · Meshless method · Kronecker product · Fractional advection–diffusion equation

1 Introduction

There is a long history on the study of fractional calculus as an extension of classical calculus. At the initial stage, the development process of fractional calculus was slow and it was highly concentrated on the field of pure mathematics. In the last few decades, fractional calculus gained considerable attention; during this time, it has been implemented in numerous areas like applied mathematics, science, engineering, finance and so on [1, 2]. A massive quantity of works in technology and engineering copes with dynamical systems which can be described via fractional-order equations that include integrals and derivatives of fractional order. These new fractional models are more suitable than the formerly used models of integer order; therefore, fractional calculus is considered as a more practical technique nowadays [3].

H. Bansu (✉) · S. Kumar
S. V. National Institute of Technology, Surat, India
e-mail: hiteshbansu@gmail.com

S. Kumar
e-mail: skumar.iitr@gmail.com

S. Bhattacharyya et al. (eds.), *Mathematical Modeling and Computational Tools*, Springer Proceedings in Mathematics & Statistics 320,
https://doi.org/10.1007/978-981-15-3615-1_16

Many phenomena in various fields can be modelled more accurately by fractional differential equations because of their nonlocal property. Above all, one of the most vital mathematical models observed in a wide range of engineering and industrial applications is the fractional advection–diffusion equation. For instance, it can be used to describe water transfer in soil, dispersion of dissolved salts in groundwater, transport in fluids [2, 4, 5].

In the present study, time and space fractional advection–diffusion equation is considered as

$$\frac{\partial^{\alpha} u}{\partial t^{\alpha}} + p(x)\frac{\partial^{\beta} u}{\partial x^{\beta}} = q(x)\frac{\partial^{1+\beta} u}{\partial x^{1+\beta}} + f(x,t), \quad 0 < x, t < 1, \quad 0 < \alpha, \beta \leq 1 \tag{1}$$

and initial and boundary conditions are taken as

$$\left.\begin{aligned} u(x,0) = f_1(x), \\ u(0,t) = g_1(t), \; u(1,t) = g_2(t). \end{aligned}\right\} \tag{2}$$

Due to its importance and applicability, many researchers have considered this model from the perspective of numerical and analytic solutions. Gómez et al. [6] derived analytic solution for fractional-order advection–diffusion equation by using Mittag-Leffler functions. Agarwal et al. [7] investigated the analytic solution for the time–space fractional-order advection–dispersion equation by applying the technique of Laplace and Fourier transforms. Safari and Danesh [8] implemented the Adomian decomposition method (ADM) to present the analytic solution of space fractional-order diffusion equations. Variable separation method was employed by Zhang et al. [9] to find an analytical solution for the time fractional-order advection–dispersion equation with variable coefficient. Xu et al. [2] used a new generalized fractional derivative in the finite difference method for the solution of fractional advection–diffusion equation numerically. Javadi et al. [10] developed a numerical scheme based on the spectral–collocation method by using the Bernstein polynomial approximation for the solution of space–time fractional advection–dispersion equation. Jacobi collocation method was used by Parvizi et al. [11] for the numerical solution of fractional-order advection–diffusion equation. Cao et al. [12] constructed an improved difference scheme to solve the Caputo-type fractional advection–diffusion equation numerically. Arshad et al. [13] formulated a numerical technique for the solution of the space–time fractional-order advection–diffusion equation where Riesz and the Caputo derivative were considered in space and time, respectively. Meerschaert and Tadjeran [5] solved the fractional advection–diffusion equation applied on groundwater hydrology by finite difference method. Jafari and Tajadodi [14] employed the homotopy analysis method (HAM) to obtain the solution of the space–time fractional advection–dispersion equation. Lian et al. [15] presented a study on meshfree method to solve the space fractional-order advection–diffusion equation via the reproducing kernel particle method (RKPM). Different techniques have been applied by Zhuang et al. [16] to find an approximate solution of variable-order fractional advection–diffusion equation with a nonlinear source term. Also, they have compared the results for various techniques like implicit and explicit Euler approximation, matrix transfer technique and fractional method of lines. The fractional advection–dispersion equation derived from Fick's first law has been solved with the finite difference method by Deng et al. [17].

In the present study, we have applied a new numerical meshless technique of collocation with radial basis function and Chebyshev polynomials to solve fractional advection–diffusion equation because whilst dealing with fractional models numerical techniques are given higher preference. The key feature of this developed RBF collocation technique is that it is truly meshless hence does not require generation of any mesh or grid. Also, we have used two different and independent domain discretization for space and time.

The layout of the current article is as follows. After a brief introduction, Sect. 2 deals with preliminaries about fractional derivatives, Chebyshev polynomials and radial basis functions. In Sect. 3, we have presented the layout of the new technique. Section 4 shows the applicability of the proposed technique with a numerical example. Lastly, Sect. 5 leads to the conclusion.

2 Preliminaries

We will start with a few important definitions and preliminaries about fractional derivatives, the notations about Chebyshev polynomials and radial basis functions (RBFs) [18, 19].

Definition 1 The Riemann–Liouville fractional derivative of order α of function $f(x)$ is defined as [20]

$$ {}_{a}^{\mathrm{RL}}D_x^{\alpha} f(x) = \frac{1}{\Gamma(n-\alpha)} \frac{\mathrm{d}^n}{\mathrm{d}x^n} \int_a^x (x-\tau)^{n-\alpha-1} f(\tau)\, d\tau, $$

$$ x > a,\ n-1 < \alpha \leq n \in N. $$

Definition 2 The Caputo fractional derivative of order α of function $f(x)$ for $\alpha > 0,\ t > a,\ (\alpha, a, t \in \mathbb{R})$ is defined as [20]

$$ {}_{a}^{C}D_t^{\alpha} f(t) = \frac{1}{\Gamma(n-\alpha)} \int_a^t \frac{f^{(n)}(\tau)}{(t-\tau)^{\alpha+1-n}} \mathrm{d}\tau, \quad t > a,\ n-1 < \alpha \leq n \in N. $$

Definition 3 Caputo fractional derivative of a basic power function $x^k,\ k \geq 0$ is defined as

$$ D^{\alpha} x^k = \begin{cases} \frac{\Gamma(k+1)}{\Gamma(k-\alpha+1)} x^{k-\alpha}, & \text{for } k \geq \alpha \\ 0, & \text{for } k < \alpha. \end{cases} $$

2.1 Radial Basis Functions

In the last four decades, RBFs have enjoyed considerable success and became a powerful tool for interpolating scattered data. Furthermore, their theoretical and convergence properties have been well established [21]. RBFs were widely imposed inside the subject of multivariate interpolation as many applications resulted in the problem of interpolating data at scattered locations. According to the process of interpolation utilizing radial basis functions, the approximation of $u(x)$ can be expressed as a linear combination of N radial basis functions as

$$u(x) = \sum_{i=1}^{N} \lambda_i \phi_i(r),$$

where N is the number of data points. $\{\lambda_i\}_{i=1}^{N}$ are unknown coefficients to be determined. $\phi(r)$ indicates some radial basis function. and $r = \|x - x_i\|$ is the Euclidean norm between points x and x_i. The big advantage of RBF is that it contains Euclidean distance as an independent variable irrespective of the dimension of the problem.

Most commonly used RBFs are the Gaussian $\phi(r) = \mathrm{e}^{-(\epsilon r)^2}$, the multiquadric $\phi(r) = (r^2 + \epsilon^2)^{\beta/2}$, $\beta = -1, 1, 3, 5, \ldots$, the polyharmonic splines $\phi(r) = r^n \log r$, $n = 2, 4, 6, \ldots$ and the conical type $\phi(r) = r^n$, $n = 1, 3, 5, \ldots$ In our study, we have used conical type RBF with $n = 3$. For more knowledge about RBF interpolation, reader is advised to refer [22, 23].

2.2 Chebyshev Polynomials

The Chebyshev polynomials $T_n(x)$; $n = 0, 1, \ldots,$ defined on the interval $[-1, 1]$, are one of the solutions of the differential equation [18]

$$(1 - x^2)y'' - xy' + n^2 y = 0.$$

The Chebyshev polynomials $T_n(x)$ satisfy the following recurrence relation [18, 19]

$$T_{n+1}(x) = 2xT_n(x) - T_{n-1}(x),\ n \geq 1,$$
$$T_0(x) = 1, \quad T_1(x) = x.$$

They are orthogonal with respect to the weight function $w(x) = 1/\sqrt{1 - x^2}$ i.e. [18, 19]

$$\int_{-1}^{1} \frac{T_m(x)T_n(x)}{\sqrt{1-x^2}} \mathrm{d}x = \begin{cases} 0, & \text{if } m \neq n, \\ \pi/2, & \text{if } m = n \neq 0, \\ \pi, & \text{if } m = n = 0. \end{cases}$$

One of the unique features of Chebyshev polynomials is their explicit relationship with trigonometric function [18]

$$T_n(x) = \cos\left(n \cos^{-1}(x)\right).$$

3 Proposed Scheme

In order to solve the problem in Eqs. (1)–(2), the function $u(x, t)$ can be expressed and approximated in terms of Chebyshev polynomials basis and radial basis function as [24]

$$\begin{aligned} u(x,t) = u_{Nn}(x,t) &\approx \sum_{i=1}^{N} \sum_{j=1}^{n} T_j^*(t) c_{ji} \Phi_i(x) \\ &= \mathbb{T}(t) C \Phi(x), \end{aligned} \tag{3}$$

where $\mathbb{T}(t) = \left[T_1^*(t), T_2^*(t), T_3^*(t), \ldots, T_n^*(x)\right]$, $\Phi(x) = [\phi_1(x), \phi_2(x), \phi_3(x), \ldots, \phi_N(x)]^t$ are Chebyshev polynomials and cubic radial basis functions, respectively.

The positive integers N and n are discretization parameters corresponding to space and time, respectively. The unknowns c_{ji}s are of the form

$$C = \begin{bmatrix} c_{11} & c_{12} & \cdots & c_{1N} \\ c_{21} & c_{22} & \cdots & c_{2N} \\ \vdots & \vdots & \ddots & \vdots \\ c_{n1} & c_{n2} & \cdots & c_{nN} \end{bmatrix}.$$

In general, for time discretization, we have used n Chebyshev nodes in any interval $[p, q]$ as

$$t_k = \frac{1}{2}(p+q) + \frac{1}{2}(q-p)\cos\left(\frac{2(n-k)-1}{2n}\pi\right); \; k = 1, 2, \ldots, n,$$

and for space discretization, we have followed m uniform nodes in any interval $[p, q]$ as

$$x_m = x_{m-1} + \frac{q-p}{n-1};\ m = 1, 2, \ldots, N,\ x_0 = p.$$

It is important to note that here space and time discretization are totally independent of each other.

From Eq. (3), we can write

$$ {}_0^C D_t^{\alpha} u(x,t) = {}_0^C D_t^{\alpha}(\mathbb{T}C\Phi) = \left[{}^C D_t^{\alpha}\mathbb{T}\right]C\Phi = \mathbb{T}^{\alpha}C\Phi, \tag{4}$$

$$ {}_0^C D_t^{\beta} u(x,t) = {}_0^C D_t^{\beta}(\mathbb{T}C\Phi) = \mathbb{T}C\left[{}^C D_t^{\beta}\Phi\right] = \mathbb{T}C\Phi^{\beta}. \tag{5}$$

Substituting Eqs. (4) and (5) in Eq. (1), we will have

$$\mathbb{T}^{\alpha}C\Phi + p(x)\left\{\mathbb{T}C\Phi^{\beta}\right\} = q(x)\left\{\mathbb{T}C\Phi^{1+\beta}\right\} + f(x,t). \tag{6}$$

Collocating (6) in $N-2$ uniform nodes, i.e. $x_m,\ m = 2, 3, \ldots N-1$ and $n-1$ Chebyshev nodes, i.e. $t_k,\ k = 2, 3, \ldots, n$, it will give $(N-2)(n-1)$ equations of the form

$$M_1 CL + p(x)\{MCL_1\} - q(x)\{MCL_2\} = f(x,t), \tag{7}$$

where

$$L_1 = \begin{bmatrix} {}_0^C D_x^{\beta}\phi_1(x_2) & {}_0^C D_x^{\beta}\phi_1(x_2) & \ldots & {}_0^C D_x^{\beta}\phi_1(x_2) \\ {}_0^C D_x^{\beta}\phi_2(x_3) & {}_0^C D_x^{\beta}\phi_2(x_3) & \ldots & {}_0^C D_x^{\beta}\phi_2(x_3) \\ \vdots & \vdots & \ldots & \vdots \\ {}_0^C D_x^{\beta}\phi_N(x_{N-1}) & {}_0^C D_x^{\beta}\phi_N(x_{N-1}) & \ldots & {}_0^C D_x^{\beta}\phi_N(x_{N-1}) \end{bmatrix},$$

$$M = \begin{bmatrix} T_1(t_2) & T_2(t_2) & \ldots & T_n(t_2) \\ T_1(t_3) & T_2(t_3) & \ldots & T_n(t_3) \\ \vdots & \vdots & \ldots & \vdots \\ T_1(t_n) & T_2(t_n) & \ldots & T_n(t_n) \end{bmatrix},$$

$$L_2 = \begin{bmatrix} {}_0^C D_x^{1+\beta}\phi_1(x_2) & {}_0^C D_x^{1+\beta}\phi_2(x_2) & \ldots & {}_0^C D_x^{1+\beta}\phi_N(x_2) \\ {}_0^C D_x^{1+\beta}\phi_1(x_3) & {}_0^C D_x^{1+\beta}\phi_2(x_3) & \ldots & {}_0^C D_x^{1+\beta}\phi_N(x_3) \\ \vdots & \vdots & \ldots & \vdots \\ {}_0^C D_x^{1+\beta}\phi_1(x_{N-1}) & {}_0^C D_x^{1+\beta}\phi_2(x_{N-1}) & \ldots & {}_0^C D_x^{1+\beta}\phi_N(x_{N-1}) \end{bmatrix},$$

$$M_1 = \begin{bmatrix} {}_0^C D_x^{\alpha}T_1(t_2) & {}_0^C D_x^{\alpha}T_2(t_2) & \ldots & {}_0^C D_x^{\alpha}T_n(t_2) \\ {}_0^C D_x^{\alpha}T_1(t_3) & {}_0^C D_x^{\alpha}T_2(t_3) & \ldots & {}_0^C D_x^{\alpha}T_n(t_3) \\ \vdots & \vdots & \ldots & \vdots \\ {}_0^C D_x^{\alpha}T_1(t_n) & {}_0^C D_x^{\alpha}T_2(t_n) & \ldots & {}_0^C D_x^{\alpha}T_n(t_n) \end{bmatrix}.$$

Implementing Eq. (3) on the initial and boundary conditions given in Eq. (2)

$$\begin{aligned} M_2CL_3 &= f(x), \\ MCL_4 &= g_1(t), \\ MCL_5 &= g_2(t), \end{aligned} \tag{8}$$

where

$$L_3 = \begin{bmatrix} \phi_1(x_1) & \phi_2(x_1) & \dots & \phi_N(x_1) \\ \phi_1(x_2) & \phi_2(x_2) & \dots & \phi_N(x_2) \\ \vdots & \vdots & \dots & \vdots \\ \phi_1(x_N) & \phi_2(x_N) & \dots & \phi_N(x_N) \end{bmatrix},$$

$L_4 = \left[\phi_1(x_1)\ \phi_2(x_1)\ \dots\ \phi_N(x_1)\right]^t, L_5 = \left[\phi_1(x_N)\ \phi_2(x_N)\ \dots\ \phi_N(x_N)\right]^t$ and $M_2 = \left[T_1(t_1)\ T_2(t_1)\ \dots\ T_n(t_1)\right]$.

By collocating Eq. (8), we get $(N + 2n - 2)$ equations. These equations with Eq. (7) will give Nn equations.

To solve Eq. (7), we will first modify it in a more simplified form. To accomplish that task, we will use Kronecker product (indicated by $\otimes$) to express equation as follows

$$\left\{L^t \otimes M_1 + p(x)\left(L_1^t \otimes M\right) - q(x)\left(L_2^t \otimes T\right)\right\}\text{vec}(c) = \text{vec}(f(x,t)),$$

which can be formed as

$$A_1C = F_1 \tag{9}$$

where A_1 is a matrix of size $(N-2)(n-1) \times Nn$. vec(c) can be obtained by stacking the columns of C on top of one another and is of size $Nn \times 1$ [25, 26].

F_1 is vector of size $(N-2)(n-1) \times 1$. Superscript "t" stands for transpose of the matrix.

Initial and boundary conditions can be expressed as

$$\begin{aligned} \left(L_3^t \otimes M2\right)\text{vec}(c) &= \text{vec}(f(x)), \\ \left(L_4^t \otimes M\right)\text{vec}(c) &= \text{vec}(g_1(t)), \\ \left(L_5^t \otimes M\right)\text{vec}(c) &= \text{vec}(g_2(t)), \end{aligned}$$

which can be written as

$$\begin{aligned} A_2C &= F_2, \\ A_3C &= F_3, \\ A_4C &= F_4, \end{aligned} \tag{10}$$

where dimension of A_2 is $N \times Nn$. Vector F_2 is of size $N \times 1$. A_3 and A_4 are of the same dimension, i.e. $(n-1) \times Nn$. Similarly, F_3 and F_4 are of the size $(n-1) \times 1$.

The resulting system of equation can be described from collecting Eqs. (9) and (10)

$$AC = F \tag{11}$$

where the dimension of A is $Nn \times Nn$, and it has the form $A = [A_1, A_2, A_3, A_4]^t$. F is of the form $F = [F_1, F_2, F_3, F_4]^t$ and of the size $Nn \times 1$.

After solving the linear system of Eq. (11), we can find the values of unknown coefficients C. Putting C in Eq. (3), we will get the desired approximate solution $u(x, t)$ from (3) for the given problem (1).

4 Numerical Example

Example 1 To test the efficiency for the new technique, consider the following time fractional advection–diffusion equation [27]

$$\begin{aligned} {}^{C}D_t^{\alpha}u(x,t) + D_x u(x,t) - D_x^2 u(x,t) = f(x,t) \qquad 0 < \alpha \le 1 \\ 0 < x < 1, \quad 0 < t \le 1, \end{aligned} \tag{12}$$

the initial and boundary conditions as

$$\begin{aligned} &u(x,0) = 0 && 0 < x < 1, \\ &u(0,t) = 0 \quad u(1,t) = t^3, && 0 < t \le 1, \end{aligned} \tag{13}$$

where source term is given by

$$f(x,t) = \frac{6}{\Gamma(4-\alpha)} x^2 t^{3-\alpha} + 2t^3(x-1).$$

The exact solution of the above problem is $u(x,t) = x^2 t^3$ and $p(x) = q(x) = 1$.

This problem has been solved by Fazio et al. [27] using the finite difference method. We have solved this problem by the scheme proposed in Sect. 3 and compared the results with the results in [27]. Table 1 shows the comparison of the scheme proposed in [27] with the current scheme. Results say that our scheme gives better accuracy that is too with less number of points and less computational cost compared to the scheme in [27].

Table 1 Comparison of error for (12)

α	Method in [27]		Proposed method	
	N	L_∞	L_∞	CPU time (s)
0.1		$n = 100$	$n = 10$	
	10	3.7869×10^{-5}	2.9458×10^{-4}	0.06
	20	9.6542×10^{-5}	6.7613×10^{-5}	0.06
	40	2.4674×10^{-5}	1.5559×10^{-5}	0.08
	80	6.2843×10^{-6}	2.2691×10^{-5}	0.013
0.5	10	4.4597×10^{-4}	2.8335×10^{-4}	0.06
	20	1.3436×10^{-4}	6.4846×10^{-5}	0.06
	40	4.1920×10^{-4}	1.4915×10^{-5}	0.08
	80	1.3435×10^{-4}	3.4032×10^{-6}	0.13
0.9	10	3.3229×10^{-3}	2.6825×10^{-4}	0.06
	20	1.4844×10^{-3}	6.1127×10^{-5}	0.06
	40	6.7617×10^{-4}	1.4076×10^{-5}	0.08
	80	3.1119×10^{-4}	3.3415×10^{-6}	0.15

5 Conclusion

The computational results obtained from the technique proposed in Sect. 3 using MATLAB® are shown in Table 1.

The results obtained from the proposed technique have been compared with the results in [27]. We note that the proposed method gives superior results with a very less number of points in the time direction (only 10) and that reduces the computational cost effectively compared to [27]. Also, the scheme proposed in the current study can be implemented to solve other partial differential equations with appropriate initial and boundary conditions.

References

1. Li, W., Li, C.: Second-order explicit difference schemes for the space fractional advection diffusion equation. Appl. Math. Comput. **257**, 446–457 (2015)
2. Xu, Y., He, Z., Xu, Q.: Numerical solutions of fractional advection–diffusion equations with a kind of new generalized fractional derivative. Int. J. Comput. Math. **91**, 588–600 (2014)
3. Garg, M., Manohar, P.: Numerical solution of fractional diffusion-wave equation with two space variables by matrix method. Fract. Calc. Appl. Anal. **13**, 191–207 (2010)
4. Ahmed, S.: A numerical algorithm for solving advection-diffusion equation with constant and variable coefficients. J. Open Numer. Methods **4**, 1–7 (2012)
5. Meerschaert, M.M., Tadjeran, C.: Finite difference approximations for fractional advection–dispersion flow equations. J. Comput. Appl. Math. **172**, 65–77 (2004)

6. Gómez, F., Escalante, E., Calderón, C., Morales, L., González, M., Laguna, R.: Analytical solutions for the fractional diffusion-advection equation describing super-diffusion. Open Phys. **14**, 668–675 (2016)
7. Agarwal, R., Jain, S., Agarwal, R.: Analytic solution of generalized space time advection-dispersion equation with fractional Laplace operator. J. Nonlinear Sci. Appl. **9**, 3545–3554 (2016)
8. Safari, M., Danesh, M.: Application of Adomians decomposition method for the analytical solution of space fractional diffusion equation. Adv. Pure Math. **1**, 345–350 (2011)
9. Zhang, S., Liu, M., Zhang, L.: Variable separation for time fractional advection-dispersion equation with initial and boundary conditions. Therm. Sci. **20**, 789–792 (2016)
10. Javadi, S., Jani, M., Babolian, E.: A numerical scheme for space-time fractional advection-dispersion equation. Int. J. Nonlinear Anal. Appl. **7**, 331–343 (2015)
11. Parvizi, M., Eslahchi, M., Dehghan, M.: Numerical solution of fractional advection-diffusion equation with a nonlinear source term. Numer. Algorithms **68**, 601–629 (2015)
12. Cao, J., Li, C., Chen, Y.: High-order approximation to Caputo derivatives and Caputo-type advection-diffusion equations (II). Fract. Calc. Appl. Anal. **18**, 735–761 (2015)
13. Arshad, S., Baleanu, D., Huang, J., Al Qurashi, M.M., Tang, Y., Zhao, Y.: Finite difference method for time-space fractional advection-diffusion equations with Riesz derivative. Entropy **20**, 321 (2018)
14. Jafari, H., Tajadodi, H.: Numerical solutions of the fractional advection-dispersion equation. Prog. Fract. Differ. Appl **1**, 37–45 (2015)
15. Lian, Y., Wagner, G.J., Liu, W.K.: A meshfree method for the fractional advection-diffusion equation. In: Meshfree Methods for Partial Differential Equations VIII, vol. 115, pp. 53–66. Springer (2017)
16. Zhuang, P., Liu, F., Anh, V., Turner, I.: Numerical methods for the variable-order fractional advection-diffusion equation with a nonlinear source term. SIAM J. Numer. Anal. **47**, 1760–1781 (2009)
17. Deng, Z.Q., Singh, V.P., Bengtsson, L.: Numerical solution of fractional advection-dispersion equation. J. Hydraul. Eng. **130**, 422–431 (2004)
18. Jain, M.K., Iyengar, S.R., Jain, R.K.: Numerical Methods: Problems and Solutions. New Age International (2007)
19. El-Baghdady, G.I., El-Azab, M.: Chebyshev–Gauss–Lobatto pseudo-spectral method for one-dimensional advection–diffusion equation with variable coefficients. Sohag J. Math. **3**, 1–8 (2016)
20. Podlubny, I.: Fractional Differential Equations: An Introduction to Fractional Derivatives, Fractional Differential Equations, to Methods of Their Solution and Some of Their Applications, vol. 198. Elsevier (1998)
21. Schaback, R.: Improved error bounds for scattered data interpolation by radial basis functions. Math. Comput. 201–216 (1999)
22. Powell, M.: The Theory of Radial Basis Function Approximation in 1990. Clarendon (1992)
23. Fornberg, B., Flyer, N.: Accuracy of radial basis function interpolation and derivative approximations on 1-D infinite grids. Adv. Comput. Math. **23**, 5–20 (2005)
24. Bansu, H., Kumar, S.: Numerical solution of space and time fractional telegraph equation: a meshless approach. Int. J. Nonlinear Sci. Numer. Simul. **20**(3–4), 325–337 (2019)
25. Hanert, E., Piret, C., et al.: Numerical solution of the space-time fractional diffusion equation: alternatives to finite differences. In: 5th IFAC Symposium on Fractional Differentiation and Its Applications-FDA2012 (2012)
26. Laub, A.J.: Matrix Analysis for Scientists and Engineers, vol. 91. Siam (2005)
27. Fazio, R., Jannelli, A., Agreste, S.: A finite difference method on non-uniform meshes for time-fractional advection–diffusion equations with a source term. Appl. Sci. **8**, 960 (2018)

Numerical Studies of Blockage in Human Heart

Akansh Kumar, Vikash Kumar, Milan Kumar, Aman Kumar, Vivek Kumar Srivastav, R. Pandey and M. Kumar

Abstract In the present paper, computational fluid dynamics (CFD) simulation of blood flow in the human heart is performed using angiography images. The angiography was taken from CT scan images of a healthy person. The two-dimensional model is created using the Ansys Workbench software. Three inlet velocities (blood flow) of 0.15, 0.3, and 0.65 m/s corresponding to normal, moderately, and exercise (running) conditions are considered in this study. The CFD prediction of blood flow in the coronary artery is useful for diagnosis, prognosis, and prevention from coronary diseases.

Keywords Human heart · Tumorous heart · Computational fluid dynamics

1 Introduction

Coronary arteries are the blood vessels that branch off from the ascending aorta. The aorta is the largest artery in the body that transports precious oxygen blood to all the arteries. The primary function of coronary arteries is to supply oxygenated and nutrient-filled blood to the heart muscle. The coronary artery bifurcates into the left and right coronary artery [1]. The left main coronary artery is further divided into two parts: the left anterior descending (LAD) and left circumflex coronary artery (LCX) [2]. The accumulation of cholesterol causes the narrowing of the coronary artery, also termed as atherosclerotic plaques. The oxygen-rich blood flows into a restricted path because of narrowed coronary arteries [3]. Plaque deposition is the primary reason for the evolution of coronary artery disease (CAD). The yearly report indicates that CAD is the sole reason behind the 47% of the deaths in Europe [4].

Coronary artery (LCA) has more complex branching as compared to right coronary artery (RCA); this is why it is more prone to atherosclerosis plaque formation

A. Kumar · V. Kumar · M. Kumar · A. Kumar · V. K. Srivastav (✉)
Motihari College of Engineering, Motihari, Bihar, India
e-mail: vivekapril@gmail.com

R. Pandey · M. Kumar
Motilal Nehru National Institute of Technology Allahabad, Prayagraj, Uttar Pradesh, India

S. Bhattacharyya et al. (eds.), *Mathematical Modeling and Computational Tools*, Springer Proceedings in Mathematics & Statistics 320,
https://doi.org/10.1007/978-981-15-3615-1_17

to RCA [5, 6]. Hemodynamic of blood is an eminent prospect to judge the plaque formation in arteries. Hemodynamic factors include the density of blood, viscosity, vorticity, wall shear stress (WSS), inlet velocity, oscillatory shear stress (OSI), and operating pressure at the wall of arteries [7, 8]. Wall stress is most oscillatory during the cardiac cycle in the left coronary artery. Taking these factors into consideration, we analyze the hemodynamic of blood using a vital tool called computational fluid (CFD). Thus, in the medical sector, CFD results contribute to a good approximation of reality in available time duration [9].

In this paper, we attempt to highlight the blood flow mechanism in different levels of blockage of the human coronary artery (human heart).

2 Geometry of the Human Heart Model (Left Coronary Artery)

The 2D reconstruction of the human heart is done based on the three-dimensional model constructed using CT scan data. After the construction of the 3D model, it was converted into a 2D model using the image of the 3D picture. The human heart model is demonstrated in Fig. 1.

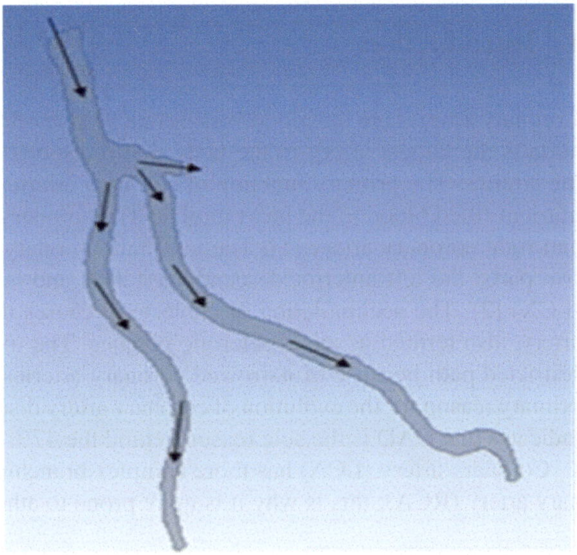

Fig. 1 Human left coronary artery

3 Grid Generation

The grid generation of the two-dimensional human heart model (Fig. 2) was done using the quadrilateral and triangular elements. The triangular elements fit the curved surfaces with minimum skewness, therefore used in the present study.

The human heart models of different blockage percentages (normal model or 0, 25, 50, 75%) are shown in Fig. 3.

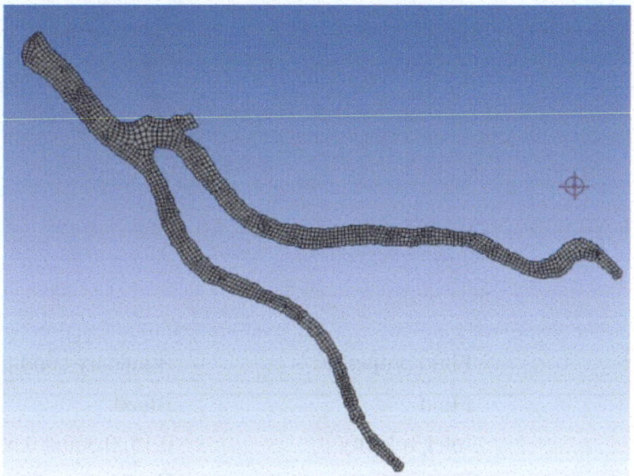

Fig. 2 Grid generation of human heart model

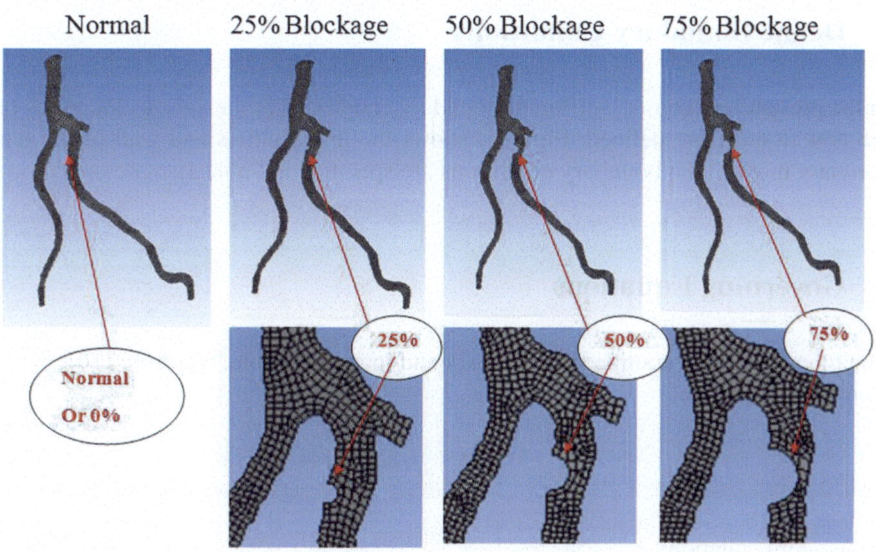

Fig. 3 Grid generation of different blockage models of human heart

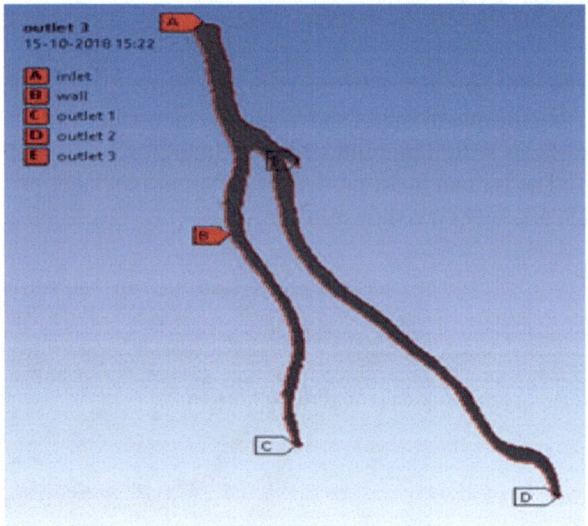

Fig. 4 Name selection for boundary conditions

Table 1 Boundary conditions

Fluid properties	Boundary conditions
Fluid	Blood
Inlet velocity	0.15, 0.3 and 0.65 m/s
Pressure outlet	Outflow condition
Density	1000 kg/m^3

4 Define Boundary Conditions

In the present heart model, different boundary conditions at the various locations of the flow domain are defined. Figure 4 shows the inlet, outlets and wall of the left coronary model. The boundary conditions are specified in Table 1.

5 Governing Equations

The blood flow was assumed to be steady and incompressible, therefore [10]
Continuity equation:

$$\frac{\partial u_j}{\partial x_j} = 0 \tag{1}$$

Momentum equation:

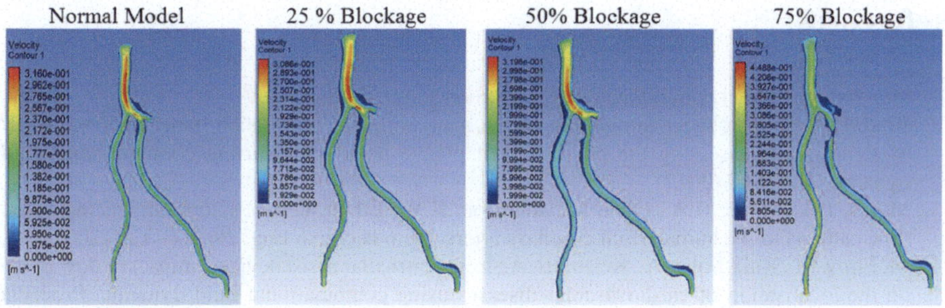

Fig. 5 Velocity contours for different tumorous models (normal, 25, 50 and 75%)

$$\frac{\partial(u_i u_j)}{\partial x_j} = -\frac{1}{\rho}\frac{\partial p}{\partial x_i} + \frac{\mu}{\rho}\frac{\partial^2 u_i}{\partial x_i \partial x_j} \tag{2}$$

μ	Viscosity coefficient
$u_i,\ u_j\ (i,\ j = 1, 2, 3)$	are the velocity component in *x*-, *y*-, and *z*-direction
P	Pressure
ρ	Density of fluid.

6 Results and Discussion

The blood flow of the 2D human heart is carried out for two different flow rates, namely regular, moderate, and heavy blood flow conditions. An in-depth analysis of velocity contours performed in the following flow conditions.

Velocity Contours

The velocity contours for normal blood (Inlet velocity = 0.15 m/s) flow condition of different blockage models are shown in Fig. 5. It is found that as the blockage increases from 25 to 75%, then velocity gradients also increase near the blockage.

Acknowledgements The authors are grateful to the Department of Biotechnology (DBT), New Delhi, Government of India, for providing financial support through its project, BT/PR15126/BID/7/546/2015, received-August 2017, which was used extensively to carry out the present study. The authors are also thankful to TEQIP-III (AICTE, CRS Project) for financial support through its project entitled "Computational Fluid Dynamics Studies of Blood flow in human coronary artery of diabetic patient".

References

1. http://biology.about.com/od/anatomy/ss/Coronary-Arteries.htm
2. Binu, L.S., Kumar, A.S.: Simulation of left main coronary bifurcation under different cases of stenosis and assessing the possibility of plaque proliferation using computational fluid dynamics. In: ISCI (2012)
3. Myers, J.G., Moore, J.A., Ojha, M., Johnston, K.W., Ethier, C.R.: Factors influencing blood flow patterns in the human right coronary artery. Ann. Biomed. Eng. **29**, 109–120 (2001)
4. McElroy, M., Ruiz-Soler, A., Keshmiri, A.: Left ventricular assist devices: impact of flow ratios on the localisation of cardiovascular diseases using computational fluid dynamic. Procedia CIRP **49**, 163–169 (2016)
5. Ramaswamy, S., Vigmostad, S., Wahle, A., Lai, Y., Olszewski, M., Braddy, K., Brennan, T., Rossen, J., Sonka, M., Chandran, K.B.: Fluid dynamic analysis in a human left anterior descending coronary artery with arterial motion. Ann. Biomed. Eng. **32**, 1628–1641 (2004)
6. Olgac, U., Knight, J., Poulikakos, D., Saur, S.C., Alkadhi, H., Desbiolles, L.M., Cattin, P.C., Kurtcuoglu, V.: Computed high concentrations of low-density lipoprotein correlate with plaque locations in human coronary arteries. J. Biomech. **44**, 2466–2471 (2011)
7. Skiadopoulos, A., Neofytou, P., Housiadas, C.: Comparison of blood rheological models in patient specific cardiovascular system simulations. J. Hydrodyn. **29**(2), 293–304 (2017)
8. Karimi, A., Razaghi, R.: Interaction of the blood components and plaque in a stenotic coronary artery. Artery Res. **24**, 47–61 (2018)
9. Huberts, W., Heinen, S.G.H., Zonnebeld, N., Heuvel, D.A.F., Vries, J.P., Tordoir, J.H.M., Hose, D.R., Delhaas, T., Vosse, F.N.: What is needed to make cardiovascular models suitable for clinical decision support? A viewpoint paper. J. Comput. Sci. **24**, 68–84 (2018)
10. Johnston, B.M., Johnston, P.R., Corney, S., Kilpatrick, D.: Non-Newtonian blood flow in human right coronary arteries: steady state simulations. J. Biomech. **37**, 709–720 (2004)

Numerical Analysis of Partition Clustering in a High-Temperature Gradient Region for Suppression of Heat Transfer in Porous Enclosure

Jayesh Subhash Chordiya and Ram Vinoy Sharma

Abstract Subdual of heat transfer rate across a porous medium is an important aspect of many engineering applications like thermal insulations, energy storage and contemporary building walls. One effective way is to employ diathermal partitions within the porous enclosure. Yet, the literature is scarce with the knowledge on the effect of partition orientation and configuration on free convection in porous enclosures. The objective of current paper is to suppress the rate of heat transfer across a differentially heated porous enclosure with the help of horizontally and vertically orientated partition clustering and to assess the best combination of cluster that yields the least value of the Nusselt number. The Darcy model is solved using successive accelerated replacement (SAR) scheme with second-order finite difference method. Streamlines and isotherms are observed for qualitative analysis while the Nusselt number is evaluated for quantitative analysis. The computational code is validated against the benchmark solutions available in the literature. The novelty of present work is the approach of obstructing the fluid flow, which is targeted at only those regions where temperature gradient is high.

Keywords Porous medium · Natural convection · Partition · Clustering

1 Introduction

Porous medium can be encountered in numerous engineering applications to curtail or enhance the rate of heat transfer. This study primarily focuses on decreasing the heat transfer rate across a differentially heated porous medium with the help of clustered partition orientated horizontally and/or vertically and positioned in the regions of higher thermal gradients which are obstructed. As thermal gradient within the fluid-saturated porous enclosure rises, convection dominates. In these conditions, the sole dependency on porous insulation to reduce the rate of heat transfer across it may be fairly unreliable. Thus, a need to further lessen the convection heat transfer

J. S. Chordiya (✉) · R. V. Sharma
National Institute of Technology Jamshedpur, Jamshedpur, Jharkhand 831013, India
e-mail: jayesh.subhash@gmail.com

S. Bhattacharyya et al. (eds.), *Mathematical Modeling and Computational Tools*,
Springer Proceedings in Mathematics & Statistics 320,
https://doi.org/10.1007/978-981-15-3615-1_18

rate arises. Anderson and Bejan [3] reported that use of partitions decreases the Nusselt number. Further, Anderson and Bejan [5] also employed baffles to examine their effect on natural convection heat transfer. This was further explored by several researchers, viz. Tatsuo et al. [15] studied the free convection in a rectangular porous cavity with horizontal fluid and porous regions. Analysis of natural convection in a fluid and heat-generating porous bed was numerically performed by Chen and Lin [6]. Shu and Pop [14] used the Kármán–Pohlhausen theory to analyse the time-varying exchange of heat between the boundary layer convection and vertical flat plate within a porous enclosure. Baytas et al. [2] studied the horizontal conductive thick walls at dissimilar temperatures in porous medium. Varol et al. [18] employed a thin fin in porous cavity of triangular shape and reported that obstructions can act as a control parameter for transport phenomena within porous enclosures. He extended this study, Varol et al. [17], and analysed the free convection flow when a porous enclosure is diagonally divided. It was reported that heat transfer rate is dropped if the plate is inclined at 45°, and even lesser at 135°. A study on free convection in porous media by Saha and Gu [13] with triangle-shaped enclosure with baffles reported that heat transfer due to natural convection in the enclosure was reduced if the length of baffle is increased.

In the current paper, partitions are in the form of clusters; this sort of study has not been found in the literature. The clustering of partition increases the obstruction degree and area. Fully extended partitions may not be feasible in all applications, and therefore, grouping smaller partitions seems to be one of the best alternatives to occupy smaller space with greater area of obstruction. Moreover, the orientation and location of the clustered partitions are investigated to evaluate its effect on natural convection using streamlines, isotherms and the Nusselt number.

2 Mathematical Formulation

Consider a laminar, 2D, laminar incompressible and steady flow in a square-shaped enclosure of length L as depicted in Fig. 1. It is comprised of a pair of grouped partitions, three in each pair, with distance dy between them, length L_p each and middle partition placed at a distance of H_p from the top face. The left wall is at high uniform temperature T_h, and the top and bottom wall are insulated. The boundaries are impermeable. The Boussinesq approximation is assumed valid. The solid matrix of the porous media is assumed rigid; porous media are considered homogenous, isotropic and saturated. Thermal equilibrium exists locally between porous medium and fluid.

The governing equations for the Darcy flow model of mass, momentum and energy are,

$$\frac{\partial u}{\partial x} + \frac{\partial v}{\partial y} = 0 \tag{1}$$

Fig. 1 Physical domain

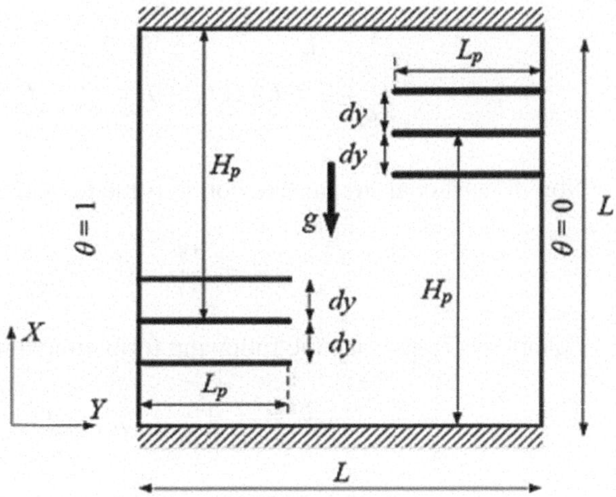

$$u = -\frac{K}{\mu}\left(\frac{\partial p}{\partial x}\right) \tag{2}$$

$$v = -\frac{K}{\mu}\left(\frac{\partial p}{\partial y} + \rho g\right) \tag{3}$$

$$(\rho c_{\mathrm{p}})_f\left(u\frac{\partial T}{\partial x} + v\frac{\partial T}{\partial y}\right) = k_{\mathrm{p}}\left(\frac{\partial^2 T}{\partial x^2} + \frac{\partial^2 T}{\partial y^2}\right) \tag{4}$$

$$\rho = \rho_f[1 - \beta(T - T_{\mathrm{c}})] \tag{5}$$

Subject to following boundary conditions,

$$T = T_{\mathrm{h}},\ u = 0, \quad \text{at}\, x = 0$$

$$T = T_{\mathrm{c}},\ u = 0, \quad \text{at}\ x = L$$

$$\frac{\partial T}{\partial y} = 0,\ v = 0, \quad \text{at}\, y = 0, L \tag{6}$$

Conditions at the partitions, we have,

$$\frac{\partial T^-}{\partial n} = \frac{\partial T^+}{\partial n} \quad \text{and} \quad u = 0, v = 0.$$

Above equations are normalized using following the non-dimensional variables and parameters,

$$X = \frac{x}{L} \quad Y = \frac{y}{L} \quad U = \frac{u}{\alpha/L} \quad V = \frac{v}{\alpha/L} \quad \theta = \frac{T - T_{\mathrm{c}}}{T_{\mathrm{h}} - T_{\mathrm{c}}}$$

$$Ra^* = \frac{KLg\beta(T_{\mathrm{h}} - T_{\mathrm{c}})}{\alpha\nu} \quad \lambda = \frac{L_{\mathrm{p}}}{L} \quad \delta = \frac{H_{\mathrm{p}}}{L} \tag{7}$$

Non-dimensional stream function ψ is mathematically described as,

$$U = \frac{\partial\psi}{\partial Y};\ V = -\frac{\partial\psi}{\partial X} \tag{8}$$

Equations (7)–(8) take the following form after simplification,

$$\frac{\partial^2\psi}{\partial X^2} + \frac{\partial^2\psi}{\partial Y^2} + Ra * \frac{\partial\theta}{\partial X} = 0 \tag{9}$$

$$\frac{\partial\theta}{\partial\tau} + \frac{\partial\psi}{\partial Y}\frac{\partial\theta}{\partial X} - \frac{\partial\psi}{\partial X}\frac{\partial\theta}{\partial Y} = \frac{\partial^2\theta}{\partial X^2} + \frac{\partial^2\theta}{\partial Y^2} \tag{10}$$

Boundary conditions

$$\theta = 1, \psi = 0 \quad \text{at} \quad X = 0$$

$$\theta = 0, \psi = 0, \quad \text{at} \quad X = 1$$

$$\frac{\partial\theta}{\partial Y} = 0, \psi = 0, \quad \text{at} \quad Y = 0, 1 \tag{11}$$

Thermal condition at partitions is,

$$\frac{\partial\theta}{\partial n}^{-} = \frac{\partial\theta}{\partial n}^{+} \quad \text{and} \quad \psi = 0$$

To manifest the heat transfer rate, the mean Nusselt number is calculated as,

$$\overline{\mathrm{Nu}} = \int_0^1 -\left.\frac{\partial\theta}{\partial X}\right|_{X=1,0} \mathrm{d}Y \tag{12}$$

3 Numerical Procedure

Governing equations, boundary conditions and partition condition are discretized using finite difference method. Successive accelerated replacement (SAR) scheme is used to solve the stream function and temperature equation until the convergence is achieved.

SAR Scheme

Chordiya and Sharma [7–10] and Mishra et al. [11] have discussed its capability to solve such two-dimensional free convection in porous media. If the error in equation at (i, j) node of nth iteration is $\widetilde{\psi}_{ij}^{n}$, then in $(n+1)$th iteration, the variable ψ is obtained as,

$$\psi_{ij}^{n+1} = \psi_{ij}^{n} - \omega \frac{\widetilde{\psi}_{ij}^{n}}{\partial \widetilde{\psi}_{ij}^{n} / \partial \psi_{ij}^{n}} \tag{13}$$

The accelerating factor ω varies from 0 to 2. The criterion for convergence of stream function and temperature at all grid points is,

$$\frac{\sum_{i=2}^{i\max-1} \sum_{j=2}^{j\max-1} \left| \psi_{ij}^{n+1} - \psi_{ij}^{n} \right|}{\sum_{i=2}^{i\max-1} \sum_{j=2}^{j\max-1} \left| \psi_{ij}^{n+1} \right|} < \varepsilon \tag{14}$$

Here, the value of ε is the tolerance error limit of 10^{-5}.

4 Results and Discussions

Influence of clustered, diathermal partitions is examined by investigating the streamlines and temperature distribution for modified $Ra^* = 100$ and 500, and N_p value is fixed at 3 while L_p and H_p are varied to change the orientation and position of partition clustering within the enclosure. The value of the acceleration factor is set to 0.3. By performing grid sensitivity test, the grid size of 80×80 is chosen based on both computational cost and precision. For validation, the length and height of partitions, L_p and H_p, are set to 0 to remove the partition. The values of the mean Nusselt number are compared with several studies found in literature as shown in Table 1. It can be seen that the difference in values of the Nusselt number is smaller for smaller Ra^*. The validation results show good agreement with the results reported by other authors. The developed code can be thus used with greater confidence to investigate the problem stated in the current paper.

Figure 2 shows streamline contours and isotherms in porous enclosure without any partition. Maximum absolute stream function $|\psi|_{max}$ value is 4.5. It may be noted that the isotherm lines are extremely steep and grouped in the north-east and south-west part of the square enclosure.

Figure 3 illustrates streamline contours and isotherm lines for various partition clustering orientations having $N_p = 3$, $L_p = 0.3$ and $H_p = 0.3$ for $Ra^* = 100$. Four types of orientations are under consideration, namely

Table 1 Comparison of the Nusselt number with results available in literature

Authors	Ra^*		
	10	100	1000
Walker and Homsy [19]		3.097	
Bejan [4]		4.200	12.96
Moya et al. [12]	1.065	2.801	15.800
Baytas and Pop [1]	1.079	3.160	14.060
Trevisan and Bejan [16]	1.080	3.270	18.380
Present study	1.079	3.279	16.913

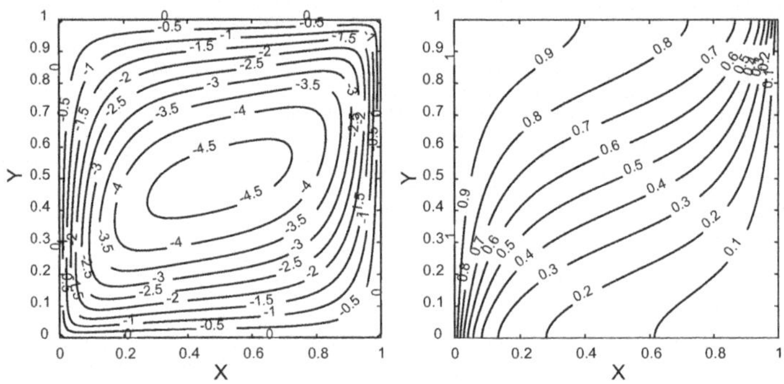

Fig. 2 Streamlines (left) and isotherms (right) for no partition enclosure ($Ra^* = 100$; $L_p = 0$; and $H_p = 0$)

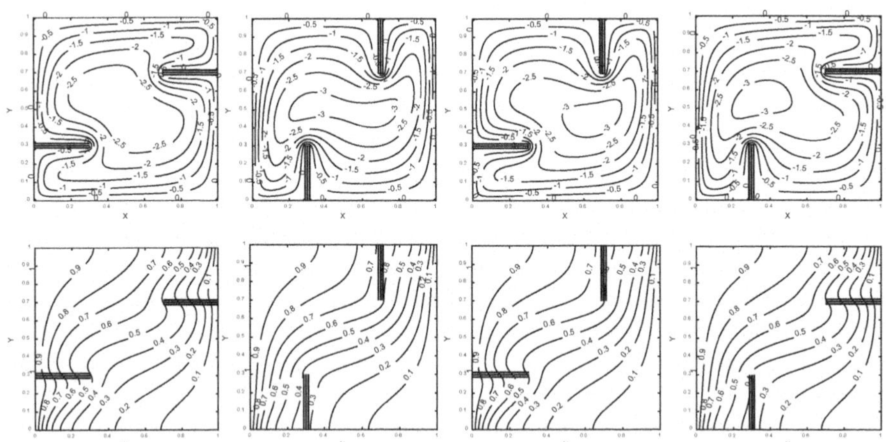

Fig. 3 Streamline (up) and isotherms for H-H, V-V, H-V and V-H type of clustering ($Ra^* = 100$; $L_p = 0.3$; $H_p = 0.3$)

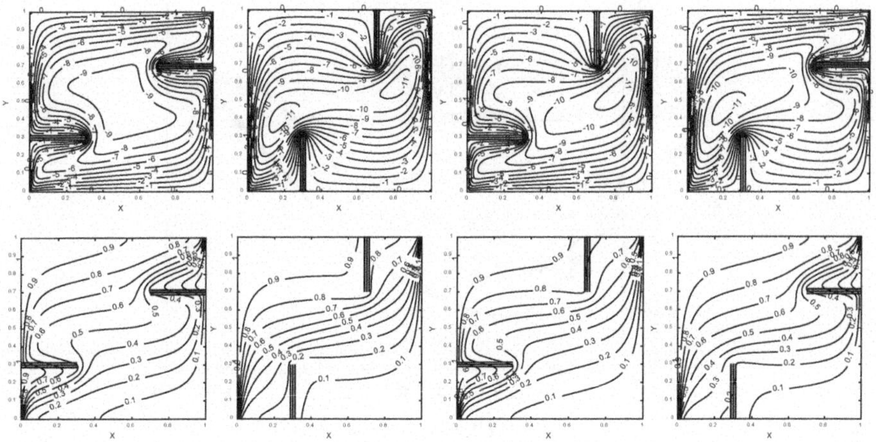

Fig. 4 Streamline (up) and isotherms for H-H, V-V, H-V and V-H type of clustering ($Ra^* = 500$; $L_p = 0.3$; $H_p = 0.3$)

1. *H-H type*: both clusterings are horizontal.
2. *V-V type*: both clusterings are vertical.
3. *H-V type*: Left-side clustering is horizontal while the right side is vertical.
4. *V-H type*: Right-side clustering is horizontal while the left side is vertical.

The stagnant inner portion of the streamlines can be seen from Fig. 1 to orient differently in different cases. In all the cases, it can be seen that the value of $|\psi|_{max}$ is lower than 4.5, which was the case for enclosure having no partition in Fig. 2. The least value is found in H-H type. Further, the thermal gradients in Fig. 3 are not clubbed as closely as that in Fig. 2. This is the indication of the fact that heat flux is relieved considerably from this region. Higher amount of deviation can be found in H-H type of partition.

Figure 4 demonstrates streamline contours and isotherm lines in various partition-clustering orientations having $N_p = 3$, $L_p = 0.3$ and $H_p = 0.3$ for $Ra^* = 500$. Since, the Darcy-modified Rayleigh number is higher, the buoyancy strength is higher. The lowest value of $|\psi|_{max}$ is again for the H-H type. Also, the deviation in isotherms is more for horizontally oriented partitions in all the cases considered individually.

Figure 5 shows the effect of position of clustered partition on the mean Nusselt number values for all types of clustering for $Ra^* = 100$; $L_p = 0.3$; and $N_p = 3$. It is clear from the figure that at the position of the cluster at around 0.3, all the types of cluster yield the lowest value of the Nusselt number, with the lowest for H-H type of clustering. The reason behind this might be the behaviour of free convection flow within the enclosure. The effect of rising cold air from the bottom and falling warm air from the top is more predominant in the one-third portion of the staring length. In other words, the difference in temperature is higher in the initial part of the length which then starts to decrease with increase in length. Higher the temperature difference, higher is the rate of heat transfer. Placing the clustered partitions in these

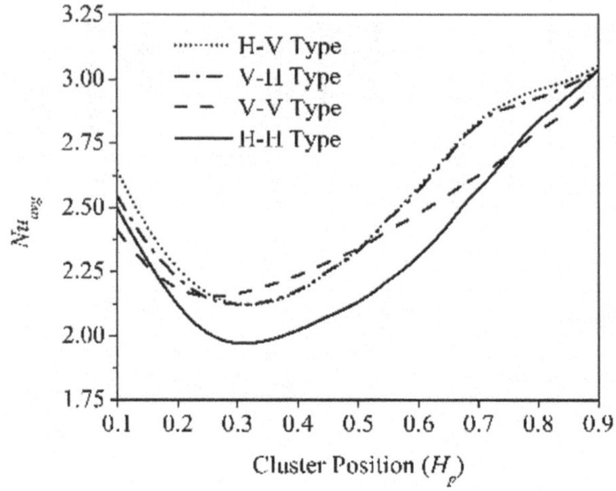

Fig. 5 Variation of the mean Nusselt number with H_p for various partition clustering ($Ra^* = 100$; $L_p = 0.3$; $N_p = 3$)

regions affect the rate of heat transfer by obstructing the flow. Hence, the rate of heat transfer drops higher at the location of one-third of the length.

5 Conclusions

The influence of a pair of clustered diathermal partitions on natural convection flow in a differentially heated square fluid-saturated porous enclosure is investigated in this paper. Four types of orientations were considered and studied for modified Rayleigh number 100 and 500. Streamlines and isotherms were carefully noticed in all the types of orientation, and value of the Nusselt number was calculated for quantitative analysis.

It may be concluded that:

1. As compared to porous enclosure without any partition the flow obstruction is greater and temperature distribution is not clubbed or less clubbed in case of enclosure with clustered partition. The degree of flow obstruction depends upon its orientation and position.
2. Least value of Nu is obtained for $H_p \sim 0.3$ for all types of clustering.
3. The H-H type of clustering yields the highest reduction in Nu of about 42% relative to enclosure without partition

References

1. Baytas, A.C., Pop, I.: Free convection in oblique enclosures filled with a porous medium. Int. J. Heat Mass Transf. **42**(6), 1047–1057 (1999)
2. Baytaş, A.C., Liaqat, A., Groşan, T., Pop, I.: Conjugate natural convection in a square porous cavity. Heat Mass Transf. **37**(4–5), 467–473 (2001)
3. Bejan, A., Anderson, R.: Heat transfer across a vertical impermeable partition imbedded in porous medium. Int. J. Heat Mass Transf. **24**(7), 1237–1245 (1981)
4. Bejan, A.: On the boundary layer regime in a vertical enclosure filled with a porous medium. Lett. Heat Mass Transf. **6**(2), 93–102 (1979)
5. Bejan, A.: Natural convection heat transfers in a porous layer with internal flow obstructions. Int. J. Heat Mass Transf. **26**(6), 815–822 (1983)
6. Chen, Y.H., Lin, H.T.: Natural convection in an inclined enclosure with a fluid layer and a heat-generating porous bed. Heat Mass Transf. **33**(3), 247–255 (1997)
7. Chordiya, J.S., Sharma, R.V.: Conjugate natural convection in a fluid-saturated porous enclosure with two solid vertical partitions. Heat Transf. Asian Res. **47**(8), 1031–1047 (2018a)
8. Chordiya, J.S., Sharma, R.V.: Numerical study on the effects of multiple internal diathermal obstructions on natural convection in a fluid-saturated porous enclosure. Arch. Mech. Eng. **65**(4) (2018b)
9. Chordiya, J.S., Sharma, R.V.: Numerical study on effect of corrugated diathermal partition on natural convection in a square porous cavity. J. Mech. Sci. Technol. **33**(5), 2481–2491 (2019a)
10. Chordiya, J.S., Sharma, R.V.: Natural convection in a fluid-saturated porous enclosure with a pair of vertical diathermal partition. Int. J. Therm. Sci. **144**, 42–49 (2019b)
11. Mishra, A.K., Kumar, S., Sharma, R.V.: Non-Darcy effects on three-dimensional natural convection in a rectangular box containing a heat-generating porous medium. J. Porous Media **19**(12) (2016)
12. Moya, S.L., Ramos, E., Sen, M.: Numerical study of natural convection in a tilted rectangular porous material. Int. J. Heat Mass Transf. **30**(4), 741–756 (1987)
13. Saha, S.C., Gu, Y.: Free convection in a triangular enclosure with fluid-saturated porous medium and internal heat generation. ANZIAM J. **53**, 127–141 (2012)
14. Shu, J.J., Pop, I.: Transient conjugate free convection from a vertical flat plate in a porous medium subjected to a sudden change in surface heat flux. Int. J. Eng. Sci. **36**(2), 207–214 (1998)
15. Tatsuo, N., Toru, T., Mitsuhiro, S., Yuji, K., Hiroyuki, O.: Numerical analysis of natural convection in a rectangular enclosure horizontally divided into fluid and porous regions. Int. J. Heat Mass Transf. **29**(6), 889–898 (1986)
16. Trevisan, O.V., Bejan, A.: Natural convection with combined heat and mass transfer buoyancy effects in a porous medium. Int. J. Heat Mass Transf. **28**(8), 1597–1611 (1985)
17. Varol, Y., Oztop, H.F., Pop, I.: Natural convection in a diagonally divided square cavity filled with a porous medium. Int. J. Therm. Sci. **48**(7), 1405–1415 (2009)
18. Varol, Y., Oztop, H.F., Varol, A.: Natural convection in porous triangular enclosures with a solid adiabatic fin attached to the horizontal wall. Int. Commun. Heat Mass Transf. **34**(1), 19–27 (2007)
19. Walker, K.L., Homsy, G.M.: Convection in a porous cavity. J. Fluid Mech. **87**(3), 449–474 (1978)

Real-Time Numerical Scheme for Crater Geometry Simulation in Micro-EDM Process

Nithin Allwayin, Deepak G. Dilip, Satyananda Panda and Jose Mathew

Abstract In this era of miniaturization, micro-EDM process plays a significant role. Micro-EDM due to its characteristic non-contact nature and ability to machine any material irrespective of its mechanical properties is ideal for the high precise micro-machining operations. The model describes the transient machining process using the two-dimensional heat conduction equation in cylindrical coordinates with flux boundary conditions. It also incorporates the different process elements like Gaussian distribution of heat flux and temperature-independent specific heat and thermal conductivity. A novel numerical scheme for the simulation of the crater shape formed on the workpiece during the micro-EDM process is introduced. This numerical scheme based on the finite volume method in cylindrical coordinates is developed for the real-time simulation of the process dynamics. The existing numerical schemes describe the material removal phenomenon without taking into effect the actual material removal mechanism. The proposed scheme is designed to replicate the anode erosion mechanism, where the phase change in the material, once the temperature exceeds the threshold value, is included. Single-spark micro-EDM experiments are conducted for the same simulation process parameter. The predicted crater shapes obtained from the real-time numerical scheme agree well with the experimental results with a relative error of less than 3%.

Keywords Micro-EDM · Inconel 718 · Single-spark crater · Dynamic crater simulation · 3D optical profilometer

1 Introduction

In the early 1950s, Lazarenko and Lazarenko studied the effectiveness of electrical discharges as a material removal mechanism. Electrical discharge machining (EDM) is a non-conventional material removal mechanism which removes material based

N. Allwayin · D. G. Dilip · S. Panda (✉) · J. Mathew
National Institute of Technology Calicut, Kozhikode, Kerala, India
e-mail: satyanand@nitc.ac.in

D. G. Dilip
Mar Baselios College of Engineering and Technology, Trivandrum, Kerala, India

S. Bhattacharyya et al. (eds.), *Mathematical Modeling and Computational Tools*,
Springer Proceedings in Mathematics & Statistics 320,
https://doi.org/10.1007/978-981-15-3615-1_19

on the heat generated between tool and workpiece by electrical discharges [1]. A schematic of the EDM process is shown in Fig. 1. The tool is moved towards the workpiece submerged in a dielectric fluid. Once the optimum gap is reached, the spark occurs and machining takes place. EDM has the ability to machine all electrically conductive materials with zero process forces.

In the modern era, the advancements in material development and the enormous demands for miniaturization have led the manufacturing industries to go for micro-machining. Micro-machining is the methodology for manufacturing products in the range of 1–500 μm. The 'difficult to machine' nature of these modern materials makes the traditional machining techniques cumbersome. Thus, micro-EDM, a miniaturized form of EDM proves to be an ideal manufacturing technique. Before making any improvements in a process, understanding the process mechanism is of paramount importance. Due to the stochastic nature of micro-EDM, a comprehensive model able to explain the entire process has not yet been developed. Many attempts have been made in this regard, and the major findings are discussed below.

Researchers have used different approaches in EDM/micro-EDM modelling. Some aimed at finding out the exact phenomenon behind the spark formation in the plasma between the tool and the workpiece. However, others strived towards finding the material removal mechanism, which can explain the material removal at the tool and/or workpiece.

Patel et al. [2] considered a constant percentage of heat input and input heat flux in Gaussian form to formulate an anode erosion model. The qualitative features which are related to anode erosion were discussed. Dhanik and Joshi [3] predicted the crater radius and plasma temperature by considering the plasma as a time variable source of energy. The predicted results were in good agreement with previously published experimental results. Joshi and Pande's model [4] incorporated latent heat

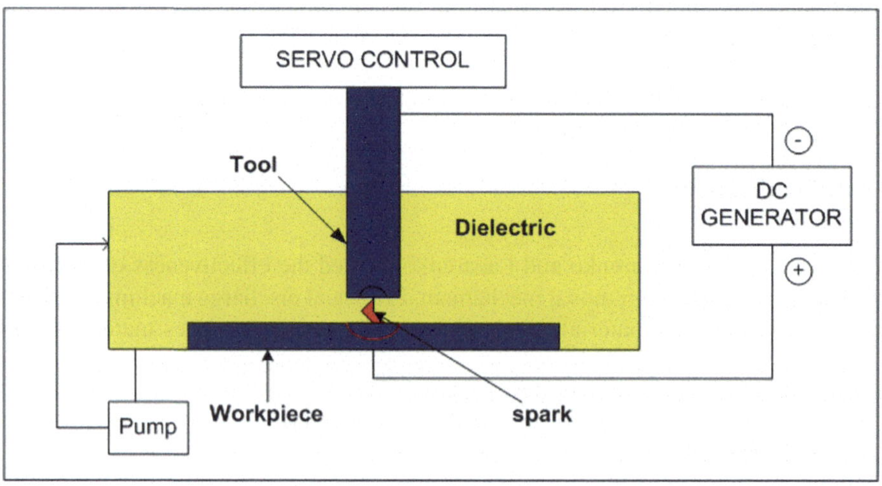

Fig. 1 Schematic of EDM process

of melting, discharge duration and current-based spark radius equation and Gaussian distribution of heat flux to their model. The predicted crater shape was similar to the experimentally obtained one. Yeo et al. [5] analytically modelled the material removal from the anode and cathode in micro-EDM. They were able to predict the crater volume to an error of less than 10%. Allen and Chen [6] used temperature-independent material properties and constant heat flux to analyse the material removal in molybdenum using micro-EDM. The predicted and experimental results were in good agreement.

Murali and Yeo [7] were able to predict the diameter-to-depth ratio of the crater to an error of less than 15% by considering Gaussian heat input and temperature-dependent material properties in the model. Zhang et al. [8] investigated different heat source models in relation to the EDM plasma characteristics and inferred that the Gaussian heat source is the most ideal as a heat source input while considering EDM. Weingartner et al. [9] showed in the thermal modelling of the wire EDM process that latent heat of fusion and vaporization had a significant influence on simulation results.

Singh [10] studied experimentally that as current and pulse duration increased, the input energy distribution to the workpiece varied between 6.1 and 26.82%. Bigot et al. [11] presented a new approach for the calculation of quantity of energy distributed to the tool, workpiece and dielectric during the micro-EDM process. They found that approximately 18% of the input energy goes to the anode for a rectangular tool electrode. Shao and Rajurkar [12] proposed a model incorporating machining conditions like Gaussian-distributed heat flux, temperature-dependent thermal properties, expanding plasma radius, etc., and it was able to predict the energy distribution to anode and cathode as 7.37% and 6.78%, respectively. Somashekhar et al. [13] proposed an electro-thermal theory approach for numerical approximation of the micro-EDM process. The diameter-to-depth ratio observed numerically was 2.92, which is in close agreement with the experimentally observed value of 2.67. Kuriachen et al. [14] developed a predictive thermal model for the simulation of single-spark micro-electric discharge machining using the finite volume approach for Ti-6Al-4V. The numerical results were compared with experiments for the crater geometries, and the results were in very close agreement.

From the literature review, it can be seen that a model which can comprehensively describe the erosion mechanism in EDM has not been developed. In most of the models, the predicted crater geometry is calculated based on the temperature distribution on the electrode. The major issue associated with this approach is that in most cases, the regions where the temperature has exceeded the melting point are treated as solids during the simulation and the material removal is done after the entire time period. This, in turn, results in an increased rate of conduction and extremely high-temperature prediction, which in turn enhances the crater dimensions.

In the proposed model, a real-time simulation of the process dynamics is undertaken where the region whose temperature has transcended the melting point is treated as a fluid. The interaction between the fluid and the neighbouring solid region by Newton's law of coöling and conduction occurs within the liquid phase.

The obtained crater dimensions were compared with the craters obtained from static crater simulation scheme and experimental results.

2 Real-Time Numerical Scheme for Micro-EDM Process

2.1 Mathematical Formulation

The physical phenomenon of the EDM process can be better explained in 2D using cylindrical coordinates rather than Cartesian. Before discussing the governing equation and the boundary conditions used, the assumptions taken in the numerical modelling are:

1. Material is isotropic and homogeneous
2. The capacitor is fully charged and discharged during a spark
3. Heat transfer along the workpiece is governed by conduction and convection
4. The entire workpiece is at room temperature before sparking
5. Gaussian input heat distribution at the top of the workpiece
6. 100% dielectric flushing efficiency
7. Fixed fraction of heat energy to workpiece
8. The model is axisymmetric with respect to an axis normal to the workpiece surface.

Fourier heat conduction equation in cylindrical coordinates, which was used as the governing equation, is given as:

$$\frac{\partial}{\partial t}(\rho C_{\mathrm{p}} T) = \frac{1}{r}\frac{\partial}{\partial r}\left(rk\frac{\partial T}{\partial r}\right) + \frac{\partial}{\partial z}\left(k\frac{\partial T}{\partial z}\right) \tag{1}$$

with T (r, z, t) being the temperature variable defined at position (r, z) and at time t, and ρ, k and C_{p} are the material density, thermal conductivity and specific heat, respectively. The heat energy used by the material to change its phase from solid to liquid at the melting temperature is represented by the latent heat of fusion (L).

In order to incorporate the effect of latent heat of fusion (L) in the model, effective specific heat was considered [15] which is given by

$$C_{\mathrm{peff}} = C_{\mathrm{p}} + \frac{L}{T_{\mathrm{melt}}}, \tag{2}$$

where T_{melt} is the melting temperature of Inconel 718 (1609 K). Initially, at $t = 0$, the workpiece, placed at room temperature, T_{a} is given by

$$T(r, z, t = 0) = T_{\mathrm{a}} = 293\,\mathrm{K}. \tag{3}$$

The boundary conditions for the model are as shown in Fig. 2. The boundary condition for the top surface where the spark occurs is given as:

Fig. 2 Boundary conditions for 2D cylindrical model

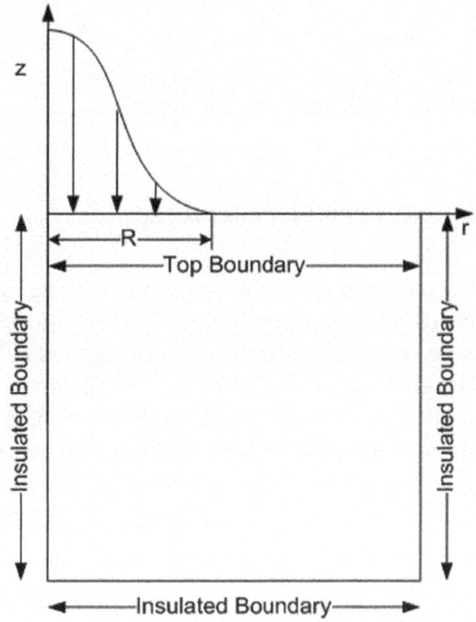

$$-k\frac{\partial T}{\partial z} = \begin{cases} q_{\mathrm{r}}, & r \le R \\ h(T - T_{\mathrm{a}}), & r > R \end{cases} \quad (4)$$

Here, R is the radius of the spark. During t_{off} time, the value of q_{r} is zero and the entire top surface is subjected to convection.

The heat flux q_{r} for micro-EDM [7, 14] is defined as

$$q_{\mathrm{r}} = 3.157 q_0 \mathrm{e}^{-3\left(\frac{r}{R}\right)^2}, \quad (5)$$

where q_0 is the amount of heat energy reaching the workpiece given by

$$q_0 = \frac{\eta E}{\pi R^2 t_{\mathrm{on}}}, \quad (6)$$

where η is the percentage of heat transferred to the workpiece, t_{on} is the spark on time and E is the input energy. In the case of an RC circuit-based micro-EDM, the input energy per spark [13, 14, 16] is represented as

$$E = \frac{1}{2} C V^2, \quad (7)$$

where the capacitance is represented by C and the discharge voltage by V. All other faces are insulated and given by

$$k\frac{\partial T}{\partial \hat{\mathbf{n}}} = 0, \tag{8}$$

where $\hat{\mathbf{n}}$ is the unit normal vector.

3 Numerical Procedure

The micro-EDM model consists of solving Eq. (1) with boundary conditions' Eqs. (4) and (8) and initial condition Eq. (3). The governing equations in Cartesian coordinates were solved using finite volume method (FVM) inspired by Kuriachen et al. [14]. The governing equation under consideration is in cylindrical coordinates, and special treatment is needed for the discretization. In order to ease the finite volume method discretization, we first recast Eq. (1) in conservative form as follows

$$r\frac{\partial}{\partial t}(\rho C_{\mathrm{p}}T) = \frac{\partial}{\partial r}\left(rk\frac{\partial T}{\partial r}\right) + \frac{\partial}{\partial z}\left(kr\frac{\partial T}{\partial z}\right). \tag{9}$$

The given domain $[0, L] \times [0, L]$ is discretized into $N \times N$ equal grid cells of size $\Delta r \times \Delta z = \frac{L}{N} \times \frac{L}{N}$. We define $r_i = \frac{\Delta r}{2} + i\Delta r,\ i = 0, 1, 2 \ldots, N-1$, so that (r_i, z_j) is the centre of the cell (Fig. 3). The edges of the cell (r_i, z_j) are located at $(r_{i-1/2}, z_{j-1/2})$ and $(r_{i+1/2}, z_{j+1/2})$ where

$$r_{i-1/2} = r_i - \frac{\Delta r}{2} \text{ and } z_{j-\frac{1}{2}} = z_j - \frac{\Delta z}{2}.$$

In FVM, the unknown is approximated as the average of the solution over the control volume $\left[r_{i-\frac{1}{2}}, r_{i+\frac{1}{2}}\right] \times \left[z_{j-\frac{1}{2}}, z_{j+\frac{1}{2}}\right]$. An exact formula for temperature of the internal nodes, i.e., $i, j = 1, 2, \ldots N-2$ is derived by integrating the governing Eq. (9) over the interval $\left[r_{i-\frac{1}{2}}, r_{i+\frac{1}{2}}\right] \times \left[z_{j-\frac{1}{2}}, z_{j+\frac{1}{2}}\right]$, i.e.,

$$\int\limits_{r_{i-\frac{1}{2}}}^{r_{i+\frac{1}{2}}}\int\limits_{z_{j-\frac{1}{2}}}^{z_{j+\frac{1}{2}}} r\frac{\partial}{\partial t}(\rho C_{\mathrm{p}}T)\mathrm{d}r\mathrm{d}z = \int\limits_{r_{i-\frac{1}{2}}}^{r_{i+\frac{1}{2}}}\int\limits_{z_{j-\frac{1}{2}}}^{z_{j+\frac{1}{2}}} \left(\frac{\partial}{\partial r}\left(kr\frac{\partial T}{\partial r}\right) + \frac{\partial}{\partial z}\left(kr\frac{\partial T}{\partial z}\right)\right)\mathrm{d}r\mathrm{d}z \tag{10}$$

Following the works of Sellier and Panda [17], who discretized the 1D partial differential equation in cylindrical coordinates using FVM, Eq. (10) is discretized assuming constant material properties. Applying the Taylor series expansion and neglecting higher-order terms, the LHS of Eq. (10) can be written as

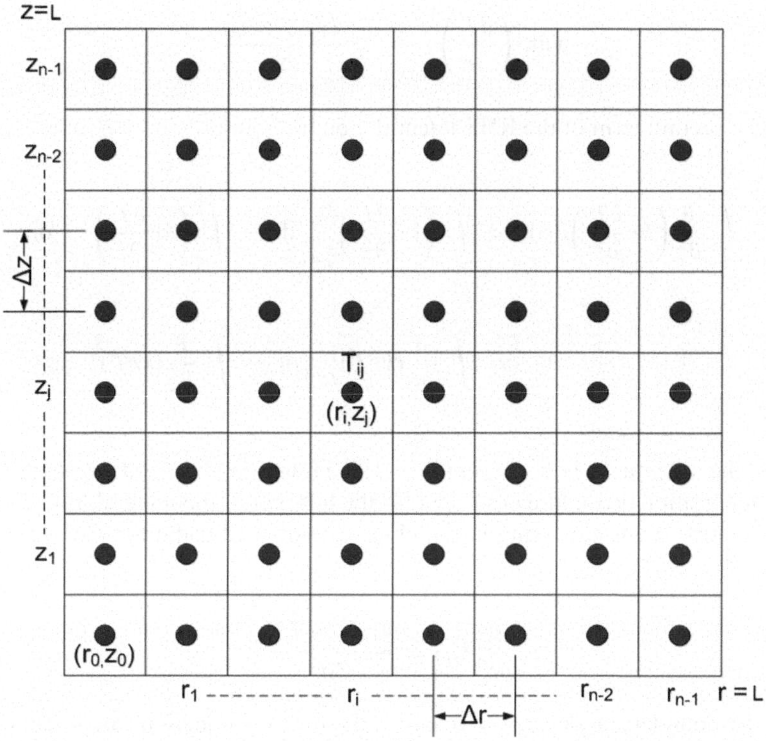

Fig. 3 Finite volume discretization (the blue dots are the nodes, and the lines are cell faces)

$$\int_{r_{i-\frac{1}{2}}}^{r_{i+\frac{1}{2}}}\int_{z_{j-\frac{1}{2}}}^{z_{j+\frac{1}{2}}} \frac{\partial}{\partial t}(rC_{\mathrm{p}}\rho T)\mathrm{d}r\mathrm{d}z = \rho C_{\mathrm{p}}\frac{\partial}{\partial t}\left[\frac{1}{8}r_{i+1}T_{i+1j} + \frac{6}{8}r_iT_{ij} + \frac{1}{8}r_{i-1}T_{i-1j}\right]\Delta r\Delta z \tag{11}$$

The right-hand side of the integral of Eq. (10) can be integrated in the following way. The first integral of the RHS is

$$\int_{r_{i-\frac{1}{2}}}^{r_{i+\frac{1}{2}}}\int_{z_{j-\frac{1}{2}}}^{z_{j+\frac{1}{2}}} \frac{\partial}{\partial r}\left(rk\frac{\partial T}{\partial r}\right)\mathrm{d}r\mathrm{d}z = F^*_{i+\frac{1}{2}j} - F^*_{i-\frac{1}{2}j}, \tag{12}$$

where the discrete flux function $F^*_{i+\frac{1}{2}j}$ is given by

$$F^*_{i+\frac{1}{2}j} = F\left(r_i + \frac{1}{2}\Delta r, z_j, t^*\right) = kr_{i+\frac{1}{2}}\left(\frac{\partial T}{\partial r}\right)^*_{r_{i+1/2,j}}$$

$$\text{with} \left(\frac{\partial T}{\partial r}\right)^*_{r_{i+1/2,j}} = \frac{T^*_{i+1j} - T^*_{ij}}{\Delta r}.$$

For the second term of the RHS integral, i.e.,

$$\int_{r_{i-\frac{1}{2}}}^{r_{i+\frac{1}{2}}} \int_{z_{j-\frac{1}{2}}}^{z_{j+\frac{1}{2}}} \frac{\partial}{\partial z}\left(kr\frac{\partial T}{\partial z}\right) \mathrm{d}r\mathrm{d}z = \int_{r_{i-\frac{1}{2}}}^{r_{i+\frac{1}{2}}} \left(kr\frac{\partial T}{\partial z}\right)^*_{j+\frac{1}{2}} \mathrm{d}r - \int_{r_{i-\frac{1}{2}}}^{r_{i+\frac{1}{2}}} \left(kr\frac{\partial T}{\partial z}\right)^*_{j-\frac{1}{2}} \mathrm{d}r$$

$$= \int_{r_{i-\frac{1}{2}}}^{r_{i+\frac{1}{2}}} \frac{\partial}{\partial z}(krT)^*_{j+\frac{1}{2}} \mathrm{d}r - \int_{r_{i-\frac{1}{2}}}^{r_{i+\frac{1}{2}}} \frac{\partial}{\partial z}(krT)^*_{j-\frac{1}{2}} \mathrm{d}r \quad (13)$$

Since the integrand $g\,(r, z, t) = krT\,(r, z, t)$ is a function of r, z and time t, we follow similar integration procedure described for the left part of the integral, Eq. (11). The time derivative terms appearing in Eq. (11) are estimated using forward difference, e.g.,

$$\frac{\partial}{\partial t}(T_{ij}) = \frac{T^{n+1}_{ij} - T^{n}_{ij}}{\Delta t}.$$

For the boundary nodes, $i, j = 0$ and N, the discrete equations are obtained in a similar way using boundary conditions' Eqs. (4) and (8).

The symbol $* \in \{n, n+1\}$ appearing in Eqs. (12) and (13) represents the time step. We can obtain three distinct schemes depending on which time we evaluate the terms of Eqs. (12) and (13). The explicit first-order scheme can be obtained by evaluating all terms from the old time step, i.e., $* = n$. A fully first-order implicit scheme can be derived by approximating all terms at a new time step, i.e., $* = n + 1$. In this work, we formulate a second-order Crank–Nicolson scheme by arithmetic averaging of the explicit and fully implicit scheme. The entire function is discretized, and the aforementioned initial and boundary conditions are applied using the numerical parameters (Table 1). The temperature distribution is obtained, and the temperature contour is plotted.

4 Crater Dimension Prediction Using Static Crater Simulation Scheme

In this method, the implicit equations obtained after discretizing Eq. (9) is solved using the *fsolve* routine in MATLAB. In this methodology, the program is made to run for the entire time step, and the temperature contour at the end is plotted. The material removal and re-initialization of region whose temperature has exceeded

Table 1 Numerical simulation parameters

Voltage (V)	100 V
Capacitance (C)	0.4 μF
Convective heat transfer coefficient (h)	1000 W/m^{2}K
Density (ρ)	8190 kg/m^3
Latent heat of fusion (L)	250 kJ/kg
Specific heat (C_p)	435 kJ/kgK
Thermal conductivity (k)	11.2 W/mK
Melting temperature (T_{melt})	1609 K
T_{on}	3 μs
T_{off}	10 μs

the melting temperature are not taken into account in this model. The temperature distribution along the radius and depth of the work domain under consideration are given in Fig. 4a, b, respectively.

The contour plot (Fig. 5) is generated in the r-z plane at the end of the total time of simulation with only heat conduction throughout the workpiece as the mode of heat transfer. From the contour plot, the crater radius and depth are calculated. An assumption was taken that all points above the melting temperature (1609 K) are removed from the workpiece surface. Based on that the point corresponding to 1609 K along both the radius and depth is found by linear interpolation between the points within which the temperature corresponding to 1609 K exists. The results are compared with the crater dimensions obtained after single-spark experiments under similar input conditions given by Dilip et al. [16].

The crater was made on DT 110 micro-machining centre, and the dimensions were measured using Alicona Infinite Focus G5 non-contact 3D profilometer. The crater experimentally observed is shown in Fig. 6.

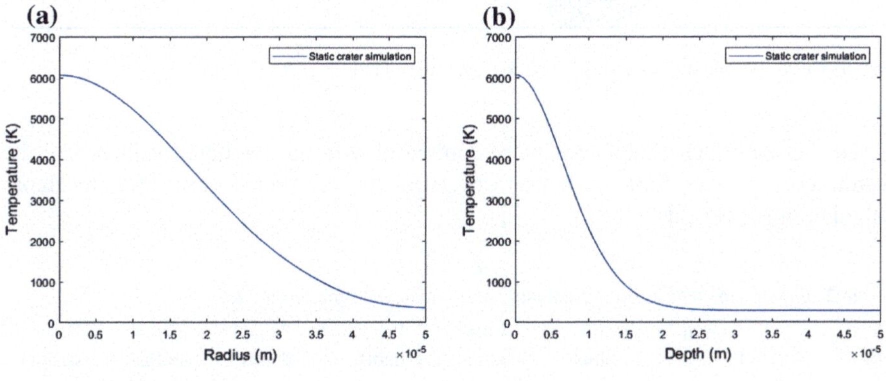

Fig. 4 Temperature distribution along (**a**) radius and (**b**) depth

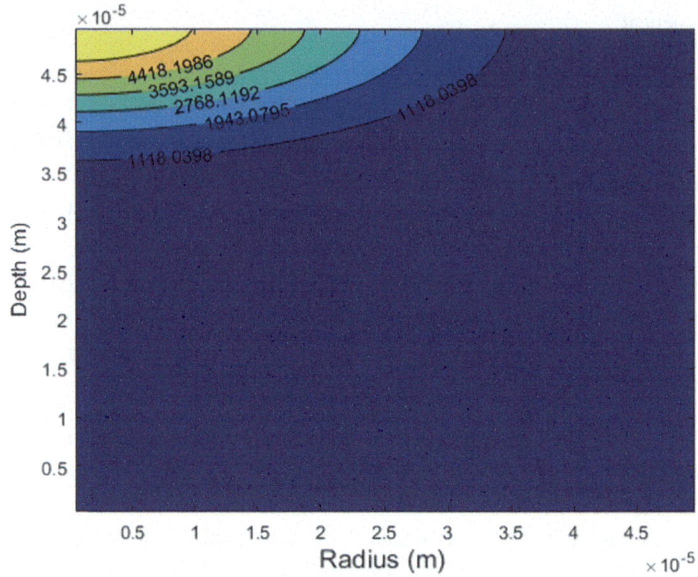

Fig. 5 Temperature contour plot for 100 V and 0.4 μF

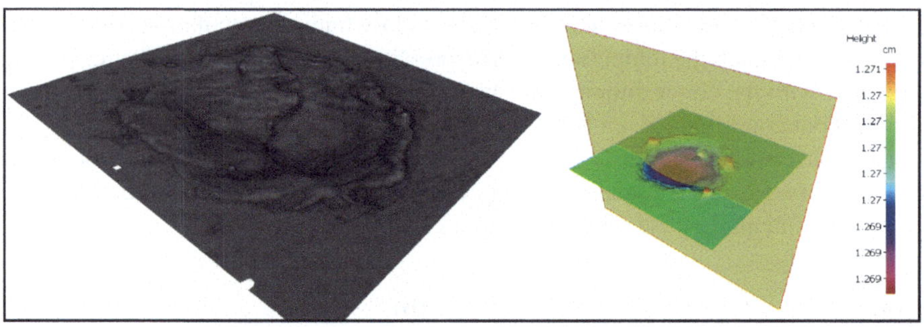

Fig. 6 Crater obtained after a single-spark experiment [16]

The actual crater dimensions were compared with the predicted values, and the results are given in Table 2. It was observed that the relative error for the depth calculation is over 20%.

Table 2 Crater dimensions predicted using static material removal model

Voltage (V)	Capacitance (μF)	Predicted radius (μm)	Actual radius (μm)	Predicted depth (μm)	Actual depth (μm)	Error radius (%)	Error depth (%)
100	0.4	30.38	27.93	11.95	9.66	8.77	23.70

In actual condition, when the temperature of the material exceeds the melting temperature, it gets removed from the surface. But in this model, the material removal of the individual nodes is not taken into consideration, and the total material removed was calculated after the entire time period based on the final simulated temperature profile. This may be the underlying reason behind this high error in prediction. In order to rectify this issue, a model which reinitializes the workpiece region whose temperature has exceeded the melting temperature as the liquid was attempted.

5 Crater Dimension Prediction with Dynamic Crater Simulation Scheme

In this methodology, the regions where the temperature exceeds the melting temperature are treated as liquid with Newton's law of cooling governing the heat transfer between the solid and liquid boundary while conduction being the source of heat transfer within the liquid and solid regions. This, in turn, helps in limiting the rapid transfer of heat through the workpiece while considering conduction alone as the form of heat transfer. The detailed description of the material removal mechanism followed in the simulation is as follows:

1. At initial time $t = 0$, initialize temperature for all nodes to the room temperature;
2. Simulate a single time step;
3. Based on the temperature plot, the temperature at the nodes which are higher than the melting temperature are found;
4. Identify the neighbouring nodes of the melting node and modify the discrete flux condition as per the Newton's law of cooling, i.e.,

$$-k\frac{\partial T}{\partial z} = h(T_2 - T_1),$$

   where T_1 and T_2 are the temperatures of the neighbouring nodes. If the neighbouring nodes are having a temperature higher than the melting temperature, then the discrete flux condition will revert to the original condition as stated in the model boundary condition;
5. Simulate for the next time step, i.e., $t = t + \mathrm{d}t$;
6. If the total time for the process is less than the t_{on} time, then go to step-2 and continue the process;
7. If the total time exceeds t_{on}, run the t_{off} time with convection boundary conditions;
8. Complete the total simulation time and calculate the crater dimensions.

The details of the procedure are also illustrated in Figs. 7, 8, 9, 10 and 11.

The results were tabulated based on the real-time crater simulation scheme, and the temperature distribution along the radius and depth after the total time of simulation is shown in Fig. 12a, b, respectively.

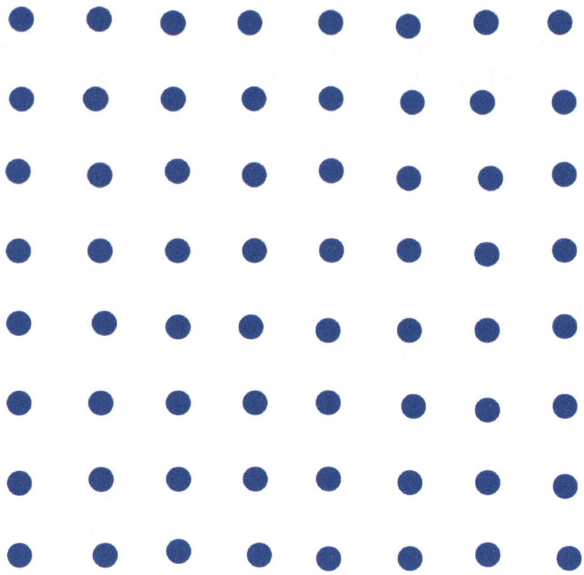

Fig. 7 Finite volume nodes at the initial time $t = 0$

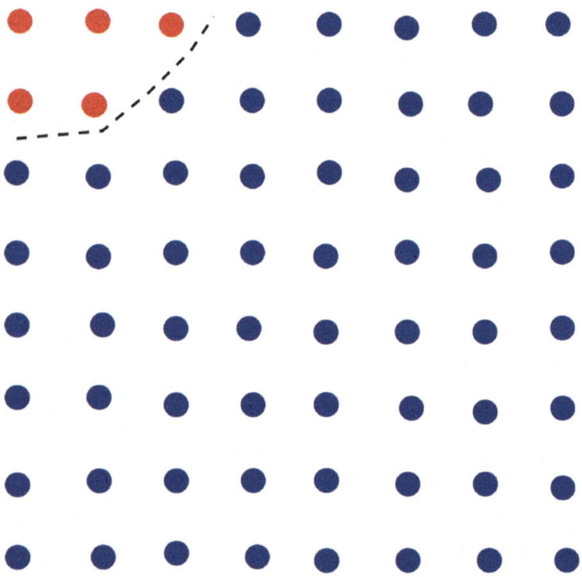

Fig. 8 After simulation at time $t = dt$, the nodes with red circles represent the temperature exceeding melting point

It can be observed that the present scheme gives much lesser and more physically realistic maximum temperature compared to the static crater simulation. In order to validate the accuracy of the model, the results are compared with the experimentally created crater at similar machining conditions. The temperature contour plot for the real-time crater simulation scheme is shown in Fig. 13.

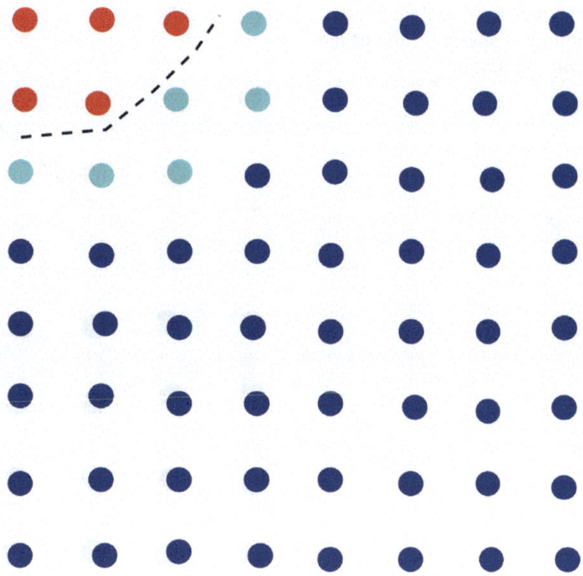

Fig. 9 At simulation time $t = \mathrm{d}t$, the neighbouring nodes are marked with cyan colour

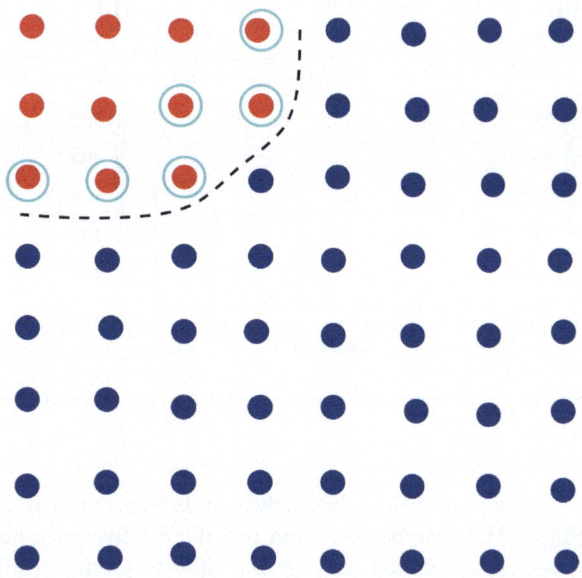

Fig. 10 After next time simulation at time $t = 2\mathrm{d}t$, the nodes which are having higher temperature than melting temperature are marked in red colour. The neighbouring nodes shown in Fig. 9 are in the melted zone

The crater dimensions were calculated and compared with the static scheme as shown in Fig. 14. It can be observed that the crater dimensions predicted were much lesser for the real-time crater prediction.

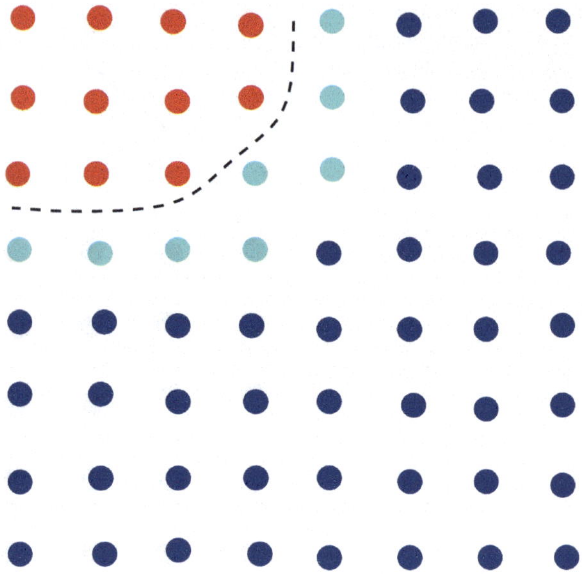

Fig. 11 Re-initialization of boundary nodes for the next time simulation

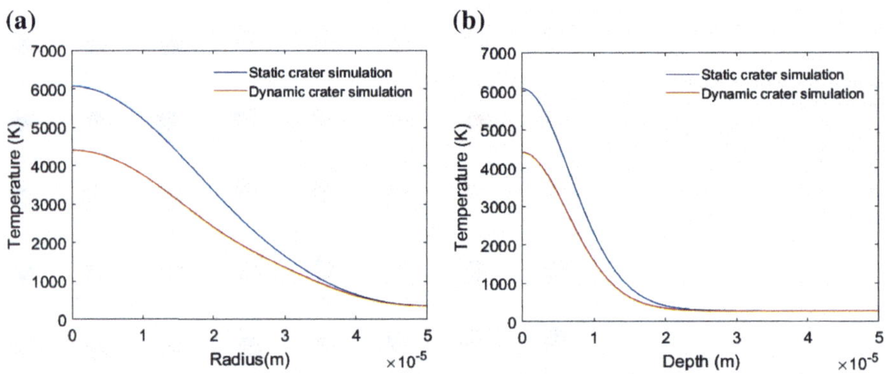

Fig. 12 Temperature distribution along the (**a**) radius and (**b**) depth for static and dynamic material removal

In order to test its validity, the results were compared with the experimental reading (Table 3). It can be perceived that the relative error has reduced drastically and the dynamic simulation scheme was able to predict results much closer to the actual value.

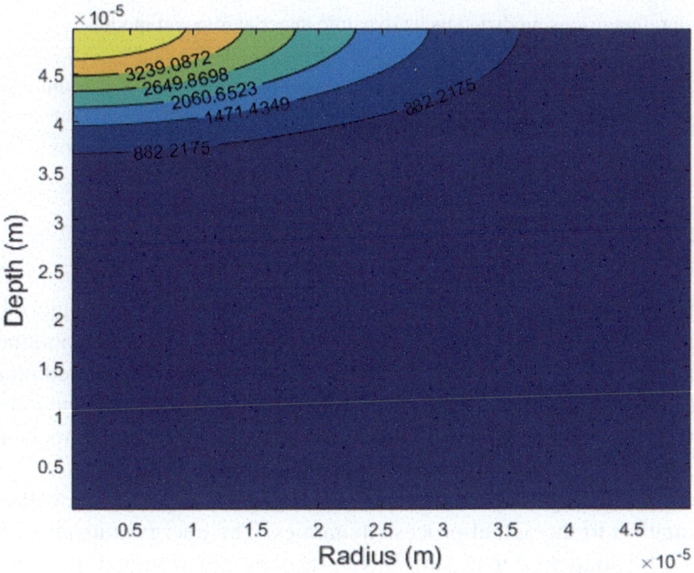

Fig. 13 Temperature contour plot at 100 V and 0.4 μF for dynamic material removal

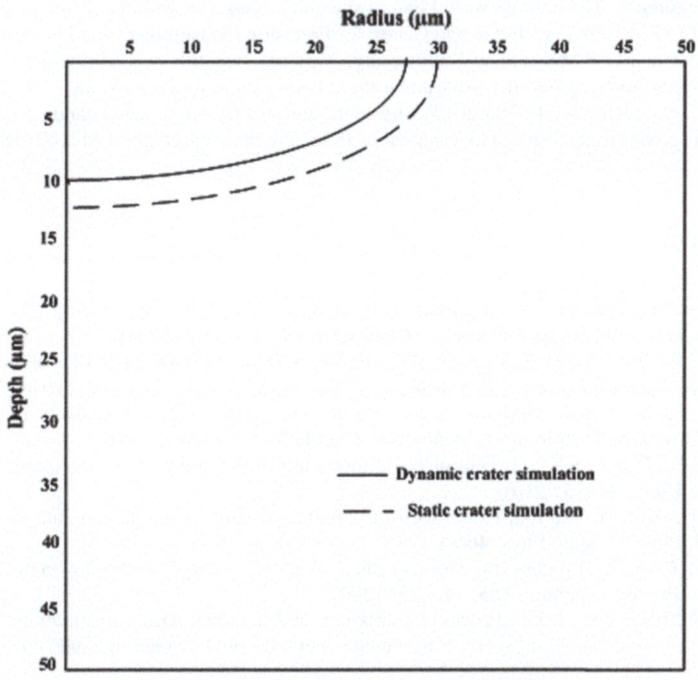

Fig. 14 Predicted crater comparison for both static and dynamic crater simulation

Table 3 Crater dimensions predicted using dynamic material removal model

Voltage (V)	Capacitance (μF)	Predicted radius (μm)	Actual radius (μm)	Predicted depth (μm)	Actual depth (μm)	Error radius (%)	Error depth (%)
100	0.4	27.35	27.93	9.89	9.66	2.08	2.38

6 Conclusions

The crater dimensions were calculated using static and dynamic material removal schemes, and the results were compared with the experimentally obtained crater. The error in prediction of the crater dimension was drastically reduced on using the dynamic material removal. During the actual machining condition, the material gets removed when the temperature exceeds the melting temperature. This is applied to the model, and results with an error of less than 3% were obtained.

In spite of predicting the crater dimensions with very high accuracy, the model is an approximation to the actual process dynamics. The energy transfer in the liquid phase should be addressed using the Navier–Stokes equation and the phase change conditions. This will be attempted as a future course of action.

Acknowledgements The authors would like to sincerely thank Department of Science and Technology (DST), Government of India, and Centre for Precision Measurements and Nanomechanical Testing, Department of Mechanical Engineering, National Institute of Technology, Calicut, for providing support to carry out this work under the scheme 'Fund for Improvement of Science and Technology' (No. SR/FST/ETI-388/2015). One of the authors, Dr. Satyananda Panda acknowledges the support received from SERB, Government of India, under research grant MTR/2018/000451.

References

1. Kuneida, M., Lauwers, B., Rajurkar, K.P., Schumacher, B.M.: Advancing EDM through fundamental insights into the process. CIRP Ann. **54**(2), 64–87 (2005)
2. Patel, M.R., Barrufet, M.A., Eubank, P.T., Dibitonto, D.D.: Theoretical models of the electrical discharge machining process. II. The anode erosion model. J. Appl. Phys. **66**, 4104–4111 (1989)
3. Dhanik, S., Joshi, S.S.: Modeling of a single resistance capacitance pulse discharge in micro-electro discharge machining. J. Manuf. Sci. Eng. **127**(4), 759–767 (2005)
4. Joshi, S.N., Pande, S.S.: Thermo-physical modeling of die-sinking EDM process. J. Manuf. Process. **12**(1), 45–56 (2010)
5. Yeo, S.H., Kurnia, W., Tan, P.C.: Electro-thermal modelling of anode and cathode in micro-EDM. J. Phys. D Appl. Phys. **40**(8), 2513–2521 (2007)
6. Allen, P., Chen, X.: Process simulation of micro electro-discharge machining on molybdenum. J. Mater. Process. Technol. **186**, 346–355 (2007)
7. Murali, M.S., Yeo, S.H.: Process simulation and residual stress estimation of micro-electrodischarge machining using finite element method. Jpn. J. Appl. Phys. **44**(7A), 5254–5263 (2005)
8. Zhang, Y., Liu, Y., Shen, Y., Li, Z., Ji, R., Wang, F.: A new method of investigation the characteristic of the heat flux of EDM plasma. Procedia CIRP **6**, 450–455 (2013)
9. Weingartner, E., Kuster, F., Wegeier, K.: Modeling and simulation of electrical discharge machining. Procedia CIRP **2**, 74–78 (2012)

10. Singh, H.: Experimental study of distribution of energy during EDM process for utilization in thermal models. Int. J. Heat Mass Transf. **55**, 5053–5064 (2012)
11. Bigot, S., D'Urso, G., Pernot, J.P., Merla, C., Surleraux, A.: Estimating the energy repartition in micro electrical discharge machining. Precis. Eng. **43**, 479–485 (2016)
12. Shao, B., Rajurkar, K.P.: Modelling of the crater formation in micro-EDM. Procedia CIRP **33**, 376–381 (2015)
13. Somashekhar, K.P., Mathew, J., Ramachandran, N.: Electrothermal theory approach for numerical approximation of the μ-EDM process. Int. J. Adv. Manuf. Technol. **61**, 1241–1246 (2012)
14. Kuriachen, B., Varghese, A., Somashekar, K.P., Panda, S., Mathew, J.: Three-dimensional numerical simulation of microelectric discharge machining of Ti-6Al-4V. Int. J. Adv. Manuf. Technol. **79**(1–4), 147–160 (2015)
15. Varghese, A., Kuriachen, B., Panda, S., Mathew, J.: Experiments and simulation of three dimensional micro EDM with single and multiple discharges. In: Proceedings of 5th International and 26th All India Manufacturing Technology, Design and Research Conference, vol. 327, pp. 1–6 (2014)
16. Dilip, D.G., Ananthan, S.P., Panda, S., Mathew, J.: Numerical simulation of the influence of fluid motion in mushy zone during micro-EDM on the crater surface profile of Inconel 718 alloy. J. Braz. Soc. Mech. Sci. Eng. **41**, 107 (2019). https://doi.org/10.1007/s40430-019-1595-0
17. Sellier, M., Panda, S.: Unraveling surfactant transport on a thin liquid film. Wave Motion **70**, 183–194 (2017)

Existence, Bifurcation, and Multiplicity Results for a Class of $n \times n$ p-Laplacian System

Mohan Mallick and Subbiah Sundar

Abstract We study positive solutions to the $n \times n$ system:

$$\begin{cases} -\Delta_{p_1} u_1 = \lambda \left(u_1^{(p_1-1-\alpha_1)} + f_1(u_2) \right) & \text{in } \Omega; \\ -\Delta_{p_2} u_2 = \lambda \left(u_2^{(p_2-1-\alpha_2)} + f_2(u_3) \right) & \text{in } \Omega; \\ \quad \vdots = \quad \vdots & \\ -\Delta_{p_{n-1}} u_{n-1} = \lambda \left(u_{n-1}^{(p_{n-1}-1-\alpha_{n-1})} + f_{n-1}(u_n) \right) & \text{in } \Omega; \\ -\Delta_{p_n} u_n = \lambda \left(u_n^{(p_n-1-\alpha_n)} + f_n(u_1) \right) & \text{in } \Omega; \\ u_1 = u_2 = \cdots = u_n = 0 & \text{on } \partial\Omega. \end{cases}$$

where Ω is a bounded domain in $\mathbb{R}^N$; $N \geq 1$ with smooth boundary $\partial\Omega$, $\lambda > 0$, $p_i > 1, \alpha_i \in (0, p_i - 1)$ for $i = 1, 2, \ldots, n$ and $\Delta_m w := \text{div}(|\nabla w|^{m-2}\nabla w)$; $m > 1$ is the m-Laplacian operator of w. Here, $f_i : [0, \infty) \to [0, \infty)$ are non-decreasing continuous functions such that $f_i(0) = 0$ for $i = 1, 2, \ldots, n$ and satisfy a combined sublinear condition at infinity. We will discuss bifurcation, existence, and multiplicity results. We establish our results via the method of sub-super solutions.

Keywords p-Laplacian · Singular system · Positive solution · Multiplicity and bifurcation

---

M. Mallick (✉)
TIFR CAM, Bangalore 560065, India
e-mail: mohan.math09@gmail.com

S. Sundar
Department of Mathematics, IIT Madras, Chennai 600036, India
e-mail: slnt@iitm.ac.in

S. Bhattacharyya et al. (eds.), *Mathematical Modeling and Computational Tools*, Springer Proceedings in Mathematics & Statistics 320,
https://doi.org/10.1007/978-981-15-3615-1_20

1 Introduction

Recently, in [1], the authors study positive solutions to the 2×2 system:

$$\begin{cases} -\Delta_{p_1} u_1 = \lambda \left(u_1^{p_1-1-\alpha_1} + f_1(u_2) \right) \text{ in } \Omega, \\ -\Delta_{p_2} u_2 = \lambda \left(u_2^{p_2-1-\alpha_2} + f_2(u_1) \right) \text{ in } \Omega, \\ \quad u_j = 0 \text{ on } \partial\Omega \, ; \quad j = 1, 2, \end{cases} \tag{1}$$

where Ω is a bounded domain in $\mathbb{R}^N$; $N \geq 1$ with smooth boundary $\partial\Omega$, $\lambda > 0$, $p_i > 1$, $\alpha_i \in (0, p_i - 1)$ for $i = 1, 2$ and $\Delta_m w := \text{div}(|\nabla w|^{m-2}\nabla w)$; $m > 1$ is the m-Laplacian operator of w. Assuming $f_i : [0, \infty) \to [0, \infty)$ are non-decreasing continuous functions such that $f_i(0) = 0$ for $i = 1, 2$, they first establish that for $\lambda \approx 0$ and there exist positive solutions of (1) bifurcating from the trivial branch $(\lambda, u_1 \equiv 0, u_2 \equiv 0)$ at $(0, 0, 0)$. Further, under additional assumptions on f_i for $i = 1, 2$, they discuss an existence result for all $\lambda > 0$ and a multiplicity result for a certain range of λ.

Motivated by these observations, in this paper, we study positive solutions to a general $n \times n$ system:

$$\begin{cases} -\Delta_{p_1} u_1 = \lambda \left(u_1^{(p_1-1-\alpha_1)} + f_1(u_2) \right) & \text{in } \Omega; \\ -\Delta_{p_2} u_2 = \lambda \left(u_2^{(p_2-1-\alpha_2)} + f_2(u_3) \right) & \text{in } \Omega; \\ \quad \vdots = \quad \vdots & \\ -\Delta_{p_{n-1}} u_{n-1} = \lambda \left(u_{n-1}^{(p_{n-1}-1-\alpha_{n-1})} + f_{n-1}(u_n) \right) & \text{in } \Omega; \\ -\Delta_{p_n} u_n = \lambda \left(u_n^{(p_n-1-\alpha_n)} + f_n(u_1) \right) & \text{in } \Omega; \\ u_1 = u_2 = \cdots = u_n = 0 & \text{on } \partial\Omega. \end{cases} \tag{2}$$

where Ω is a bounded domain in $\mathbb{R}^N$; $N \geq 1$ with smooth boundary $\partial\Omega$, $\lambda > 0$, $p_i > 1$, $\alpha_i \in (0, p_i - 1)$ for $i = 1, 2, \ldots, n$ and $\Delta_m w := \text{div}(|\nabla w|^{m-2}\nabla w)$; $m > 1$ is the m-Laplacian operator of w. Assuming $f_i : [0, \infty) \to [0, \infty)$ are non-decreasing continuous functions such that $f_i(0) = 0$ for $i = 1, 2, \ldots, n$. By a positive solution $\underline{u} = (u_1, u_2, \ldots, u_n)$, we mean $u_i \in \left[\mathbb{W}^{1,p_i}(\Omega) \cap \mathbb{C}(\bar{\Omega})\right]$ with $u_i > 0$ on Ω for $i = 1, 2, \ldots, n$. We first establish a bifurcation result at $(0, \underline{0})$ from the trivial branch $(\lambda, \underline{u} \equiv \underline{0})$. Namely, we prove:

Theorem 1.1 *There exists $\lambda_0 > 0$ such that for $\lambda \in [0, \lambda_0)$, (2) has a positive solution $\underline{u} = (u_1, u_2, \ldots, u_n)$ such that $\sum_{i=1}^{n} \|u_i\|_\infty \to 0$ as $\lambda \to 0$.*

Next we assuming a combined sublinear condition at ∞, namely

(F1) $\lim_{s\to\infty} \frac{[f_1^{[m]} \circ f_2^{[m]} \circ \ldots f_{n-1}^{[m]} \circ f_n^{[m]}(s)]^{p_1-1}}{s^{p_1-1}} = 0$ for every $m > 0$, where $f_i^{[m]}(s)$ $= f_i(ms)^{\frac{1}{p_i-1}}$, and establish.

Theorem 1.2 *Let $F1$ hold. Then, (2) has a positive solution $(u_1, u_2, \ldots u_n)$ for all $\lambda > 0$.*

Next we discuss the multiplicity of positive solutions for certain range of λ. Let assume

(F2) There exist positive constants a and $b(> a)$ such that

$$\min_{j=1,2,\ldots,n}\left\{\frac{1}{2\|e_{p_j}\|_\infty^{p_j-1}}\min\left\{a^{\alpha_j}, \frac{a^{p_j-1}}{f_j(a)}\right\}\right\} > \max_{j=1,2,\ldots,n}\left\{A_j\frac{b^{p_j-1}}{f_j(b)}\right\}$$

then we prove:

Theorem 1.3 *Let $F1$ and $F2$ hold. Then, 2 has at least three positive solutions for $\lambda \in (\lambda_*, \lambda^*)$ where $\lambda^* = \min_{i=1,2,\ldots,n}\left\{\frac{1}{2\|e_{p_i}\|_\infty^{p_i-1}}\min\left\{a^{\alpha_i}, \frac{a^{p_i-1}}{f_i(a)}\right\}\right\}$, $\lambda_* =$ $\max_{i=1,2,\ldots,n}\left\{A_i\frac{b^{p_i-1}}{f_i(b)}\right\}$.*

We establish Theorems 1.1–1.3 by the method of sub-super solution. By a subsolution of (2), we mean a function n-tuples of functions $(\psi_1, \psi_2, \ldots, \psi_n)$ such that $\psi_i \in \mathbb{W}^{1,p_j}(\Omega) \cap \mathbb{C}(\bar{\Omega})$ with $\psi_i = 0$ on $\partial\Omega$ and for $i = 1, 2, \ldots, n-1$

$$\int_\Omega |\nabla\psi_i|^{p_i-2}\nabla\psi_i.\nabla\zeta \le \int_\Omega \lambda\left(\psi_i^{(p_i-1-\alpha_i)} + f_i(\psi_{i+1})\right)\zeta, \quad \forall\zeta \in \mathbb{W}$$

and for $i = n$

$$\int_\Omega |\nabla\psi_n|^{p_n-2}\nabla\psi_n.\nabla\zeta \le \int_\Omega \lambda\left(\psi_n^{(p_n-1-\alpha_n)} + f_n(\psi_1)\right)\zeta, \quad \forall\zeta \in \mathbb{W}$$

And by a supersolution of (2), we mean a n-tuples of functions $(\phi_1, \phi_2, \ldots, \phi_n)$ such that $\phi_i = \mathbb{W}^{1,p_i}(\Omega) \cap \mathbb{C}(\bar{\Omega})$ with $\phi_i = 0$ on $\partial\Omega$ and for $i = 1, 2, \ldots, n-1$

$$\int_\Omega |\nabla\phi_i|^{p_i-2}\nabla\phi_i.\nabla\zeta \ge \int_\Omega \lambda\left(\phi_i^{(p_i-1-\alpha_i)} + f_i(\phi_{i+1})\right)\zeta, \quad \forall\zeta \in \mathbb{W}$$

and for $i = n$

$$\int_\Omega |\nabla\phi_n|^{p_n-2}\nabla\phi_n.\nabla\zeta \ge \int_\Omega \lambda\left(\phi_n^{(p_n-1-\alpha_n)} + f_n(\phi_1)\right)\zeta, \quad \forall\zeta \in \mathbb{W}$$

where $\mathbb{W} = \left\{h \in \mathbb{C}_0^\infty(\Omega) : h \ge 0\, in\, \Omega\right\}$. By a strict subsolution of (2), we mean a subsolution which is not a solution. By a strict supersolution of (2), we mean a supersolution which is not a solution. Then, the following results are well known (see [2, 3]).

Proposition 1.1 *If there exist a subsolution* $(\psi_1, \psi_2, \ldots, \psi_n)$ *and a supersolution* $(\phi_1, \phi_2, \ldots, \phi_n)$ *of (2) such that* $(\psi_1, \psi_2, \ldots, \psi_n) \leq (\phi_1, \phi_2, \ldots, \phi_n)$, *then (2) has at least one solution* $(u_1, u_2, \ldots, u_n)$ *such that* $u_i \in \mathbb{W}^{1,p_i}(\Omega) \cap \mathbb{C}(\bar{\Omega})$ *for* $i = 1, 2, \ldots n$, *satisfying*

$$(\psi_1, \psi_2, \ldots, \psi_n) \leq (u_1, u_2, \ldots, u_n) \leq (\phi_1, \phi_2, \ldots, \phi_n).$$

Proposition 1.2 *Let* f_i *be non-negative and non-decreasing for* $i = 1, 2, \ldots, n$, *and suppose there exist a subsolution* $(\psi_1, \psi_1, \ldots, \psi_1)$, *a supersolution* $(\phi_1, \phi_2, \ldots, \phi_n)$, *a strict subsolution* $\left(\tilde{\psi}_1, \tilde{\psi}_2, \ldots, \tilde{\psi}_n\right)$, *and a strict supersolution* $\left(\tilde{\phi}_1, \tilde{\phi}_2, \ldots, \tilde{\phi}_n\right)$ *for (2) such that*

$$(\psi_1, \psi_2, \ldots, \psi_n) \leq \left(\tilde{\phi}_1, \tilde{\phi}_2, \ldots, \tilde{\phi}_n\right) \leq (\phi_1, \phi_2, \ldots, \phi_n),$$

$$(\psi_1, \psi_2, \ldots, \psi_n) \leq \left(\tilde{\psi}_1, \tilde{\psi}_2, \ dots, \tilde{\psi}_n\right) \leq (\phi_1, \phi_2, \ldots, \phi_n)$$

and $\left(\tilde{\psi}_1, \tilde{\psi}_2, \ldots, \tilde{\psi}_n\right) \not< \left(\tilde{\phi}_1, \tilde{\phi}_2, \ldots, \tilde{\phi}_n\right)$. *Then, (2) has at least three distinct solutions* $\left(u_1^i, u_2^i, \ldots, u_n^i\right), i = 1, 2, 3$ *such that*

$$\left(u_1^1, u_2^1, \ldots, u_n^1\right) \in \left[(\psi_1, \psi_2, \ldots, \psi_n), \left(\tilde{\phi}_1, \tilde{\phi}_2, \ldots, \tilde{\phi}_n\right)\right],$$

$$\left(u_1^2, u_2^2, \ldots, u_n^2\right) \in \left[\left(\tilde{\psi}_1, \tilde{\psi}_2, \ldots, \tilde{\psi}_n\right), (\phi_1, \phi_2, \ldots, \phi_n)\right]$$

$$and\ \left(u_1^3, u_2^3, \ldots, u_n^3\right) \in K\ where$$

$$K := [(\psi_1, \psi_2, \ldots, \psi_n), (\phi_1, \phi_2, \ldots, \phi_n)] \setminus \left(\left[(\psi_1, \psi_2, \ldots, \psi_n), \left(\tilde{\phi}_1, \tilde{\phi}_2, \ldots, \tilde{\phi}_n\right)\right] \cup \left[\left(\tilde{\psi}_1, \tilde{\psi}_2, \ldots, \tilde{\psi}_n\right), (\phi_1, \phi_2, \ldots, \phi_n)\right]\right).$$

2 Proof of Theorem 1.1

Let e_{p_i} be the unique positive solution of equation

$$\begin{cases} -\Delta_{p_i} e = 1 & \text{on } \Omega; \\ e = 0 & \text{on } \partial\Omega. \end{cases} \tag{3}$$

Let $0 < \gamma < 1$, be such that $\gamma(p_i - 1) < 1$, for all $i = 1, 2, \dots, n$ for sufficiently small λ_0

$$\lambda_0^{1-\gamma\alpha_i} \|e_{p_i}\|_\infty^{p_i-1-\alpha_i} + \lambda_o^{1-\gamma(p_i-1)} f_i(\lambda_o^\gamma \|e_{p_{i+1}}\|_\infty) < 1 \text{ for } i = 1, 2, \dots, n-1. \quad (4)$$

$$\lambda_0^{1-\gamma\alpha_n} \|e_{p_n}\|_\infty^{p_n-1-\alpha_n} + \lambda_o^{1-\gamma(p_n-1)} f_n(\lambda_o^\gamma \|e_{p_1}\|_\infty) < 1 \text{ for } i = n. \quad (5)$$

For $\lambda < \lambda_0$, define $\phi_i = \lambda^\gamma e_{p_i}, i = 1, 2, 3, \dots, n-1$.
Then, $-\Delta_{p_i}\phi_i = -\Delta_{p_i}(\lambda^\gamma e_{p_i}) = \lambda^{\gamma(p_i-1)}(-\Delta_{p_i} e_{p_i}) = \lambda^{\gamma(p_i-1)}$

$$\begin{aligned}
-\Delta_{p_i}\phi_i &= \lambda^{\gamma(p_i-1)}.1 \\
&> \lambda^{\gamma(p_i-1)}(\lambda_0^{1-\gamma\alpha_i} \|e_{p_i}\|_\infty^{p_i-1-\alpha_i} + \lambda_o^{1-\gamma(p_i-1)} f_i(\lambda_o^\gamma \|e_{p_{i+1}}\|_\infty) \qquad [by\ (4)] \\
&> \lambda^{\gamma(p_i-1)}(\lambda^{1-\gamma\alpha_i} \|e_{p_i}\|_\infty^{p_i-1-\alpha_i} + \lambda^{1-\gamma(p_i-1)} f_i(\lambda^\gamma \|e_{p_{i+1}}\|_\infty) \\
&= \lambda\left\{(\lambda^\gamma \|e_{p_i}\|_\infty)^{p_i-1-\alpha_i} + f_i\left(\lambda^\gamma \|e_{p_{i+1}}\|_\infty\right)\right\} \\
&> \lambda\left\{(\lambda^\gamma e_{p_i})^{p_i-1-\alpha_i} + f_i\left(\lambda^\gamma e_{p_{i+1}}\right)\right\}
\end{aligned}$$

$\therefore$ for $i = 1, 2, \dots, n-1$

$$-\Delta_{p_i}\phi_i > \lambda\left\{\phi_i^{p_i-1-\alpha_i} + f_i\left(\phi_{i+1}\right)\right\}$$

similarly for $i = n$,

$$-\Delta_{p_n}\phi_n > \lambda\left\{\phi_n^{p_n-1-\alpha_n} + f_n(\phi_1)\right\}$$

and $\phi_i = 0$ on $\partial\Omega$.
$\therefore (\phi_1, \phi_2, \dots, \phi_n) = \left(\lambda^\gamma e_{p_1}, \lambda^\gamma e_{p_2}, \dots, \lambda^\gamma e_{p_n}\right)$ is a supersolution.

Next we will construct a subsolution of (2). Let $z_{p_i} > 0$; be the eigenfunction with $\|z_{p_i}\|_\infty = 1$ corresponding the principal eigenvalue λ_{1,p_i} of the problem

$$\begin{cases} -\Delta_{p_i} z = \lambda |z|^{p_i-2} z & \text{on } \Omega, \\ z = 0 & \text{on } \partial\Omega. \end{cases}$$

Let for fix λ, we can find small $m_\lambda > 0$ such that $\lambda_{1,p_i} m_\lambda^{\alpha_i} \leq \lambda$ for $i = 1, 2, \dots, n$.

Let $\psi_i = m_\lambda z_{p_i}$,

$$\begin{aligned}
-\Delta_{p_i}\psi_i =& \lambda_{1,p_i}(m_\lambda z_{p_i})^{p_i-1-\alpha_i} \leq \lambda(m_\lambda z_{p_i})^{p_i-1-\alpha_i}, \qquad (\because \|z_{p_i}\|_\infty = 1) \\
\geq& \lambda\left(\left(m_\lambda z_{p_i}\right)^{p_i-1-\alpha_i} + f_i(m_\lambda z_{p_{i+1}})\right)
\end{aligned}$$

Then, for $i = 1, 2, \dots, n-1$

$$-\Delta_{p_i}\psi_i \leq \lambda\left(\psi_i^{p_i-1-\alpha_i} + f_i(\psi_{i+1})\right)$$

and similarly for $i = n$

$$-\Delta_{p_n}\psi_n \le \lambda\left(\psi_n^{p_n-1-\alpha_n} + f_i(\psi_1)\right)$$

Therefore, $(\psi_1, \psi_2, \dots \psi_n)$ is a subsolution and $\dfrac{\partial e}{\partial n} < 0$ on $\partial\Omega$, so we can make m_λ very small such that $(\psi_1, \psi_2, \dots \psi_n) \le (\phi_1, \phi_2, \dots \phi_n)$. So by Proposition 1.1 there exists solution $(u_1, u_2, \dots u_n)$ such that $(\psi_1, \psi_2, \dots \psi_n) \le (u_1, u_2, \dots u_n) \le (\phi_1, \phi_2, \dots \phi_n)$. Since $\sum_{i=1}^{n} \|\phi_i\|_\infty = \lambda^\gamma \sum_{i=1}^{n} \|e_{p_i}\|_\infty$. Then $\sum_{i=1}^{n} \|u_i\|_\infty \le \sum_{i=1}^{n} \|\phi_i\|_\infty \to 0 \quad \left(\because \lambda \to 0, \sum_{i=1}^{n} \|\phi\|_\infty \to 0\right)$
$\therefore \sum_{i=1}^{n} \|u_i\|_\infty \to 0.$ □

3 Proof of Theorems 1.2–1.3

Proof of Theorem 1.2 Let $(\psi_1, \psi_2, \dots, \psi_n)$ as before in the previous theorem. Then, $(\psi_1, \psi_2, \dots, \psi_n)$ is a subsolution for all $\lambda > 0$, next we construct a positive supersolution $(\phi_1, \phi_2, \dots, \phi_n)$ of (2). For given $\lambda > 0$, choose $m_\lambda \gg 1$ such that for $i = 2, 3, \dots, n$

$$\left[m_\lambda f_i^{[\beta_i]} \circ f_{i+1}^{[\beta_{i+1}]} \circ \cdots \circ f_{n+1}^{[\beta_{n-1}]} \circ f_n^{[\beta_n]}\left(m_\lambda \|e_{p_1}\|_\infty\right)\right]^{\alpha_i} \ge \left((2\lambda)^{\frac{1}{p_i-1}} \|e_{p_i}\|_\infty\right)^{p_i-1-\alpha_i} \tag{6}$$

$$\frac{1}{2\lambda \|e_{p_1}\|_\infty^{p_1-1}} \ge \frac{\left[f_1^{[\beta_1]} \circ f_2^{[\beta_2]} \circ \cdots \circ f_{n-1}^{[\beta_{n-1}]} \circ f_n^{[\beta_n]}\left(m_\lambda \|e_{p_1}\|_\infty\right)\right]^{p_1-1}}{(m_\lambda \|e_{p_1}\|_\infty)^{p_1-1}} \tag{7}$$

$$\frac{m_\lambda^{\alpha_1}}{2} \ge \lambda \|e_{p_1}\|_\infty^{p_1-1-\alpha_1} \tag{8}$$

for $i = 1, 2, \dots, n$

$$m_\lambda^{p_i-1} \gg 1 \tag{9}$$

where

$$\beta_i = \begin{cases} (2\lambda)^{\frac{1}{p_{i+1}-1}} m_\lambda \|e_{p_{i+1}}\|_\infty; & i = 1, 2, \dots, n-1 \\ 1; & i = n. \end{cases} \tag{10}$$

Then choose

$$\phi_i = \begin{cases} m_\lambda e_{p_1}; \ i = 1, \\ \left((2\lambda)^{\frac{1}{p_i-1}} m_\lambda f_i^{[\beta_i]} \circ f_{i+1}^{[\beta_{i+1}]} \circ \cdots \circ f_{n-1}^{[\beta_{n-1}]} \circ f_n^{[\beta_n]}\left(m_\lambda \|e_{p_1}\|_\infty\right)\right) e_{p_i}; \ i = 2, \dots, n. \end{cases} \tag{11}$$

where e_{p_i} is the solution of 3. Now, by using (5), (7), (8), (9), (10), and (F2)

$$\begin{aligned}
-\Delta_{p_1}\phi_1 &= \frac{m_\lambda^{p_1-1}}{2} + \frac{m_\lambda^{p_1-1}}{2} \\
&\geq m_\lambda^{p_1-1-\alpha_1}\frac{m_\lambda^{\alpha_1}}{2} + \lambda\left[f_1^{[\beta_1]}\circ f_2^{[\beta_2]}\circ\cdots\circ f_{n-1}^{[\beta_{n-1}]}\circ f_n^{[\beta_n]}\left(m_\lambda\|e_{p_1}\|_\infty\right)\right]^{p_1-1} \\
&\geq \lambda\left[\left(m_\lambda\|e_{p_1}\|_\infty\right)^{p_1-1-\alpha_1} + f_1\left((2\lambda)^{\frac{1}{p_2-1}}m_\lambda\|e_{p_2}\|_\infty f_2^{[\beta_2]}\circ\cdots\circ f_{n-1}^{[\beta_{n-1}]}\circ f_n^{[\beta_n]}\left(m_\lambda\|e_{p_1}\|_\infty\right)\right)\right] \\
&\geq \lambda\left[\left(m_\lambda e_{p_1}\right)^{p_1-1-\alpha_1} + f_1\left((2\lambda)^{\frac{1}{p_2-1}}m_\lambda f_2^{[\beta_2]}\circ\cdots\circ f_{n-1}^{[\beta_{n-1}]}\circ f_n^{[\beta_n]}\left(m_\lambda\|e_{p_2}\|_\infty\right)e\right)\right] [\because f_1\uparrow] \\
&= \lambda\left[\phi_1^{p_1-1-\alpha_1} + f_1(\phi_2)\right]
\end{aligned}$$

So we have,

$$-\Delta\phi_1 \geq \lambda\left[\phi_1^{p_1-1-\alpha_1} + f_1(\phi_2)\right]$$

For $i = 2, 3, \ldots, n-1$,

$$\begin{aligned}
-\Delta_{p_i}\phi_i &= \left[(2\lambda)^{\frac{1}{p_i-1}}m_\lambda f_i^{[\beta_i]}\circ f_{i+1}^{[\beta_{i+1}]}\circ\cdots\circ f_{n-1}^{[\beta_{n-1}]}\circ f_n^{[\beta_n]}(m_\lambda\|e_1\|_\infty)\right]^{p_i-1} \\
&= \lambda\left[m_\lambda f_i^{[\beta_i]}\circ f_{i+1}^{[\beta_{i+1}]}\circ\cdots\circ f_{n-1}^{[\beta_{n-1}]}\circ f_n^{[\beta_n]}(m_\lambda\|e_{p_1}\|_\infty)\right]^{\alpha_i} \\
&\quad\times\left[m_\lambda f_i^{[\beta_i]}\circ f_{i+1}^{[\beta_{i+1}]}\circ\cdots\circ f_{n-1}^{[\beta_{n-1}]}\circ f_n^{[\beta_n]}(m_\lambda\|e_{p_1}\|_\infty)\right]^{p_i-1-\alpha_i} \\
&\quad+\lambda\left[m_\lambda f_i^{[\beta_i]}\circ f_{i+1}^{[\beta_{i+1}]}\circ\cdots\circ f_{n-1}^{[\beta_{n-1}]}\circ f_n^{[\beta_n]}(m_\lambda\|e_{p_1}\|_\infty)\right]^{p_i-1} \\
&\geq \lambda\left((2\lambda)^{\frac{1}{p_i-1}}\|e_{p_i}\|_\infty\right)^{p_i-1-\alpha_i}\left[m_\lambda f_i^{[\beta_i]}\circ f_{i+1}^{[\beta_{i+1}]}\circ\cdots\circ f_{n-1}^{[\beta_{n-1}]}\circ f_n^{[\beta_{n-1}]}(m_\lambda\|e_{p_1}\|_\infty)\right]^{p_i-1-\alpha_i} \\
&\quad+\lambda f_i\left((2\lambda)^{\frac{1}{p_{i+1}-1}}m_\lambda\|e_{p_{i+1}}\|_\infty f_{i+1}^{[\beta_{i+1}]}\circ\cdots\circ f_{n-1}^{[\beta_{n-1}]}\circ f_n^{[\beta_n]}(m_\lambda\|e_{p_1}\|_\infty)\right) \quad \left[\because m_\lambda^{p_i-1}\gg 1\right] \\
&\geq \lambda\left((2\lambda)^{\frac{1}{p_i-1}}m_\lambda f_i^{[\beta_i]}\circ f_{i+1}^{[\beta_{i+1}]}\circ\cdots\circ f_{n-1}^{[\beta_{n-1}]}\circ f_n^{[\beta_n]}(m_\lambda\|e_1\|_\infty)e_{p_i}\right)^{p_i-1-\alpha_i} \\
&\quad+\lambda f_i\left((2\lambda)^{\frac{1}{p_{i+1}-1}}m_\lambda f_{i+1}^{[\beta_{i+1}]} f_{i+2}^{[\beta_{i+2}]}\circ\cdots\circ f_{n-1}^{[\beta_{n-1}]}\circ f_n^{[\beta_n]}(m_\lambda\|e_{p_1}\|_\infty)e_{p_{i+1}}\right) \quad [\because f_i\uparrow] \\
&\geq \lambda\left(\phi_i^{p_i-1-\alpha_i} + f_i\left(\phi_{i+1}\right)\right)
\end{aligned}$$

$$\Rightarrow -\Delta_{p_i}\phi_i \geq \lambda\left(\phi_i^{p_i-1-\alpha_i} + f_i\left(\phi_{i+1}\right)\right).$$

For $i = n$,

$$
\begin{aligned}
-\Delta_{p_n}\phi_n &= \left((2\lambda)^{\frac{1}{p_n-1}} m_\lambda f_n^{[\beta_n]}(m_\lambda \|e_{p_1}\|_\infty)\right)^{p_n-1} \\
&= \lambda\left\{\left(m_\lambda f_n^{[\beta_n]}(m_\lambda\|e_{p_1}\|_\infty)\right)^{p_n-1} + \left(m_\lambda f_n^{[\beta_n]}(m_\lambda\|e_{p_1}\|_\infty)\right)^{p_n-1}\right\} \\
&= \lambda\left\{\left(m_\lambda f_n^{[\beta_n]}(m_\lambda\|e_{p_1}\|_\infty)\right)^{\alpha_n}\left(m_\lambda f_n^{[\beta_n]}(m_\lambda\|e_{p_1}\|_\infty)\right)^{p_n-1-\alpha_n} + m_\lambda^{p_n-1} f_n(m_\lambda\|e_{p_1}\|_\infty)\right\} \\
&\geq \lambda\left\{\left((2\lambda)^{\frac{1}{p_n-1}}\|e_{p_n}\|_\infty\right)^{p_n-1-\alpha_n}\left(m_\lambda f_n^{[\beta_n]}(m_\lambda\|e\|_\infty)\right)^{p_n-1-\alpha_n} + m_\lambda^{p_n-1} f_n(m_\lambda\|e\|_\infty)\right\} \\
&\geq \lambda\left\{\left((2\lambda)^{\frac{1}{p_n-1}} m_\lambda f_n^{[\beta_n]}(m_\lambda\|e\|_\infty)\, e_{p_n}\right)^{p_n-1-\alpha_n} + f_n(m_\lambda e)\right\}\left(\because f_n \uparrow \text{ and } m_\lambda^{p_n-1} \gg 1\right) \\
&= \lambda\left\{\phi_n^{p_n-1-\alpha_n} + f_n(\phi_1)\right\}.
\end{aligned}
$$

$$\Rightarrow -\Delta_{p_n}\phi_n \geq \lambda\left\{\phi_n^{p_n-1-\alpha_n} + f_n(\phi_1)\right\}.$$

Therefore, (11) is a supersolution of (2), for all $\lambda > 0$. Since $\frac{\partial e_{p_i}}{\partial n} < 0$, and $m_\lambda \gg 1$. So, we can have $(\psi_1, \psi_2, \ldots, \psi_n) \leq (\phi_1, \phi_2, \ldots, \phi_n)$. So for $\lambda > 0$, $\exists$ a solution $(u_1, u_2, \ldots, u_n)$ of (2) with $(\psi_1, \psi_2, \ldots, \psi_n) \leq (u_1, u_2, \ldots, u_n) \leq (\phi_1, \phi_2, \ldots, \phi_n)$. □

Proof of Theorem 1.3 Let establish the result when Ω is a ball of radius R. Let

$$\lambda^* = \min_{i=1,2,\ldots,n}\left\{\frac{1}{2\|e_{p_i}\|_\infty^{p_i-1}}\min\left\{a^{\alpha_i}, \frac{a^{p_i-1}}{f_i(a)}\right\}\right\}$$

$$\left(\tilde{\phi}_1, \tilde{\phi}_2, \ldots, \tilde{\phi}_n\right) = \left(\frac{a}{\|e_{p_1}\|_\infty}e_{p_1}, \frac{a}{\|e_{p_2}\|_\infty}e_{p_2}, \ldots, \frac{a}{\|e_{p_n}\|_\infty}e_{p_n}\right) \tag{12}$$

for $\lambda < \lambda^*$

$$
\begin{aligned}
-\Delta_{p_i}\tilde{\phi}_i &= \frac{a^{p_i-1}}{2\|e\|_\infty^{p_i-1}} + \frac{a^{p_i-1}}{2\|e\|_\infty^{p_i-1}} \\
&\geq \lambda a^{p_i-1-\alpha_i} + \lambda f_i(a) \\
&\geq \lambda\left(\left(\frac{a}{\|e_{p_i}\|_\infty}e_{p_i}\right)^{p_i-1-\alpha_i} + f_i\left(\frac{a}{\|e_{p_{i+1}}\|_\infty}e_{p_{i+1}}\right)\right)
\end{aligned}
$$

$\therefore$ for $i = 1, 2, \ldots, n-1$,

$$\Rightarrow -\Delta_{p_i}\tilde{\phi}_i \geq \lambda\left(\tilde{\phi}_i^{p_i-1-\alpha_i} + f_i(\tilde{\phi}_{i+1})\right)$$

similarly, for $i = n$

$$-\Delta_{p_i}\tilde{\phi}_n \geq \lambda\left(\tilde{\phi}_n^{p_n-1-\alpha_n} + f_n(\tilde{\phi}_1)\right)$$

$\therefore$ (12) is a supersolution of (2) for $\lambda < \lambda^*$.

Now, we construct a positive strict subsolution $(\tilde{\psi}_1, \tilde{\psi}_2, \ldots, \tilde{\psi}_n)$ of (2) when $\lambda > \lambda_*$.

Where $\lambda_* = \max\limits_{i=1,2,\ldots,n}\left\{\frac{b^{p_i-1}}{f(b)}A_{p_i}\right\}$

and $A_{p_i} = \inf\limits_{\epsilon}\frac{NR^{N-1}}{\epsilon^N(R-\epsilon)^{p_i-1}} = \frac{(N+p_i-1)^{(N+p_i-1)}}{R^{p_i}N^{N-1}(p_i-1)^{(p_i-1)}}$; *and* $\epsilon_i = \frac{NR}{N+p_i-1}$.

For $0 < \epsilon < R$; $\alpha, \beta > 1$ define

$\rho : [0, R] \to [0, 1]$ by

$$\rho(r) = \begin{cases} 1 & 0 \leq r \leq \epsilon, \\ 1 - \left(1 - \left(\frac{R-r}{R-\epsilon}\right)^{\beta}\right)^{\alpha} & \epsilon < r \leq R. \end{cases}$$

Then

$$\rho'(r) = \begin{cases} 0 & 0 \leq r \leq \epsilon, \\ -\frac{\alpha\beta}{R-\epsilon}\left(1 - \left(\frac{R-r}{R-\epsilon}\right)^{\beta}\right)^{\alpha-1}\left(\frac{R-r}{R-\epsilon}\right)^{\beta-1} & \epsilon < r \leq R. \end{cases}$$

And hence, $|\rho'(r)| \leq \frac{\alpha\beta}{R-\epsilon}$. Let $d(r) = b\rho(r)$, then

$$|d'(r)| \leq \frac{b\alpha\beta}{R-\epsilon} \tag{13}$$

Define $\left(\tilde{\psi}_1(r), \tilde{\psi}_2(r), \ldots, \tilde{\psi}_n(r)\right)$ as the radially symmetric $\mathbb{C}^2(\Omega)$ solution of

$$\begin{cases} -\Delta_{p_1}\tilde{\psi}_1 & = \lambda\left(f_1(d(r))\right) \quad in \ \ B(0, R); \\ -\Delta_{p_2}\tilde{\psi}_2 & = \lambda\left(f_2((d(r))\right) \quad in \ \ B(0, R); \\ \ \vdots & = \ \ \vdots \\ -\Delta_{p_{n-1}}\tilde{\psi}_{n-1} & = \lambda\left(f_{n-1}((d(r))\right) \quad in \ \ B(0, R); \\ -\Delta_{p_n}\tilde{\psi}_n & = \lambda\left(f_n((d(r))\right) \quad in \ \ B(0, R); \\ \tilde{\psi}_1 = \tilde{\psi}_2 & = \cdots = \tilde{\psi}_n = 0 \quad on \ \ \partial B(0, R); \\ \tilde{\psi}_1'(0) = \tilde{\psi}_2'(0) & = \cdots = \tilde{\psi}_n'(0) = 0. \end{cases} \tag{14}$$

By changing variable we have,

for $i = 1, 2, \ldots, n$ *and for* $t \in (0, R)$.

$$-\left(r^{N-1}\varphi_{p_i}(\tilde{\psi}_i'(r))\right)' = \lambda r^{N-1} f_i(d(r))$$

where $\varphi_{p_i}(r) = |r|^{p_i-2}r$ for all $r \in \mathbb{R}$. Integrating from 0 to r, we have

$$-\varphi_{p_i}(\tilde{\psi}_i') = \frac{\lambda}{r^{N-1}} \int_0^r s^{N-1} f_i(d(s))ds.$$

Since φ_{p_i} is monotone, $\varphi_{p_i}^{-1}$ is also continuous and monotone . Hence, we have $-\tilde{\psi}_i' = \varphi_{p_i}^{-1}\left(\frac{\lambda}{r^{N-1}} \int_0^r s^{N-1} f_i(d(s))ds\right)$, for $i = 1, 2, \ldots, n$.
for $\lambda > \lambda_*$, we claim that

$$\tilde{\psi}_i(r) > d(r), \quad 0 \le r < R \tag{15}$$

If our claim is true, $\left(\tilde{\psi}_1, \tilde{\psi}_2, \ldots, \tilde{\psi}_n\right)$ is a strict subsolution of (2) since

$$-\Delta_{p_i}\tilde{\psi}_i = \lambda f_i(d) < \lambda\left(\tilde{\psi}_i^{p_i-1-\alpha_i} + f(\tilde{\psi}_{i+1})\right), i = 1, 2, \ldots, n-1 \text{ in } B_R \text{ and}$$

$$-\Delta\tilde{\psi}_n = \lambda f_n(d) < \lambda\left(\tilde{\psi}_n^{p_n-1-\alpha_n} + f(\tilde{\psi}_1)\right) \text{ in } B_R$$

It suffices to prove that $\tilde{\psi}_i'(r) < d'(r)$ on $(0, R)$. Note that for $0 \le r < \epsilon$, for $i = 1, 2, \ldots, n \tilde{\psi}_i'(r) < d'(r) \quad (\because d'(r) = 0$ for $0 \le r < \epsilon$ and $\tilde{\psi}_i' < 0, \ \forall r)$
Now for $r > \epsilon$

$$\begin{aligned}
-\tilde{\psi}_i' &= \varphi_{p_i}^{-1}\left(\frac{\lambda}{r^{N-1}} \int_0^r s^{N-1} f_i(d(s))ds\right) \\
&\ge \varphi_{p_i}^{-1}\left(\frac{\lambda}{r^{N-1}} \int_0^\epsilon s^{N-1} f_i(d(s))ds\right) \\
&= \varphi_{p_i}^{-1}\left(\frac{\lambda}{r^{N-1}} \int_0^\epsilon s^{N-1} f_i(b)ds\right) \quad \because d(s) = b \text{ for } s \in (0, \epsilon) \\
&= \varphi_{p_i}^{-1}\left(\frac{\lambda}{R^{N-1}} f_i(b) \int_0^\epsilon s^{N-1}ds\right) = \varphi_{p_i}^{-1}\left(\frac{\lambda\epsilon^N f_i(b)}{R^{N-1}N}\right).
\end{aligned} \tag{16}$$

Noting that from (13), it is easy to see that $\tilde{\psi}_i'(r) < d'(r)$ *in* (ϵ, R) provided

$$\varphi_{p_i}^{-1}\left(\frac{\lambda\epsilon^N f_i(b)}{R^{N-1}N}\right) > \frac{\alpha\beta b}{R-\epsilon}, \quad \text{for } i = 1, 2, \ldots, n.$$

Equivalently, if

$$\lambda > \max_{i=1,2,\ldots,n}\left\{(\alpha\beta)^{p_i-1}\frac{NR^{N-1}}{\epsilon^N(R-\epsilon)^{p_i-1}}\frac{b^{p_i-1}}{f_i(b)}\right\} \tag{17}$$

Now if $\lambda_* = \max\limits_{1,2,\ldots,n}\left\{A_{p_i}\dfrac{b}{f_i(b)}\right\}$, maximum is taken over finite number of term so maximum value will be for some $i = j$ choose $\epsilon_j = \dfrac{NR}{N-p_j-1}$, in the definition of ρ, (17) reduce to showing

$$\lambda > \max_{i=1,2,\ldots,n}\left\{(\alpha\beta)^{p_i-1}A_{p_i}\frac{b^{p_i-1}}{f_i(b)}\right\} \tag{18}$$

Again since $\lambda > \lambda_*$, we can choose $\alpha > 1$, $\beta > 1$ s.t. (18) satisfies, hence (15) hold for $\lambda > \lambda_*$. Thus $\left(\tilde{\psi}_1, \tilde{\psi}_2, \ldots, \tilde{\psi}_n\right)$ is a strict subsolution of (2), from the Theorem 1.2, we have a sufficiently small positive subsolution $(\psi_1, \psi_2, \ldots, \psi_n)$ and a sufficiently large supersolution $(\phi_1, \phi_2, \ldots, \phi_n)$, s.t.

$$(\psi_1, \psi_2, \ldots, \psi_n) \le \left(\tilde{\phi}_1, \tilde{\phi}_2, \ldots, \tilde{\phi}_n\right) \le (\phi_1, \phi_2, \ldots, \phi_n)\,, \text{ and}$$

$$(\psi_1, \psi_2, \ldots, \psi_n) \le \left(\tilde{\psi}_1, \tilde{\psi}_2, \ldots, \tilde{\psi}_n\right) \le (\phi_1, \phi_2, \ldots, \phi_n)\,.$$

Since $\|\tilde{\psi}_i\|_\infty \ge \|d\|_\infty = b$ and $\|\tilde{\phi}_i\|_\infty = a$.

$$\left(\tilde{\psi}_1, \tilde{\psi}_2, \ldots, \tilde{\psi}_n\right) \not< \left(\tilde{\phi}_1, \tilde{\phi}_2, \ldots, \tilde{\phi}_n\right).$$

By Proposition 1.2, (2) has atleast three distinct solution for $\lambda \in (\lambda_*, \lambda^*)$. Next, when Ω is a general bounded open subset of $\mathbb{R}^N$ let B_R be the largest inscribed ball in Ω. Define

$$\chi_i(x) = \begin{cases} \tilde{\psi}_i & x \in B_R, \\ 0 & x \in \Omega \backslash B_R. \end{cases}$$

where $\left(\tilde{\psi}_1, \tilde{\psi}_2, \ldots, \tilde{\psi}_n\right)$ is a second subsolution (2) constructed above when $\Omega = B_R$. Then, $\chi_i \in W^{1,p_i}(\Omega)\mathbb{C}(\bar{\Omega})$, and further on B_R we have, for $i = 1, 2, \ldots, n-1$

$$-\Delta_{p_i}\chi_i = -\Delta_{p_i}\tilde{\psi}_i \le \lambda\{\tilde{\psi}_i^{P_i-1-\alpha_i} + f_i(\tilde{\psi}_{i+1})\} = \lambda\{\chi^{p_i-1-\alpha_i} + f_i(\chi_{i+1})\}$$

for $i = n$

$$-\Delta_{p_n}\chi_n = -\Delta_{p_n}\tilde{\psi}_n \le \lambda\{\tilde{\psi}_i^{p_n-1-\alpha_n} + f_n(\tilde{\psi}_1)\} = \lambda\{\chi^{p_n-1-\alpha_n} + f_n(\chi_1)\}$$

While outside B_R, we have for $i = 1, 2, \ldots, n-1$

$$-\Delta_{p_i}\chi_i = 0 = \lambda\{\tilde{\psi}_i^{p_n-1-\alpha_i} + f_i(\tilde{\psi}_{i+1})\} = \lambda\{\chi^{p_n-1-\alpha_i} + f_i(\chi_{i+1})\}$$

for $i = n$

$$-\Delta_{p_n}\chi_n = 0 = \lambda\{\tilde{\psi}_i^{p_n-1-\alpha_n} + f_n(\tilde{\psi}_1)\} = \lambda\{\chi^{p_n-1-\alpha_n} + f_n(\chi_1)\}.$$

Hence, $(\chi_1, \chi_2, \ldots, \chi_n)$ is a strict subsolution to the previous case except that here for the second subsolution we will use $(\chi_1, \chi_2, \ldots, \chi_n)$ describe above. □

4 Example

We give an example that satisfy the hypothesis in Theorems 1.2 and 1.3. Consider the system:

$$\begin{cases} -\Delta_{p_1}u_1 = \lambda\left(u_1^{(p_1-1-\alpha_1)} + e^{\frac{\tau u_2}{\tau+u_2}} - 1\right) & \text{in } \Omega; \\ -\Delta_{p_2}u_2 = \lambda\left(u_2^{(p_2-1-\alpha_2)} + u_3^{\zeta_3}\right) & \text{in } \Omega; \\ \quad\vdots = \quad\vdots & \\ -\Delta_{p_{n-1}}u_{n-1} = \lambda\left(u_{n-1}^{(p_{n-1}-1-\alpha_{n-1})} + u_n^{\zeta_n}\right) & \text{in } \Omega; \\ -\Delta_{p_n}u_n = \lambda\left(u_n^{(p_n-1-\alpha_n)} + u_1^{\zeta_1}\right) & \text{in } \Omega; \\ u_1 = u_2 = \cdots = u_n = 0 & \text{on } \partial\Omega. \end{cases} \tag{19}$$

where $\tau > 0$ and $\zeta_i > 0$, for $i = 1, 3, 4, \ldots, n$. Clearly, $f_i(0) = 0$ and since f_1 is bounded for each $\tau > 0$, then (H_1) holds. Hence, Theorems 1.1–1.2 hold for all $\tau > 0$ and $\zeta > 0$. Next by choosing $a = 1$ and $b = \tau$, we have

$$\frac{\min\limits_i\left\{\frac{1}{2\|w_{p_i}\|_\infty^{p_i-1}}\min\left\{a^{\alpha_i}, \frac{a^{p_i-1}}{f_i(a)}\right\}\right\}}{\max_i\left\{A_i\frac{b^{p_i-1}}{f_i(b)}\right\}}$$

$$\geq \frac{\min\left\{\frac{1}{2\|e_{p_1}\|_\infty^{p_1-1}(e^{\frac{\tau}{\tau+1}}-1)}, \frac{1}{2\|e_{p_2}\|_\infty^{p_2-1}}, \ldots, \frac{1}{2\|e_{p_n}\|_\infty^{p_n-1}}\right\}}{\max\left\{A_{p_i}\frac{\tau^{p_1-1}}{e^{\tau/2}-1}, A_{p_2}\tau^{p_2-1-\zeta_3}, \ldots, A_{p_n}\tau^{p_n-1-\zeta_1}\right\}}$$

which is bigger than one if $\tau \gg 1$ and $\min_{1,3,4,\ldots,n} \{\zeta_i\} > \max_{2,3,\ldots,n} \{p_i - 1\}$. Hence, (H_2) satisfied. Therefore, (19) has at least three positive solutions for $\lambda \in (\lambda_*, \lambda^*)$ where $\lambda_* = \max \left\{ A_{p_i} \frac{\tau^{p_1-1}}{e^{\tau/2}-1}, A_{p_2} \tau^{p_2-1-\zeta_3}, \ldots, A_{p_n} \tau^{p_n-1-\zeta_1} \right\}$ and

$$\lambda^* = \min \left\{ \frac{1}{2\|w_{p_1}\|_\infty^{p_1-1}(e^{\frac{\tau}{\tau+1}} - 1)}, \frac{1}{2\|w_{p_2}\|_\infty^{p_2-1}}, \ldots, \frac{1}{2\|w_{p_n}\|_\infty^{p_n-1}} \right\}.$$

References

1. Shivaji, R., Son, B.: Bifurcation and multiplicity results for classes of p, q Laplacian systems. Topol. Methods Nonlinear Anal. **48**, 103–114 (2016)
2. Amann, H.: Fixed point equations and nonlinear eigen value problems in order Banach space. SIAM Rev. **18**(4), 620–709 (1976)
3. Lee, E.K., Shivaji, R., Ye, J.: Subsolutions: a journey from positone to infinite semipositone problems. In: Proceedings of the 7th Mississippi State UAB Conference for Differential Equations and Computational Simulations. Electron. J. Differ. Equ. Conf. **17**, 123–131 (2009)
4. Ali, J., Brown, K.J., Shivaji, R.: Positive solutions for $n \times n$ elliptic systems with combined nonlinear effects. Differ. Integr. Equ. **24**, 307–324 (2011)

Uniqueness and Asymptotic Behavior of the Solutions to a Singular Coagulation–Fragmentation Equation

Debdulal Ghosh and Jitendra Kumar

Abstract In this paper, we demonstrate the uniqueness and asymptotic property of the solutions of a coagulation–fragmentation equation. We take into account coagulation kernels with singularities and fragmentation kernels of the kind which influences breaking of a particle into multiple ones. A numerical example of stability behavior of the time-dependent solution for coagulation–fragmentation equation is given.

Keywords Coagulation–fragmentation process · Coagulation kernels · Fragmentation kernels · Uniqueness · Singularity

1 Introduction

Coagulation and fragmentation is a particulate process that describes the time evolution of a system in which clusters react in either coagulate together or break. This is first studied by Smoluchowski [1]. It concerns about Brownian motion. The model involves a set of differential equations. After that, Muller [2] introduced its continuous version. Melzak [3] derived the coagulation–fragmentation equation which is formulated as

$$\begin{aligned}\frac{\partial w(x,t)}{\partial t} =& - w(x,t)\int_0^x \frac{y}{x}\Gamma(x,y)dy - \int_x^\infty \Gamma(y,x)w(y,t)\ dy\\ &- w(x,t)\int_0^\infty K(x,y)w(y,t)\,dy\\ &+\frac{1}{2}\int_0^x K(x-y,y)w(x-y,t)w(y,t)\,dy\end{aligned} \tag{1}$$

D. Ghosh (✉) · J. Kumar
Department of Mathematics, Indian Institute of Technology Kharagpur, Kharagpur, West Bengal 721 302, India
e-mail: debdulal.email@gmail.com

J. Kumar
e-mail: jkumar@maths.iitkgp.ac.in

S. Bhattacharyya et al. (eds.), *Mathematical Modeling and Computational Tools*, Springer Proceedings in Mathematics & Statistics 320,
https://doi.org/10.1007/978-981-15-3615-1_21

In Eq. (1), $w(x,t)$ represents the density of x-size clusters at time t. The term $w(x,t)dx$ denotes the average number of particle that lies in $(x, x+dx)$ at time t. The function $\Gamma(x, y)$ is the multiple fragmentation kernel which shows the rate at which y-sized particles are produced by the fragmentation of x-sized particle. The function $K(x, y)$, known as the coagulation kernel, gives the rate at which x-sized and y-sized particles coalesce. The kernel Γ is known as a multiple fragmentation kernel as a particle splits into many pieces at each fragmentation process.

In this study, we consider the following equation of coagulation–fragmentation (C-F equation):

$$\left.\begin{aligned} \frac{\partial f(x,t)}{\partial t} &= \int_x^\infty b(x,y)S(y)f(y,t)\,dy + \frac{1}{2}\int_0^x K(x-y,y)f(x-y,t)f(y,t)\,dy \\ &\quad - S(x)f(x,t) - f(x,t)\int_0^\infty K(x,y)f(y,t)\,dy \\ &\text{with the initial condition } f(x,0) = f_0(x), \end{aligned}\right\} \tag{2}$$

where f_0 is a non-negative function in $[0, \infty)$. In Eq. (2), $S(x)$ provides a description of the overall breaking frequency of a particle of size x. The function $b(x, y)$ is the distribution function corresponding to formation of x-sized particles and the breakage of y-sized particle. It is nonzero for $x < y$. The function $b(x, y)$ further satisfies

$$\int_0^y b(x,y)\,dx = N(y) \quad \text{for } y > 0, \tag{3}$$

where $N(y)$ indicates the number of pieces from the y-sized particle breakage. Throughout this paper, we assume

(i) $N(y)$ is size dependent,
(ii) $N(y) \le N$, a constant, and
(iii) by fragmentation, number of particles is increased but mass remains same, i.e., b obeys the following relation

$$\int_0^y x b(x,y)\,dx = y \quad \text{for all } y > 0. \tag{4}$$

The interrelations between the multiple fragmentation kernel, the breakage function, and the selection function are:

$$\Gamma(x,y) = S(y)b(x,y) \quad \text{and} \quad S(x) = \int_0^x \frac{y}{x}\Gamma(x,y)\,dy.$$

The model equation (2) is referred to as a continuous form of C-F equation. Applications of this model equation arise in aerosol physics [4], population dynamics of animal grouping [5], hematological red blood cell aggregation [6], astrophysics [7], polymer science, colloidal chemistry [8, 9], etc.

1.1 Literature on Eq. (2)

Aizenman and Bak [10] have analyzed an equation similar to (2) in the study of chemical kinetics of system of reacting polymers. They have considered the Boltzman equation and shown uniqueness result in the function space

$$\mathfrak{F} := \left\{ \phi : [0, \infty) \to \mathbb{R} \;\middle|\; \|\phi\| = \int_0^\infty (1+x)|\phi(x)|dx < \infty \right\}.$$

Under the assumptions on the coagulation kernel that $K(x, y) \leq \psi(x)\psi(y)$, for all $x, y \in (0, \infty)$, $\psi : (0, \infty) \to (0, \infty)$ being a continuous function, Norris [11] has shown that there is a unique solution to (2).

Banasiak [12] analyzed a fragmentation model and described the existence of multiple solutions. The reason behind the non-uniqueness is also given in [12]. Melzak [3] investigated a coagulation fragmentation equation and showed that there exists a unique solution under the following assumption on kernels

(i) $0 \leq K(x, y) \leq A$, a constant, and
(ii) $0 \leq F(x, y) \leq B$, $\int_0^x yF(x, y) \leq x$ and $\int_0^x F(x, y)dy < \infty$.

For constant kernels, Aizenman and Bak [10] showed the uniqueness of solutions to (2). For a class of bounded kernels, Melzak [3] has proved the existence and uniqueness of solutions.

Under a sufficient condition, Norris [11] investigated the unique solutions to the problem (2) with a coagulation kernel that obeys $K(x, y) \leq \phi_1(x)\phi_2(y)$ where ϕ_1 and ϕ_2 are sublinear functions.

Banasiak [12] demonstrated the presence of several solutions and showed that non-unique solutions hold for a wide range of sensible physical alternatives.

Giri et al. [13] have discussed the uniqueness of weak solution for the problem (2). The coagulation kernel under consideration in [13] is bounded by $\psi(x)\psi(y)$, for $x > 0$ and $y > 0$, where ψ satisfies

$$\psi(x) \leq k_1(1 + x^\mu), \; \mu \in [0, 1),$$

and the selection function obeys

$$S(x) \leq k_2(1 + x)^\nu, \quad \nu \in [0, 1).$$

Dubovski and Stewart [14] proved the global existence and uniqueness for (2) with a linear K and an unbounded b.

It is to observe that the existing study on Eq. (2) with singular kernels is very limited. The analysis of (2) with singular kernels can be found in the recent papers [15, 16]. In this work, we show the uniqueness of the solutions to (2) with a singular kernel in the function space that is defined in [16].

The paper is demonstrated in the following sequence. Section 2 states some preliminaries which are used in this paper. In Sect. 3, we derive the uniqueness of the solutions. A numerical example on asymptotic behavior of the solutions is presented in Sect. 4. Finally, in Sect. 5, we conclude and give future scopes.

2 Preliminaries

We use the function space $\Omega_{\lambda,r_2}(T)$. Which is defined as follows

(i) a function $\phi \in \Omega_{\lambda,r_2}(T)$ implies it is continuous, and
(ii) for an r_2 in (0, 1),

$$\|\phi\|_{\lambda,r_2} := \sup_{t\in[0,T]} \int_0^\infty \left(\frac{1}{x^{r_2}} + \exp(\lambda x)\right) |\phi(x,t)| dx, \text{ a finite quantity.}$$

For a given $T > 0$, let

$$\Omega_{.,r_2}(T) = \bigcup_{\lambda>0} \Omega_{\lambda,r_2}(T).$$

We denote cones of non-negative functions in $\Omega_{\lambda,r_2}(T)$ and $\Omega_{.,r_2}(T)$ by $\Omega^+_{\lambda,r_2}(T)$ and $\Omega^+_{.,r_2}(T)$, respectively. We also use the following notation in the sequel

$$\Pi = \{(x,t) : 0 \le t \le T, 0 < x < \infty\}$$

3 Uniqueness Theorem

In [16], the existence of a solution to (2) is given. In this section, we demonstrate the uniqueness of the solution to (2), within the function sphere $\Omega_{.,r_2}(T)$, under the hypothesis in Theorem 1 of [16]. The following lemma is used to derive the uniqueness.

Lemma 1 (See *[14]*) *Let $w(\lambda, t)$ be a real-valued continuous function and w_λ and $w_{\lambda\lambda}$ are continuous on $\mathcal{D} = \{(\lambda, t) : t \in [0, T], \lambda \in [0, \lambda_0]\}$. Moreover, we assume that the real-valued functions $\vartheta(\lambda, t)$, $\eta(\lambda)$, $\tau(\lambda, t)$ and $\rho(\lambda, t)$ are continuous on $\mathcal{D}$. Also, let their partial derivatives in λ are continuous and the function w, w_λ, ϑ, ρ are non-negative. Suppose in the region $\mathcal{D}$ that the following inequalities hold*

$$w(\lambda,t) \le \eta(\lambda) + \int_0^t (\rho(\lambda,s)v(\lambda,s) + \vartheta(\lambda,s)w_\lambda(\lambda,s) + \tau(\lambda,s))ds$$

and

$$w_\lambda(\lambda,t) \le \eta_\lambda(\lambda) + \int_0^t \frac{\partial}{\partial \lambda}(\vartheta(\lambda,s)w_\lambda(\lambda,s) + \rho(\lambda,s)w(\lambda,s) + \tau(\lambda,s))ds.$$

Let $\mathcal{C}_0 = \sup_{\lambda\in[0,\lambda_0]} \eta$, $\mathcal{C}_1 = \sup_{\mathcal{D}} \vartheta$ *and* $\mathcal{C}_3 = \sup_{\mathcal{D}} \tau$. *Then,*

$$w(\lambda,t) \le \tfrac{\mathcal{C}_3}{\mathcal{C}_2}(\exp(\mathcal{C}_2 t) - 1) + \mathcal{C}_0 \exp(\mathcal{C}_2 t)$$

in a region $\mathcal{R} \subset \mathcal{D}$:

$$\mathcal{R} = \{(\lambda,t) : \lambda \in [\lambda_1 - \mathcal{C}_1 t,\ \lambda_0 - \mathcal{C}_1 t],\ 0 \le t \le t' < T',\ \lambda_1 \in (0,\lambda_0)\},$$

where $T' = \min\{(\lambda_1/\mathcal{C}_1), T\}$.

Theorem 1 (Uniqueness result) *Suppose* $b(x,y)$ *and* $K(x,y)$ *are continuous and non-negative in* $(0,\infty)\times(0,\infty)$ *and* $K(x,y)$ *is symmetric in* $(0,\infty)\times(0,\infty)$. *Let* $S(x)$ *be a continuous and non-negative function in* $(0,\infty)$. *Furthermore, we assume that*

(*i*) $K(x,y) \le k\,\frac{1}{(xy)^\mu}$ $\forall x,y \in (0,\infty)$, *where* $\mu \in \left[0,\frac{1}{2}\right)$ *and* k *is a positive constant,*
(*ii*) *there exists* $S_1 > 0$ *such that* $S(x) \le S_1\, x^\beta$ $\forall x \in (0,\infty)$, *where* β *is a positive real number,*
(*iii*) *for some* $\gamma \in (0,1)$, *and a constant* $n_0 > 0$, $\int_0^y \frac{1}{x^\gamma} b(x,y)\,dx \le \frac{n_0}{y^\gamma}$, *and*
(*iv*) *for* $0 < x_1 < x_2$, $\lim_{y\to\infty} \sup_{x\in[x_1,x_2]} b(x,y) \le \bar{b}$, *a constant.*

Then, the solution to C-F equation (2) is unique in the function space $\Omega_{.,r_2}(T)$.

Proof If possible let there exit two different solutions c and g, in $\Omega_{.,r_2}(T)$, to the initial value problem (2).
Let $u(x,t) = c(x,t) - g(x,t)$ and $\psi(x,t) = c(x,t) + g(x,t)$.
Since $c, g \in \Omega_{.,r_2}(T)$, there exists a $\hat{\lambda} > 0$ such that the following inequalities hold uniformly in $0 \le t \le T$:

$$\left.\begin{aligned} &\int_0^\infty \left(\frac{1}{x^\nu} + \exp(\lambda x)\right) u(x,t)\,dx < \infty \\ \text{and } &\int_0^\infty \left(\frac{1}{x^\nu} + \exp(\lambda x)\right) \psi(x,t)\,dx < \infty. \end{aligned}\right\} \tag{5}$$

Let

$$0 \le \lambda < \hat{\lambda}. \tag{6}$$

Therefore, by the definition of u, we obtain

$$\begin{aligned}\frac{\partial u(x,t)}{\partial t} &= \int_x^\infty b(x,y)S(y)\{c(y,t)-g(y,t)\}\,dy - S(x)\{c(x,t)-g(x,t)\}\\ &\quad -\int_0^\infty K(x,y)\{c(x,t)c(y,t)-g(x,t)g(y,t)\}\,dy\\ &\quad +\frac{1}{2}\int_0^x K(x-y,y)\{c(x-y,t)c(y,t)-g(x-y,t)g(y,t)\}\,dy\end{aligned} \tag{7}$$

By the definition of signum function, we note that

$$\frac{d|Q(\xi)|}{d\xi} = \operatorname{sgn}(Q(\xi))\frac{d}{d\xi}Q(\xi).$$

We define

$$\Psi(\lambda,t) = \int_0^\infty \left(\exp(\lambda x)+\frac{1}{x^\nu}\right)|\psi(x,t)|\,dx, \tag{8}$$

and

$$U(\lambda,t) = \int_0^\infty \left(\exp(\lambda x)+\frac{1}{x^\nu}\right)|u(x,t)|\,dx, \tag{9}$$

where we choose ν such that $0<\nu\le r_2-\mu$.

By the integration after multiplying both sides of (7) by $\left(\frac{1}{x^\nu}+\exp(\lambda x)\right)$, we get

$$\begin{aligned}U(\lambda,t) &= \int_0^t\int_0^\infty \left(\exp(\lambda x)+\frac{1}{x^\nu}\right)\operatorname{sgn}(u(x,s))\\ &\quad\times\left[\frac{1}{2}\int_0^x K(x-y,y)\{c(x-y,s)c(y,s)-g(x-y,s)g(y,s)\}\,dy\right.\\ &\quad+\int_x^\infty b(x,y)S(y)\{c(y,s)-g(y,s)\}\,dy - S(x)\{c(x,s)-g(x,s)\}\\ &\quad\left.-\int_0^\infty K(x,y)\{c(x,s)c(y,s)-g(x,s)g(y,s)\}\,dy\right]dx\,ds.\end{aligned}$$

By simplification, we get

$$\begin{aligned}U(\lambda,t) &= \int_0^t\int_0^\infty\int_0^\infty\left[\frac{1}{2}\left(\exp(\lambda(x+y))+\frac{1}{(x+y)^\nu}\right)\operatorname{sgn}(u(x+y,s))\right.\\ &\quad\left.-\left(\exp(\lambda x)+\frac{1}{x^\nu}\right)\operatorname{sgn}(u(x,s))\right]\\ &\quad\times K(x,y)\{c(x,s)c(y,s)-g(x,s)g(y,s)\}\,dy\,dx\,ds \qquad (10)\\ &\quad+\int_0^t\int_0^\infty\left(\exp(\lambda x)+\frac{1}{x^\nu}\right)\operatorname{sgn}(u(x,s))\\ &\quad\times\left[\int_x^\infty b(x,y)S(y)\{c(y,s)-g(y,s)\}\,dy - S(x)\{c(x,s)-g(x,s)\}\right]dx\,ds. \qquad (11)\end{aligned}$$

We note that

$$c(x,s)c(y,s) - g(x,s)g(y,s) = u(x,s)c(y,s) + u(y,s)g(x,s).$$

We observe that

$$\begin{aligned}
&\int_0^t \int_0^\infty \int_0^\infty \Bigg[\frac{1}{2}\left(\exp(\lambda(x+y)) + \frac{1}{(x+y)^\nu}\right) \mathrm{sgn}\,(u(x+y,s)) \\
&\quad - \left(\exp(\lambda x) + \frac{1}{x^\nu}\right) \mathrm{sgn}\,(u(x,s))\Bigg] c(y,s)K(x,y)u(x,s)dy\,dx\,ds \\
&\le k \int_0^t \int_0^\infty \int_0^\infty \frac{1}{2}\left(\exp(\lambda y) + \frac{1}{y^\nu}\right) \exp(\lambda x) \frac{1}{(xy)^\mu} c(y,s)|u(x,s)|\,dy\,dx\,ds.
\end{aligned} \tag{12}$$

In the next, we evaluate a few inequalities.

$$\begin{aligned}
\int_0^\infty \exp(\lambda x)\frac{1}{x^\mu}|u(x,t)|dx \le\ & \exp(\lambda) \int_0^1 \left(\frac{1}{x^\nu} + \exp(\lambda x)\right) |u(x,t)|dx \\
& + \int_1^\infty \left(\frac{1}{x^\nu} + \exp(\lambda x)\right) |u(x,t)|dx \\
=\ & U(\lambda,t)(1+\exp(\lambda)).
\end{aligned} \tag{13}$$

By a similar approach,

$$\int_0^\infty \left(\exp(\lambda y) + \frac{1}{y^\nu}\right) \frac{1}{y^\mu} c(y,t)dy \le (\exp(\lambda)+1)\,\bar{N}_{-\nu-\mu} + \Psi = \Gamma_1, \text{ say.} \tag{14}$$

By similar analysis of the expression (2.5) in [16], we note that

$$\int_0^\infty x^k \left[-S(x)\big|U(x,s)\big| + \int_x^\infty b(x,y)S(y)\big|U(y,s)\big|\,dy\right] dx \le 0,$$

for $k = 1, 2, 3, \ldots$.

With the help of the hypothesis (iii) of Theorem 1 and get from Eq. (11) that

$$
\begin{aligned}
&\int_0^t \int_0^\infty \left(1 + \frac{1}{x^\nu}\right)\left[-|U(x,s)|S(x) + \int_x^\infty S(y)b(x,y)|U(y,s)|\,dy\right] dx\,ds \\
&\quad \le (n_0 - 1)\int_0^t \int_0^\infty \left(1 + \frac{1}{y^\nu}\right) S(y)|U(y,s)|\,dy\,ds \\
&\quad \le (n_0 - 1)S_1 \int_0^t \int_0^\infty \left(1 + \frac{1}{y^\nu}\right) y^\beta |U(y,s)|\,dy\,ds \\
&\quad \le (n_0 - 1)S_1 \int_0^t \left[\int_0^1 \left(1 + \frac{1}{y^\nu}\right) y^\beta |U(y,s)|\,dy\,ds \right.\\
&\qquad \left. + \int_1^\infty \left(1 + \frac{1}{y^\nu}\right) y^\beta |U(y,s)|\,dy\,ds\right] \\
&\quad \le (n_0 - 1)S_1 \int_0^t \left[\int_0^1 \left(1 + \frac{1}{y^\nu}\right) |U(y,s)|\,dy\,ds \right.\\
&\qquad \left. + \int_1^\infty (1+1) y^\beta |U(y,s)|\,dy\,ds\right] \\
&\quad \le \Gamma_3 \int_0^t U(\lambda, s)ds. \qquad (15)
\end{aligned}
$$

By the inequalities (13)–(14), we obtain from Eqs. (10) and (11) that

$$
\begin{aligned}
U(\lambda, t) &\le 2\int_0^t [\Gamma_1 U(1 + \exp(\lambda)) + \Gamma_3 U]ds \\
&= 2\int_0^t [(\chi_0 + \Psi)\chi_1 U + \chi_2 U]ds, \qquad (16)
\end{aligned}
$$

where $\chi_0 + \Psi = (\exp(\hat{\lambda}) + 1)\bar{N}_{-\nu-\mu} + \Psi \ge \Gamma_1$, $\chi_1 = 1 + \exp(\hat{\lambda})$ and $\chi_2 = \Gamma_3$. Till now we have attempted to obtain a bound for the function $U(\lambda, t)$. In the next, we endeavor to obtain an upper bound of the partial derivative function $U_\lambda(\lambda, t)$.

We recall from (9) that

$$
U_\lambda(\lambda, t) = \int_0^\infty \left(\frac{1}{x^\nu} + x\exp(\lambda x)\right) |u(x,t)|\, dx,
$$

where we choose ν to be $0 < \nu \le r_2 - \mu$. To obtain the expression of U_λ, we multiply (7) by $\left(x\exp(\lambda x) + \frac{1}{x^\nu}\right)$ after that by integrating we obtain

$$
\begin{aligned}
&U_\lambda(\lambda, t)\\
&= \int_0^t \int_0^\infty \int_0^\infty \Bigg[\frac{1}{2}\left((x+y)\exp(\lambda(x+y)) + \frac{1}{(x+y)^\nu}\right)\operatorname{sgn}(u(x+y,s))\\
&\quad - \left(x\exp(\lambda x) + \frac{1}{x^\nu}\right)\operatorname{sgn}(u(x,s))\Bigg]K(x,y)\\
&\quad \times \{c(x,s)c(y,s) - g(x,s)g(y,s)\}\,dy\,dx\,ds \qquad (17)\\
&\quad + \int_0^t \int_0^\infty \left(x\exp(\lambda x) + \frac{1}{x^\nu}\right)\operatorname{sgn}(u(x,s))\\
&\quad \times \left[\int_x^\infty b(x,y)S(y)\{c(y,s)-g(y,s)\}\,dy - S(x)\{c(x,s)-g(x,s)\}\right]dx\,ds. \qquad (18)
\end{aligned}
$$

We next proceed after executing the following inequalities:

$$
\int_0^\infty \exp(\lambda y)\frac{1}{y^\mu}c(y,s)dy \leq [\exp(\lambda)+1]\Psi(\lambda,s) \qquad (19)
$$

$$
\text{and} \quad \int_0^\infty x\exp(\lambda x)\frac{1}{x^\mu}|u(x,s)|dx \leq \exp(\lambda)\,U_\lambda. \qquad (20)
$$

Here, we note that

$$
\left.
\begin{aligned}
&\int_0^\infty \frac{1}{x^\mu}\exp(\lambda x)|u(x,s)|dx \leq U(\exp(\lambda)+1),\\
\text{and} \quad &\int_0^\infty x^{1-\mu}\exp(\lambda x)|u(x,s)|dx \leq U_\lambda(\exp(\lambda)+1).
\end{aligned}
\right\} \qquad (21)
$$

Further,

$$
\left.
\begin{aligned}
&\int_0^\infty \frac{1}{x^\mu}\exp(\lambda x)c(x,s)dx \leq \Psi(\exp(\lambda)+1),\\
\text{and} \quad &\int_0^\infty x^{1-\mu}\exp(\lambda x)g(x,s)dx \leq \Psi,
\end{aligned}
\right\} \qquad (22)
$$

With the help of (21) and (22), the equation in (17) and (18) yields

$$
\begin{aligned}
U_\lambda(\lambda,t) &\leq \int_0^t \left[U\Big((\exp(\lambda)+1)\Psi + \Gamma_3\Big) + U_\lambda\Big((\exp(\lambda)+1)^2\Psi\Big)\right]ds\\
&= \int_0^t \left[U(\chi_1\Psi + \chi_2) + U_\lambda(\chi_1^2\Psi)\right]ds. \qquad (23)
\end{aligned}
$$

The functions U and Ψ, defined in (9) and (8), respectively, are analytic for $\lambda \in (0, \hat{\lambda})$ and for any fixed values of t such that $0 \leq t \leq T$.

Let us choose λ that satisfies

$$0 \leq \lambda \leq \lambda_0 < \hat{\lambda}. \tag{24}$$

Then, the inequality (5) ensures that for $i \geq 1$,

$$\sup_{0 \leq t \leq T,\ 0 \leq \lambda \leq \lambda_0} \left\{ \frac{\partial^i}{\partial \lambda^i} U(\lambda, t),\ \frac{\partial^i}{\partial \lambda^i} \Psi(\lambda, t) \right\} < \infty. \tag{25}$$

Due to continuity of the functions $\psi(x, t)$ and $u(x, t)$ on Π, from (5), for any given $\epsilon > 0$, there exist $\delta(\epsilon) > 0$ and $\delta_i(\epsilon) > 0$ so that for any $i \geq 1$, we have the following for $|t' - t| < \delta$ with $t \geq 0$ and $t' \leq T$,

$$\left.\begin{aligned} &\sup_{0 \leq \lambda \leq \lambda_0} \left\{ |\Psi(\lambda, t) - \Psi(\lambda, t')|, |U(\lambda, t) - U(\lambda, t')| \right\} < \epsilon \\ \text{and}\ &\sup_{0 \leq \lambda \leq \lambda_0} \left\{ \left| \frac{\partial^i}{\partial \lambda^i} \Psi(\lambda, t') - \frac{\partial^i}{\partial \lambda^i} \Psi(\lambda, t) \right|, \left| \frac{\partial^i}{\partial \lambda^i} U(\lambda, t') - \frac{\partial^i}{\partial \lambda^i} U(\lambda, t) \right| \right\} < \epsilon \end{aligned}\right\} \tag{26}$$

To show the inequalities (26), we note from (5) for a sufficiently large $\xi > 0$ that the term $\int_\xi^\infty \left(\exp(\lambda x) + \frac{1}{x^\nu}\right) |u(x, t') - u(x, t)|\, dx$ can be made arbitrarily small. Thus, there exists a $\delta_1(\epsilon) > 0$ such that

$$\sup_{0 \leq \lambda \leq \lambda_0} |U(\lambda, t) - U(\lambda, t')| < \epsilon$$

for $|t' - t| < \delta$ with $t \geq 0$ and $t' \leq T$. Similarly, the other three terms in (26) involving Ψ, $\frac{\partial^i}{\partial \lambda^i} U$ and $\frac{\partial^i}{\partial \lambda^i} \Psi$ are arbitrarily small in a range of t.

It follows from (25) and (26) that U and Ψ and their partial derivatives are continuous on λ in $D = \{(\lambda, t) \mid 0 \leq \lambda \leq \lambda_0, 0 \leq t \leq T\}$. Inequalities (16) and (23) imply the existence a function $c_1(\lambda) = 2(\chi_1^2 + \chi_2)\Psi \exp(\hat{\lambda}) + \chi_0 \chi_1$ such that

$$\left.\begin{aligned} U(\lambda, t) &\leq \int_0^t U(\lambda, s) c_1(\lambda, s) ds \\ \text{and}\ \frac{\partial}{\partial \lambda} U(\lambda, t) &\leq \int_0^t \left\{ \frac{\partial c_1}{\partial \lambda} U(\lambda, s) + U_\lambda(\lambda, t) c_1(\lambda, s) \right\} ds, \end{aligned}\right\} \tag{27}$$

and U, Ψ and their partial derivatives are non-negative in $\mathcal{D}$. Then, by applying Lemma 1 in $\mathcal{D}$, we have for the region $\mathcal{R}$, $U(\lambda, t) = 0$.

As $u(x, t)$ belongs to the set of all continuous function, for $t \in [0, t]$, $x \in (0, \infty)$, we have $u(x, t) = 0$. Thus, $U(\lambda, t) = 0$ is not only true on $\mathcal{R}$, but also for all $\lambda \in [0, \lambda_0]$, $t \in [0, t']$. Hence, $u(x, t) = 0$ for $x \in (0, \infty)$.

Applying an identical logic for $t' \leq t \leq 2t'$, we observe that $u(x,t) = 0$ where $0 \leq t \leq 2t'$, and $x \in (0, \infty)$. Repeating same procedure, we can conclude that for $(x,t) \in \Pi$, $u(x,t) = 0$, i.e., $c(x,t) = g(x,t)$ for $(x,t) \in \Pi$. Hence, the result follows.

4 Asymptotic Behavior of Time-Dependent Solution

In the mathematical study of a model equation, such as coagulation–fragmentation equation, we often come across the problem to find its explicit solution. In many instances, it is known that the model equation has a unique solution, but often a precise closed form solution is difficult to find. In this circumstance, an important point of analysis is to find the essential properties, such as the existence of a self-similar solution, gel formation, shattering, and asymptotic behavior of time-dependent solution of the solutions.

In this section, we provide a numerical example where time-dependent solution approaches to equilibrium. Though analytical proof is not given, researcher can get help to investigate analysis on this problem, i.e., stability property of time-dependent solution.

For the numerical computations, we have used the numerical scheme that is established in [17, 18]. The computational range under consideration is $[10^{-9}, 512]$ and it is broken into 20 non-uniform intervals $\Lambda_i := [x_{i-1/2}, x_{i+1/2}]$, $i = 1, 2, \ldots, 20$, where the end points satisfy $x_{i+1/2} = rx_{i-1/2}$; $r > 1$ being the geometric ratio. The mid-point of Λi is considered to be the cell representative or the pivot. The system of ODEs is solved in MATLAB-R2015 software by adaptive Runge-Kutta 4(5) solver.

4.1 *Example 1*

In this example, we take

$$K(x, y) = (1 + x^{1.3} + y^{1.3})(xy)^{-0.15}, \quad F(x, y) = 1, \quad \text{and} \quad c_0 = \exp(-x).$$

The expression of the moment M_i is $M_i(t) = \int_0^\infty x^i c(x,t)dx$. In Fig. 1, we plot the moments. And in Fig. 2, the number density function is plotted with respect to the pivots at four different times. Figure 2 shows that the time-dependent solution is stable after $t = 3$, since $c(x,t)$ has fixed value for $t = 3$, 5, and 8. If look closely at Fig. 1, we see that all the moments $M_0(t)$, $M_2(t)$, and $M_{-\sigma}(t)$ are constants after $t = 3$. Hence, the system is stable after $t = 3$.

Thus, with $c_0 = \exp(-x)$, the time-dependent solution $c(x,t)$ converges to the steady-state solution.

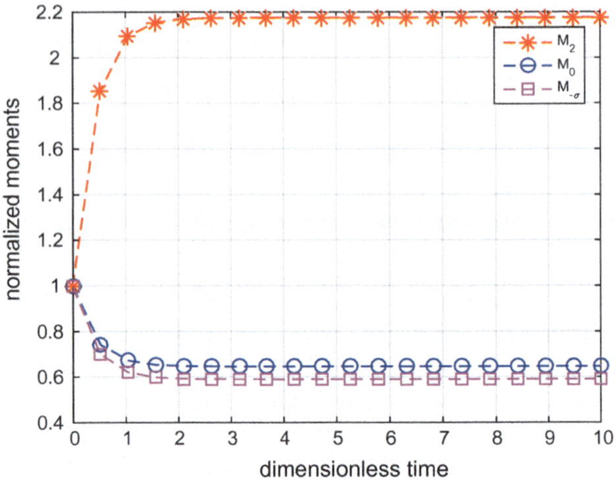

Fig. 1 Normalized moments

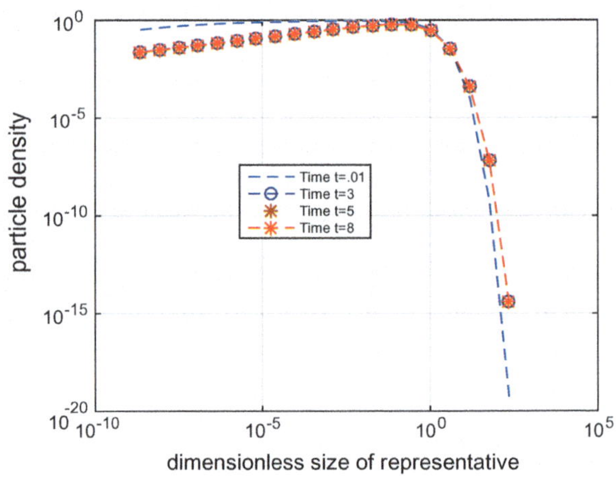

Fig. 2 Particle number density

5 Conclusion

In this paper, it has been showed that the solutions to C-F equation with a singular coagulation kernel are unique. For the considered kernel, we note that it has singularity in both the axes. In future, we will focus to prove uniqueness property for the coagulation kernel in the form considered in [16]. Also, in this article, we do not show the analytical proof of stability analysis. In the future, we will try to analyze the convergence property of time-dependent solutions to a steady state solution.

References

1. Smoluchowski, M.V.: An experiment on mathematical theorization of coagulation kinetics of the colloidal solutions. Z. Phys. Chem. **92**, 129–168 (1917)
2. Muller, H.: To the general theory of rapid coagulation. Progr. Rep. Colloid. Polym. **27**(6), 223–250 (1928)
3. Melzak, Z.A.: A scalar transport equation. Trans. Am. Math. Soc. **85**(2), 547–560 (1957)
4. Drake, R.L.: A general mathematical survey of the coagulation equation. Top. Curr. Aerosol Res. **3**(Part 2), 201–376 (1972)
5. Okubo, A.: Dynamical aspects of animal grouping: swarms, schools, flocks, andherds. Adv. Biophys. **22**, 1–94 (1986)
6. Perelson, A.S., Samsel, R.W.: Kinetics of red blood cell aggregation: an example of geometric polymerization. In: Family, F., Landau, D.P. (eds.) Kinetics of Aggregation and Gelation. Elsevier (1984)
7. Safronov, V.S.: Evolution of the Protoplanetary Cloud and Formation of the Earth and Planets, by Safronov, V.S. Translated from Russian, vol. 1, 212 p. Israel Program for Scientific Translations, Keter Publishing House, Jerusalem, Israel (1972)
8. Smoluchowski, M.: Drei vortrage uber diffusion. Brownsche bewegung und koagulation von kolloidteilchen. Z. Phys. **17**, 557–585 (1916)
9. Smoluchowski, M.: Grundriß der koagulationskinetik kolloider löosungen. Coll. Polym. Sci. **21**(3), 98–104 (1917)
10. Aizenman, M., Bak, T.A.: Convergence to equilibrium in a system of reacting polymers. Commun. Math. Phys. **65**(3), 203–230 (1979)
11. Norris, J.R.: Smoluchowskis coagulation equation: uniqueness, nonuniqueness and a hydrodynamic limit for the stochastic coalescent. Ann. Appl. Probab. **9**(1), 78–109 (1999)
12. Banasiak, J.: On a non-uniqueness in fragmentation models. Math. Methods Appl. Sci. **25**(7), 541–556 (2002)
13. Giri, A.K., Kumar, J., Warnecke, G.: The continuous coagulation equation with multiple fragmentation. J. Math. Anal. Appl. **374**(1), 71–87 (2011)
14. Dubovskiĭ, P.B., Stewart, I.W.: Existence, uniqueness and mass conservation for the coagulation-fragmentation equation. Math. Methods Appl. Sci. **19**(7), 571–591 (1996)
15. Camejo, C.C., Gropler, R., Warnecke, G.: Regular solutions to the coagulation equations with singular kernels. Math. Methods Appl. Sci. **38**(11), 2171–2184 (2014)
16. Ghosh, D., Kumar, J.: Existence of mass conserving solution for the coagulation-fragmentation equation with singular kernel. Jpn. J. Ind. Appl. Math. **35**(3), 1283–1302 (2018)
17. Kumar, J., Kaur, G., Tsotsas, E.: An accurate and efficient discrete formulation of aggregation population balance equation. Kinet. Relat. Model. **9**(2), 373–391 (2016)
18. Kumar, J., Saha, J., Tsotsas, E.: Development and convergence analysis of a finite volume scheme for solving breakage equation. SIAM J. Numer. Anal. **53**(4), 1672–1689 (2015)

Natural Convection Melting of PCM: Numerical Simulation Techniques and Applications

Nadezhda S. Bondareva and Mikhail A. Sheremet

Abstract Creation of electronic equipment, heat exchangers, and thermal insulation of buildings is related to the development of effective cooling systems or heat storage systems. One of the solutions to the considered problem is the usage of phase change materials (PCMs) that can essentially enhance the characteristics of the developed system. Phase change materials are characterized by high phase transition heat at a fixed temperature, and these materials have a thermal capacity higher than the typical heat storage media. The aim of this study is a numerical simulation of free convection melting of PCM within a chamber with a heat-generating element of time-dependent volumetric thermal production and finned radiator system. The presented new numerical results for the effective cooling system for the heat-generating unit including the copper heat sink, *n*-octadecane as PCM have been analyzed.

Keywords Phase change material · Melting · Numerical simulation

1 Introduction

Creation of electronic equipment and thermal power technology is related to the development of effective cooling systems [1–4]. For this purpose, it is possible to use active or passive cooling techniques. In the case of active systems, the presence of external forced loading is necessary. Such approach demands an additional energy, and therefore, it cannot be implemented in microelectronics and some energy systems. Nowadays, one of the most perspective cooling systems is the usage of phase change material that allows to remove extra heating from the elements and to support the temperature in a working range.

In spite of wide applications, numerical and experimental analysis of PCM free convection melting is not so widely spread [5–20]. Thus, Naaktgeboren et al. [5] studied analytically the natural convection melting of PCM within an electronic cabinet with heat sinks under the influence of external periodic temperature using the

N. S. Bondareva · M. A. Sheremet (✉)
Tomsk State University, 36 Lenin Avenue, Tomsk 634050, Russia
e-mail: sheremet@math.tsu.ru

S. Bhattacharyya et al. (eds.), *Mathematical Modeling and Computational Tools*,
Springer Proceedings in Mathematics & Statistics 320,
https://doi.org/10.1007/978-981-15-3615-1_22

zero-phase formulation approach. Experimental and numerical analysis of PCM-assisted heat pipe for electronics cooling was performed by Behi et al. [6]. It was ascertained that the considered system can promote 86.7% to the cooling performance and 11.7% reduction of the thermal dissipation due to a supplementary thermal absorption. Dinesh and Bhattacharya [7] analyzed computationally the energy transport properties of PCM-based system enhanced with the metal foam. Authors showed that the energy transport strength enhances with a diminution of the pore dimensions owing to large surface areas for the energy transport between the metal foam and PCM. Rehman et al. [8] examined experimentally the heat sink behavior with the copper foam enhanced by the phase change material and without PCM. They ascertained that a combination of the metal foam and phase change material allows reducing the maximum temperature of the system. Krishna et al. [9] performed an experimental analysis of an opportunity to employ the heat pipe with PCM enhanced or not by the nanoparticles. Authors studied a wide range of governing characteristics including the thermal inputs, PCM, and nanoparticle concentration. It was found that tricosane (PCM) with alumina nanoparticles (1%) can save 53% of the fan power consumption. Ali et al. [10] conducted an experimental analysis of the pin-fin configuration influence on energy transport performance in PCM for electronics cooling systems. Authors showed that pin fins of triangular shape have strong advantages for the thermal transmission within the considered system. Computational analysis of the energy transport in a cooling system using the heat sink with pin fins and phase change material was performed by Xie et al. [11]. The obtained results demonstrated that the optimized tree-shaped configuration of fins can decrease essentially the heat source temperature. Moreover, the upward orientation of the heat sink system is more effective in comparison with downward orientation. Ashraf et al. [12] studied experimentally the pin-fin configuration effect combined with PCM on the passive cooling system performance. The optimal configuration and PCM were defined in dependence on the power level. Rakotondrandisa et al. [13] numerically considered the phase transition cycle of PCM within a differentially heated chamber. The finite element technique of the second-order accuracy combined with dynamically adaptive mesh was used. Authors showed that convective energy transport is the major mechanism for the melting phenomenon, thus intensifying the thermal transmission, while heat conduction is the major energy transport mechanism for the solidification process, illustrating the slower mode. Lin et al. [14] on the basis of the lattice Boltzmann technique studied numerically the free convection melting of PCM within a spherical capsule under the impacts of region size, thermal diffusivity ratio, and Stefan number. Authors revealed that the dimensionless fully melting time reduced when rising of the region size. Computational analysis of the free convection melting of PCM within the horizontal sleeve tube with longitudinal fins was conducted by Wang et al. [15] under the effects of the fins configuration. They found that the low fin ratio allows decreasing the melting duration, and the angle between neighbor fins characterizes by a weak influence on the melting phenomenon. Tasnim et al. [16] conducted the mathematical modeling of the free convection melting in a differentially heated porous chamber saturated with nano-enhanced PCM. Authors considered the impacts of the buoyancy force and nanoparticles concentration on the melting process. It was ascertained that energy transport within the enclosure degrades with nanoparticles, and the position of the phase transition line reflects the melting phenomenon prolongation in the presence of nanoparticles.

The presented brief review illustrates the high level of applications for PCM and the presence of experimental and numerical works for the considered topic. Unfortunately, there are no papers concerning the periodical heat generation of the element under the effects of PCM in a cavity with finned heat sink. Therefore, the aim of this research is a computational study of 2D free convection melting of PCM inside a chamber with a local heater of the time-dependent internal volumetric thermal production under the influence of the finned heat sink and external cooling of the chamber.

2 Mathematical Model and Numerical Technique

Figure 1 demonstrates the analyzed region filled with PCM having heat-conducting fins and a local heat element of periodic volumetric thermal production. Local energy element of time-dependent heat generation mounted in the bottom wall is placed under the heat-conducting fins of the heat sink. At the beginning of the phenomenon, the considered region includes solid PCM (pure *n*-octadecane). Vertical borders and the upper horizontal border are assumed to be cooling from outside, while the external bottom wall is adiabatic. For an amplification of the heat thermal dissipation, the heat sink with heat-conducting fins is located over the energy element. Melt, appeared during the phenomenon, is satisfied with the Boussinesq approach. The volumetric heat generation of the energy source is defined by the following function $Q = Q_0\{1 - \sin(ft)\}$.

The liquid motion and thermal transmission within the considered domain of interest (see Fig. 1) are described by the Oberbeck–Boussinesq partial differential equations with an energy equation formulated using the enthalpy variable. The heat

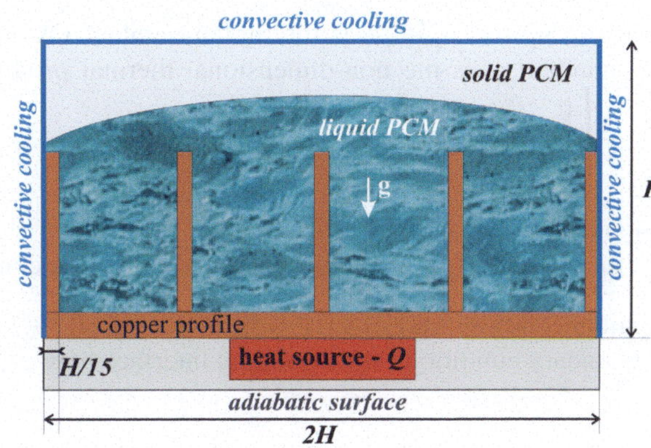

Fig. 1 Analyzed region with boundary conditions

conduction equations within the heat sink and heat-generating element are added to the mathematical model. The non-dimensional partial differential equations written using the stream function, vorticity, and temperature are the following [17, 18]:

$$\frac{\partial^2 \psi}{\partial x^2} + \frac{\partial^2 \psi}{\partial y^2} = -\omega \tag{1}$$

$$\frac{\partial \omega}{\partial \tau} + \frac{\partial \psi}{\partial y}\frac{\partial \omega}{\partial x} - \frac{\partial \psi}{\partial x}\frac{\partial \omega}{\partial y} = \sqrt{\frac{\mathrm{Pr}}{\mathrm{Ra}}}\left(\frac{\partial^2 \omega}{\partial x^2} + \frac{\partial^2 \omega}{\partial y^2}\right) + \frac{\partial \theta}{\partial x} \tag{2}$$

$$\zeta(\varphi)\left[\frac{\partial \theta}{\partial \tau} + \frac{\partial \psi}{\partial y}\frac{\partial \theta}{\partial x} - \frac{\partial \psi}{\partial x}\frac{\partial \theta}{\partial y}\right] + \mathrm{Ste}\left[\frac{\partial \varphi}{\partial \tau} + \frac{\partial \psi}{\partial y}\frac{\partial \varphi}{\partial x} - \frac{\partial \psi}{\partial x}\frac{\partial \varphi}{\partial y}\right]$$
$$= \frac{\xi(\varphi)}{\sqrt{\mathrm{Ra}\cdot\mathrm{Pr}}}\left(\frac{\partial^2 \theta}{\partial x^2} + \frac{\partial^2 \theta}{\partial y^2}\right) \tag{3}$$

The thermal conduction equations for the thermal radiator and the local energy element are:

- for the energy source

$$\frac{\partial \theta}{\partial \tau} = \frac{\alpha_{\mathrm{hs,m}}}{\sqrt{\mathrm{Ra}\cdot\mathrm{Pr}}}\left(\nabla^2 \theta + \mathrm{Os}\{1 - \sin(\gamma\tau)\}\right) \tag{4}$$

- for the heat sink

$$\frac{\partial \theta}{\partial \tau} = \frac{\alpha_{\mathrm{pl,m}}}{\sqrt{\mathrm{Ra}\cdot\mathrm{Pr}}}\nabla^2 \theta \tag{5}$$

Here $\zeta(\varphi) = \frac{(\rho c)_s}{(\rho c)_m} + \varphi\left(1 - \frac{(\rho c)_s}{(\rho c)_m}\right)$, $\xi(\varphi) = \frac{k_s}{k_m} + \varphi\left(1 - \frac{k_s}{k_m}\right)$ are the additional functions; $\mathrm{Pr} = \frac{\mu_m c_m}{k_m}$ is the Prandtl number; $\mathrm{Ra} = \frac{g(\rho\beta)_m(\rho c)_m(T_h - T_F)L^3}{\mu_m k_m}$ is the Rayleigh number; $\mathrm{Ste} = \frac{L_F}{c_m(T_h - T_F)}$ is the Stefan number; $\mathrm{Os} = \frac{Q_0 L^2}{k_m(T_h - T_F)}$ is the Ostrogradsky number; γ is the non-dimensional thermal production oscillation frequency; $\varphi = \begin{cases} 0, & \theta < -\eta, \\ \frac{\theta+\eta}{2\eta}, & -\eta \le \theta \le \eta, \\ 1, & \theta > \eta; \end{cases}$ is smoothing function; η describes the dimensions of smoothing area having low magnitude.

Equations (1)–(5) are subjected to the following conditions:

- initial conditions are $\psi = \omega = 0$, $\theta = -\eta/(T_h - T_F)$;
- boundary conditions at the internal interface between PCM and the heat sink are

$$\theta_{\text{melt}} = \theta_{\text{heat sink}},\ k_{\text{melt}} \left.\frac{\partial \theta}{\partial \bar{n}}\right|_{\text{melt}} = k_{\text{heat sink}} \left.\frac{\partial \theta}{\partial \bar{n}}\right|_{\text{heat sink}}$$

- boundary conditions at the internal interface between the heat sink and the local heater are

$$\begin{cases} \theta_{\text{heat source}} = \theta_{\text{heat sink}}, \\ k_{\text{heat source}} \left.\frac{\partial \theta}{\partial \bar{n}}\right|_{\text{heat source}} = k_{\text{heat sink}} \left.\frac{\partial \theta}{\partial \bar{n}}\right|_{\text{heat sink}} \end{cases}$$

- convective heat transport is simulated at the vertical and upper walls: $\frac{\partial \theta}{\partial \bar{n}} = \text{Bi} \cdot \theta$;
- boundary conditions at rigid walls and heat sink surfaces are $\psi = 0, \omega = -\left(\frac{\partial^2 \psi}{\partial x^2} + \frac{\partial^2 \psi}{\partial y^2}\right)$.

The non-dimensional control Eqs. (1)–(5) with additional conditions were calculated using the developed computational code created by the finite difference technique [17–20]. Comprehensive illustration of the considered numerical technique is in [17–21].

Accuracy of the developed computational code was validated using the experimental benchmark for pure gallium natural convection melting in a chamber [22]. Figure 2 demonstrates a good accordance between the calculated phase change line location and experimental results [22].

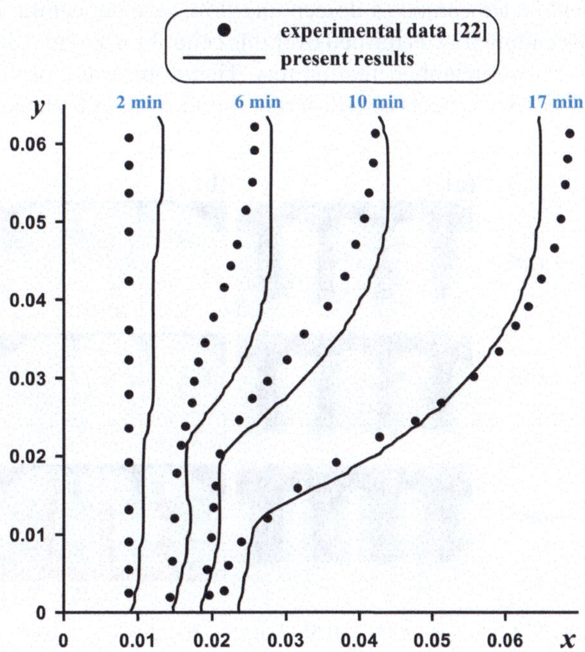

Fig. 2 Experimental and numerical phase change line location

3 Results and Discussion

Numerical analysis was performed for the Rayleigh number (Ra = 1.19×10^6), Prandtl number (Pr = 48.36), Stefan number (Ste = 1.84), Biot number (Bi = 10), Ostrogradsky number (Os = 0.3515, 0.703), and heat generation oscillation frequency ($\gamma = 0.02$–0.0025). The impacts of oscillation frequency and non-dimensional time on the melt circulation and energy transport performance were examined.

Figure 3 demonstrates an evolution of isotherms within the enclosure for different values of the oscillation frequency at Os = 0.3515. An initial time ($\tau = 636.3$) illustrates a weak melting of PCM where the essential heating can be found near the fins due to the heat conduction process from the energy source. At the same time, in gaps between fins one can find a location of solid PCM due to the formation of descending flows in these zones. Significant melting can be found for high magnitudes of the oscillation frequency. An increment of the time ($\tau = 1060.5$) characterizes more essential melting of PCM and the formation of thermal plumes over the fins. The formed temperature distribution is symmetrical relative to the middle vertical line. The solid PCM is melted in zones between the fins, and some volume of solid PCM can be found in the upper part near the upper horizontal wall. Taking into account of these distributions, one can conclude that a rise of γ results in the strongest melting of PCM. Further raise of non-dimensional time ($\tau = 1696.8$) reflects an essential melting and a formation of asymmetrical temperature distributions due to high Ra value. It is interesting to highlight that for $\gamma = 0.005\pi$ and $\gamma = 0.01\pi$, one can find an appearance a descending flow over the central fin; while for $\gamma = 0.02\pi$, an ascending flow is formed over this central fin and two descending flows can be found over two neighbor internal fins. Therefore, value of the heat generation oscillation frequency reflects also different liquid circulation behavior.

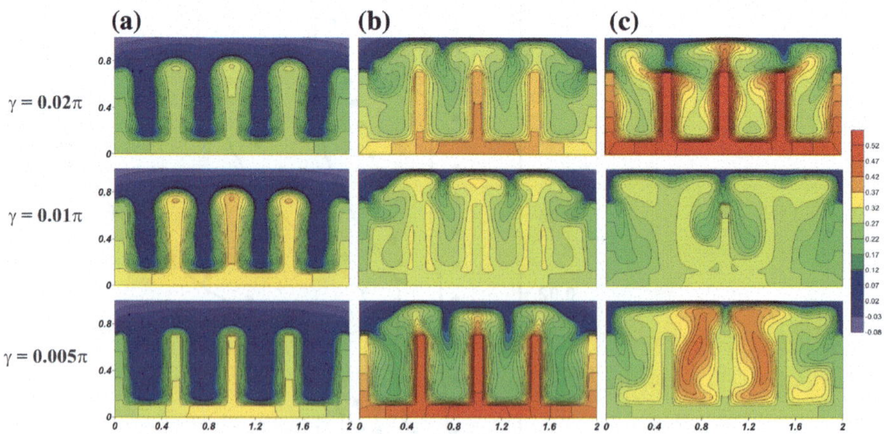

Fig. 3 Isotherms for Os = 0.3515 at: $\tau = 636.3$ (**a**), $\tau = 1060.5$ (**b**), $\tau = 1696.8$ (**c**)

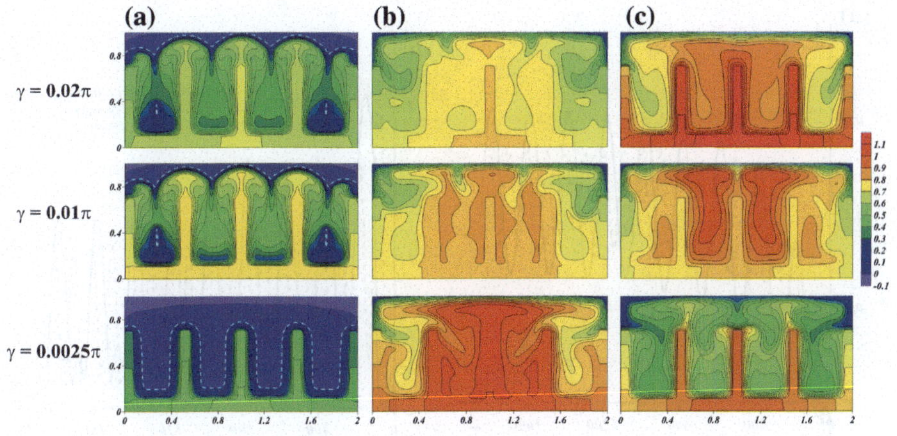

Fig. 4 Isotherms for Os = 0.703 at: $\tau = 424.2$ (**a**), $\tau = 848.4$ (**b**), $\tau = 1272.6$ (**c**)

Figure 4 demonstrates the temperature isolines inside the chamber for Os = 0.703, various magnitudes of γ and τ. A rise of the Ostrogradsky number illustrates an increment of the volumetric heat generation of the element; therefore, the melting process occurs rapidly. As it was mentioned above, low value of γ reflects less intensive PCM melting within the chamber (see Fig. 4a). An appearance of the un-melting zones between the solid fins for $\gamma = 0.01\pi$ and $\gamma = 0.02\pi$ is explained by the influence of intensive cold descending flows in these zones. More intensive circulation of the melt for $\tau \geq 848.4$ illustrates asymmetrical temperature distributions and various liquid behaviors within the cavity. For the considered cases, the presence of external convective cooling from the upper and vertical walls does not allow to suppress the intensive melting of PCM.

Figure 5 presents the time profiles of the mean Nu and mean heated unit temperature for various magnitudes of Os and heat generation oscillation frequency. For the considered case, one can find that the analyzed non-dimensional time range is enough for the formation of periodical variations, and this periodicity depends on the oscillation frequency. As it is expected, a rise of the Ostrogradsky number results in an amplification of the average Nu and average heater temperature and the time for reaching the periodical mode increases also. An increase in the oscillation frequency reflects a diminution of the oscillation amplitude and a decrease of the oscillation period in Nu and average heater temperature.

4 Conclusions

Numerical modeling of PCM free convection melting within the enclosure having the energy element of time-dependent volumetric heat generation and finned heat sink under the Newtonian cooling from the upper and vertical walls was performed.

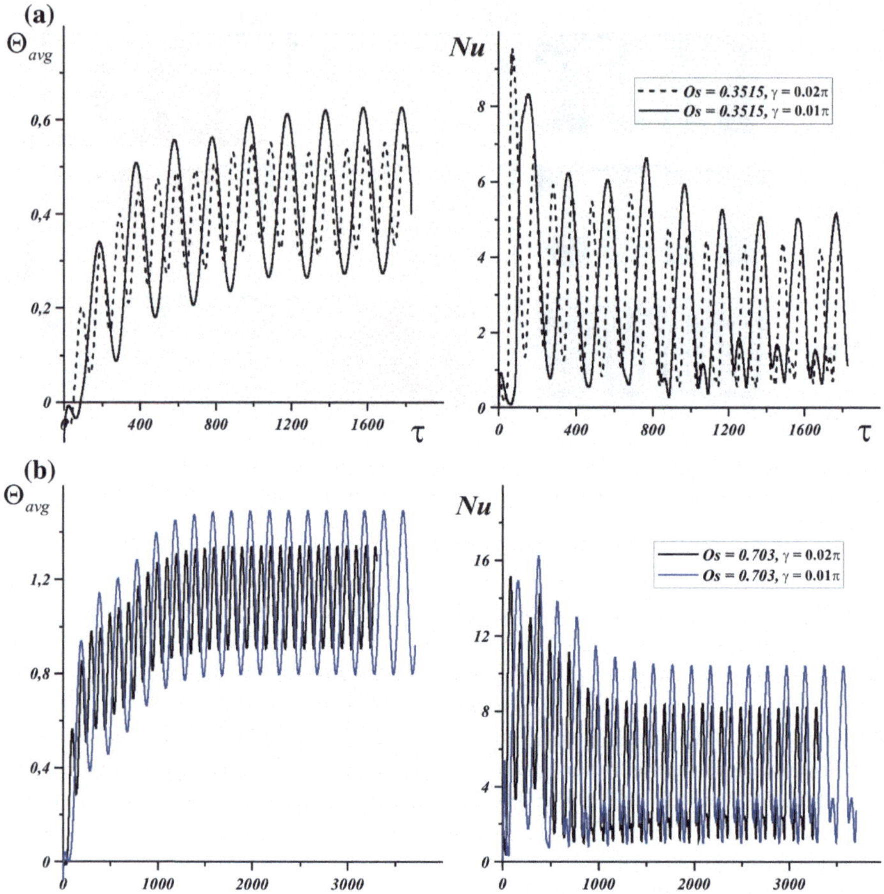

Fig. 5 Time profiles of the mean heater temperature and mean Nu for various magnitudes of the Ostrogradsky number and volumetric heat generation oscillation frequency: Os = 0.3515 (**a**), Os = 0.703 (**b**)

The analysis was conducted for various magnitudes of the Ostrogradsky number and volumetric heat generation oscillation frequency. Distributions of isotherms within the cavity and time profiles for the mean Nusselt number and mean heated element temperature were studied. It was ascertained, that a rise of Os characterizes significant heating of the chamber with a rise of the mean Nu and mean heated element temperature while a decrease in the oscillation frequency illustrates the less intensive melting of PCM within the enclosure and a growth of the oscillation amplitude for Nu and Θ_{avg}.

Acknowledgements This work was supported by the Russian Science Foundation (Project No. 17-79-20141).

References

1. Liang, K., Li, Z., Chen, M., Jiang, H.: Comparisons between heat pipe, thermoelectric system, and vapour compression refrigeration system for electronics cooling. Appl. Therm. Eng. **146**, 260–267 (2019)
2. Bahiraei, M., Heshmatian, S.: Electronics cooling with nanofluids: a critical review. Energy Convers. Manag. **172**, 438–456 (2018)
3. Wu, R., Hong, T., Cheng, Q., Zou, H., Fan, Y., Luo, X.: Thermal modeling and comparative analysis of jet impingement liquid cooling for high power electronics. Int. J. Heat Mass Transf. **137**, 42–51 (2019)
4. Sohel Murshed, S.M., Nieto de Castro, C.A.: A critical review of traditional and emerging techniques and fluids for electronics cooling. Renew. Sustain. Energy Rev. **78**, 821–833 (2017)
5. Naaktgeboren, C., Franco, A.T., Junqueira, S.L.M.: On a theory for system-level cooling of close electronics enclosures by PCM-filled heat sinks—exact solution and second law performance limits. Int. J. Heat Mass Transf. **127**, 535–543 (2018)
6. Behi, H., Ghanbarpour, M., Behi, M.: Investigation of PCM-assisted heat pipe for electronic cooling. Appl. Therm. Eng. **127**, 1132–1142 (2017)
7. Dinesh, B.V.S., Bhattacharya, A.: Effect of foam geometry on heat absorption characteristics of PCM-metal foam composite thermal energy storage systems. Int. J. Heat Mass Transf. **134**, 866–883 (2019)
8. Rehman, T., Ali, H.M., Saieed, A., Pao, W., Ali, M.: Copper foam/PCMs based heat sinks: an experimental study for electronic cooling systems. Int. J. Heat Mass Transf. **127**, 381–393 (2018)
9. Krishna, J., Kishore, P.S., Solomon, A.B.: Heat pipe with nano enhanced-PCM for electronic cooling application. Exp. Thermal Fluid Sci. **81**, 84–92 (2017)
10. Ali, H.M., Ashraf, M.J., Giovannelli, A., Irfan, M., Irshad, T.B., Hamid, H.M., Hassan, F., Arshad, A.: Thermal management of electronics: an experimental analysis of triangular, rectangular and circular pin-fin heat sinks for various PCMs. Int. J. Heat Mass Transf. **123**, 272–284 (2018)
11. Xie, J., Lee, H.M., Xiang, J.: Numerical study of thermally optimized metal structures in a phase change material (PCM) enclosure. Appl. Therm. Eng. **148**, 825–837 (2019)
12. Ashraf, M.J., Ali, H.M., Usman, H., Arshad, A.: Experimental passive electronics cooling: parametric investigation of pin-fin geometries and efficient phase change materials. Int. J. Heat Mass Transf. **115**, 251–263 (2017)
13. Rakotondrandisa, A., Danaila, I., Danaila, L.: Numerical modelling of a melting-solidification cycle of a phase-change material with complete or partial melting. Int. J. Heat Fluid Flow **76**, 57–71 (2019)
14. Lin, Q., Wang, S., Ma, Z., Wang, J., Zhang, T.: Lattice Boltzmann simulation of flow and heat transfer evolution inside encapsulated phase change materials due to natural convection melting. Chem. Eng. Sci. **189**, 154–164 (2018)
15. Wang, P., Yao, H., Lan, Z., Peng, Z., Huang, Y., Ding, Y.: Numerical investigation of PCM melting process in sleeve tube with internal fins. Energy Convers. Manag. **110**, 428–435 (2016)
16. Tasnim, S.H., Hossain, R., Mahmud, S., Dutta, A.: Convection effect on the melting process of nano-PCM inside porous enclosure. Int. J. Heat Mass Transf. **85**, 206–220 (2015)
17. Bondareva, N.S., Sheremet, M.A.: Conjugate heat transfer in the PCM-based heat storage system with finned copper profile: application in electronics cooling. Int. J. Heat Mass Transf. **124**, 1275–1284 (2018)
18. Bondareva, N.S., Buonomo, B., Manca, O., Sheremet, M.A.: Heat transfer inside cooling system based on phase change material with alumina nanoparticles. Appl. Therm. Eng. **144**, 972–981 (2018)
19. Bondareva, N.S., Sheremet, M.A.: Numerical simulation of natural convection melting in 2D and 3D enclosures. J. Therm. Eng. **5**(1), 51–61 (2019)

20. Bondareva, N.S., Buonomo, B., Manca, O., Sheremet, M.A.: Heat transfer performance of the finned nano-enhanced phase change material system under the inclination influence. Int. J. Heat Mass Transf. **135**, 1063–1072 (2019)
21. Shenoy, A., Sheremet, M., Pop, I.: Convective Flow and Heat Transfer from Wavy Surfaces: Viscous Fluids, Porous Media and Nanofluids. CRC Press, Boca Raton, USA (2016)
22. Gau, C., Viskanta, R.: Melting and solidification of pure melting on a vertical wall. J. Heat Transf. **108**, 174–181 (1986)

Hypersingular Integral Equation Approach for Hydroelastic Analysis of a Submerged Elastic Plate

Santanu Koley

Abstract In this paper, obliquely incident surface ocean waves interaction with a horizontal submerged thin floating elastic plate is investigated in ocean water of finite depth. Firstly, a proper Green's function associated with the physical problem is developed. Applying Green's second identity on the upper plate and lower plate regions and using the plate conditions, the BVP is converted into a hypersingular integral equation. Most of the time, these kinds of hypersingular integral equations are solved by using some standard numerical solution techniques. But in the present case, this hypersingular integral equation is directly solved using the plate deflection in terms of summations of horizontal components of eigenfunctions related to the flexural gravity waves. In this way, a system of linear algebraic equations is obtained from the hypersingular integral equation. Further, using the plate edge conditions, some more equations involving the unknowns are obtained and solved to get the required unknowns. Variations of reflection and transmission coefficients for a wide range of physical parameters are evaluated, plotted, and analyzed.

Keywords Elastic plate · Green's function · Hypersingular integral equation

1 Introduction

Recently, there is an increasing interest to use submerged wave barriers to protect various marine structures by dissipating a major portion of incoming ocean wave energy. The durability of these kinds of structures is more compared to the vertical counterpart as the horizontal wave loads acting on these structures are almost negligible. Further, these horizontal plate structures are environmentally friendly, also lightweight, easily handled, and reusable in nature.

The interaction of free surface ocean waves by submerged barriers has started since the classical work of [1]. In [1], a Wiener–Hopf solution technique is applied to solve

S. Koley (✉)
Department of Mathematics, Birla Institute of Technology and Science Pilani, Hyderabad Campus, Hyderabad 500078, India
e-mail: santanu@hyderabad.bits-pilani.ac.in

S. Bhattacharyya et al. (eds.), *Mathematical Modeling and Computational Tools*, Springer Proceedings in Mathematics & Statistics 320,
https://doi.org/10.1007/978-981-15-3615-1_23

the water waves scattering by a rigid thin wave barrier in finite water depth. Durgin and Shiau [2] used a vortex sheet-based theory to calculate the wave loads on a submerged plate floating in water waves. Patarapanich [3] studied the wave energy fluxes across the regions around a rigid horizontal submerged plate and found the conditions for the occurrences of zero wave reflections. Later on, [4] developed a numerical solution technique to investigate the trapped modes above a submerged impermeable submerged plate. Parsons and Martin [5] used a solution methodology based on hypersingular integral equation approach to study the wave trapping by a submerged curved and inclined rigid plates. Using the potential flow theory-based approach, [6] studied the utility of multiple submerged impermeable plates placed parallel to each other vertically in the water wave regime. Recently, [7] used Galerkin method to study the scattering and radiation problems involving forced motion by thin horizontal plates. In the aforementioned studies, the plate was considered impermeable and rigid in nature.

On the other hand, nowadays, flexible plates and membranes are used as wave barriers. One of the benefits in using these kinds of structures is that these can dissipate a substantial portion of incoming ocean wave energy, and in this process, a tranquility zone is created at the lee side of the structures. Moreover, this will effectively increase the durability of the structures. Meylan and Squire [8] used Fredholm integral equation-based solution approach to investigate the interaction of ocean surface wave with a floating elastic sheet. Sahoo et al. [9] applied eigenfunction expansion method to obtain the hydroelastic response of a semi-infinite floating horizontally inclined elastic plate. A Wiener–Hopf-based solution technique is used by [10] to model the wave scattering in the presence of a horizontally placed semi-infinite elastic floating plate in deepwater case. Wang et al. [11] used a coupling between boundary element method and eigenfunction expansion method to study the wave diffraction by a thin elastic plate floating over undulated seabed. Andrianov and Hermans [12] used integro-differential equation-based techniques to perform the hydroelastic analysis of a flexible floating barrier in water waves. By constructing suitable Green's function associated with the BVP, [13] studied the water wave scattering by an array of flexible floating plates placed in a periodic manner. Williams and Meylan [14] used Wiener–Hopf technique to analyze the hydroelastic behavior of a submerged horizontal floating plate in water domain. Recently, [15] used eigenfunction expansion technique to study the oblique incident ocean surface waves by an elastic submerged permeable barrier.

In this paper, the wave scattering by a floating flexible submerged horizontal sheet under the action of obliquely incident surface gravity ocean waves is studied. The solution methodology is based on hypersingular integral equation approach. The overall structure of this paper is the following. Section 2 contains the mathematical formulation of the associated BVP. In Sect. 3, the detailed solution procedure is provided. Section 4 contains the results and discussions part. Finally, in Sect. 5, the conclusion of the present study is briefly highlighted.

2 Mathematical Formulation

Here, the governing equation and related boundary conditions obliquely impinge on ocean surface wave scattering by submerged elastic sheet, provided under the assumption of linearized potential water wave theory. In Cartesian coordinate system, the horizontal plane coincides with the xy-plane the z-axis is considered vertically upward positive with the plane $z = 0$ represents the mean free water surface. The water having density ρ occupies the domain $-\infty < x, y < \infty$, $-h < z < 0$ as in Fig. 1. A flexible plate of small thickness having width b is horizontally situated at $z = -d$ and occupies the domain $0 < x < b, -\infty < y < \infty$ in the water domain. It is assumed that the water flow follows the potential wave theory. Further, the water flow is simple harmonic in time with circular frequency ω. The incident gravity waves impinge on the horizontal elastic plate at an angle θ with the x-axis. These assumptions ensure the total velocity potential will take the form $\Phi(x, y, z, t) = \text{Re}\{\phi(x, z)e^{i(\beta_0 y - \omega t)}\}$ with $\beta_0 = k_0 \sin\theta$. It is to be noted that k_0 is the real and positive root of the dispersion equation $\omega^2 = gk \tanh kh$. Thus, $\phi(x, z)$ satisfy the governing equation

$$(\nabla^2 - \beta_0^2)\phi = 0 \tag{1}$$

with $\nabla^2 \equiv (\partial^2/\partial x^2 + \partial^2/\partial z^2)$. Now, the free surface boundary conditions are provided as

$$\frac{\partial \phi}{\partial z} - K\phi = 0, \text{ on } z = 0 \tag{2}$$

Here $K = \omega^2/g$. The boundary condition for rigid impermeable bottom bed takes the form

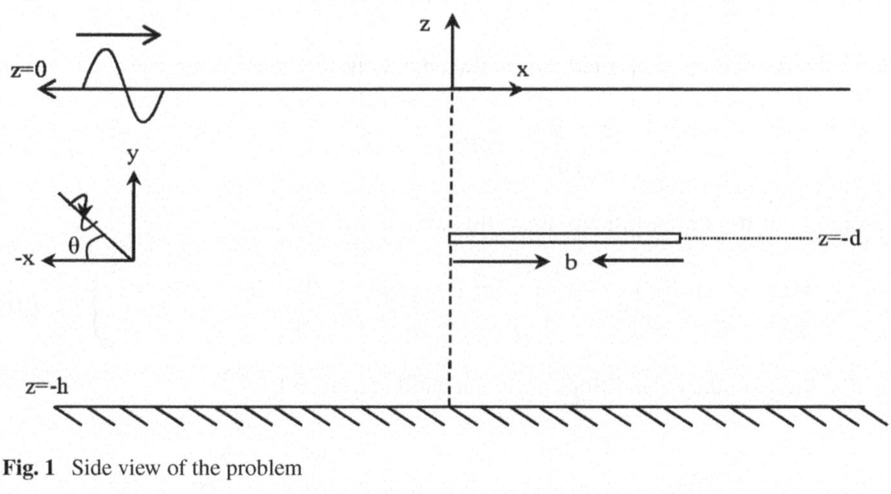

Fig. 1 Side view of the problem

$$\frac{\partial \phi}{\partial z} = 0, \text{ on } z = -h \tag{3}$$

Elastic plate motion is assumed uniform in the y-direction and so the plate deflection $\chi(x, y, t)$ is expressed as $\chi(x, y, t) = \mathrm{Re}\{\zeta(x)e^{i(\beta_0 y - \omega t)}\}$ with $\zeta(x)$ represents the deflection amplitude. Thus, the equation of motion for the flexible plate is given by (for $0 < x < b$)

$$\mathrm{EI}\left(\frac{\mathrm{d}^2}{\mathrm{d}x^2} - \beta_0^2\right)^2 \zeta + Q\left(\frac{\mathrm{d}^2}{\mathrm{d}x^2} - \beta_0^2\right)\zeta - m_{\mathrm{p}}\omega^2\zeta = -i\rho\omega(\phi(x, -d+) - \phi(x, -d-)) \tag{4}$$

where EI represents the flexural rigidity of the elastic plate. It is to be noted that in Eq. (4), $m_{\mathrm{p}} = \rho_{\mathrm{p}} d_{\mathrm{p}}$ represents the plate mass/length. Further, ρ_{p} represents the plate material density and d_{p} is the plate thickness (negligible). The linearized version of the kinematic boundary condition at the surface of the elastic plate is given by

$$-i\omega\zeta = \left.\frac{\partial \phi}{\partial z}\right|_{z=-d-} = \left.\frac{\partial \phi}{\partial z}\right|_{z=-d+} \tag{5}$$

For fixed edge plate, the edge conditions are provided

$$\left(\frac{\mathrm{d}^2}{\mathrm{d}x^2} - \upsilon\beta_0^2\right)\zeta = 0, \quad \left\{\mathrm{EI}\left(\frac{\mathrm{d}^2}{\mathrm{d}x^2} - (2-\upsilon)\beta_0^2\right)\frac{\mathrm{d}}{\mathrm{d}x} + Q\frac{\mathrm{d}}{\mathrm{d}x}\right\}\zeta = 0 \text{ at } x = 0, b \tag{6}$$

whereas, for fixed edge plates, the plate edges conditions give

$$\zeta = 0, \ \frac{\mathrm{d}\zeta}{\mathrm{d}x} = 0 \text{ at } x = 0, b \tag{7}$$

Similarly, for simply supported edges, the edge conditions are given by

$$\zeta = 0, \left(\frac{\mathrm{d}^2}{\mathrm{d}x^2} - \upsilon\beta_0^2\right)\zeta = 0 \text{ at } x = 0, b \tag{8}$$

Continuity of fluid pressure and mass flux at $z = -d$ yields

$$\left.\begin{array}{l} \phi(x, -d-) = \phi(x, -d+) \quad \text{for } \{-\infty < x < 0\} \cup \{b < x < \infty\}, \\ \frac{\partial \phi}{\partial z}(x, -d-) = \frac{\partial \phi}{\partial z}(x, -d+) \text{ for } -\infty < x < \infty \end{array}\right\} \tag{9}$$

Finally, the boundary conditions at the far-field are given by

$$\phi(x, z) \approx \begin{cases} T\phi^I(x, z), & \text{as } x \to \infty \\ \phi^I(x, z) + R\phi^I(-x, z), & \text{as } x \to -\infty \end{cases} \tag{10}$$

where $|R|$ and $|T|$ are the coefficients that represent the reflected and transmitted wave heights, respectively, w.r.t. to the incident wave height. In Eq. (10), the incident wave velocity potential $\phi^I(x,z)$ is given by

$$\phi^I(x,z) = \frac{\cosh k_0(h+z)}{\cosh k_0 h} e^{i\alpha_0 x}, \tag{11}$$

It may be noted that in Eq. (11), $\alpha_0 = k_0 \cos\theta$. The solution procedure of the aforementioned BVP is discussed subsequently.

3 Solution Methodology

In this section, using suitably derived Green's function, the above BVP is converted into hypersingular integral equations. For the same, we have to construct appropriate Green's function. Now, the free surface Green's function $G(\vec{x}_\mathrm{r}; \vec{x}_\mathrm{s})$ corresponding to the boundary values problem described in Sect. 2 will satisfy

$$\left(\nabla^2 - \beta_0^2\right) G(\vec{x}_\mathrm{r}; \vec{x}_\mathrm{s}) = 2\pi\delta(\vec{x}_\mathrm{r} - \vec{x}_\mathrm{s}) \tag{12}$$

along with the boundary conditions (2) and (3) takes the form

$$G(\vec{x}_\mathrm{r}; \vec{x}_\mathrm{s}) = \begin{cases} \frac{1}{\gamma'} \frac{\gamma' \cosh \zeta\gamma' + K \sinh \zeta\gamma'}{K \cosh h\gamma' - \gamma' \sinh h\gamma'} \cosh \gamma'(h+z) e^{i(x-\xi)\gamma} & \text{for } z < \zeta \\ \frac{1}{\gamma'} \frac{\gamma' \cosh z\gamma' + K \sinh z\gamma'}{K \cosh h\gamma' - \gamma' \sinh h\gamma'} \cosh \gamma'(h+\zeta) e^{i(x-\xi)\gamma} & \text{for } z > \zeta \end{cases} \tag{13}$$

where $\gamma'^2 = \gamma^2 + \beta_0^2$. For notational convenience, in the rest of the discussion, $\phi^{\pm}(x,z)$ denotes the velocity potential for the regions $z > -d$ and $z < -d$, respectively. Applying Green's second identity on the functions $\phi^+(\vec{x}_\mathrm{r}) - \phi^I(\vec{x}_\mathrm{r})$ and $G(\vec{x}_\mathrm{r}; \vec{x}_\mathrm{s})$ on a domain of (x,z) plane bounded the contour Γ^+ which consists of external boundary $\{z = 0, -X \le x \le X;\ x = -X, -d+0 \le z \le 0;$ $z = -d+0, -X \le x \le X;\ x = X, -d+0 \le z \le 0\}$ and internal boundary (a circle having small radius ε with center (ξ,ζ)), we get

$$2\pi\phi^+(\vec{x}_\mathrm{s}) = 2\pi\phi^{\mathrm{inc}}(\vec{x}_\mathrm{s}) - \int_0^b \left(\phi^+(\vec{x}_r)\frac{\partial G}{\partial z}(\vec{x}_\mathrm{r}; \vec{x}_\mathrm{s}) - G(\vec{x}_\mathrm{r}; \vec{x}_\mathrm{s})\frac{\partial \phi^+}{\partial z}(\vec{x}_\mathrm{r})\right)\Bigg|_{z=-d+} \mathrm{d}x \tag{14}$$

where $\vec{x}_\mathrm{r} = (x,z)$ and $\vec{x}_\mathrm{s} = (\xi,\zeta)$. Similarly, using Green's second identity to $\phi^-(\vec{x}_\mathrm{r}) - \phi^I(\vec{x}_\mathrm{r})$ and $G(\vec{x}_\mathrm{r}; \vec{x}_\mathrm{s})$ in a region of the $(\vec{x}_\mathrm{r})$ plane which is closed by Γ^+ as described above, it is derived that

$$0 = \int_0^b \left(\phi^-(\vec{x}_\mathrm{r}) \frac{\partial G}{\partial z}(\vec{x}_\mathrm{r}; \vec{x}_\mathrm{s}) - G(\vec{x}_\mathrm{r}; \vec{x}_\mathrm{s}) \frac{\partial \phi^-}{\partial z}(\vec{x}_\mathrm{r}) \right)\Bigg|_{z=-d-0} \mathrm{d}x \tag{15}$$

Adding, Eqs. (14) and (15), we get

$$\begin{aligned} 2\pi\phi^+(\vec{x}_\mathrm{s}) = 2\pi\phi^{\mathrm{inc}}(\vec{x}_\mathrm{s}) &- \int_0^b \left(\phi^+(\vec{x}_\mathrm{r}) \frac{\partial G}{\partial z}(\vec{x}_\mathrm{r}; \vec{x}_\mathrm{s}) - G(\vec{x}_\mathrm{r}; \vec{x}_\mathrm{s}) \frac{\partial \phi^+}{\partial z}(\vec{x}_\mathrm{r}) \right)\Bigg|_{z=-d+} \mathrm{d}x \\ &+ \int_0^b \left(\phi^-(\vec{x}_\mathrm{r}) \frac{\partial G}{\partial z}(\vec{x}_\mathrm{r}; \vec{x}_\mathrm{s}) - G(\vec{x}_\mathrm{r}; \vec{x}_\mathrm{s}) \frac{\partial \phi^-}{\partial z}(\vec{x}_\mathrm{r}) \right)\Bigg|_{z=-d-} \mathrm{d}x \end{aligned} \tag{16}$$

Proceedings in a similar way as in Eq. (16), we get

$$\begin{aligned} 2\pi\phi^-(\vec{x}_\mathrm{s}) = 2\pi\phi^{\mathrm{inc}}(\vec{x}_\mathrm{s}) &- \int_0^b \left(\phi^-(\vec{x}_\mathrm{r}) \frac{\partial G}{\partial z}(\vec{x}_\mathrm{r}; \vec{x}_\mathrm{s}) - G(\vec{x}_\mathrm{r}; \vec{x}_\mathrm{s}) \frac{\partial \phi^-}{\partial z}(\vec{x}_\mathrm{r}) \right)\Bigg|_{z=-d-} \mathrm{d}x \\ &+ \int_0^b \left(\phi^+(\vec{x}_\mathrm{r}) \frac{\partial G}{\partial z}(\vec{x}_\mathrm{r}; \vec{x}_\mathrm{s}) - G(\vec{x}_\mathrm{r}; \vec{x}_\mathrm{s}) \frac{\partial \phi^+}{\partial z}(\vec{x}_\mathrm{r}) \right)\Bigg|_{z=-d+} \mathrm{d}x \end{aligned} \tag{17}$$

It is to be noted that to derive (16) and (17), the edge conditions of the plate are not utilized. Now, utilizing Green's function properties and using conditions (9), we get

$$\begin{aligned} 2\pi\phi^\pm(\vec{x}_\mathrm{s}) = 2\pi\phi^{\mathrm{inc}}(\vec{x}_\mathrm{s}) &- \int_0^b \left(\phi^+(\vec{x}_\mathrm{r}) \frac{\partial G^\mp}{\partial z}(\vec{x}_\mathrm{r}; \vec{x}_\mathrm{s}) - G^\mp(\vec{x}_\mathrm{r}; \vec{x}_\mathrm{s}) \frac{\partial \phi^+}{\partial z}(\vec{x}_\mathrm{r}) \right)\Bigg|_{z=-d+} \mathrm{d}x \\ &+ \int_0^b \left(\phi^-(\vec{x}_\mathrm{r}) \frac{\partial G^\mp}{\partial z}(\vec{x}_\mathrm{r}; \vec{x}_\mathrm{s}) - G^\mp(\vec{x}_\mathrm{r}; \vec{x}_\mathrm{s}) \frac{\partial \phi^-}{\partial z}(\vec{x}_\mathrm{r}) \right)\Bigg|_{z=-d-} \mathrm{d}x \end{aligned} \tag{18}$$

Now, using (4) and (5), the plate boundary condition is written as

$$\frac{\partial^5 \phi}{\partial x^4 \partial z} + A \frac{\partial^3 \phi}{\partial x^2 \partial z} + B \frac{\partial \phi}{\partial z} = C(\phi(x, -d+) - \phi(x, -d-)) \tag{19}$$

where $A = -2\beta_0^2$, $B = \beta_0^4 - \frac{\rho_\mathrm{p} d_\mathrm{p} \omega^2}{\mathrm{EI}}$, $C = -\frac{\rho\omega^2}{\mathrm{EI}}$. Substituting (19) into (18) and differentiate with respect to ζ, we get the following hypersingular integral equation

$$\frac{\partial \phi}{\partial \zeta}(\xi, \zeta) = \frac{\partial \phi^{\mathrm{inc}}}{\partial \zeta} + \frac{1}{2\pi C} \int_0^b \left\{ \left(\frac{\partial^4}{\partial x^4} + A \frac{\partial^2}{\partial x^2} + B \right) \frac{\partial \phi}{\partial z} \right\} \frac{\partial^2 G}{\partial z \partial \zeta}(x, z; \xi, \zeta) \Bigg|_{z=-d} \mathrm{d}x \tag{20}$$

where the expression for $\partial^2 G / \partial z \partial \zeta$ can be easily obtained from (13). Now to solve (20), the vertical fluid velocity at $z = -d$, i.e., at the plate boundary, is expressed as the following

$$\frac{\partial \phi}{\partial \zeta} = \sum_{n=0}^{N} a_n e^{ip_n \xi} + b_n e^{ip_n (b-\xi)} \tag{21}$$

It is to be noted that the p_n's are the roots of the dispersion equation

$$p\left(p^4 + Ap^2 + B\right) \sinh(p(d+h)) = K \frac{K \cosh ph - p \sinh ph}{K \cosh pd + p \sinh pd} \tag{22}$$

Substituting (21) into (20), as well as equating the coefficients of $e^{\pm ip_n \xi}$, we get the following equations

$$\sum_{n=0}^{N} \left(p_n^4 + Ap_n^2 + B\right) \left[\frac{a_n}{p_n - k_i} - \frac{b_n e^{ip_n b}}{p_n + k_i} \right] = \delta_{0i} \frac{h\left(K^2 - k_0^2\right) - K}{k_0 K} \frac{\sinh(k_0 h)}{\sinh(k_0(h+\zeta))} \tag{23}$$

$$\sum_{n=0}^{N} \left(p_n^4 + Ap_n^2 + B\right) \left[\frac{a_n e^{ip_n b}}{p_n + k_i} - \frac{b_n}{p_n - k_i} \right] = 0 \tag{24}$$

where $i = 0, 1, 2, \ldots, N-1$. The remaining set of four equations are obtained by substituting (21) into the edge conditions, i.e., into (6), (7), or (8). Finally, these set of $2N+2$ equations are solved to get the unknowns a_n and b_n's. The expressions for R and T can be easily obtained from (18) by taking $x \to \pm\infty$ and comparing with (10).

4 Results and Related Discussions

For the computation part, different physical parameters are chosen as: $d = h/2$, $E = 5$ GPa, $\rho_p/\rho = 0.95$, $\rho = 1025$ kgm^{-3}, $h = 20$ m, $\upsilon = 0.3$ unless it is stated explicitly. Further, the fixed edge plate is considered. In Fig. 2, the reflection coefficient $K_r = |R|$ versus incident angle θ and non-dimensional wave number $k_0 h$ is plotted. It is seen that K_r increases for higher $k_0 h$. Further, the wave reflection initially decreases as oblique angle θ increases. However, after reach a minimum, K_r will increase for higher θ. In Fig. 3, $K_t = |T|$ versus incident angle θ and non-dimensional wave number $k_0 h$ is plotted. The pattern of the transmission coefficient K_t is reverse to that of K_r. Now, in Fig. 4, the vertical wave force K_v versus incident angle θ and non-dimensional wave number $k_0 h$ is plotted. It is seen that the wave force K_v will take higher values for suitable combinations of $k_0 h$ and θ. A comparison

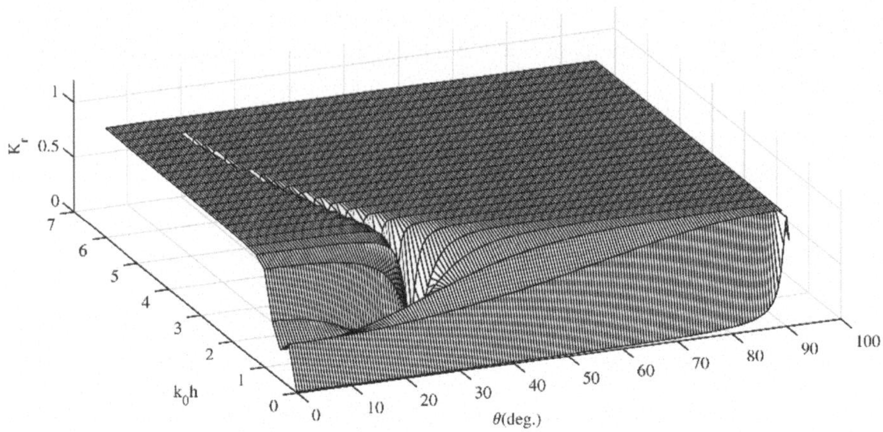

Fig. 2 K_r versus θ and k_0h

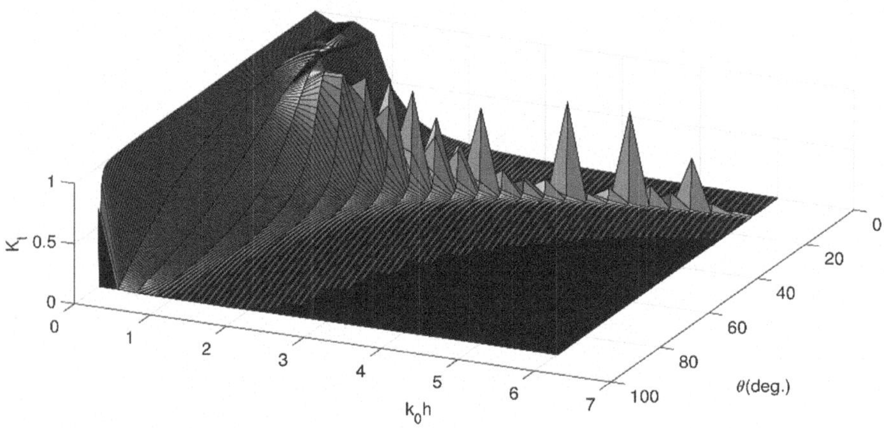

Fig. 3 K_t versus θ and k_0h

reveals that for the values of k_0h and θ, for which K_r is minimum, the wave force K_v takes maximum.

5 Conclusion

A hypersingular integral equation-based solution technique is used for analyzing the hydroelastic responses of a floating submerged and horizontal elastic barrier/plate in finite water depth. This solution technique is useful to get very accurate results and is

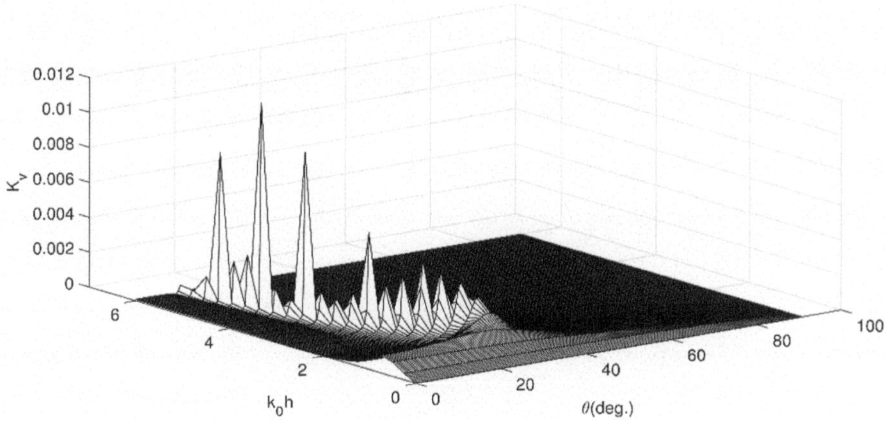

Fig. 4 K_v versus θ and k_0h

also computationally efficient. The same can be used to solve a number of problems that appear in the broad area of applied mathematics and engineering.

References

1. Heins, A.E.: Water waves over a channel of finite depth with a submerged plane barrier. Can. J. Math. **2**(2), 210 (1950)
2. Durgin, W.W., Shiau, J.C.: Wave induced pressures on submerged plates. J. Waterw. Harb. Coast Eng. **101**, 59 (1975)
3. Patarapanich, Mana: Maximum and zero reflection from submerged plate. J. Waterw. Port, Coast. Ocean Eng. **110**(2), 171–181 (1984)
4. Linton, C.M., Evans, D.V.: Trapped modes above a submerged horizontal plate. Q. J. Mech. Appl. Math. **44**(3), 487–506 (1991)
5. Parsons, N.F., Martin, P.A.: Trapping of water waves by submerged plates using hypersingular integral equations. J. Fluid Mech. **284**, 359–375 (1995)
6. Wang, Keh-Han, Shen, Qiang: Wave motion over a group of submerged horizontal plates. Int. J. Eng. Sci. **37**(6), 703–715 (1999)
7. Porter, R.: Linearised water wave problems involving submerged horizontal plates. Appl. Ocean Res. **50**, 91–109 (2015)
8. Meylan, M., Squire, V.A.: The response of ice floes to ocean waves. J. Geophys. Res. Oceans (1978–2012), **99**, 891–891 (1994)
9. Sahoo, T., Yip, T.L., Chwang, A.T.: Scattering of surface waves by a semi-infinite floating elastic plate. Phys. Fluids (1994-present) **13**(11), 3215–3222 (2001)
10. Tkacheva, L.A.: Surface wave diffraction on a floating elastic plate. Fluid Dyn. **36**(5), 776–789 (2001)
11. Wang, C.D., Meylan, M.H.: The linear wave response of a floating thin plate on water of variable depth. Appl. Ocean Res. **24**(3), 163–174 (2002)
12. Andrianov, A.I., Hermans, A.J.: The influence of water depth on the hydroelastic response of a very large floating platform. Mar. Struct. **16**(5), 355–371 (2003)
13. Wang, C.D., Meylan, M.H., Porter, R.: The linear-wave response of a periodic array of floating elastic plates. J. Eng. Math. **57**(1), 23–40 (2007)

14. Williams, T.D., Meylan, M.H.: The wiener–hopf and residue calculus solutions for a submerged semi-infinite elastic plate. J. Eng. Math. **75**(1), 81–106 (2012)
15. Behera, H., Sahoo, T.: Hydroelastic analysis of gravity wave interaction with submerged horizontal flexible porous plate. J. Fluids Struct. **54**, 643–660 (2015)

Dynamics of Bleustein–Gulyaev (BG) Waves in Smart Composite Structure

Juhi Baroi and Sanjeev Anand Sahu

Abstract The Bleustein–Gulyaev (BG) waves propagation in bedded composite structure is studied to calculate the dispersion relation by Liouville–Green (LG) method. The composite structure is made of functionally graded piezoelectric material (FGPM) layer over a dielectric substrate immersed in viscous liquid. The variation of material variables are taken quadratic in nature for FGPM layer. The method of separation of variables is employed in viscous liquid as well as dielectric medium. Dispersion relations are obtained for electrically open and short circuit cases. To portray the dependencies of different material variables on the phase velocity of the considered wave, numerical examples have been taken into account. The proposed work bestows a theoretical model for the purpose of designing of surface acoustic wave (SAW) devices and sensors.

Keywords Functionally graded piezoelectric material (FGPM) · Viscous liquid · Liouville–Green (LG) method · Dielectric material · BG waves · Saw devices

1 Introduction

The materials with linear electro-mechanical coupling are familiar as piezoelectric materials. Because of its piezoelectric effect (i.e., existence of electric field in contact with mechanical force and deformation of material when excited electrically), it has tremendous outcome on implementation of acoustic devices such as sensors as well as in the field of bio-medical, electrical and mechanical engineering [4, 6].

To heighten the sensitivity of such device, a new type of materials has been introduced with varying property along thickness known as functionally graded materials (FGM). The FGM combined with piezoelectric effect is called functionally graded piezoelectric materials [3, 7]. Dielectric medium works as an electric insulator when combined with materials which generates an electric field. Nie et al. [5] studied the

J. Baroi (✉) · S. A. Sahu
Department of Mathematics and Computing, IIT (ISM), Dhanbad, Jharkhand 826004, India
e-mail: juhibaroi@gmail.com

S. Bhattacharyya et al. (eds.), *Mathematical Modeling and Computational Tools*, Springer Proceedings in Mathematics & Statistics 320,
https://doi.org/10.1007/978-981-15-3615-1_24

Rayleigh-type wave in A Rotated Piezoelectric Crystal Imperfectly Bonded on a Dielectric Substrate. In order to recognize the different compounds in liquids, the SAW sensors are used and immersed in liquids for better results [1, 2].

The present paper deals with the significance of layer width of the FGPM material and viscous liquid on the BG waves propagation in composite material. Dispersion matrix is obtained applying appropriate boundary conditions for both electrically open and short cases using the Liouville–Green (LG) method.

2 Mathematical Formulation of the Problem

Propagation of BG waves in a composite material is considered (Fig. 1). The composite material consists of a functionally graded piezoelectric material (FGPM) over a dielectric substrate immersed in a viscous liquid. The width of the FGPM layer is taken as h_f and for liquid as h_L. Along positive y-axis direction, the substrate is considered and the wave is transferring through x-axis and the interface is taken as $y = 0$. The polarization direction is taken along z-axis. The FGPM material properties are varying along y-axis.

2.1 *For the FGPM Layer*

In the absence of body force, the field equation for the layer is

$$\begin{aligned} \sigma^f_{ij,j} &= \rho_f \ddot{u}^f_i \\ D^f_{i,i} &= 0 \end{aligned} \tag{1}$$

where ρ_f is the density of the layer and $i, j = 1, 2, 3$.

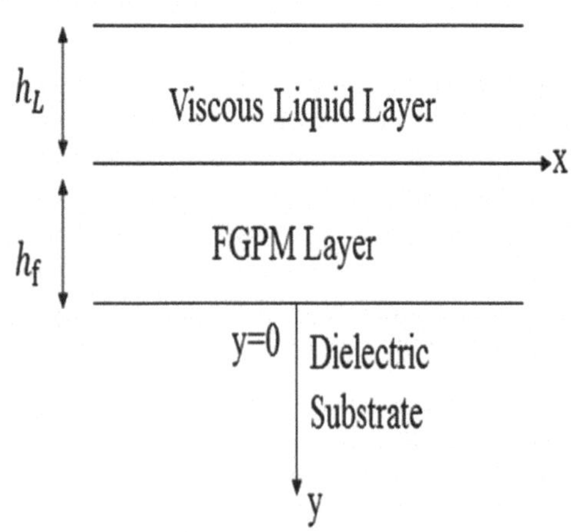

Fig. 1 Schematic diagram of the problem

The FGPM constitutive equations are

$$\begin{aligned} \sigma^f_{ij} &= c^f_{ijkl}\, F_{k\,l} - e^f_{kij}\, E^f_k \\ D^f_j &= e^f_{jkl}\, F_{k\,l} + \varepsilon^f_{jk}\, E^f_k \end{aligned} \tag{2}$$

where σ^f_{ij}, e^f_{jkl}, ε^f_{jk}, E^f_k, D^f_j and F_{kl} are stress tensor, FGPM coefficients, dielectric coefficients, electric field, electrical displacement and strain tensor, respectively.

The relation between strain, electric field, displacement component and electric potential can be written as

$$\begin{aligned} F_{k\,l} &= \frac{1}{2}\left(u^f_{k,\,l} + u^f_{l,\,k}\right) \\ E^f_i &= -\phi^f_{,i} \end{aligned} \tag{3}$$

The wave propagation direction is along x-axis for the proposed model, so we have

$$u^f = v^f = 0, \quad w^f = w^f\,(x, y, t), \quad \phi^f = \phi^f\,(x, y, t) \tag{4}$$

From Eqs. (2), (3) and (4), we gain

$$\begin{aligned} \sigma^f_{xz} &= c^f_{44} w^f_{,\,1} + e^f_{15}\phi^f_{,\,1} \\ \sigma^f_{yz} &= c^f_{44} w^f_{,\,2} + e^f_{15}\phi^f_{,\,2} \\ D^f_1 &= e^f_{15} w^f_{,\,1} - \varepsilon^f_{11}\phi^f_{,1} \\ D^f_2 &= e^f_{15} w^f_{,\,2} - \varepsilon^f_{11}\phi^f_{,2} \end{aligned} \tag{5}$$

Using Eq. (5) into Eq. (1), we have

$$\begin{aligned} & c^f_{44}\,(y)\left(\frac{\partial^2 w^f}{\partial x^2} + \frac{\partial^2 w^f}{\partial y^2}\right) + e^f_{15}\,(y)\left(\frac{\partial^2 \phi^f}{\partial x^2} + \frac{\partial^2 \phi^f}{\partial y^2}\right) \\ & \quad + \frac{\partial c^f_{44}\,(y)}{\partial y}\frac{\partial w^f}{\partial y} + \frac{\partial e^f_{15}\,(y)}{\partial y}\frac{\partial \phi^f}{\partial y} = \rho_f\,(y)\,\frac{\partial^2 w^f}{\partial t^2} \\ & e^f_{15}\,(y)\left(\frac{\partial^2 w^f}{\partial x^2} + \frac{\partial^2 w^f}{\partial y^2}\right) - \varepsilon^f_{11}\,(y)\left(\frac{\partial^2 \phi^f}{\partial x^2} + \frac{\partial^2 \phi^f}{\partial y^2}\right) \\ & \quad + \frac{\partial e^f_{15}\,(y)}{\partial y}\frac{\partial w^f}{\partial y} - \frac{\partial \varepsilon^f_{11}\,(y)}{\partial y}\frac{\partial \phi^f}{\partial y} = 0 \end{aligned} \tag{6}$$

2.2 For the Substrate

The governing equations are

$$c_{44}^{DE}\nabla^2 w_{DE} = \rho_{DE}\frac{\partial^2 w_{DE}}{\partial t^2} \tag{7a}$$

$$\nabla^2 \phi_{DE} = 0 \tag{7b}$$

The electrical displacement and stress component are given by

$$\sigma_{yz}^{DE} = c_{44}^{DE}\frac{\partial w_{DE}}{\partial y} \tag{8a}$$

$$D_y^{DE} = -\varepsilon_{11}^{DE}\phi_{DE,2} \tag{8b}$$

2.3 For the Liquid Layer

The governing equations are

$$\mu_L \nabla^2 w_L = \rho_L \frac{\partial w_L}{\partial t} \tag{9a}$$

$$\nabla^2 \phi_L = 0 \tag{9b}$$

where w_L, μ_L and ρ_L denotes velocity of liquid particle, viscous coefficient and mass density.

The only shear stress and electrical displacement are written as

$$\left(\tau_{yz}\right)_L = \mu_L \frac{\partial w_L}{\partial y} \tag{10a}$$

$$D_y^L = -\varepsilon_{11}^L \phi_{L,2} \tag{10b}$$

3 Problem Solution

3.1 For the Layer by Liouville–Green (LG) Method

To solve Eq. (6), assume

$$w^f\left(x, y, t\right) = W_f\left(y\right)\exp\left[ik\left(x - ct\right)\right] \tag{11a}$$

$$\phi^f\left(x, y, t\right) = \phi_f\left(y\right)\exp\left[ik\left(x - ct\right)\right] \tag{11b}$$

Equations (6), (11a) and (11b) give

$$\begin{aligned}
&c_{44}^{f}(y)\,W_f'' + \left(c_{44}^{f}\right)' W_f' + \left[\rho_f(y)\,c^2 - c_{44}^{f}(y)\right] k^2 W_f \\
&\quad + e_{15}^{f}(y)\,\phi_f'' + \left(e_{15}^{f}\right)' \phi_f' - k^2 e_{15}^{f}(y)\,\phi_f = 0 \\
&e_{15}^{f}(y)\,W_f'' + \left(e_{15}^{f}\right)' W_f' - k^2 e_{15}^{f}(y)\,W_f \\
&\quad - \varepsilon_{11}^{f}(y)\,\phi_f'' - \left(\varepsilon_{11}^{f}\right)' \phi_f' + k^2 \varepsilon_{11}^{f}(y)\,\phi_f = 0
\end{aligned} \tag{12}$$

The FGPM material properties are varying quadratically, so we have

$$\begin{aligned}
e_{15}^{f}(y) &= e_{15}^{fp}\left[1 + \zeta_f\left(h_f + y\right)\right]^2 \\
c_{44}^{f}(y) &= c_{44}^{fp}\left[1 + \zeta_f\left(h_f + y\right)\right]^2 \\
\varepsilon_{11}^{f}(y) &= \varepsilon_{11}^{fp}\left[1 + \zeta_f\left(h_f + y\right)\right]^2 \\
\rho_f(y) &= \rho^{fp}\left[1 + \zeta_f\left(h_f + y\right)\right]^2
\end{aligned} \tag{13}$$

From Eqs. (12) and (13), we get

$$\begin{aligned}
&c_{44}^{f}(y)\,W_f'' + \left[1 + \zeta_f\left(h_f + y\right)\right] c_{44}^{fp}\zeta_f W_f' + \left[\rho_f(y)\,c^2 - c_{44}^{f}(y)\right] k^2 W_f \\
&\quad + e_{15}^{f}(y)\,\phi_f'' + \left[1 + \zeta_f\left(h_f + y\right)\right] e_{15}^{fp}\zeta_f \phi_f' - k^2 e_{15}^{f}(y)\,\phi_f = 0 \\
&e_{15}^{f}(y)\,W_f'' + \left[1 + \zeta_f\left(h_f + y\right)\right] e_{15}^{fp}\zeta_f W_f' - k^2 e_{15}^{f}(y)\,W_f \\
&\quad - \varepsilon_{11}^{f}(y)\,\phi_f'' - \left[1 + \zeta_f\left(h_f + y\right)\right] \varepsilon_{11}^{fp}\zeta_f \phi_f' + k^2 \varepsilon_{11}^{f}(y)\,\phi_f = 0
\end{aligned} \tag{14}$$

Consider, $c_{f\,gp} = c_{44}^{fp} + \frac{\left(e_{15}^{fp}\right)^2}{\varepsilon_{11}^{fp}}$ and $p(y) = 1 + \zeta_{fp}\left(h_f + y\right)$, finally we have Eq. (14) in rearranged form as

$$W_f'' + \frac{2\zeta_f}{p} W_f' + k^2\left(\frac{\rho^{fp} c^2}{c_{f\,gp}} - 1\right) W_f = 0 \tag{15a}$$

$$\phi_f'' + \frac{2\zeta_f}{p}\phi_f' - k^2\phi_f = \frac{e_{15}^{fp}}{\varepsilon_{11}^{fp}}\left(W_f'' + \frac{2\zeta_f}{p} W_f' - k^2 W_f\right) \tag{15b}$$

Adopt the transformation,

$$W_f = e^{\int \gamma(y)dy} \tag{16}$$

Substituting Eq. (16) into Eq. (15a), we get

$$\gamma^2 + \gamma' + \frac{2\zeta_f}{p}\gamma + \left(\frac{\rho^{fp} c^2}{c_{f\,gp}} - 1\right) k^2 = 0 \tag{17}$$

The asymptotic series expansion of γ as inverse power of k is given by

$$\gamma\,(y) = \gamma_0\,(y)\,k + \gamma_1\,(y) + \frac{\gamma_2\,(y)}{k} + \cdots \tag{18}$$

From Eqs. (17) and (18), we obtain

$$\begin{aligned} \gamma_0^2 + \left(\frac{\rho^{fp} c^2}{c_{f\,gp}} - 1\right) &= 0 \\ 2\gamma_0\gamma_1 + \gamma_0{}' + \frac{2\zeta_f}{p}\gamma_0 &= 0 \\ \gamma_1^2 + 2\gamma_0\gamma_2 + \gamma_1{}' + \frac{2\zeta_f}{p}\gamma_1 &= 0 \end{aligned} \tag{19}$$

Solving Eq. (19), we obtain

$$\begin{aligned} \gamma_0^{(1)} = i\sqrt{\frac{\rho^{fp} c^2}{c_{f\,gp}} - 1}, \quad \gamma_0^{(2)} &= -i\sqrt{\frac{\rho^{fp} c^2}{c_{f\,gp}} - 1} \\ \gamma_1^{(1)} = \gamma_1^{(2)} &= -\frac{\zeta_f}{p} \\ \gamma_2^{(1)} = -\frac{i\zeta_f^2}{2p^2}\sqrt{\frac{c_{f\,gp}}{\rho^{fp} c^2 - c_{f\,gp}}}, \quad \gamma_2^{(2)} &= \frac{i\zeta_f^2}{2p^2}\sqrt{\frac{c_{f\,gp}}{\rho^{fp} c^2 - c_{f\,gp}}} \end{aligned} \tag{20}$$

Using Eq. (20) into Eq. (18), we get

$$\begin{aligned} \gamma^{(1)} &= ik\sqrt{\frac{\rho^{fp} c^2}{c_{f\,gp}} - 1} - \frac{\zeta_f}{p} - \frac{i\zeta_f^2}{2kp^2}\sqrt{\frac{c_{f\,gp}}{\rho^{fp} c^2 - c_{f\,gp}}} + \cdots \\ \gamma^{(2)} &= -ik\sqrt{\frac{\rho^{fp} c^2}{c_{f\,gp}} - 1} - \frac{\zeta_f}{p} + \frac{i\zeta_f^2}{2kp^2}\sqrt{\frac{c_{f\,gp}}{\rho^{fp} c^2 - c_{f\,gp}}} + \cdots \end{aligned} \tag{21}$$

Again, Eqs. (16) and (21) give

$$\begin{aligned} & w^f\,(x, y, t) = \left[1 + \zeta_f\left(h_f + y\right)\right]^{-1}\left[e^{it_1(y)}C_1 + e^{-it_1(y)}C_2\right] \\ & \exp\left[ik\,(x - ct)\right] \end{aligned} \tag{22}$$

where $t_1\,(y) = ky\sqrt{\frac{\rho^{fp} c^2}{c_{f\,gp}} - 1} + \frac{\zeta_f}{2kp}\sqrt{\frac{c_{f\,gp}}{\rho^{fp} c^2 - c_{f\,gp}}}$.

Equations (15b), (22) give

$$\phi^f(x, y, t) = \left[1 + \zeta_f(h_f + y)\right]^{-1}\left[e^{t_2(y)}C_3 + e^{-t_2(y)}C_4\right]\exp[ik(x - ct)] + \frac{e_{15}^{fp}}{\varepsilon_{11}^{fp}} w^f(x, y, t) \tag{23}$$

where $t_2(y) = ky - \frac{\zeta_f}{2kp}$.

3.2 For the Substrate

Suppose,

$$w_{DE}(x, y, t) = W_{DE}(y)\exp[ik(x - ct)] \tag{24a}$$

$$\phi_{DE}(x, y, t) = \overline{\phi_{DE}}(y)\exp[ik(x - ct)] \tag{24b}$$

Equations (24a) and (24b) give the solution of Eqs. (7a) and (7b) as

$$w_{DE} = C_5\exp(-k\lambda_{DE}y)\exp[ik(x - ct)] \tag{25a}$$

$$\phi_{DE} = C_6\exp(-ky)\exp[ik(x - ct)] \tag{25b}$$

where $\lambda_{DE}^2 = \left(1 - \frac{\rho_{DE}}{c_{44}^{DE}}c^2\right)$.

3.3 For Liquid Layer

Adopt,

$$w_L = W_L(y)\,e^{ik(x-ct)} \tag{26a}$$

$$\phi_L = \psi_L(y)\,e^{ik(x-ct)} \tag{26b}$$

Replacing the above into Eqs. (9a) and (9b), we gain

$$W_L''(y) - \varepsilon_L^2 W_L = 0 \tag{27a}$$

$$\psi_L'' - k^2\psi_L = 0 \tag{27b}$$

Manipulation of Eqs. (26a), (26b), (27a) and (27b) gives

$$w_L = \left(Ae^{\varepsilon_L y} + Be^{-\varepsilon_L y}\right)e^{ik_1(x-ct)} \tag{28a}$$

$$\phi_L = \left(A_1e^{ky} + B_1e^{-ky}\right)e^{ik(x-ct)} \tag{28b}$$

where $\varepsilon_L^2 = \left(k^2 - ikc\frac{\rho_L}{\mu_L}\right)$.

4 Boundary Conditions

At $y = -(h_L + h_f)$,

$$\left(\tau_{yz}\right)_L = 0 \tag{29a}$$

$$D_y^L = 0 \,(\text{Electrically open case}) \tag{29b}$$

$$\phi_L = 0 \,(\text{Electrically short case}) \tag{29c}$$

At $y = -(h_f)$,

$$\left(\tau_{yz}\right)_L = \sigma_{yz}^f \tag{29d}$$

$$w_L = \dot{w}^f \tag{29e}$$

$$D_y^L = D_2^f \tag{29f}$$

$$\phi_L = \phi^f \tag{29g}$$

At $y = 0$,

$$\sigma_{yz}^f = \sigma_{yz}^{DE} \tag{29h}$$

$$D_2^f = D_2^{DE} \tag{29i}$$

$$\phi^f = \phi_{DE} \tag{29j}$$

$$w^f = w_{DE} \tag{29k}$$

Using the solutions derived above (5), (8a), (8b), (10a), (10b), (22), (23), (25a), (25b), (28a) and (28b) and the boundary conditions (29a)–(29k), we have

$$SL = 0 \quad \text{and} \quad RL = 0$$

where $L = [L_1, L_2, L_3, L_4, L_5, L_6, L_7, L_8, L_9, L_{10}]^T$ and S and R are the non-zero 10×10 matrix.

Where $S_{11} = R_{11} = \mu_L \varepsilon_L e^{-\varepsilon_L (h_L + h_f)}$, $S_{12} = R_{12} = -\mu_L \varepsilon_L e^{\varepsilon_L (h_L + h_f)}$, $S_{23} = -k\varepsilon_{11}^L e^{-k(h_L + h_f)}$, $S_{24} = k\varepsilon_{11}^L e^{k(h_L + h_f)}$, $S_{31} = R_{31} = \varepsilon_L \mu_L e^{-\varepsilon_L h_f}$, $S_{32} = R_{32} = -\varepsilon_L \mu_L e^{\varepsilon_L h_f}$, $S_{35} = R_{35} = -c_{fgp}(il_1 - \zeta_f)e^{id_{11}}$, $S_{36} = R_{36} = c_{fgp}(il_1 + \zeta_f)e^{-id_{11}}$, $S_{37} = R_{37} = -e_{15}^{fp}(p_1 - \zeta_f)e^{d_{21}}$, $S_{38} = R_{38} = e_{15}^{fp}(p_1 + \zeta_f)e^{-d_{21}}$, $S_{41} = R_{41} = e^{-\varepsilon_L h_f}$, $S_{42} = R_{42} = e^{\varepsilon_L h_f}$, $S_{45} = R_{45} = ikce^{id_{11}}$, $S_{46} = R_{46} = ikce^{-id_{11}}$, $S_{53} = R_{53} = -k\varepsilon_{11}^L e^{-kh_f}$, $S_{54} = R_{54} = k\varepsilon_{11}^L e^{kh_f}$, $S_{57} = R_{57} = -\varepsilon_{11}^{fp}(p_1 - \zeta_f)e^{d_{21}}$, $S_{58} = R_{58} = \varepsilon_{11}^{fp}(p_1 + \zeta_f)e^{-d_{21}}$, $S_{65} = R_{65} = \frac{e_{15}^{fp}}{\varepsilon_{11}^{fp}} e^{id_{11}}$, $S_{66} = R_{66} = \frac{e_{15}^{fp}}{\varepsilon_{11}^{fp}} e^{-id_{11}}$, $S_{67} = R_{67} = e^{d_{21}}$, $S_{68} = R_{68} = e^{-d_{21}}$, $S_{75} = R_{75} = \left[1 + \zeta_f h_f\right]^{-1} c_{fgp}(il_{11} - \frac{\zeta_f}{1+\zeta_f h_f})e^{id_{12}}$, $S_{76} = R_{76} = -\left[1 + \zeta_f h_f\right]^{-1} c_{fgp}(il_{11} + \frac{\zeta_f}{1+\zeta_f h_f})e^{-id_{12}}$, $S_{77} = R_{77} = \left[1 + \zeta_f h_f\right]^{-1} e_{15}^{fp}(p_{11} - \frac{\zeta_f}{1+\zeta_f h_f})e^{d_{22}}$, $S_{78} = R_{78} = -\left[1 + \zeta_f h_f\right]^{-1} e_{15}^{fp}(p_{11} + \frac{\zeta_f}{1+\zeta_f h_f})e^{-d_{22}}$, $S_{79} = R_{79} = c_{44}^{DE} k \lambda_{DE}$, $S_{87} = R_{87} = -$

$\left[1+\zeta_f h_f\right]^{-1}\varepsilon_{11}^{fp}(p_{11}-\frac{\zeta_f}{1+\zeta_f h_f})e^{d_{22}}, S_{88}=R_{88}=\left[1+\zeta_f h_f\right]^{-1}\varepsilon_{11}^{fp}(p_{11}+\frac{\zeta_f}{1+\zeta_f h_f})e^{-d_{22}}$, $S_{89}=R_{89}=-\varepsilon_{11}^{DE}k, S_{95}=R_{95}=\frac{e_{15}^{fp}}{\varepsilon_{11}^{fp}}\left[1+\zeta_f h_f\right]^{-1}e^{id_{12}}, S_{96}=R_{96}=\frac{e_{15}^{fp}}{\varepsilon_{11}^{fp}}\left[1+\zeta_f h_f\right]^{-1}$ $e^{-id_{12}}$, $S_{97}=R_{97}=\left[1+\zeta_f h_f\right]^{-1}e^{d_{22}}$, $S_{98}=R_{98}=\left[1+\zeta_f h_f\right]^{-1}e^{-d_{22}}$, $S_{99}=R_{99}=-1$, $S_{105}=T_{105}=\left[1+\zeta_f h_f\right]^{-1}e^{id_{12}}$, $S_{106}=R_{106}=\left[1+\zeta_f h_f\right]^{-1}e^{-id_{12}}$, $S_{1010}=R_{1010}=-1$, $d_{11}=-kh_f\sqrt{\frac{\rho^{fp}c^2}{c_{f\,gp}}-1}+\frac{\zeta_f}{2k}\sqrt{\frac{c_{f\,gp}}{\rho^{fp}c^2-c_{f\,gp}}}$, $d_{12}=\frac{\zeta_f}{2k(1+\zeta_f h_f)}\sqrt{\frac{c_{f\,gp}}{\rho^{fp}c^2-c_{f\,gp}}}$, $d_{21}=-kh_f-\frac{\zeta_f}{2k}$, $d_{22}=-\frac{\zeta_f}{2k(1+\zeta_f h_f)}$, $l_1=k\sqrt{\frac{\rho^{fp}c^2}{c_{f\,gp}}-1}-\frac{\zeta_f^2}{2k}\sqrt{\frac{c_{f\,gp}}{\rho^{fp}c^2-c_{f\,gp}}}$, $l_{11}=k\sqrt{\frac{\rho^{fp}c^2}{c_{f\,gp}}-1}-\frac{\zeta_f^2}{2k(1+\zeta_f h_f)^2}\sqrt{\frac{c_{f\,gp}}{\rho^{fp}c^2-c_{f\,gp}}}$, $p_1=k+\frac{\zeta_f^2}{2k}$, $p_{11}=k+\frac{\zeta_f^2}{2k(1+\zeta_f h_f)^2}$.

For non-trivial L_i, the determinant of the coefficients matrix L_i must vanish, i.e.,

$$\det(S)=0 \quad \text{and} \quad \det(R)=0 \tag{30}$$

Equation (30) gives the dispersion equation for the considered problem for both electrically open and short cases, respectively.

4.1 Particular Case

When $h_L=0, e_{15}^f=0, \varepsilon_{11}^f=0, c_{44}^f=g, c_{44}^{DE}=g_1$ and $\varepsilon_{11}^{DE}=0$, i.e., when the structure reduces homogeneous isotropic layer lying over a homogeneous isotropic half-space, then the dispersion relation becomes

$$\tan\left(kh_f\sqrt{\frac{\rho^{fp}c^2}{g}-1}\right)=\frac{g_1\sqrt{1-\frac{\rho_{DE}c^2}{g_1}}}{g\sqrt{\frac{\rho^{fp}c^2}{g}-1}} \tag{31}$$

Equation (31) is the classical Love wave equation.

5 Numerical Examples and Discussions

For graphical explanation, the following examples are taken into consideration

1. SiO_2 is considered as dielectric medium and the respective material constants are [7] $c_{44}^{DE}=3.12\times10^{10}\,(\mathrm{N/m^2})$, $\varepsilon_{11}^{DE}=0.336\times10^{-10}\,(\mathrm{NS^2/C^2})$, $\rho_{DE}=2200\,(\mathrm{kg/m^3})$
2. FGPM layer material constants of $BaTiO_3$ are [7] $c_{44}^{fp}=4.40\times10^{10}\,(\mathrm{N/m^2})$, $e_{15}^{fp}=11.4\,(\mathrm{c/m^2})$, $\varepsilon_{11}^{fp}=128\times10^{-10}\,(\mathrm{NS^2/C^2})$, $\rho^{fp}=7.28\times10^3\,(\mathrm{kg/m^3})$
3. We have considered glycerin as viscous liquid layer, the constants are [2] $\mu_L=1.5\,(\mathrm{NS/m^2})$, $\rho_L=1.2613\times10^3\,(\mathrm{kg/m^3})$. Figs. 2 and 3 shows the impact of FGPM layer width on the phase velocity. For increasing values of FGPM width

Fig. 2 Variation of dimensionless phase velocity (c/β) against dimensionless wave number (kH) for different values of FGPM layer width (h_f) in electrically open case

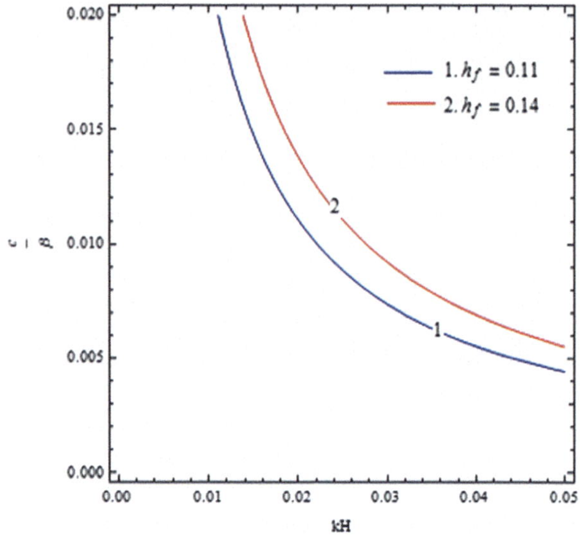

Fig. 3 Variation of dimensionless phase velocity (c/β) against dimensionless wave number (kH) for different values of FGPM layer width (h_f) in electrically short case

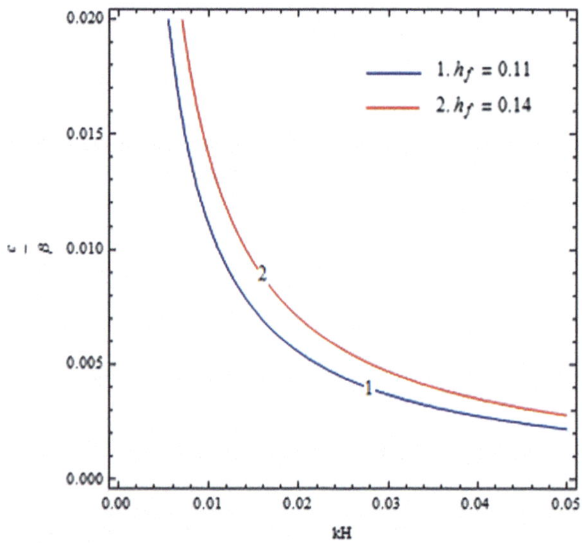

the phase velocity increases. Similarly, Figs. 4 and 5 describes the effect of liquid layer width on the phase velocity. The phase velocity decreases for increasing values of liquid layer width. Also, increment in gradient factor increases the phase velocity in both Figs. 6 and 7.

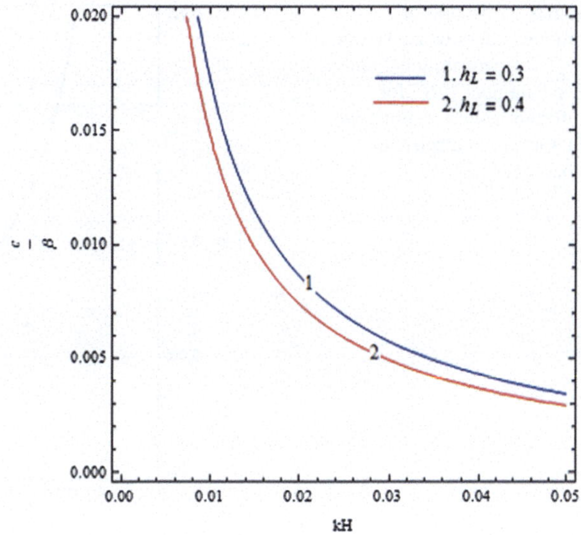

Fig. 4 Variation of dimensionless phase velocity (c/β) against dimensionless wave number (kH) for different values of liquid layer width (h_L) in electrically open case

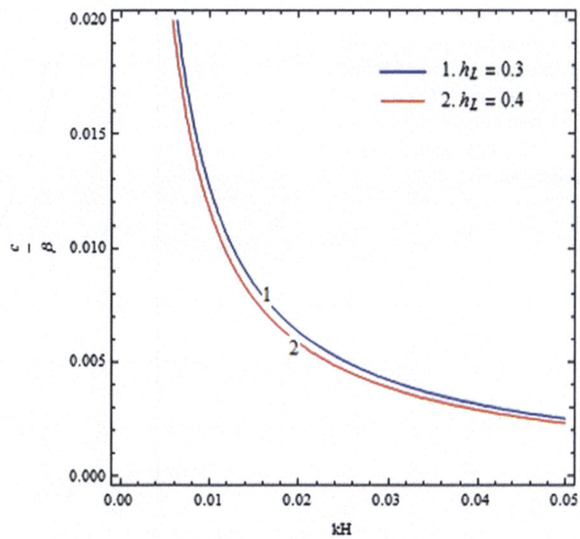

Fig. 5 Variation of dimensionless phase velocity (c/β) against dimensionless wave number (kH) for different values of liquid layer width (h_L) in electrically short case

6 Conclusions

From the study, the following conclusions may be observed

- Increment in FGPM layer width increases the phase velocity of the wave.
- As the liquid layer width increases, the phase velocity decreases. The phase velocity increases with increasing values of gradient factor.

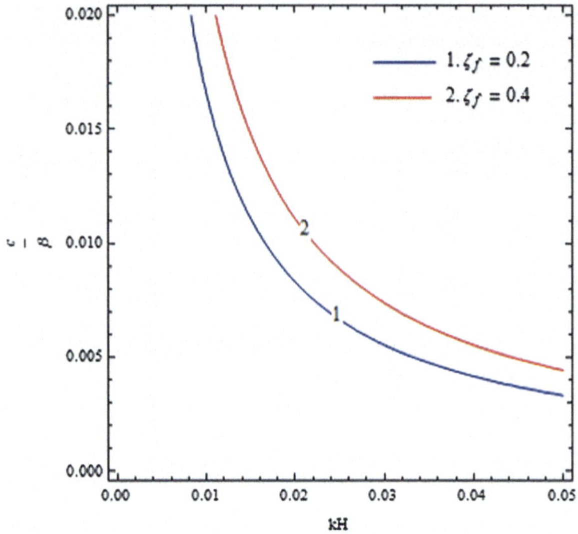

Fig. 6 Variation of dimensionless phase velocity (c/β) against dimensionless wave number (kH) for different values of gradient factor (ζ_f) in electrically open case

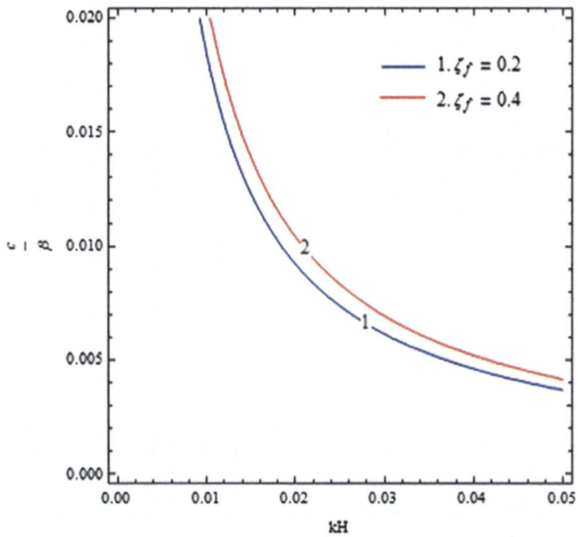

Fig. 7 Variation of dimensionless phase velocity (c/β) against dimensionless wave number (kH) for different values of gradient factor (ζ_f) in electrically short case

- The results of the present study may be utilized for designing and implementation of SAW devices and sensors.

Acknowledgements Authors convey their sincere thanks to IIT (ISM), Dhanbad, India for providing fellowship to Ms. Juhi Baroi and facilitating her with best research facilities.

References

1. Baroi, J., Sahu, S.A., Singh, M.K.: Dispersion of polarized shear waves in viscous liquid over a porous piezoelectric substrate. J. Intell. Mater. Syst. Struct. **29**(9), 2040–2048 (2018)
2. Guo, F.L., Sun, R.: Propagation of Bleustein-Gulyaev wave in 6 mm piezoelectric materials loaded with viscous liquid. Int. J. Solids Struct. **45**(13), 3699–3710 (2008)
3. Mondal, S., Anand, Sahu S.: Propagation of SH waves in corrugated FGPM layer lying over a piezomagnetic half-space. Mech. Adv. Mater. Struct. **26**(1), 29–34 (2019)
4. Nie, G.Q., Liu, J.X., An, Z.J.: Elastic wave propagation in piezoelectric/piezomagnetic bi-material plate. Eng. Mech. **27**(2), 30–36 (2010)
5. Nie, G., Wang, M.: Rayleigh-type wave in a rotated piezoelectric crystal imperfectly bonded on a dielectric substrate. CMC-Comput. Mater. Con. **59**(1), 257–274 (2019)
6. Sahu, S.A., Nirwal, S.: An asymptotic approximation of Love wave frequency in a piezo-composite structure: WKB approach. Waves Random Complex Media, 1–29 (2019)
7. Saroj, P.K., Sahu, S.A., Chaudhary, S., Chattopadhyay, A.: Love-type waves in functionally graded piezoelectric material (FGPM) sandwiched between initially stressed layer and elastic substrate. Waves Random Complex Media **25**(4), 608–627 (2015)

Graph Theory and Optimization

The Inverse Sum Indeg Index for *R*-Sum of Graphs

Amitav Doley and A. Bharali

Abstract The inverse sum indeg (ISI) index of a graph $G = (V, E)$ is defined as

$$\mathrm{ISI}(G) = \sum_{pq \in E} \frac{d_p d_q}{d_p + d_q},$$

where d_p and d_q are the degrees of the vertices p and q in G, respectively. This index is found to be useful in predicting total surface area (TSA) of octane isomers. In this paper, we investigate ISI index of *R*-sum of graphs. We also discuss the extremal cases.

Keywords Degree of vertex · Inverse sum indeg index · *R*-sum of graphs

AMS Classifications 05C76 · 05C07

1 Introduction

A topological index (TI) is a real-valued function whose domain is a collection of graphs, and it is computed based on various graph parameters like degree, distance, eccentricity, status, etc. In recent years, these indices draw considerable attention from scientist and researchers because of its usefulness in predicting various physicochemical properties of a molecule. Sometimes it is difficult to analyze these properties of a molecule by laboratory experiments due to financial constraints, time, or involvement of risk. Hence, TIs can be very helpful in drawing inferences without actual laboratory experiments. In last few decades, these indices are also studied as graph invariants by mathematicians. Thousands of topological indices are proposed and studied over the years. An account of some degree-based topological indices

A. Doley (✉) · A. Bharali
Dibrugarh University, Dibrugarh 786004, India
e-mail: amitav1987doley@gmail.com

A. Bharali
e-mail: a.bharali@dibru.ac.in

S. Bhattacharyya et al. (eds.), *Mathematical Modeling and Computational Tools*, Springer Proceedings in Mathematics & Statistics 320,
https://doi.org/10.1007/978-981-15-3615-1_25

may be found in [1]. Some of them are also found to have very limited importance. ISI index is found to be very efficient in many QSAR studies such as predicting TSA of octane isomers. In fact, this index was in the list of most significant twenty (20) indices out of the list of 148 adriatic indices studied in 2010 [2]. Few recent contributions related to ISI index may be found in [3–9].

Throughout the paper, the graph G is considered to be simple, connected, and finite. The sets $V(G)$ and $E(G)$ denote the vertex set and the edge set of the graph G, respectively. By $G \in \Im(n, m)$, we mean G is a graph with n vertices and m edges. The degree of a vertex $p \in V(G)$ is denoted by $d_G(p)$ or simply d_p. If there is an edge between the vertices p and q, then the edge is written as pq. The null graph of k vertices is denoted by N_k (for $k = 1$, it can be considered as a connected graph with no edge). The notations and terminologies used but not clearly stated will conform to those in [10].

In this paper, we compute ISI index of vertex semi-total graph and R-sums. We establish some bounds of ISI index for these graph operations.

2 Preliminaries

In this section, we formally present some topological indices and the graph operations under consideration.

Zagreb indices Let G be a graph. Then, the Zagreb indices [11] are defined as

$$M_1(G) = \sum_{p \in V(G)} d_p^2 = \sum_{pq \in E(G)} (d_p + d_q)$$

and

$$M_2(G) = \sum_{pq \in E(G)} d_p d_q.$$

Inverse degree index The inverse degree (ID) index [12] of a graph G with no isolated vertex is defined as

$$ID(G) = \sum_{p \in V(G)} \frac{1}{d_p}.$$

Definition 2.1 The subdivision graph [13] $S(G)$ is obtained by replacing each edge of G by a path of length 2.

The graph operations defined below are depicted in Fig. 1.

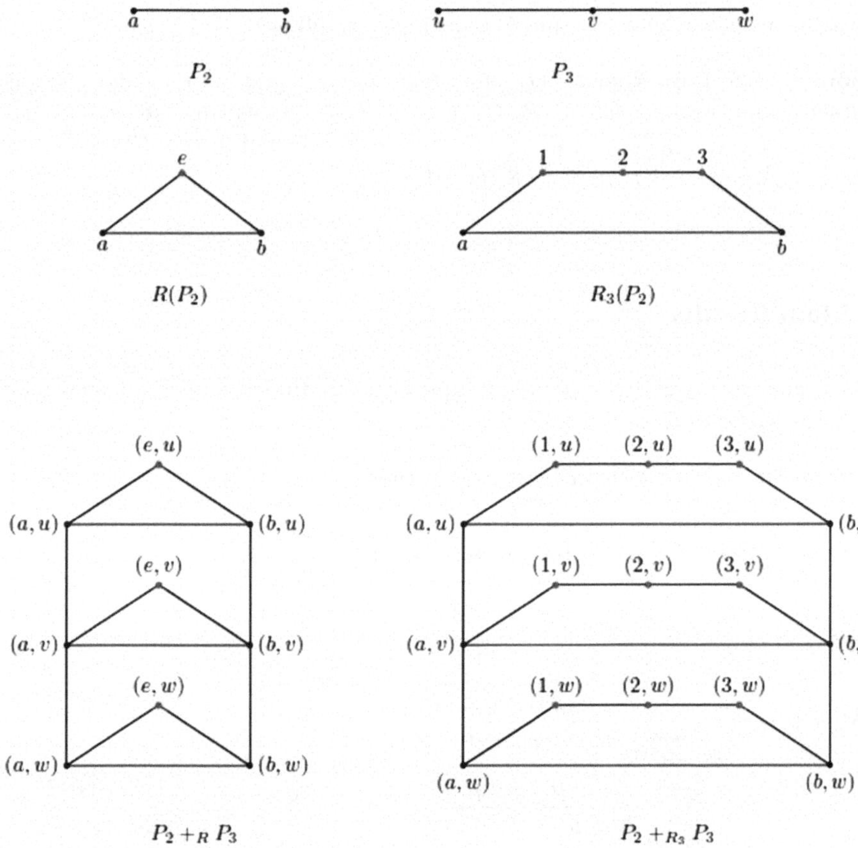

Fig. 1 Graph operations

Definition 2.2 The vertex semi-total graph [13] $R(G)$ is obtained by adding a path of length 2 parallel to each of the edges of G. The set of additional vertices is denoted by $I(G)$.

Now we extend this operation and propose a generalized operation $R_t(G)$ of the graph G as follows.

Definition 2.3 The graph $R_t(G)$ is obtained by adding a path of length $t+1$ parallel to each edge pq in G, with p and q as the end vertices of the path.

In 2009, *Eliasi* and *Taeri* propose four new sums of graphs [14]. One of them is based on vertex semi-total graph, popularly known as R-sum.

Definition 2.4 The R-sum [14] $G_1 +_R G_2$ of the graphs G_1 and G_2 is a graph with vertex set $V(R(G_1)) \times V(G_2)$ in which $(p_1, q_1)(p_2, q_2)$ is an edge iff $[p_1 = p_2 \in V(G_1)$ and $q_1q_2 \in E(G_2)]$ or $[q_1 = q_2 \in V(G_2)$ and $p_1p_2 \in E(R(G_1))]$.

Analogously, we define R_t-sum of two graphs as follows.

Definition 2.5 The R_t-sum $G_1 +_{R_t} G_2$ of the graphs G_1 and G_2 is a graph with vertex set $V(R_t(G_1)) \times V(G_2)$ in which $(p_1, q_1)(p_2, q_2)$ is in $E\big(G_1 +_{R_t} G_2\big)$ iff $[p_1 = p_2 \in V(G_1)$ and $q_1 q_2 \in E(G_2)]$ or $[q_1 = q_2 \in V(G_2)$ and $p_1 p_2 \in E(R_t(G_1))]$.

3 Main Results

In this section, we establish two explicit expressions for ISI index of vertex semi-total graph and $R_t(G)$ of G.

Theorem 3.1 *Let $G \in \Im(n, m)$ with $n \geq 2$. Then*

$$\mathrm{ISI}(R(G)) = 2\mathrm{ISI}(G) + 4m - 2n + 2 \sum_{p \in V(G)} \frac{1}{d_G(p) + 1}.$$

Proof

$$\begin{aligned}
\mathrm{ISI}(R(G)) &= \sum_{pq \in E(R(G))} \frac{d_{R(G)}(p) d_{R(G)}(q)}{d_{R(G)}(p) + d_{R(G)}(q)} \\
&= \sum_{pq \in E(G)} \frac{2d_G(p) 2d_G(q)}{2d_G(p) + 2d_G(q)} + \sum_{pe \in E(R(G)), p \in V(G), e \in I(G)} \frac{2d_G(p)2}{2d_G(p) + 2} \\
&= 2\mathrm{ISI}(G) + 2 \sum_{pe \in E(R(G)), p \in V(G), e \in I(G)} \frac{d_G(p)}{d_G(p) + 1} \\
&= 2\mathrm{ISI}(G) + 2 \sum_{pq \in E(G)} \left[\frac{d_G(p)}{d_G(p) + 1} + \frac{d_G(q)}{d_G(q) + 1} \right] \\
&= 2\mathrm{ISI}(G) + 2 \sum_{p \in V(G)} \frac{d_G^2(p)}{d_G(p) + 1} \\
&= 2\mathrm{ISI}(G) + 4m - 2n + 2 \sum_{p \in V(G)} \frac{1}{d_G(p) + 1},
\end{aligned}$$

which completes the proof. ■

Theorem 3.2 *Let $G \in \Im(n, m)$ with $n \geq 2$. Then*

$$\mathrm{ISI}(R_t(G)) = 2\mathrm{ISI}(G) + (t + 3)m - 2n + 2 \sum_{p \in V(G)} \frac{1}{d_G(p) + 1}.$$

Proof Partition $E(R_t(G))$ into E_1, E_2, and E_3 where $E_1 = \{pq \in E(R_t(G)) | p, q \in V(G)\}$, $E_2 = \{pe \in E(R_t(G)) | p \in V(G), e \in I(G)\}$, and $E_3 = \{ef \in E(R_t(G)) | e, f \in I(G)\}$. Now,

$$\begin{aligned}
\mathrm{ISI}(R_t(G)) &= \sum_{pq\in E_1} \frac{2d_G(p)2d_G(q)}{2d_G(p)+2d_G(q)} + \sum_{pe\in E_2} \frac{2d_G(p)2}{2d_G(p)+2} + \sum_{ef\in E_3} 1 \\
&= 2\mathrm{ISI}(G) + 2 \sum_{pq\in E(G)} \left[\frac{d_G(p)}{d_G(p)+1} + \frac{d_G(q)}{d_G(q)+1}\right] + m(t-1) \\
&= 2\mathrm{ISI}(G) + 2\left[2m - n + \sum_{p\in V(G)} \frac{1}{d_G(p)+1}\right] + m(t-1) \\
&= 2\mathrm{ISI}(G) + 4m - 2n + m(t-1) + 2\sum_{p\in V(G)} \frac{1}{d_G(p)+1}
\end{aligned}$$

3.1 *Some Lower Bounds on ISI Index of Vertex Semi-total Graphs*

Lemma 3.3 (Jensen's inequality) *[15] Let $y_1, \ldots, y_k$ be in the interval I and let ψ be convex on I. Then*

$$\psi\left(\frac{y_1 + \ldots + y_k}{k}\right) \le \frac{\psi(y_1) + \ldots + \psi(y_k)}{k}$$

with equality iff $y_1 = \ldots = y_k$.

Theorem 3.4 *Let $G \in \Im(n, m)$ with $n \ge 2$. Then*

$$\mathrm{ISI}(R(G)) \ge 2\mathrm{ISI}(G) + 3m - \frac{n}{2},$$

with equality iff $G = K_2$.

Proof Note that,

$$\begin{aligned}
\sum_{pq\in E(G)} \left[\frac{d_G(p)}{d_G(p)+1} + \frac{d_G(q)}{d_G(q)+1}\right] &= \sum_{pq\in E(G)} \left[1 - \frac{1}{d_G(p)+1} + 1 - \frac{1}{d_G(q)+1}\right] \\
&= 2m - \sum_{p\in V(G)} \frac{d_G(p)}{d_G(p)+1} \\
&\ge 2m - \frac{1}{4} \sum_{p\in V(G)} [d_G(p)+1]
\end{aligned}$$

by *Jensen*'s inequality. Now, by Theorem 3.1,

$$\mathrm{ISI}(R(G)) \geq 2\mathrm{ISI}(G) + 2\left[2m - \frac{1}{4}(2m+n)\right] = 2\mathrm{ISI}(G) + 3m - \frac{n}{2}.$$

Equality holds iff $G = K_2$. ■

Corollary 3.5 *Let $G \in \Im(n, m)$ with $n \geq 2$. Then*

$$\mathrm{ISI}(R_t(G)) \geq 2\mathrm{ISI}(G) + m(t+2) - \frac{n}{2},$$

with equality iff $G = K_2$.

A better lower bound can be found by using the following well-known inequality which is also satisfied by graphs more than that of the above lower bounds.

Lemma 3.6 (Cauchy–Schwarz inequality) *[15] Let c_j and d_j, $(j = 1, 2, \ldots, k)$, are real numbers. Then*

$$\left(\sum_{j=1}^{k} c_j d_j\right)^2 \leq \sum_{j=1}^{k} c_j^2 \sum_{j=1}^{k} d_j^2$$

with equality iff $\frac{c_j}{d_j}$ is constant for $j = 1, 2, \ldots, k$.

Theorem 3.7 *Let $G \in \Im(n, m)$ with $n \geq 2$. Then*

$$\mathrm{ISI}(R(G)) \geq 2\mathrm{ISI}(G) + \frac{8m^2}{2m+n},$$

with equality iff G is regular.

Proof By *Cauchy–Schwarz* inequality,

$$\sum_{p\in V(G)} \left(\sqrt{d_G(p)+1}\right)^2 \sum_{p\in V(G)} \left(\frac{1}{\sqrt{d_G(p)+1}}\right)^2$$
$$\geq \left[\sum_{p\in V(G)} \sqrt{d_G(p)+1}\frac{1}{\sqrt{d_G(p)+1}}\right]^2$$

whence $\sum_{p\in V(G)} \frac{1}{d_G(p)+1} \geq \frac{n^2}{(2m+n)}$. The desired inequality follows from Theorem 3.1 with equality iff $d_G(p) + 1 =$ a constant, i.e., iff G is regular. This completes the proof. ■

Corollary 3.8 *Let $G \in \Im(n, m)$ with $n \geq 2$. Then*

$$\mathrm{ISI}(R_t(G)) \geq 2\mathrm{ISI}(G) + \frac{8m^2}{2m+n} + m(t-1),$$

with equality iff G is regular.

3.2 Some Upper Bounds on ISI Index of Vertex Semi-total Graphs

Theorem 3.9 *Let $G \in \Im(n, m)$ with $n \geq 2$. Then*

$$\mathrm{ISI}(R(G)) \leq 2\mathrm{ISI}(G) + 4m - \frac{3}{2}n + \frac{1}{2}ID(G),$$

with equality iff $G = K_2$.

Proof By *Jensen's* inequality,

$$\sum_{p \in V(G)} \frac{1}{d_G(p)+1} \leq \frac{1}{4} \sum_{p \in V(G)} \left[\frac{1}{d_G(p)} + 1\right] = \frac{1}{4}[ID(G) + n].$$

Now, by Theorem 3.1,

$$\begin{aligned}\mathrm{ISI}(R(G)) &\leq 2\mathrm{ISI}(G) + 4m - 2n + \frac{2}{4} \sum_{p \in V(G)} \left[\frac{1}{d_G(p)} + 1\right] \\ &= 2\mathrm{ISI}(G) + 4m - \frac{3}{2}n + \frac{1}{2}ID(G),\end{aligned}$$

with equality iff $d_G(p) = 1$, i.e., iff $G = K_2$. ■

Corollary 3.10 *Let $G \in \Im(n, m)$ with $n \geq 2$. Then*

$$\mathrm{ISI}(R_t(G)) \leq 2\mathrm{ISI}(G) - \frac{3}{2}n + \frac{1}{2}ID(G) + m(t+3),$$

with equality iff $G = K_2$.

Theorem 3.11 *Let $G \in \Im(n, m)$ with $n \geq 2$. Then*

$$\mathrm{ISI}(R(G)) \leq 2\mathrm{ISI}(G) + m + \frac{1}{2}M_1(G),$$

with equality iff $G = K_2$.

Proof By *Jensen's* inequality,

$$\sum_{p\in V(G)} \frac{d_G^2(p)}{d_G(p)+1} \le \frac{1}{4} \sum_{p\in V(G)} \left[d_G(p)+d_G^2(p)\right]$$

Again $\mathrm{ISI}(G) = 2\mathrm{ISI}(G) + 2 \sum_{p\in V(G)} \frac{d_G^2(p)}{d_G(p)+1}$ by Theorem 3.1. Hence,

$$\begin{aligned}\mathrm{ISI}(R(G)) &\le 2\mathrm{ISI}(G) + \frac{2}{4} \sum_{p\in V(G)} \left[d_G(p)+d_G^2(p)\right] \\ &= 2\mathrm{ISI}(G) + m + \frac{1}{2} M_1(G),\end{aligned}$$

with equality iff $d_G(p) = d_G^2(p)$, i.e., iff $G = K_2$. ■

Corollary 3.12 *Let* $G \in \Im(n, m)$ *with* $n \ge 2$. *Then*

$$\mathrm{ISI}(R_t(G)) \le 2\mathrm{ISI}(G) + \frac{1}{2} M_1(G) + mt,$$

with equality iff $G = K_2$.

Lemma 3.13 (Schweitzer's inequality) *[15] Let* $b \le b_j \le B$, $b_j s$ *are positive real numbers* ($j = 1, \ldots, k$). *Then*

$$\left(\sum_{j=1}^{k} b_j\right)\left(\sum_{j=1}^{k} \frac{1}{b_j}\right) \le \frac{k^2(b+B)^2}{4bB},$$

with equality iff $b_1 = \ldots = b_k = b = B$ or k is even, $b_1 = \ldots = b_{\frac{k}{2}} = b$ and $b_{\frac{k}{2}+1} = \ldots = b_k = B$, where $b < B$ and $b_1 \le \ldots \le b_k$.

Hereafter, we use the notations δ and Δ for $\min\{d_p | p \in V(G)\}$ and $\max\{d_p | p \in V(G)\}$, respectively.

Theorem 3.14 *Let* $G \in \Im(n, m)$ *with* $n \ge 2$. *Then*

$$\mathrm{ISI}(R(G)) \le 2\mathrm{ISI}(G) + 4m - 2n + \frac{n^2(\delta+\Delta+2)^2}{2(2m+n)(\delta+1)(\Delta+1)},$$

with equality iff G is regular or (δ, Δ)-biregular.

Proof As $\delta + 1 \le d_G(p) + 1 \le \Delta + 1$ so by *Schweitzer's* inequality,

$$\sum_{p\in V(G)} [d_G(p)+1] \sum_{p\in V(G)} \frac{1}{d_G(p)+1} \le \frac{n^2(\delta+1+\Delta+1)^2}{4(\delta+1)(\Delta+1)}$$

$$\Rightarrow \sum_{p\in V(G)} \frac{1}{d_G(p)+1} \le \frac{n^2(\delta+\Delta+2)^2}{4(2m+n)(\delta+1)(\Delta+1)}.$$

Using this inequality in Theorem 3.1, we get the desired result with equality iff G is regular or half of the vertices of G are of degree δ and the remaining vertices are of degree Δ, i.e., iff G is regular or (δ, Δ)-biregular. ■

Corollary 3.15 *Let $G \in \Im(n, m)$ with $n \ge 2$. Then*

$$\mathrm{ISI}(R_t(G)) \le 2\mathrm{ISI}(G) - 2n + m(t+3) + \frac{n^2(\delta+\Delta+2)^2}{2(2m+n)(\delta+1)(\Delta+1)}.$$

Equality holds iff G is regular or (δ, Δ)-biregular.

3.3 *ISI Index for* R*-Sum and* R$_t$*-Sum of Graphs*

Theorem 3.16 *Let $G_i \in \Im(n_i, m_i)$, $i = 1, 2$. Then*

$$\mathrm{ISI}(G_1 +_R G_2) \le 4m_1m_2 + n_2M_1(G_1) + m_1n_2 + \frac{n_1}{4}M_1(G_2).$$

Equality holds iff $G_1 = N_1$ and $G_2 = C_{n_2}$ or $G_1 = K_2$ and $G_2 = N_1$.

Proof Partitioning $E(G_1 +_R G_2)$ into E_1 and E_2 where $E_1 = \{(p_i, q_k)(p_j, q_l) | p_i, p_j \in V(G_1),\ q_k, q_l \in V(G_2)\}$, and $E_2 = \{(p_i, q_k)(e_r, q_k) | p_i \in V(G_1),\ q_k \in V(G_2),\ e_r \in I(G_1)\}$, we obtain,

$$\begin{aligned}\mathrm{ISI}(G_1 +_R G_2) &= \sum_{(p_i,q_k)(p_j,q_l)\in E_1} \frac{[2d_{G_1}(p_i) + d_{G_2}(q_k)][2d_{G_1}(p_j) + d_{G_2}(q_l)]}{[2d_{G_1}(p_i) + d_{G_2}(q_k)]+[2d_{G_1}(p_j) + d_{G_2}(q_l)]}\\ &\quad + \sum_{(p_i,q_k)(e_r,q_k)\in E_2} \frac{[2d_{G_1}(p_i) + d_{G_2}(q_k)].2}{[2d_{G_1}(p_i) + d_{G_2}(q_k)]+2}\\ &= S_1 + S_2\end{aligned}$$

Now, by *Jensen's* inequality,

$$\begin{aligned}S_1 &\le \frac{1}{4} \sum_{(p_i,q_k)(p_j,q_l)\in E(G)} [2\{d_{G_1}(p_i) + d_{G_1}(p_j)\} + \{d_{G_2}(q_k) + d_{G_2}(q_l)\}]\\ &= \frac{1}{4} \sum_{p_i\in V(G_1)} \sum_{q_kq_l\in E(G_2)} [4d_{G_1}(p_i) + \{d_{G_2}(q_k) + d_{G_2}(q_l)\}]\end{aligned}$$

$$+\frac{1}{4}\sum_{q_k\in V(G_2)}\sum_{p_ip_j\in E(G_1)}\left[2d_{G_2}(q_k)+2\left\{d_{G_1}(p_i)+d_{G_1}\left(p_j\right)\right\}\right]$$
$$=\frac{1}{4}[8m_1m_2+n_1M_1(G_2)+2n_2M_1(G_1)+4m_1m_2]$$
$$=\frac{1}{4}[12m_1m_2+n_1M_1(G_2)+2n_2M_1(G_2)],$$

with equality iff $2d_{G_1}(p_i)+d_{G_2}(q_k)=2d_{G_1}\left(p_j\right)+d_{G_2}(q_l)$, i.e., iff both G_1 and G_2 are regular.

Similarly,

$$S_2\leq\frac{1}{4}\sum_{(p_i,q_k)(e_r,q_k)\in E(G)}\left[2d_{G_1}(p_i)+d_{G_2}(q_k)+2\right]$$
$$=\frac{1}{4}\sum_{q_k\in V(G_2)}\sum_{p_ie_r\in E(S(G_1))}\left[2d_{G_1}(p_i)+d_{G_2}(q_k)+2\right]$$
$$=\frac{1}{4}\sum_{q_k\in V(G_2)}\left[2\sum_{p_i\in V(G_1)}d^2_{G_1}(p_i)+2m_1\left(2+d_{G_2}(q_k)\right)\right]$$
$$=\frac{1}{2}n_2M_1(G_1)+m_1n_2+m_1m_2,$$

with equality iff $2d_{G_1}(p_i)+d_{G_2}(q_k)=2$, i.e., iff $d_{G_2}(q_k)=2-2d_{G_1}(p_i)$, i.e., iff $G_1=N_1$ and $G_2=C_{n_2}$ or $G_1=K_2$ and $G_2=N_1$.

Therefore, $\mathrm{ISI}(G_1+_R G_2)\leq 4m_1m_2+n_2M_1(G_1)+m_1n_2+\frac{1}{4}n_1M_1(G_2)$ with equality iff $G_1=N_1$ and $G_2=C_{n_2}$ or $G_1=K_2$ and $G_2=N_1$. ■

Corollary 3.17 *Let* $G_i\in\Im(n_i,m_i)$, $i=1,2$. *Then*

$$\mathrm{ISI}\left(G_1+_{R_t}G_2\right)\leq 4m_1m_2+n_2M_1(G_1)+\frac{n_1}{4}M_1(G_2)+tm_1n_2,$$

with equality iff $G_1=N_1$ and $G_2=C_{n_2}$ or $G_1=K_2$ and $G_2=N_1$.

4 Conclusion

The study of ISI index for various operations of graphs is found to be limited in the literature. In this paper, we compute the ISI index of vertex semi-total graph and R-sum of graphs. We also extend the R-sum of graphs to R_t-sums of graphs and obtain some bounds of ISI index for vertex semi-total graph, R-sum, and R_t-sum of graphs. The extremal cases of the bounds are also studied for their sharpness. This idea can also be applied to the rest of the four operations proposed by Eliasi and

Taeri [14]. The computation of other TIs of these graph operations may be another interesting topic for further study.

References

1. Gutman, I.: Degree-based topological indices. Croat. Chem. Acta **86**(4), 351–361 (2013)
2. Vukičević, D., Gašperov, M.: Bond additive Modeling 1. Adriatic indices. Croat. Chem. Acta **83**(3), 243–260 (2010)
3. An, M., Xiong, L.: Some results on the inverse sum indeg index of a graph. Inf. Process. Lett. **134**, 42–46 (2018)
4. Chen, H., Deng, H.: The inverse sum indeg index of graphs with some given parameters. Discret. Math., Algorithms Appl. **10**(1), 1850006 (2018)
5. Falahati-Nezhad, F., Došlić, T.: Sharp bounds on the inverse sum indeg index. Discret. Appl. Math. **217**(2), 185–195 (2017)
6. Hasani, M.: Study of inverse sum indeg index. J. Math. Nanosci. **7**(2), 103–109 (2017)
7. Matejić, M.M., Milovanović, I.Ž., Milovanović, E.I.: Upper bounds for the inverse sum indeg index of graphs. Discret. Appl. Math. **251**, 258–267 (2018)
8. Pattabiraman, K.: Inverse sum indeg index of graphs. AKCE Int. J. Graphs Comb. **15**(2), 155–167 (2018)
9. Sedlar, J., Stevanović, D., Vasilyev, A.: On the inverse sum indeg index. Discret. Appl. Math. **184**, 202–212 (2015)
10. West, D.B.: Introduction to Graph Theory, 2nd edn. Prentice Hall India, Delhi (2002)
11. Gutman, I., Trinajstić, N.: Graph theory and molecular orbitals. Total π-electron energy of alternant hydrocarbons. Chem. Phy. Lett. **17**, 535–538 (1972)
12. Fajtlowicz, S.: On conjectures of graffiti II. Congr. numer. **60**, 189–197 (1987)
13. Hammack, R., Imrich, W., Klavžar, S.: Handbook of Product Graphs, 2nd edn. CRC press, Boca Raton (2011)
14. Eliasi, M., Taeri, B.: Four new sums of graphs and their Wiener indices. Discret. Appl. Math. **157**(4), 794–803 (2009)
15. Dragomir, S.S.: A survey on Cauchy-Buyakovsky-Schwarz type discrete inequalities. J. Inequalities Pure Appl. Math. **4**(3), 63 (2003)

Neural Network-Based Fuzzy Multi-objective Optimisation for Efficiency Evaluation

Debasish Roy

Abstract Multi-objective optimisation handles the optimisation of multiple objectives on a multi-dimensional space (Lootsma in Fuzzy Multi-Objective Optimization. Springer, Boston, 1997 [1]). There are various classical methods and a wide variety of genetic algorithms for determining the Pareto-optimal front in MOOP. Most of the MOOP algorithms dealing with fuzzy systems treat fuzzy parameters (Young-Jou and Ching-Lai in Fuzzy multiple objective decision making: Methods and applications, Springer, Berlin, 1994 [2]), fuzzy inequalities (Chuntian in Hydrological Sciences Journal 44(4): 573–582, 1999 [3]) and fuzzy objective function (Young Jou and Ching-Lai in Fuzzy Sets and Systems 54(2): 135–146, 1993 [4]). In this article, an algorithm for multi-objective optimisation using neural network is presented where the variables are fuzzy. The paper deals with the core of the issue that is the fuzzy variables in multi-objective optimisation. Here, the variables are treated as triangular fuzzy variables. The arithmetic on these fuzzy variables is defined, according to the existing available work. As a numerical illustration, the new algorithm has been tested on two fractional functions. The results obtained after implementing the new algorithm using MATLAB code is presented. The algorithm uses neural network to approximate the Pareto front. This proposed algorithm is an illustration of possible optimisation technique in the fuzzy domain using Neural Network.

Keywords Fuzzy · MOOP · MOGA · VEGA · LPP

1 Introduction

Multi-objective optimisations are primarily having a number of solutions, while single-objective optimisation has one unique solution. The primary dilemma with multi-objective optimisation is a selection from alternatives of optimal solutions. However, in case a number of solutions are already worked out or derived, one can

D. Roy (✉)
CER, Mathematics Department, Indian Institute of Technology Kharagpur, Kharagpur, India
e-mail: debasishroy7@gmail.com

S. Bhattacharyya et al. (eds.), *Mathematical Modeling and Computational Tools*,
Springer Proceedings in Mathematics & Statistics 320,
https://doi.org/10.1007/978-981-15-3615-1_26

analyse every solution and make a considered selection. Thus, in multiple objectives optimisation all the objectives are treated as important and a set of solutions is derived. The solutions are to be compared on a qualitative benchmark to find the best in the context. Here a short literature review on relevant topics like fractional programming and optimisations on single and multiple objectives is presented. A new algorithm for MOOP with fuzzy variable using neural network after a brief review of fuzzy arithmetic has been given, and finally, an experiment has been conducted in MATLAB to authenticate the algorithm. The main contribution of the paper is this novel algorithm based on neural network for solving MOOP where variables are fuzzy. The algorithm proposed consists of two parts: the first part computes fuzzy dominant front using fuzzy arithmetic on the fuzzy variable. The second part demonstrates the use of neural network to evaluate this fuzzy Pareto front by first training a network and subsequently simulating to match fuzzy Pareto front with another set of fuzzy inputs with the help of the trained network.

2 Literature Review

2.1 Fractional Programming

Scholars have been working for many years on optimising ratio of linear functions. Optimisation of multiple such fractions has many practical applications [5]. Till 1985, the problem with a single ratio has ruled the arena. Among many methods which have advanced most important is LPP methods to deal fractional functions [6]. A modified simplex method to solve a function of fractional objective has been proposed by Bitran [7]. Schaible [8] used duality for finding the optimum for linear fractional programming. Multi-criteria linear programming where the efficient front is a finite number connected line segments of efficient points is dealt by Choo and Atkins [9]. Fractional interval programming is a select type which has been studied by many authors. Generalised inverses have also been used to solve such problems [10].

2.2 Single-Objective Optimisation

Random search methods comprise different algorithms ranging from pure random search to heuristic. A true random search [11] is a search method on a selected random population. These algorithms can be shown to be convergent in several way [12–14]. Box's evolutionary method has different varieties for single-objective optimisation like REVOP, EVOP, etc. These are a multi-dimensional systemic search [15]. This method is convenient as it uses optimisation method, which is free of derivative (DFO) [16–18]. Subsequently, an improvement was found by Wilson [19]. Box's method is used in many practical applications [20]. Robert Hooke and T. A Jeeves in 1961 [21] have shown that straight search method is useful for objective function which is not differentiable. The method iteratively compares current best with previous best [22]. However, convex optimisation methods define subdifferentials for non-differentiable functions as in Eq. (1).

$$\delta(\bar{\bar{\xi}}) = \{\eta \in R^n : f(\theta) - f(\xi) \geq < \eta, y - \bar{\bar{\xi}} >, \forall \theta \in R^n\} \tag{1}$$

The gradient methods [23] are efficient compared to direct search method for differentiable objective functions. Newton's method [24] is the classical method derivative-based method, and it assured convergence [25]. Conjugate direction method [26] is a variation of the Newton method. Spacer step theorem [27] is also an improved method from Newton's method.

2.3 Multi-Objective Optimisation

The difficulty in decision space is that the demands for computation increase considerably with number of variables [28, 29].

- The topological deformations is one of the methods to solve MOOP [30].
- In bounded constraint optimises single-objective, while other objectives are treated as a restrictions [31]. The boundary points found fixes the bounds of the objectives, and this is iterated till there are no new solutions left.
- The two-phase method [32] finds solutions of the affine combination of objectives in the first step, and then remaining solutions which are non-dominated are determined in phase two.

2.4 Fuzzy Multi-Objective Optimisation

Policy-makers not only contemplate "but also develop new alternatives by considering all possible situations" [2]. Some of them require multiple objectives having constraints in fuzzy domain. Many authors studied such models [4, 33, 34]. Most of the current work related to fuzzy multi-objective optimisation primarily handles by transforming fuzzy MOOP into crisp MOOP and then treating the problem in a classical way [35]. Some researcher has handled fuzzy MOOP where the constraints are fuzzy [3]. In many cases where coefficients are fuzzy, the problem is treated as fuzzy MOOP [36]. This paper handles the problem at the core by treating the variables as fuzzy. The problem has not been converted to crisp case neither the coefficients are fuzzy nor the constraints. The final non-dominant front has been proposed to be traced using neural network after due training. The algorithm has been proposed in a subsequent section. The algorithm has been implemented in MATLAB.

3 Discourse

3.1 Multi-Objective Optimisation

The type of problem this paper addresses is given in Eq. (2):

$$\begin{aligned} \text{Minimise: } & [\xi_1, \xi_2, \ldots, \xi_m] \\ \text{Subject to: } & \xi_i \in (0, 1] \\ \xi_i = & \frac{\sum_1^p c_j \gamma_j}{\sum_1^p d_i \chi_i}, \\ & \chi_i, \gamma_j \in R^+ \end{aligned} \tag{2}$$

Here, the variable space is R^p. The objective is to find the Pareto front for the function defined above.

3.2 Fuzzy Arithmetic

The problem dealt with in this paper is generalised fuzzy multi-objective optimisation which is defined in Eq. (3) :

$$\begin{aligned} \text{Minimise: } & [\tilde{\xi_1}, \tilde{\xi_2}, \ldots, \tilde{\xi_m}] \\ & \text{s.t:} \tilde{\xi_i} \leq 1, \\ \text{Where: } \tilde{\xi_j} = & \frac{\sum_{i=1}^n c_{ij} \tilde{\gamma_i}}{\sum_{i=1}^n d_{ij} \tilde{\chi_i}} \end{aligned} \tag{3}$$

Here, $\tilde{\chi}$ and $\tilde{\gamma}$ are n-dimensional fuzzy variable. Before delving into the solution procedure, there is a need to define fuzzy arithmetic of fuzzy variables. Ranks of fuzzy numbers must be established for ordering the fuzzy variables in order for a decision maker to take a call. Fuzzy sets can have non-empty intersection, and therefore, it is problematic to establish clearly as to which fuzzy number (FN) is larger. Here, a ranking function, which establishes a bijection between FN and R^+, will be used. The idea of ordering the functions for comparing normal fuzzy numbers is built in there. This paper presents a method to solve the fuzzy MOOP using **Neural Network** in which the variables are triangular fuzzy variables.

Fuzzy set is pair (Λ, m), where m: $\Lambda \rightarrow [0, 1]$ is a membership function. The set Λ is the universe of discourse, and for every $\xi \in \Lambda$, $m(\xi)$ is called membership level of ξ in (Λ, m).

TFN Λ is depicted by three real numbers κ, λ, μ whose interpretations are given in Fig. 1. TFN $\equiv$ Triangular Fuzzy Number.

Fig. 1 TFN

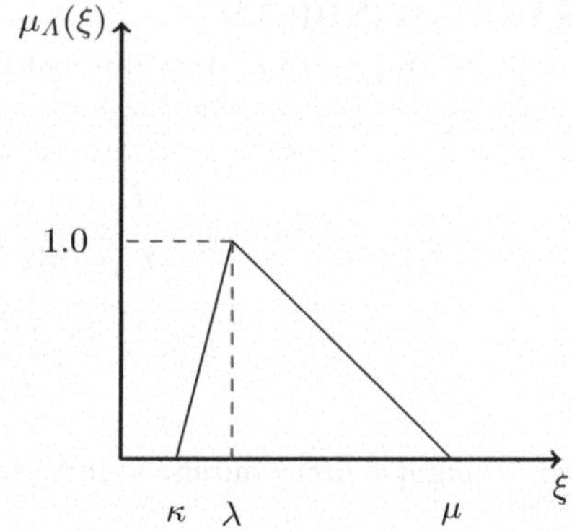

Therefore, a TFN is represented as: $\tilde{\Lambda} = (\kappa, \lambda, \mu)$.

Arithmetic on TFN

Let $\tilde{\Lambda}_1 = (\kappa_1, \lambda_1, \mu_1)$ and $\tilde{\Lambda}_2 = (\kappa_2, \lambda_2, \mu_2)$ be two triangular fuzzy numbers and let $\tilde{\Lambda}_i = (\kappa_i, \lambda_i, \mu_i)$ be a generalised fuzzy number. The arithmetic operations are defined in Eqs. (4)–(7).

ADDITION

$$\sum \tilde{\Lambda}_i = \sum \left(\kappa_i, \lambda_i, \mu_i\right) = \left(\sum \kappa_i, \sum \lambda_i, \sum \mu_i\right) \tag{4}$$

SUBTRACTION

$$\tilde{\Lambda}_1 - \tilde{\Lambda}_2 = (\kappa_1 - \kappa_2, \lambda_1 - \lambda_2, \mu_1 - \mu_2) \tag{5}$$

DIVISION

$$\frac{\tilde{\Lambda}_1}{\tilde{\Lambda}_2} = \left(\min\left(\left(\frac{\kappa_i}{\lambda_j}\right), i, j = 1, 2\right), \max\left(\left(\frac{\kappa_i}{\lambda_j}\right), i, j = 1, 2\right)\right) \tag{6}$$

SCALAR MULTIPLICATION

$$\begin{aligned} c > 0, \tilde{\Lambda}c &= (\kappa_1 c, \lambda_1 c, \mu_1 c) \\ c < 0, \tilde{\Lambda}c &= (\mu_1 c, \lambda_1 c, \kappa_1 c) \end{aligned} \tag{7}$$

PARTIAL ORDER

1. $\leq$ is defined by $\tilde{\Lambda}_1 \leq \tilde{\Lambda}_2$ iff MAX $(\Lambda_1, \Lambda_2) = \Lambda_2$
2. For any two triangular fuzzy numbers $\tilde{\Lambda}_1 \leq \tilde{\Lambda}_2$ iff $\kappa_1 - \lambda_1 \leq \kappa_2 - \lambda_2, \kappa_1 + \mu_1 \leq \kappa_2 + \mu_2$.

RANKING INDICES
Centroid (x_0, y_0) of a fuzzy number is given by a formula in Eq. (8) [37].

$$x_0 = \frac{\int_a^b xL_A(x)\mathrm{d}x + \int_b^c x\mathrm{d}x + \int_c^d xR_A(x)\mathrm{d}x}{\int_a^b L_A(x)\mathrm{d}x + \int_b^c x\mathrm{d}x + \int_c^d xR_A(x)\mathrm{d}x}$$
$$y_0 = \frac{\int_0^w yR_A^{-1}(y)\mathrm{d}y - \int_0^w yL_A^{-1}(y)\mathrm{d}y}{\int_0^w R_A^{-1}(y)\mathrm{d}y - \int_0^w yL_A^{-1}(y)\mathrm{d}y} \quad (8)$$

For triangular fuzzy numbers, this yields as stated in Eq. (9).

$$x_0 = \frac{1}{2}(a+b+c),\ y_0 = \frac{w}{3} \quad (9)$$

By this method, triangular fuzzy numbers can be compared and imposed a rank calculated from their centroid.
Another idea of ranking is as in Eq. (10).

$$R(A) = \sqrt{x_0(A)^2 + y_0(A)^2} \quad (10)$$

The fuzzy numbers can be ranked based on x_0 values and then on y_0 values. The various methods of fuzzy multi-objective methodologies primarily deal with fuzzy parameters, coefficients of constraints, objective function, etc. However in this paper, the fuzzy variable in multi-objective optimisation has been dealt with using neural network to handle real-world problems. The focal point is not only fuzzy MOOP but the individual fractional functions. The fractional functions attract special attention due the fact that they clearly define efficiency of a system. But a clear solution to fractional functions in multi-dimension is not available. The specific case of multiple fractional functions is of serious interest since there are always situations which may require optimisation of the efficiency of multiple units. The problem formulation may incorporate a number of constraints. But this paper has demonstrated a way of handling the situation in a novel way with existing methodologies like neural network. Experiment section demonstrates numerical example. The fractional functions are particularly interesting due to non-availability of analytic solution for optimisation of the function.

4 A New Algorithm for MOOP with Fuzzy Variables

The proposed algorithm is presented below.

Algorithm 1 Neural Network-Based Fuzzy Multi-objective Optimisation

Step1- Select n random fuzzy numbers. Here, n=100.
Step1.1- Ordered random triplet (a,b,c) defined over [0,1] represents fuzzy numbers.
Step 1.2 - Choose 100 such ordered random triplets. These are treated as 100 random fuzzy triangular numbers.
Step 2: For each fuzzy number, compute z_i using fuzzy arithmetic described in Section 3.2 on Equation 3. Thereby, a vector of $(z_1, z_2, \ldots, z_m)$ is formed depending on number of functions to be evaluated.
Step 3: Find non-dominant set of solutions from the 100 solutions based on fuzzy genetic algorithm and fuzzy ranking. Follow subsequent steps to generate elitist.
Step 3.1- For each fuzzy variable z_i , compute the centroid. Thereby, 100 X 2 matrix is formed.
Step 3.2- Compute the ranking of Centroid for each point.
Step 3.3- Keep r proportion of dominant points.
Step 4- Repeat Step 3 to iterate subsequent steps by genetic algorithm till distance between Pareto fronts of two successive steps is more than 10^{-4}.
Step 5- Based on the non-dominant set generate Pareto front.
Step 6- Set up a feedforward network with random weights.
while Standard Deviation of Error $> 10^{-4}$ **do**
  Step 7- Train the network with the inputs defined in Step 1 after defuzzifying and non-dominant front as output. The revised weights for the network are stored.
  Step 8- Generate a set of fuzzy random values to find the non-dominated front.
  Step 9- Simulate the network output with the input.
  Step 10- Retrain the network or recompute the weight.
end while

In this algorithm, 100 ordered random triplets are chosen to initialise the population. The two-objective functions are evaluated using fuzzy arithmetic to get hundred two-dimensional FN. The ranking of the FN is done using propositions of Chu and Tsao stated in Eq. (10). The top ten ranks are kept as elitist. This is the initialisation of the algorithm. The Pareto front is generated using fuzzy genetic algorithm [38, 39]. This is the dominant front for this population. The dominant front is used as the output of a neural network, while inputs are 100 random fuzzy numbers after defuzzification [40]. The network is trained with this set. The trained neural network can be used approximate the non-dominant front. Here, a feedforward multilayer perceptron model is used to train with set of inputs generated by the precalculations stated above. Theoretically, any function can be approximated by neural network [41]. Neural networks are nonlinear function approximators. The proof is based on extension of the Weierstrass theorem [42]. This actually follows from a stronger version of Kolmogorov's construction which states that $\forall f \in \mathbb{C}_n$ can be represented as:

$$f(x_1, \ldots, x_n) = \sum_{q=1}^{2n+1} g\left\{\sum_{p=1}^{n} \lambda^{pq} \psi(x_p + q\epsilon)\right\} \tag{11}$$

where $g(\xi) \in \mathbb{C}$, λ, and ϵ are constants, $\psi(\xi) \in \mathbb{C}$ is monotonic increasing and Holder continuous, λ, ϵ, ψ being independent of f.
The presented algorithm demonstrates the use of neural network for approximation of fuzzy dominant front, which can be further used for optimisation.

5 Experiment

5.1 Set-Up

$$
\begin{aligned}
\text{Minimise: } b_1 &= \frac{3\tilde{a}_1 + 4\tilde{a}_2 + 1}{5\tilde{a}_1 + 7\tilde{x}_2 + 5}, b_2 = \frac{4\tilde{a}_1 + 5\tilde{a}_2 + 2}{7\tilde{a}_1 + 9\tilde{a}_2 + 3} \\
& 5\tilde{a}_1 + 7\tilde{a}_2 + 5 \neq 0, 7\tilde{a}_1 + 9\tilde{a}_2 + 3 \neq 0 \\
& \frac{3\tilde{a}_1 + 4\tilde{a}_2 + 1}{5\tilde{a}_1 + 7\tilde{a}_2 + 5} \leq 1, \frac{4\tilde{a}_1 + 5\tilde{a}_2 + 2}{7\tilde{a}_1 + 9\tilde{a}_2 + 3} \leq 1
\end{aligned} \tag{12}
$$

Here, $\tilde{a}_1$ and $\tilde{a}_2$ are triangular fuzzy variables.

5.2 Operation

The arithmetic and order of fuzzy numbers are already defined. MATLAB code was written to implement the algorithm.

5.3 Results

Coordinates of non-dominated fuzzy front is presented in Table 1. The non-dominant fuzzy front as computed by the proposed new algorithm due to simulation by neural network (NN) in MATLAB is presented in Fig 2. The FFNN with three layers and the training of NN in the toolbox of MATLAB are given in Figs. 3 and 4.
FFNN ≡ Feedforward Neural Network.

6 Conclusion

The non-dominated front from random triangular fuzzy variables is computed using a new proposed algorithm which has been implemented in MATLAB. A neural network is trained to derive this output from fuzzy random inputs. This network is found to generate the fuzzy dominant front from another set of fuzzy inputs at a reasonable approximation. The algorithm demonstrates the use of neural network as the first step to fuzzy multi-objective optimisation. The algorithm has been validated with numerical experiment. The graphical and tabular results are presented in the paper. The MATLAB code for the algorithm with 100 random initial fuzzy numbers and two-objective test function given in Eq. (12) is given in Sect. 7.

Table 1 Non-dominated fuzzy front simulated by neural network

X	*Y*
0.1285	0.2786
0.1387	0.2903
0.1243	0.2964
0.1242	0.3034
0.1372	0.3193
0.1215	0.3222
0.1283	0.3429
0.1283	0.3429
0.1275	0.3457
0.1252	0.3490

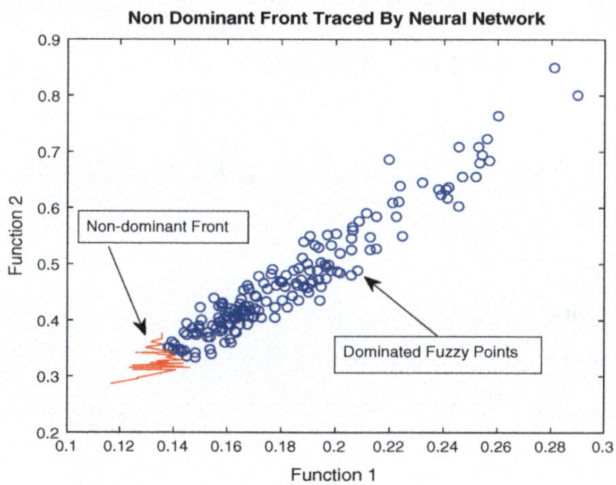

Fig. 2 Fuzzy Pareto front derived by neural network

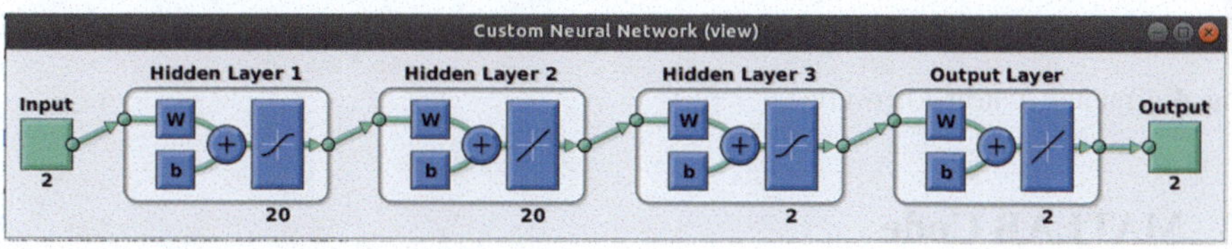

Fig. 3 Feedforward neural network

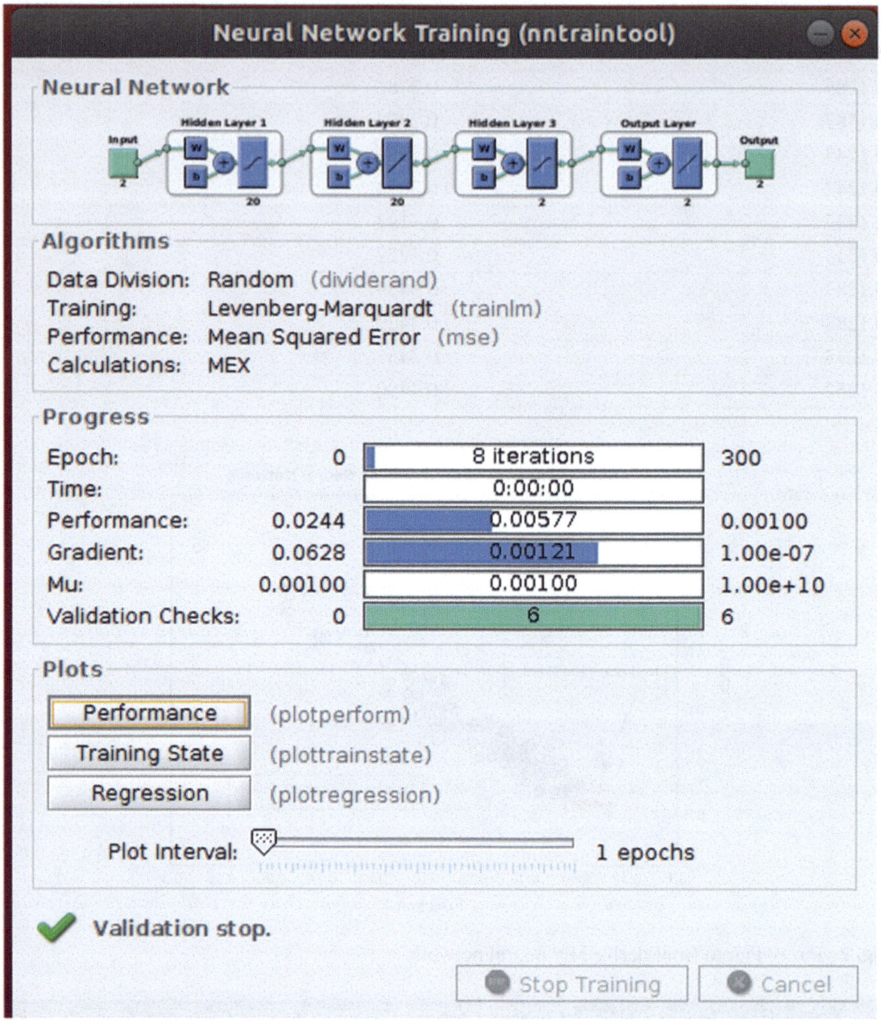

Fig. 4 Training of neural network

7 MATLAB Code

Listing 1.1 This is the MATLAB Code.

```
function []=NeuNetfuzzyMOOPLatest()
ptn=200;mnx=.001; mxx=1.001;mny=.001;mxy=1.001;dim=200;
fuzzout=ones(2,dim);
[nd_s o ii]=fuzzyMOOP(dim);
[m n]=size(nd_s);
fuzzout(:,1:n)=nd_s(:,1:n);
%disp(out');
nt=newff(ii,o,[22 22 2],{'logsig','transig'},'trainlm');
```

```
disp(net);
view(net);
nt.trainParam.show=60;
nt.trainParam.lr=0.06;
nt.trainParam.epochs=350;
nt.trainParam.goal=1.1e-3;
nt1=train(nt,ii,o);
sim_out=sim(nt1,ii);
[sim_dm sim_ndm]=evalDom(sim_out);
[k l]=size(sim_ndm);
[k1 l1]=size(nd_s);
l1=min(l,l1);
err=nd_s(:,1:l1)-sim_ndm(1:2,1:l1);
disp('err');disp(err');
% First Plot
f=figure;
set(f,'name','1st Plot Simulated and Actual Output for testing','numbertitle','off');
plot(o(1,:),o(2,:),'g*',sim_out(1,:),sim_out(2,:),'bo');
title('Plot of simulated output and actual output');
%err=sim_out-o;
disp('err');disp(err');
%disp(' non dominated');disp(');
%disp('sim_out');disp(sim_out(:,1:n)');
% SECOND RUN FOR TESTING THE NETWORK
[nd_s1 o1 ii1]=fuzzyMOOP(dim);
sim_out1=sim(nt1,ii1);
[sim_dm1 sim_ndm1]=evalDom(sim_out1);
[k2 l2]=size(sim_ndm1);
[k3 l3]=size(nd_s1);
l11=min(l2,l3);
err1=nd_s1(:,1:l11)-sim_ndm1(1:2,1:l11);
disp('nd_s1');
disp(size(nd_s1(:,1:l11)));
disp(size(sim_ndm1(1:2,1:l11)));
figure;
set(f,'name','2nd PlotActual and Simulated Non Dominated Set','numbertitle','off');
plot(nd_s1(1,1:l11),nd_s1(2,1:l11),'-r',sim_ndm1(1,1:l11),sim_ndm(2,1:l11),'-b');
title('Plot of Actual values and Simulated values');
disp('err1');disp(err1');
% REDUCING DISTANCE FROM THE IDEAL POINT
[f1 x1 f2 x2]=idealPoint()
end

function []=distanceEst()
end
function [f1 x1 f2 x2]=idealPoint()
clc; clear data;
param1=[3 4 1 5 7 5];
param2=[4 5 2 7 9 3];
[f1 x1 i1 t1]=gradDescMod([1 1],param1);
[f2 x2 i2 t2]=gradDescMod([1 1],param2);

end

function [nd_s o ii]=fuzzyMOOP(dim)
o=ones(2,dim);
ii=ones(2,dim);
for i=1:dim
[o1 o2 i1 i2]=subFuzzyMOOP();
o(:,i)=[o1 o2];
ii(:,i)=[i1 i2];
end
[dm ndm]=evalDom(o);
[nd_s]=sortFND(ndm);
% disp('dm'); disp(dm');
% disp('ndm'); disp(nd_s');
figure;
```

```
plot(dm(1,:),dm(2,:),'bo',nd_s(1,:),nd_s(2,:),'-r');
end

function [nd_s]=sortFND(ndm)
[m n]=size(ndm);
[ynd_s p]=sort(ndm(2,:));
xnd_s=ones(1,n);
nd_s=ones(2,n);
for i=1:n
    xnd_s(i)=ndm(1,p(i));
    nd_s(:,i)=[xnd_s(i) ynd_s(i)];
end
end

function [dm ndm]=evalDom(o)
% Here Domination of values is checked
 [m n]=size(o);
 DN=zeros(3, n);
 dmi=zeros(3,n);
 ndmi=zeros(3,n);
   k=1;l=1;
   Mx=max(DN(3,:));
   disp('Max Val');
   disp(Mx);
  for i=1:n
      if DN(3,i) <Mx/10-1
          ndmi(:,k)=DN(:,i);
          k=k+1;
      end
      if DN(3,i) > Mx/10
          dmi(:,l)=DN(:,i);
          l=l+1;
      end
  end
  dm=dmi(:,1:l-1);
  ndm=ndmi(:,1:k-1);

  %end of function
end

function [o1 i1 i2]=subFuzzyMOOP()
[xfuzzy,l1,m1,n1]=triang(a1,b1,c1,x);
[yfuzzy,l2,m2,n2]=triang(a2,b2,c2,y);
[ix1 iy1]=Centroid(xfuzzy);
i1=ix1*iy1;
[ix2 iy2]=Centroid(yfuzzy);
i2=ix2*iy2;
[z1]=fuzzyFn1(xfuzzy,yfuzzy);
[z2]=fuzzyFn2(xfuzzy,yfuzzy);
[NFz1 NFz2]=NonZeroExtract(z1,z2);
[x1 y1]=Centroid(NFz1);
o1=x1*y1;
[x2 y2]=Centroid(NFz2);
o2=x2*y2;
figure;
plot(NFz1(1,:),NFz1(2,:),'g*',NFz2(1,:),NFz2(2,:),'bo',x1,y1,'g+',x2,y2,'b+');
end

[m n]=size(z);
maxVal=max(z(2,:));
a=z(1,1);
c=z(1,n);
for i=1:n
    if maxVal==z(2,i)
        b=z(1,i);
    end
```

```
end
x=(a+b+c)/3;
y=maxVal/3;
end

function [NFz1 NFz2]=NonZeroExtract(z1,z2)
global point_n;
k=0;l=0;Nz1=ones(3,point_n);Nz2=ones(3,point_n);
for i=1:point_n
    if z2(2,i) ~=0
        l=l+1;
        Nz2(1:2,l)=z2(1:2,i);Nz2(3,l)=i;
    end
end
kk=k;ll=l;
NFz1=Nz1(:,1:kk);NFz2=Nz2(:,1:ll);
end
function [z]=fuzzyFn1(xfuzzy,yfuzzy)
[z1,l1,m1,n1]=fuzzScalarMult(xfuzzy);
[z2,l2,m2,n2]=fuzzScalarMult(yfuzzy);
[z3,l3,m3,n3]=fuzzScalarMult(xfuzzy);
[z4,l4,m4,n4]=fuzzScalarMult(xfuzzy);
[nm1,ln1,mn1,nn1]=fuzzAdd(z1(1,:),l1,m1,n1,z2(1,:),l2,m2,n2);
[dm1,ld1,md1,nd1]=fuzzAdd(z3(1,:),l3,m3,n3,z4(1,:),l4,m4,n4);
[dm,ld,md,nd]=fuzzScalarAdd(dm1(1,:),ld1,md1,nd1,dm1(1,:),3);
[nm,ln,mn,nn]=fuzzScalarAdd(nm1(1,:),ln1,mn1,nn1,nm1(1,:),2);
[z,lfinal,mfinal,nfinal]=fuzzDiv(nm,ln,mn,nn,dm,ld,md,nd);
end
function [z]=fuzzyFn2(xfuzzy,yfuzzy)
 [z1,l1,m1,n1]=fuzzScalarMult(xfuzzy,l1,m1,n1,3);
[z2,l2,m2,n2]=fuzzScalarMult(yfuzzy,l2,m2,n2,4);
[z3,l3,m3,n3]=fuzzScalarMult(xfuzzy,l1,m1,n1,5);
[z4,l4,m4,n4]=fuzzScalarMult(xfuzzy,l2,m2,n2,7);
[nm1,ln1,mn1,nn1]=fuzzAdd(z1(1,:),l1,m1,n1,z2(1,:),l2,m2,n2);
[dm1,ld1,md1,nd1]=fuzzAdd(z3(1,:),l3,m3,n3,z4(1,:),l4,m4,n4);
[dm,ld,md,nd]=fuzzScalarAdd(dm1(1,:),ld1,md1,nd1,dm1(1,:),1);
[nm,ln,mn,nn]=fuzzScalarAdd(nm1(1,:),ln1,mn1,nn1,nm1(1,:),5);
[z,lfinal,mfinal,nfinal]=fuzzDiv(nm,ln,mn,nn,dm,ld,md,nd);
end


function [fuzzyScalarAddxk,l3,m3,n3]=fuzzScalarAdd(xfuzzy,l1,m1,n1,x,k)
l3=l1+k;m3=m1+k;n3=n1+k;xk=x+k;
[fuzzyScalarAddxk,l3,m3,n3]=triang(l3,m3,n3,xk);
end

function [fuzzyScalarMultxy,l3,m3,n3]=fuzzScalarMult(xfuzzy,l1,m1,n1,k)
l3=k*l1;
m3=k*m1;
n3=k*n1;
xk=k*xfuzzy(1,:);
[fuzzyScalarMultxy,l3,m3,n3]=triang(l3,m3,n3,xk);
end

function [fuzzyDivxy,l3,m3,n3]=fuzzDiv(xfuzzy,yfuzzy)
% Range of the fuzzy variable is to be worked out
n3=max(a);
deltal=(l3-((l1+l2)/2));
deltau=1-((n1+n2)/2);
if deltal < 0
    lb=0;
else
    lb=deltal;
end
ub=n3+abs(deltal);
xy=linspace(lb,ub,point_n);
[fuzzyDivxy,l3,m3,n3]=triang(l3,m3,n3,xy);
```

```
end

function [fuzzyMultxy,l3,m3,n3]=fuzzMult(xfuzzy,yfuzzy)
l3=min(a);
m3=m1*m2;
n3=max(a);
avg=(l1+l2)/2;
delta=l3-avg;
lb=delta;
ub=1+lb;
Multxy=linspace(lb,ub,point_n);
[fuzzyMultxy,l3,m3,n3]=triang(l3,m3,n3,Multxy);
end

function [fuzzySubxy,l3,m3,n3]=fuzzSub(xfuzzy,yfuzzy)
n3=n1-n2;
[fuzzySubxy,l3,m3,n3]=triang(l3,m3,n3,xfuzzy(1,:));
disp('inside fuzz sub');
end

function [fuzzyAddxy,l3,m3,n3]=fuzzAdd(xfuzzy,l1,m1,n1,yfuzzy,l2,m2,n2)
global point_n;
l3=l1+l2;
m3=m1+m2;
n3=n1+n2;
delta=l3-((l1+l2)/2);
lb=delta;
ub=n3+abs(1-((n1+n2)/2));
% 100 is to be parameterised
addxy=linspace(lb,ub,point_n);
[fuzzyAddxy,l3,m3,n3]=triang(l3,m3,n3,addxy(1,:));
end

function [xfuzzy,l1,m1,n1]=triang(a,b,c,x)
l1=a;m1=b;n1=c;
[p q]=size(x);
xfuzzy=ones(2,q);
xfuzzy(1,:)=x;
for i=1:q
    if x(i)<a
        l=i;
    end;
    if  x(i)<b
        m=i;
     end;
    if x(i)<c
        n=i;
    end;
end
   uslope=1.0/(b-a);
    lslope=1.0/(c-b);
   for i=1:l
       xfuzzy(2,i)=0;
   end
   for i=l+1:m
       xfuzzy(2,i)=uslope*(x(i)-x(l));
   end
   for i=m+1:n
       xfuzzy(2,i)=lslope*(x(n)-x(i));
   end
   for i=n+1:q
       xfuzzy(2,i)=0;
  end
  end
```

References

1. Lootsma, F.A.: Fuzzy Multi-Objective Optimization. Springer, Boston, MA (1997). https://doi.org/10.1007/978-1-4757-2618-3_7
2. Young-Jou, L., Ching-Lai, H.: Fuzzy multiple objective decision making: methods and applications (1994)
3. Chuntian, C.: Fuzzy optimal model for the flood control system of the upper and middle reaches of the yangtze river. Hydrol. Sci. J. **44**(4), 573–582 (1999)
4. Young Jou Lai CLH: Possibilistic linear programming for managing interest rate risk. Fuzzy Sets Syst. **54**(2), 135–146 (1993)
5. Cohon, J.L.: Multicriteria programming: brief review and application. In: Design Optimization, pp. 163–191 (1985)
6. Charnes, A., Cooper, W.W.: An explicit general solution in linear fractional programming. Nav. Res. Logist. Q. **20**(3), 449–467 (1973)
7. Bitran, G.R., Novaes, A.G.: Linear programming with a fractional objective function. Oper. Res. **21**(1), 22–29 (1973). https://doi.org/10.1287/opre.21.1.22
8. Schaible, S.: Fractional programming. I, duality. Manage. Sci. **22**(8), 858–867 (1976). https://doi.org/10.1287/mnsc.22.8.858
9. Choo, E.U., Atkins, D.R.: Bicriteria linear fractional programming. J. Optim. Theory Appl. **36**(2), 203–220 (1982). https://doi.org/10.1007/BF00933830
10. Buhler, W.: A note on fractional interval programming. Oper. Res. A B **19**, 29–36 (1975)
11. Banks, J.: Handbook of Simulation: Principles, Methodology, Advances, Applications, and Practice. Wiley, Hoboken (1998)
12. Billingsley, P.: Convergence of Probability Measures. John, Hoboken (2013)
13. Cabo, M., Possani, E.: Considerations on applying cross entropy methods to the vehicle routing problem. Int. J. Comb. Optim. Probl. Inform. **6**(3), 22 (2015)
14. Grefenstette, J.J.: Optimization of control parameters for genetic algorithms. IEEE Trans. Syst. Man Cybern. **16**(1), 122–128 (1986)
15. Box GE.: Evolutionary operation: a method for increasing industrial productivity. Appl. Stat. 81–101 (1957)
16. Brent, R.P.: Algorithms for Minimization Without Derivatives. Courier Corporation (2013)
17. Mifflin JJS Robert: A bracketing technique to ensure desirable convergence in univariate minimization. Math. Program. **43**(1–3), 117–130 (1989)
18. Robert Mifflin JJS: A rapidly convergent five-point algorithm for univariate minimization. Math. Program. **62**(1–3), 299–319 (1993)
19. Box, G.: Wkb on the experimental attainment of optimum condition. J. R. Stat. Soc. Ser. B **13**(1), 20 (1951)
20. George, E.P., Box, N.R.D.: Evolutionary Operation: A Statistical Method for Process Improvement, vol. 67. Wiley, Hoboken (1998)
21. Xiaoli Zhang, Y.W., Zhou, Qinghua: An efficient pattern search method. J. Appl. Math. Phys. **1**(04), 68 (2013)
22. Swan, W.J.: Report on Development of New Direct Search Method of Optimisation. Tech. Rep, ICI Ltd. (1964)
23. Fletcher, R.: Practical Methods of Optimization. Wiley, Hoboken (2013)
24. Gill, P.E., Murray, W., Wright, M.H.: Practical optimization. Academic press (1981)
25. Gabay, D.: Reduced quasi-newton methods with feasibility improvement for nonlinearly constrained optimization. In: Algorithms for Constrained Minimization of Smooth Nonlinear Functions, pp. 18–44. Springer, New York (1982)
26. Adams, L.M., Nazareth, J.L., et al. (1996) Linear and Nonlinear Conjugate Gradient-Related Methods, vol. 85. Siam
27. Zangwill, W.I.: Nonlinear programming: a unified approach. Prentice-Hall (1969)
28. Engau, A.: Interactive decomposition-coordination methods for complex decision problems. In: Handbook of Multicriteria Analysis, pp. 329–365. Springer, New York (2010)

29. Geue, F.: An improved n-tree algorithm for the enumeration of all neighbors of a degenerate vertex. Ann. Oper. Res. **46**(2), 361–391 (1993)
30. Maeda, T.: Second order conditions for efficiency non-smooth multi objective optimisation. J. Optim. Theory Appl. **122**(3), 139–153 (2004)
31. Ricardo Feced, M.A.M., Zervas, Michalis N.: An efficient inverse scattering algorithm for the design of nonuniform fiber bragg gratings. IEEE J. Quantum Electron. **35**(8), 1105–1115 (1999)
32. Ulungu, E.L. Teghem, J.: The two phases method- an efficient process to solve bi-objective combinatorial optimisation problems. Foundaions Comput. Decis. Sci. **20**(2), 149–165 (1995)
33. Lai, J.Y.: Imost: interactive multiple objective system technique. J. Oper. Res. Soc. **46**(8), 958–976 (1995)
34. Zimmermann, H.J.: Fuzzy programming and linear programming with several objective functions. Fuzzy Sets Syst. **1**(1), 45–55 (1978)
35. Kannan, D., Khodaverdi, R., Olfat, L., Jafarian, A., Khodaverdi, A..: Integrated fuzzy multi criteria decision making method and multi-objective programming approach for supplier selection and order allocation in a green supply chain. J. Clean. **47**, 355–367 (2013). https://www.sciencedirect.com/science/article/pii/S0959652613000590
36. Carlsson, C.: Fuzzy multiple criteria decision making: recent developments. Fuzzy Sets Syst. **78**(2), 139–153 (1996). https://www.sciencedirect.com/science/article/pii/0165011495001654
37. Cheng, C.H.: A new approach for ranking fuzzy numbers by distance method. Fuzzy Sets Syst. **95**(3), 307–317 (1998). https://doi.org/10.1016/S0165-0114(96)00272-2
38. Herrera, F., Lozano, M.: Fuzzy genetic algorithms: issues and models. Tech. Rep. (1994) https://pdfs.semanticscholar.org/8595/aedf2e923018a1d1fac85bec28c0c309445a.pdf
39. Schaefer, G., Nakashima, T.: Michigan vs. pittsburgh style ga optimisation of fuzzy rule bases for gene expression analysis. Int. J. Fuzzy. Syst. Appl. **3**(4), 60–72 (2013). https://doi.org/10.4018/ijfsa.2013100105
40. Fortemps MR (1996) Ranking and defuzzification methods based on area compensation. https://www.sciencedirect.com/science/article/pii/0165011495002731
41. Nielsen, M.: Neural networks and deep learning (2015). http://static.latexstudio.net/article/2018/0912/neuralnetworksanddeeplearning.pdf
42. Barron, A.: Universal approximation bounds for superpositions of a sigmoidal function. IEEE Trans. Inf. Theory (1993)

Multi-choice Chance-Constrained Programming Problems Using Genetic Algorithm

D. K. Mohanty, R. K. Jana and M. P. Biswal

Abstract Multi-choice programming (MCP) problem is a type of combinatorial optimization problem where the decision maker has to choose a value for a parameter from many alternative values. Genetic algorithm (GA) is a very popular approach used for solving combinatorial optimization problems. If some or all parameters present in the MCP problem are random, then it is known as multi-choice stochastic programming or multi-choice probabilistic programming (MCPP) problem. Chance-constrained programming (CCP) and two-stage stochastic programming (TSSP) are widely used to solve problems involving randomness. In this paper, we have considered an MCPP problem where some parameters are multi-choice types, and some are random variables. First, we apply the CCP technique to convert it to a deterministic MCP problem. While solving MCP problems, generally, some transformation techniques are used to transform the MCP problem into a mixed-integer programming (MIP) problem. After that, a standard mathematical programming approach is followed to solve the transformed MIP problem. These transformation techniques generate some extra variables and extra constraints which complicates the problem. But here we have proposed a GA to solve the MCP problem directly (without using any transformation technique). At last, a numerical example is provided to demonstrate the proposed algorithm and the solution approach.

Keywords Stochastic programming · Chance-constrained programming · Multi-choice programming · Genetic algorithm

---

D. K. Mohanty (✉) · M. P. Biswal
Indian Institute of Technology Kharagpur, Kharagpur 721 302, India
e-mail: dkmohanty.iitkgp@gmail.com

R. K. Jana
Indian Institute of Management Raipur, GEC Campus, Sejbahar 492 015, India

S. Bhattacharyya et al. (eds.), *Mathematical Modeling and Computational Tools*, Springer Proceedings in Mathematics & Statistics 320,
https://doi.org/10.1007/978-981-15-3615-1_27

1 Introduction

While solving many real-life decision-making problems, the decision maker (DM) has often to take decisions where some or all input parameters are uncertain.These uncertainties of the parameters can be expressed by using fuzzy numbers or random variables or intervals. Probabilistic programming or stochastic programming (SP) is a class of uncertain programming where the parameters present in the objective function and/or in the constraints are considered as random variables. Many methodologies and techniques have been developed in the area of SP; among them, two very popular approaches are widely used to solve SP problems, these are,

(i) Chance-constrained programming (CCP) and
(ii) Two-stage stochastic programming (TSSP).

The CCP technique is used to solve the problems where constraints are allowed to violate up to certain probability levels. This technique was initially introduced by Charnes and Cooper [1]. Several models and methodologies used to solve SP have been proposed by many researchers [2–4]. Stancu and Wets [5] presented a nice literature review of CCP . In most of the SP models, the uncertain parameters are assumed to follow normal distributions. In some cases, the decision makers used other non-normal distributions for their models. Goicoechea et al. [6] have presented deterministic equivalents to multi-objective SP models where random variables follow different continuous distributions. Later, Goicoechea and Duckstein [7] presented an equivalent deterministic model for a SP model where the cost coefficients are considered as random variables following uniform distributions. Miller and Wagner [8, 9] have presented a procedure to find deterministic equivalent of chance-constrained models with joint constraints where the right-hand side parameters are independent random variables. Further, Jagannathan [9] presented an equivalent deterministic model of a joint CCP problem where the technological coefficients are normally distributed where right-hand side constants are treated as dependent random variables. Later, Sahoo and Biswal [10] have presented the solution procedure of some SP problems with joint constraints where the parameters follow normal and log-normal random distribution.

In some chance-constrained programming problems, the DM is allowed to set multiple values for some or all parameters to handle uncertainties; these types of problems are called multi-choice chance-constrained programming (MCCCP) problems. Healey [11] first introduced multi-choice programming technique to solve problems under uncertainty. A survey of multi-choice programming (MCP) and its different solution procedures have been presented by [12]. Chang [13] proposed different methods to solve goal programming (GP) problems where the aspiration levels are considered to be of multi-choice types. They have used a binary variable to tackle multi-choiceness of each goal. Later, Liao [14] used the method provided by Chang [13] to solve multi-segment GP problem where aspirations levels are multi-segments.

Further, Chang et al. [15] have proposed a new method to solve multi-coefficient GP, for multi-group pricing problem. Biswal and Acharya [16] have presented a new technique to solve MCP problems; they have used interpolating polynomials to handle multi-choice parameters. Later, Acharya and Biswal [17] presented a method to solve multi-choice SP problems where parameters present in the right-hand side of the constraints have multiple choices, and technological coefficients are random variables.

Genetic algorithm (GA) is a population-based stochastic search technique that is inspired by the laws of natural evolution and selection. It was introduced by John Holland [18] as a computer-based model to solve the problems whose deterministic models are very costly. GA is very useful to solve optimization problems, particularly nonlinear programming problems. Unlike classical optimization methods, GA does not require derivatives and does not stuck at local optima during solving nonlinear programming problems. Several researchers have applied GAs to solve many optimization problems [19–21]. Homaifar et al. [22] developed a special GA to solve nonlinear constrained optimization problems; he used a penalty function to handle the constraints. Later, a new constraint handling technique had been developed by Deb [23] where no penalty parameters are required. Further, Jana and Biswal [24] proposed a GA based on stochastic simulation to solve CCP problems where some parameters are random. Nazario and Ruggiero [25] presented a heuristic algorithm for solving a mixed-integer programming problem, and they successfully applied this algorithm in designing a production planning. Yokota et al. [26] presented a GA to solve a nonlinear mixed-integer problem; they used penalty function to evaluate chromosomes and applied this algorithm to solve several problems involving system reliability. Later, Wasanapradit et al. [27] proposed an improved genetic algorithm to solve nonlinear mixed-integer programming problem by improving on the work of Yokota et al. [26].They have used secant method with bisection method for converting chromosomes from infeasible to feasible chromosomes. Recently, Mohanty et al. [28] proposed a GA to solve multi-choice integer linear programming problems.

In this study, we have considered a CCP problem in which right-hand side parameters of the constraints are multi-choice type and left-hand side parameters are normal random variables. First, we apply CCP technique to convert the problem to a MCP problem which is also nonlinear and then we use our proposed genetic algorithm to solve the MCP directly and without using any transformation techniques.

2 Multi-choice Chance-Constrained Programming Model

The mathematical formulation of a MCCCP problem is given by:

$$\min : z = \sum_{j=1}^{n} c_j x_j \tag{1}$$

subject to

$$\text{Prob}\Big(\sum_{j=1}^{n} a_{ij}x_j \geq b_i\Big) \geq (1-\beta_i),\ b_i \in \{b_i^{(1)}, b_i^{(2)}, \ldots, b_i^{(t_i)}\},\quad i = 1, 2, \ldots, m \quad (2)$$

$$0 < \beta_i < 1, \qquad i = 1, 2 \ldots, m \quad (3)$$

$$x_j \geq 0, \quad j = 1, 2, 3, \ldots, n. \quad (4)$$

where $x_1, x_2, \ldots, x_n$ are n decision variables, right-hand side parameter b_i $(i = 1, 2, \ldots, m)$ of the i-th constraint is considered to be multi-choice types. Each b_i $(i = 1, 2, \ldots, m)$ has t_i number of different choices. Only the left-hand side parameters a_{ij} $(i = 1, 2, \ldots, m;\ j = 1, 2, \ldots, n)$ of the constraints are considered as random variables following some continuous distributions. Here, $Prob$ stands for the probability, β_i is the probability level up to which i-th constraint violation is permitted. The inequalities presented by (2) are known as probabilistic constraints or chance constraints. Charnes and Cooper [1] developed CCP technique to solve the optimization problems involving chance constraints. Here, we assume all the random variables a_{ij} $(i = 1, 2, \ldots, m;\ j = 1, 2, \ldots, n)$ as normal independent random variables. Using CCP technique, we will first convert MCCCP problem to an equivalent deterministic MCP problem.

2.1 Conversion of MCCCP to Deterministic MCP

For establishing the equivalent deterministic model of the problem (1)–(4) by using CCP technique, we consider ith constraint of the problem,

$$\text{Prob}\Big(\sum_{j=1}^{n} a_{ij}x_j \geq b_i\Big) \geq (1-\beta_i),\ b_i \in \{b_i^{(1)}, b_i^{(2)}, \ldots, b_i^{(t_i)}\}$$

Here, the parameters a_{ij} $(i = 1, 2, \ldots, m;\ j = 1, 2, \ldots, n)$ are considered to be independent random variables and are distributed normally with means μ_{ij} and variances σ_{ij}^2, i.e.,

$$a_{ij} \sim \mathcal{N}(\mu_{ij}, \sigma_{ij}^2)\ (i = 1, 2, \ldots, m;\ j = 1, 2, \ldots, n)$$

Let $h_i = \sum_{j=1}^{n} a_{ij}x_j$ $(i = 1, 2, \ldots, m)$ are linear combinations of random variables a_{ij} $(j = 1, 2, \ldots, n)$. As a_{ij} $(j = 1, 2, \ldots, n)$ are independent normal random variables then their linear combinations h_i, $(i = 1, 2, \ldots, m)$ are also independent normal random variables.
So, we have

$$E(h_i) = E\Big(\sum_{j=1}^{n} a_{ij}x_j\Big) = \sum_{j=1}^{n} \mu_{ij}x_j,$$

and

$$\mathrm{Var}(h_i) = \sum_{j=1}^{n} \sigma_{ij}^2 x_j^2$$

Now from (2.1), we have

$$\mathrm{Prob}\Big(\sum_{j=1}^{n} a_{ij}x_j \geq b_i\Big) \geq (1-\beta_i),\ b_i \in \{b_i^{(1)}, b_i^{(2)}, \ldots, b_i^{(t_i)}\},\quad i = 1, 2, \ldots, m$$

$$\text{i.e., Prob}\ (h_i \geq b_i) \geq (1-\beta_i)$$

$$\text{i.e., Prob}\Big(\frac{h_i - E(h_i)}{\sqrt{\mathrm{Var}(h_i)}} \geq \frac{b_i - E(h_i)}{\sqrt{\mathrm{Var}(h_i)}}\Big) \geq (1-\beta_i)$$

$$\text{i.e.,Prob}\Big(Z_i \geq \frac{b_i - E(h_i)}{\sqrt{\mathrm{Var}(h_i)}}\Big) \geq (1-\beta_i)\ \text{ where }\ Z_i = \frac{h_i - E(h_i)}{\sqrt{\mathrm{Var}(h_i)}}$$

$$\text{i.e., Prob}\Big(Z_i \leq \frac{b_i - E(h_i)}{\sqrt{\mathrm{Var}(h_i)}}\Big) \leq \beta_i$$

$$\text{i.e., }\Phi\Big(\frac{b_i - E(h_i)}{\sqrt{\mathrm{Var}(h_i)}}\Big) \leq \Phi(-Z_{\beta_i})$$

$$\text{i.e., } E(h_i) - Z_{\beta_i}\sqrt{\mathrm{Var}(h_i)} \geq b_i$$

$$\text{i.e., }\sum_{j=1}^{n} \mu_{ij}x_j - Z_{\beta_i}\sqrt{\sum_{j=1}^{n} \sigma_{ij}^2 x_j^2} \geq, b_i\ \ b_i \in \{b_i^{(1)}, b_i^{(2)}, \ldots, b_i^{(t_i)}\},\quad i = 1, 2, \ldots, m$$

Hence, the equivalent deterministic model of the MCCCP problem (1)–(4) is a MCP problem written as

$$\min : z = \sum_{j=1}^{n} c_j x_j \tag{5}$$

subject to

$$\sum_{j=1}^{n} \mu_{ij}x_j - Z_{\beta_i}\sqrt{\sum_{j=1}^{n} \sigma_{ij}^2 x_j^2} \geq b_i, \tag{6}$$

$$b_i \in \{b_i^{(1)}, b_i^{(2)}, \ldots, b_i^{(t_i)}\},\quad i = 1, 2, \ldots, m \tag{7}$$

$$x_j \geq 0,\quad j = 1, 2, 3, \ldots, n. \tag{8}$$

The above model is a nonlinear MCP programming model, and to solve above problem MCP directly, $\prod_{i=1}^{m} t_i$ number of nonlinear programming problems have to be solved, and the whole procedure is generally very complex and time-consuming. Several models and transformation techniques have been developed to tackle the presence of multi-choice parameters in the above model. Some important transformation techniques have been briefly discussed below.

2.2 Transformation Techniques for MCP Problem

Here, we discuss different transformation techniques used generally for transforming a MCP problem into a corresponding optimization problem.

(i) **Auxiliary Variable Technique:**
This approach has been developed by Ravindran et al. [29]. In this approach, one binary variable is used for each alternative choices of a multi-choice parameter, and one extra constraint will be added for each multi-choice parameter. For example, if the multi-choice parameter b_i has t_i number of multi-choice values, $b_i^{(1)}, b_i^{(2)}, \ldots, b_i^{(t_i)}$, then we will have t_i number of binary variables. So,for the ith constraint of the problem (5)–(7), the equivalent constraints will be,

$$\sum_{j=1}^{n} \mu_{ij} x_j - Z_{\beta_i} \sqrt{\sum_{j=1}^{n} \sigma_{ij}^2 x_j^2} \geq s_i^{(1)} b_i^{(1)} + s_i^{(2)} b_i^{(2)} + \cdots + s_i^{(t_i)} b_i^{(t_i)}, \quad i = 1, 2, 3, \ldots, m \tag{9}$$

$$s_i^{(1)} + s_i^{(2)} + \cdots + s_i^{(t_i)} = 1, \quad i = 1, 2, 3, \ldots, m \tag{10}$$

where $s_i^{(1)}, s_i^{(2)}, \ldots, s_i^{(t_i)}$, $(i = 1, 2, \ldots, m)$ are t_i number of binary variables. In this technique, m-number of extra constraints, and $\sum_{i=1}^{m} t_i$ number of extra binary variables are required for transforming the MCP problem.

(ii) **Binary Variable Technique:**
Biswal and Acharya [30] proposed this approach to transform MCLP problem. Here, total $\sum_{i=1}^{m} \lceil (\frac{\ln(t_i)}{\ln 2}) \rceil$ number of binary variables are required for tackling the multi-choice parameters of the problem (5)–(7). Like the previous approach, here some additional constraints are also required related to transform the problem into an equivalent NLP model. The number of extra constraints depends on the number of different choices of multi-choice parameters. The additional constraints are used to restrict the repetition of the alternative choices of the parameter. There is no additional constraint if $t_i = 2$ or 4 or 8, if $t_i = 3$ or 7, then only one auxiliary constraint is required, we require 3 and 2 additional constraints respectively for $t_i = 5$ and 6 . Details of this technique can be found in the paper by Biswal and Acharya [30]. Here, less number of binary variables and less number of extra constraints are required in this approach than the previous approach.

Table 1 Data table for multi-choice coefficient b_i

z_i	0	1	2	…	$t_i - 1$
$f_{b_i}(z_i)$	$b_i^{(1)}$	$b_i^{(2)}$	$b_i^{(3)}$	…	$b_i^{(t_i)}$

(iii) **Interpolating Polynomial Technique:**
This approach has been also developed by Biswal and Acharya [16].Here, for each of the multi-choice parameter, an integer variable is introduced. This has been done to reduce number of extra constraints and additional variables. For ith constraint of the problem (5)–(7), an integer variable z_i is introduced for the multi-choice parameter b_i. As there are t_i number of different choices available for the multi-choice parameter b_i, we have t_i number of functional values associated with corresponding $t - i$ number of choices. The t_i number of nodes nodes and the corresponding functional values at these nodes are given in Table 1. An interpolating polynomial $f_{b_i}(z_i)$ of degree $t_i - 1$ has been constructed which interpolates the nodes and their corresponding functional values given in (Table 1). Using the Lagranges interpolation formula [31], the corresponding interpolating polynomial has been established as:

$$\begin{aligned} f_{b_i}(z_i) = & \frac{(z_i-1)(z_i-2)\cdots(z_i-t_i+1)}{(-1)^{(t_i-1)}(t_i-1)!}b_i^{(1)} \\ & + \frac{z_i(z_i-2)\cdots(z_i-t_i+1)}{(-1)^{(t_i-2)}(t_i-2)!}b_i^{(2)} \\ & + \frac{z_i(z_i-1)(z_i-3)\cdots(z_i-t_i+1)}{(-1)^{(t_i-3)}2!(t_i-3)!}b_i^{(3)} + \cdots \\ & + \frac{z_i(z_i-1)(z_i-2)\cdots(z_i-t_i+2)}{(t_i-1)!}b_i^{(t_i)}, \quad i = 1, 2, \ldots, m. \end{aligned} \tag{11}$$

Therefore, the corresponding transformed model of the problem (1)–(3) is given by:

$$\min z = \sum_{j=1}^{n} c_j x_j \tag{12}$$

subject to

$$\sum_{j=1}^{n} \mu_{ij} x_j - z_{\gamma_i} \sqrt{\sum_{j=1}^{n} \sigma_{ij}^2 x_j^2} \geq f_{b_i}(z_i), \quad i = 1, 2, 3, \ldots, m \tag{13}$$

$$x_j \geq 0, \, j = 1, 2, 3, \ldots, n; \; 0 \leq z_i \leq t_i - 1; \; z_i \in N_0 \quad i = 1, 2, 3, \ldots, m. \tag{14}$$

where $f_{b_i}(z_i)$ is given by (11). Here, the obtained model is a mixed-integer NLP model. In this approach, Lagranges interpolating polynomial has been applied for transformation of MCP problem; similarly, one can use other interpolating polynomials to handle the multi-choiceness of the parameters. This approach requires no additional constraints and less number of binary variables as compared to previous techniques.

3 Genetic Algorithm

Genetic algorithm (GA) is a stochastic search-based algorithm inspired by the process of natural evolution and selection. GA was developed by John Holland and his team in 1975 at the University of Michigan. In GA, there are possible sets of solutions known as population. Like natural genetics, these solutions have to perform mutation and crossover (recombination) operations to produce new offsprings. These processes are continued for several generations or till the favorable result is obtained.

Advantages of GA

GA has several benefits which have made it very popular. These are:

- Most of the classical optimization methods are gradient-based; they often have tendencies of getting stuck at the local optima. On contrary, GA being a population-based technique does not involve any derivative to solve the problem and avoid getting stuck during the process.
- GA is sufficient and more faster as compared to conventional optimization methods.
- It has the ability to solve single, multi-objective , linear, nonlinear optimization problems, and it can solve problems involving continuous, discrete, or mixed-integer variables.

- It provides a set of good or efficient solutions and not merely a single solution.
- GA is very useful in solving difficult problems like NP-hard problems within short time.
- It is also very efficient in solving optimization problems involving large search space.

Basic Terminology

Before starting discussion on GA, we will discuss the basic terminologies used in GA for better understanding of the algorithm.

Population—It is a set of all possible solutions involved in the search process. Size of population varies from problem to problem. The population size must be as big as possible for better result.

Chromosomes—Each solution is called a chromosome which is analogous to the chromosome in natural genetics.

Gene—A chromosome is made up of genes. Practically, when a chromosome is represented as a binary string, then each bit is represented as a gene.
Genotype—Population in the computation space is known as genotype.
Phenotype—Population in the actual real-world solution space is known as phenotype.
Encoding and Decoding—Encoding is a process of transforming from the phenotype to genotype space so that computer can process, for example, when a chromosome is transformed from decimal to its binary equivalent. Similarly, decoding is a process of converting a solution from the genotype to the phenotype space. Decoding is required for fitness evaluation. There are different types of encoding techniques available in GA; these are namely: binary encoding, octal encoding, hexadecimal encoding, permutation encoding, value encoding, etc.
Crossover—Crossover in GA is analogous to biological crossover. Here, more than one chromosomes are selected as parent to produce one or more offsprings. There are different types of crossover operations available for GA, namely single-point crossover, two-point and k-point crossover, and uniform crossover, etc.
Mutation —Mutation in genetic algorithm is used to introduce and maintain genetic diversity of populations from one generation to next generation. It changes one or more gene values of chromosomes by performing bit-by-bit basis. For different genome types, different mutation techniques are available. These are uniform, nonuniform, gaussian, shrink, boundary, etc.
Termination Condition—The execution of GA can be stopped either GA completes a fixed number of generations or the fitness values of the chromosomes are not improved after completion of a certain number of generations.

3.1 GA for MCP Problem

In previous section, we witnessed that different model formed by using many transformation techniques to MCP are generally mixed-integer nonlinear programming models, and these also involve some extra variables and/or extra constraints. We prefer genetic algorithm (GA) over traditional approaches to solve the above transformed models because GA is more robust than other traditional methods, it never get stuck at local optima, and it does not involve any derivative in it. GA also has more success rate while solving nonlinear programming problems. It also solves both continuous and discrete functions. Apart from these, our proposed GA solves MCP problems directly which does not require any transformation techniques; hence, the process does not involve or create additional variables or extra constraints.

Step-by-Step procedure for GA Here, our proposed genetic algorithm for MCP problems has been described as follows:

1. **Representation and initialization of population**
   First, we define population size P_{size} and then we represent the chromosome. Let $Y_1, Y_2, \ldots, Y_n$ be the n-number of decision variables and then each chromosome is represented as:

$$Y_P = (Y_1, Y_2, \ldots, Y_n)_P$$

   where $P = 1, 2, \ldots, P_{\text{size}}$, and all chromosomes are initialized randomly. As $Y_j \geq 0$, $(j = 1, 2, \ldots, n)$, the values of decision variables $Y_j (j = 1, 2, \ldots, n)$ are initialized uniformly between 0 and the upper limits of jth decision variable.
2. **Constraints Checking**
   In this step, constraints checking is done for all the constraints and for the different choices of multi-choice parameters present in MCP problem. For example, if the ith constraint is $G_i(x, \mu, \sigma) \geq b_i,\ b_i \in \{b_i^{(1)}, b_i^{(2)}, \ldots, b_i^{(t_i)}\},\ (i = 1, 2, \ldots, m)$ where right-hand side parameter has t_i number of alternative choices and then we check the constraints by $G_i(x, \mu, \sigma) \geq b_i^1$, or $G_i(x, \mu, \sigma) \geq b_i^2$, or,..., ,or $G_i(x, \mu, \sigma) \geq b_i^{t_i}$ for $i = 1, 2, \ldots, m$.
3. **Fitness**
   In this stage, fitness value of each chromosome is calculated. Here, we have taken objective function values as the fitness values. After he chromosomes satisfying constraint checking conditions, their corresponding fitness values are calculated.
4. **Selection**
   In this step, fittest individual chromosomes are selected as parents from a population to create offsprings for next generation. Here, we have used roulette-wheel selection strategy [18] to solve our problem.
5. **Crossover**
   Here, we have used single-point crossover in our algorithm. First crossover probability P_c is set, so that we have an expected number $P_c X P_{\text{size}}$ of chromosomes to take part in crossover operation. Then the crossover point is selected randomly. A a random number R is generated in the range (0, 1) for each pair of chromosomes in the current population, if $R < P_c$ and then given pair of chromosomes is selected to undergo crossover operation.
6. **Mutation**
   Here, we have used uniform crossover in our algorithm. First, the probability of mutation P_m is set, so that we have an expected number $P_m X P_{\text{size}}$ of chromosomes which will take part in mutation operation. A random number R is generated within (0, 1) for every bit in the population. If $R < P_m$, then the chromosome is selected to undergo mutation operation.
7. **Termination**
   This is final stage of GA where the termination condition decides when the GA run will end. It may be determined as the number of generations or when the solution of individual chromosomes meets a pre-specified fitness level. Here, we have taken number of generations as stopping or termination criteria, i.e., we have to first set the number of generations. When number of iteration becomes equal to the generation number as defined, then the execution of the algorithm will be stopped.

3.2 Summary of the Proposed GA for MCP

Step 1: First define population size P_{size}, then randomly initialize p_{size} number of chromosomes as described above.
Step 2: Check all the constraints with respective multi-choice parameters.
Step 3: Set mutation probability P_{m} and crossover probability P_{c}. Apply crossover and mutation operation as described above to update the chromosomes.
Step 4: Calculate the objective value with respect to individual chromosomes.
Step 5: Calculate the fitness value of each chromosome with respect to the calculated objective values.
Step 6: According to the selection procedure described above, select the fittest chromosomes for the next generation.
Step 7: If the termination criteria are satisfied, stop, and return the best chromosome in current population as the optimal solution.
Step 8: Repeat Steps 2–7.

4 Numerical Example

In this section, we have considered an MCSP problem given by Biswal and Acharya [32].

$$\min : z = 24.83x_1 + 28.5x_2 + 43.5x_3 + 45.21x_4 \tag{15}$$

subject to

$$2.3x_1 + 5.6x_2 + 11.1x_3 + 1.3x_4 \geq b_1, \quad b_1 \in \{5, 5.4, 5.8, 6.0, 6.2\} \tag{16}$$

$$Pr(a_{21}x_1 + a_{22}x_2 + a_{23}x_3 + a_{24}x_4 \geq b_2) \geq .95, \quad b_2 \in \{21, 21.5, 22.0\} \tag{17}$$

$$x_1 + x_2 + x_3 + x_4 \leq 1 \tag{18}$$

$$x_2 \geq 0.01 \tag{19}$$

$$x_j = 0, 1, 2, 3, 4 \tag{20}$$

where $E(a_{21}) = 12.0$, $E(a_{22}) = 11.9$, $E(a_{23}) = 41.8$, $E(a_{24}) = 52.1$
and $\text{Var}(a_{21}) = 0.53$, $\text{Var}(a_{22}) = 0.44$, $\text{Var}(a_{23}) = 4.58$, $\text{Var}(a_{21}) = 0.79$. Now using (5)–(7), the equivalent deterministic MCP model of (15)–(19) is presented as

$$\min : z = 24.83x_1 + 28.5x_2 + 43.5x_3 + 45.21x_4 \tag{21}$$

subject to

$$2.3x_1 + 5.6x_2 + 11.1x_3 + 1.3x_4 \geq b_1, \quad b_1 \in \{5, 5.4, 5.8, 6.0, 6.2\} \tag{22}$$
$$12x_1 + 11.9x_2 + 41.8x_3 + 52.1x_4 - 1.645 \tag{23}$$
$$\sqrt{0.2809x_1^2 + 0.193x_2^2 + 20.25x_3^2 + 0.6241x_4^2} \geq b_2, \tag{24}$$
$$b_2 \in \{21, 21.5, 22.0\} \tag{25}$$
$$x_1 + x_2 + x_3 + x_4 \leq 1 \tag{26}$$
$$x_2 \geq 0.01 \tag{27}$$
$$x_j = 0, 1, 2, 3, 4 \tag{28}$$

Using Interpolating polynomial approach as given in (11), the above model (21)–(28) can be transformed to a mixed-integer nonlinear programming model as

$$\min : z = 24.83x_1 + 28.5x_2 + 43.5x_3 + 45.21x_4 \tag{29}$$

subject to

$$2.3x_1 + 5.6x_2 + 11.1x_3 + 1.3x_4 \geq \tag{30}$$
$$5 - 0.2333z_1 + 0.28333z_1^2 - 0.1333z_1^3 + 0.16667z_1^4 \tag{31}$$
$$12x_1 + 11.9x_2 + 41.8x_3 + 52.1x_4 - 1.645 \tag{32}$$
$$\sqrt{0.2809x_1^2 + 0.193x_2^2 + 20.25x_3^2 + 0.6241x_4^2} \geq 21.0 + 0.5z_2, \tag{33}$$
$$x_1 + x_2 + x_3 + x_4 \leq 1 \tag{34}$$
$$x_2 \geq 0.01 \tag{35}$$
$$z_1 = 0, 1, 2, 3, 4; z_2 = 0, 1, 2 \tag{36}$$
$$x_j = 0, 1, 2, 3, 4 \tag{37}$$

The above problem is solved by using LINGO(11.0) [33] software and the optimal solutions are found as follows: $x_1 = 0$, $x_2 = 0.0100$, $x_3 = 0.6070501$, $x_4 = 0$, $z_1 = 3.000000$, $z_2 = 0.007525087$ and minimum value of $z = 26.69168$.

Again, the above model (21)–(28) is a nonlinear MCP problem which has been solved by our proposed GA. The proposed GA is coded in C programming language with population size is 100, total number of generations = 1001, crossover probability = 0.2, mutation probability = 0.01.

The result obtained after the execution of 900 number of generations using GA is shown in Table 2.

The result obtained in 900th generation is repeated in the next generations. Hence, the optimal solution obtained is as follows: $x_1 = 0.002$, $x_2 = 0.01$, $x_3 = 0.4321284$, $x_4 = 0.115492$ and minimum value of $z = 24.3$ Here, we see that our proposed model solved by genetic algorithm gives better result as compared to those obtained by using transformation techniques.

Table 2 Result using genetic algorithm

Generation No.	x_1	x_2	x_3	x_4	f
0	7.611316e−002	4.234443e−002	4.260384e−001	1.387066e−001	2.79e+001
20	7.304505e−002	2.651449e−002	4.125988e−001	1.387825e−001	2.68e+001
40	3.129231e−002	2.560024e−002	4.181380e−001	1.149749e−001	2.49e+001
60	3.000078e−002	2.535633e−002	4.181380e−001	1.144302e−001	2.48e+001
80	3.000078e−002	2.535633e−002	4.181380e−001	1.144302e−001	2.48e+001
100	3.000078e−002	2.535633e−002	4.181380e−001	1.144302e−001	2.48e+001
120	2.502138e−002	2.025904e−002	4.233396e−001	1.132713e−001	2.47e+001
140	2.502138e−002	2.025904e−002	4.233396e−001	1.132713e−001	2.47e+001
160	2.502138e−002	2.012338e−002	4.232702e−001	1.133720e−001	2.47e+001
180	2.502138e−002	2.012338e−002	4.232702e−001	1.133720e−001	2.47e+001
200	2.502138e−002	2.019909e−002	4.232091e−001	1.133720e−001	2.47e+001
220	2.502138e−002	2.019909e−002	4.232091e−001	1.133720e−001	2.47e+001
240	2.595318e−002	1.927532e−002	4.219844e−001	1.142358e−001	2.47e+001
260	2.595318e−002	1.927532e−002	4.219844e−001	1.142358e−001	2.47e+001
280	2.595318e−002	1.927532e−002	4.219844e−001	1.142358e−001	2.47e+001
300	2.595318e−002	1.925614e−002	4.219844e−001	1.142358e−001	2.47e+001
320	2.558238e−002	1.948115e−002	4.221697e−001	1.140836e−001	2.47e+001
340	2.558238e−002	1.621906e−002	4.236711e−001	1.140836e−001	2.47e+001
360	2.560271e−002	1.621906e−002	4.237245e−001	1.138546e−001	2.47e+001
380	2.560271e−002	1.607948e−002	4.237245e−001	1.138546e−001	2.47e+001
400	2.526425e−002	1.627974e−002	4.237245e−001	1.138546e−001	2.47e+001
420	2.495948e−002	1.626961e−002	4.237245e−001	1.140010e−001	2.47e+001
440	2.495948e−002	1.626961e−002	4.237245e−001	1.140010e−001	2.47e+001
460	2.495948e−002	1.626961e−002	4.237245e−001	1.140010e−001	2.47e+001
480	2.495948e−002	1.626961e−002	4.237245e−001	1.140010e−001	2.47e+001
500	7.273431e−003	1.595163e−002	4.309391e−001	1.134047e−001	2.45e+001
520	5.954036e−003	1.572137e−002	4.310767e−001	1.136155e−001	2.45e+001
540	6.130728e−003	1.572137e−002	4.310268e−001	1.135640e−001	2.45e+001
560	6.130728e−003	1.572137e−002	4.310268e−001	1.135640e−001	2.45e+001
580	6.130728e−003	1.572137e−002	4.310268e−001	1.135640e−001	2.45e+001
600	4.076472e−003	1.246111e−002	4.334690e−001	1.132719e−001	2.44e+001
620	3.549610e−003	1.246111e−002	4.331080e−001	1.135817e−001	2.44e+001
640	3.549610e−003	1.246111e−002	4.331080e−001	1.135325e−001	2.44e+001
660	1.997880e−003	1.246111e−002	4.331080e−001	1.140257e−001	2.44e+001
680	1.398539e−003	1.246111e−002	4.331080e−001	1.140257e−001	2.44e+001
700	1.385619e−003	1.246111e−002	4.331080e−001	1.140257e−001	2.44e+001
720	1.092638e−003	1.120229e−002	4.336574e−001	1.140257e−001	2.44e+001
740	1.092638e−003	1.120229e−002	4.336574e−001	1.140257e−001	2.44e+001
760	1.092638e−003	1.120229e−002	4.336574e−001	1.140257e−001	2.44e+001
780	1.092638e−003	1.120229e−002	4.336574e−001	1.140257e−001	2.44e+001
800	2.830075e−004	1.090466e−002	4.331912e−001	1.146130e−001	2.43e+001
820	2.646072e−004	1.088532e−002	4.331763e−001	1.146130e−001	2.43e+001
840	2.858449e−004	1.023446e−002	4.320443e−001	1.154921e−001	2.43e+001
860	2.858449e−004	1.004285e−002	4.321284e−001	1.154921e−001	2.43e+001
880	2.858449e−004	1.004285e−002	4.321284e−001	1.154921e−001	2.43e+001
900	2.858449e−004	1.004285e−002	4.321284e−001	1.154921e−001	2.43e+001

5 Conclusions

The stated MCCCP problem is first converted to a deterministic nonlinear MCP programming problem using chance-constrained technique. The transformed model obtained is a nonlinear MCP programming model. As GA is very useful method to solve NLP problem, our proposed GA for MCP is used to solve the nonlinear MCP programming problem without applying any transformation technique. Hence, our proposed GA does not require any extra variables or additional constraints unlike other available techniques, and also, we observed that our proposed model solved by genetic algorithm gives better result as compared to those obtained by transformation techniques.The model we consider in this study has right-hand side parameters are multi-choice type. Our proposed GA can be modified to solve MCCCP problem where cost coefficients or/and technological coefficients of the problems are multi-choice parameters. This study can be extended to multi-level or multi-objective framework with different probability distributions.

References

1. Charnes, A., Cooper, W.W.: Chance-constrained programming. Manag. Sci. **6**(1), 73–79 (1959)
2. Kall, P.: Stochastic Programming. Springer, Berlin (1976)
3. Kall, P., Wallace, S.W.: Stochastic Programming. Springer, New York (1994)
4. Infanger, G.: Planning under uncertainty solving large-scale stochastic linear programs (No. SOL-92-8). Stanford University, CA (United States). Systems Optimization Lab (1992)
5. Stancu-Minasian, I.M., Wets, M.J.: A research bibliography in stochastic programming, 1955–1975. Oper. Res. **24**(6), 1078–1119 (1976)
6. Goicoechea, A., Hansen, D.R., Duckstein, L.: Multiobjective Decision Analysis with Engineering and Business Applications. Wiley, New York (1982)
7. Goicoechea, A., Duckstein, L.: Nonnormal deterministic equivalents and a transformation in stochastic mathematical programming. Appl. Math. Comput. **21**(1), 51–72 (1987)
8. Miller, B.L., Wagner, H.M.: Chance constrained programming with joint constraints. Oper. Res. **13**(6), 930–945 (1965)
9. Jagannathan, R.: Chance-constrained programming with joint constraints. Oper. Res. **22**(2), 358–372 (1974)
10. Sahoo, N.P., Biswal, M.P.: Computation of Probabilistic linear programming problems involving normal and log-normal random variables with a joint constraint. Comput. Math. **82**(11), 1323–1338 (2005)
11. Healy Jr., W.C.: Multiple choice programming (a procedure for linear programming with zero-one variables). Oper. Res. **12**(1), 122–138 (1964)
12. Lin, E.Y.H.: Multiple choice programming: a state-of-the-art review. Int. Trans. Oper. Res. **1**(4), 409–421 (1994)
13. Chang, C.T.: Multi-choice goal programming. Omega **35**(4), 389–396 (2007)
14. Liao, C.N.: Formulating the multi-segment goal programming. Comput. Ind. Eng. **56**(1), 138–141 (2009)
15. Chang, C.T., Chen, H.M., Zhuang, Z.Y.: Multicoefficients goal programming. Comput. Ind. Eng. **62**, 616–623 (2012)
16. Biswal, M.P., Acharya, S.: Solving multi-choice linear programming problems by interpolating polynomials. Math. Comput. Model. **54**(5), 1405–1412 (2011)

17. Acharya, S., Biswal, M.P.: Solving probabilistic programming problems involving multi-choice parameters. Opsearch **48**(3), 217–235 (2011)
18. Holland, J.H.: Adaptation in Natural and Artificial Systems: An Introductory Analysis with Applications to Biology, Control, and Artificial Intelligence. MIT press (1992)
19. De Jong, K.: Adaptive system design: a genetic approach. IEEE Trans. Syst. Man Cybern. **10**(9), 566–574 (1980)
20. Goldberg, D.E., Richardson, J.: Genetic algorithms with sharing for multimodal function optimization. In: Genetic Algorithms and Their Applications: Proceedings of the Second International Conference on Genetic Algorithms, pp. 41–49. Lawrence Erlbaum, Hillsdale, NJ (1987)
21. Abdullah, A.R.: A robust method for linear and nonlinear optimization based on genetic algorithm. Cybernetica **34**(4), 279–287 (1991)
22. Homaifar, A., Qi, C.X., Lai, S.H.: Constrained optimization via genetic algorithms. Simulation **62**(4), 242–253 (1994)
23. Deb, K.: An efficient constraint handling method for genetic algorithms. Comput. Methods Appl. Mech. Eng. **186**(2), 311–338 (2000)
24. Jana, R.K., Biswal, M.P.: Stochastic simulation-based genetic algorithm for chance constraint programming problems with continuous random variables. Int. J. Comput. Math. **81**(9), 1069–1076 (2004)
25. Ramrez-Beltrn, N.D., Aguilar-Ruggiero, K.: Application of an geuristic procedure to solve mixed-integer programming problems. Comput. Ind. Eng. **33**(1–2), 43–46 (1997)
26. Yokota, T., Gen, M., Li, Y.X.: Genetic algorithm for non-linear mixed integer programming problems and its applications. Comput. Ind. Eng. **30**(4), 905–917 (1996)
27. Wasanapradit, T., Mukdasanit, N., Chaiyaratana, N., Srinophakun, T.: Solving mixed-integer nonlinear programming problems using improved genetic algorithms. Korean J. Chem. Eng. **28**(1), 32–40 (2011)
28. Mohanty, D.K., Jana, R.K. and Biswal, M.P.: Genetic algorithm for multi-choice integer linear programming problems. In: Soft Computing for Problem Solving, pp. 809–819. Springer, Singapore (2019)
29. Phillip, D., Revindran, A., Solberg, J.: Operations Research: Principles and Practice (1975)
30. Biswal, M.P., Acharya, S.: Transformation of a multi-choice linear programming problem. Appl. Math. Comput. **210**(1), 182–188 (2009)
31. Micha, D.A.: An introduction to numerical analysis. In: Atkinson, K.E. (ed.) (1980)
32. Biswal, M.P., Biswal, N.P., Li, D.: Probabilistic linear programming problems with exponential random variables: a technical note. Eur. J. Oper. Res. **111**(3), 589–597 (1998)
33. Schrage, L.E., LINDO Systems, Inc.: Optimization modeling with LINGO. Duxbury Press, CA (1997)

The ISI Index of Edge-Semitotal and Total Graphs

A. Mahanta, A. Bharali and J. Buragohain

Abstract We have many associated graphs when it comes to the domain of a connected graph. Vertex-semitotal graph $R(G)$, total graph $T(G)$, edge-semitotal graph $Q(G)$ and line graph $L(G)$ are some examples of such graphs. In this paper, we study the ISI index of $Q(G)$, $T(G)$, Q-sums and T-sums and obtain explicit expressions for the same. Also, the extremal cases of the index for these graphs have been investigated.

Keywords Degree of vertex · Line graph · ISI index · Edge-semitotal graph · Total graph

1 Introduction

In our discussion, we have considered only finite, simple, undirected and connected graphs. We have denoted the vertex set, edge set and the degree of a vertex u in a graph G by $V(G)$, $E(G)$ and $d_G(u)$, respectively. We have used P_n to represent a path of order n. Let $\delta = \underbrace{\min}_{u} d_G(u)$.

To obtain the edge-semitotal graph $Q(G)$ from a graph G, we can insert a new vertex into each edge of G and then join these new pairs of vertices on adjacent edges of G (see Fig. 1). The total graph $T(G)$ has the edges and vertices of G as its vertices with the adjacency of the elements of G determining the adjacency in $T(G)$. For more detail on these operations, one may refer to [1] and *Handbook of Product Graphs* by Hammack et al. [2].

A. Mahanta (✉) · A. Bharali · J. Buragohain
Dibrugarh University, Dibrugarh, Assam, India
e-mail: am02dib@gmail.com

A. Bharali
e-mail: a.bharali@dibru.ac.in

J. Buragohain
e-mail: j.bgohain75@yahoo.com

S. Bhattacharyya et al. (eds.), *Mathematical Modeling and Computational Tools*, Springer Proceedings in Mathematics & Statistics 320,
https://doi.org/10.1007/978-981-15-3615-1_28

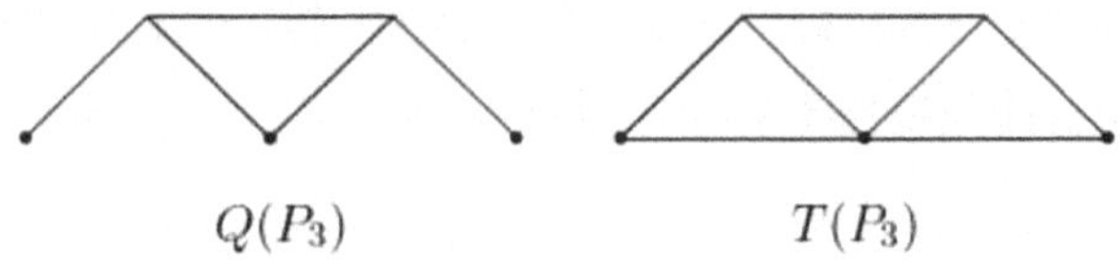

Fig. 1 Example of Q and T operation of graph

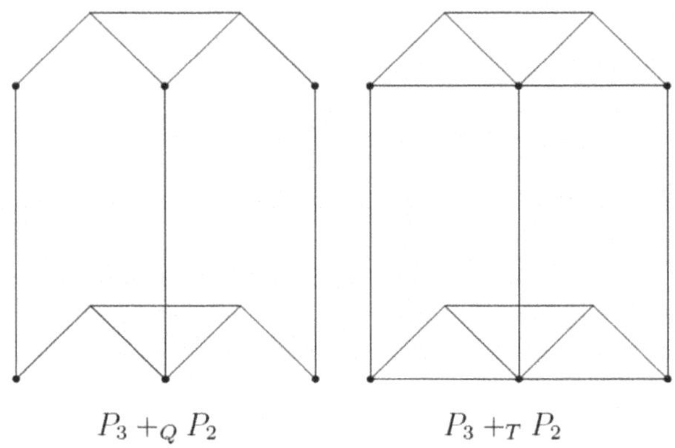

Fig. 2 $P_3 +_Q P_2$ and $P_3 +_T P_2$

Let us consider two graphs G_1 and G_2 and $F \in \{Q, T\}$. Then, the F-sum, $G_1 +_F G_2$ generates $|V(G_2)|$ copies of the graph $F(G_1)$ which can be labelled by the vertices of G_2. Here, we have two categories of vertices: the vertices in $V(G_1)$ which are denoted by black vertices and the vertices in $E(G_1)$ which are denoted by white vertices. We only join black vertices with the same name in $F(G_1)$ in which their corresponding labels are adjacent in G_2 (Fig. 2). More details into these sums can be looked up in [1].

The topological index of a molecular graph is in simple terms a number generated out of it which quantifies the graph's molecular structuring and branching pattern with various physical, chemical and biological properties of the graph. Though a lot many topological indices have been defined based on degree, distance, eccentricity and so on, yet not all of them have been found to be significant. One may refer to [3] for an account of some degree-based topological indices. On the other hand, the ISI index is found to have special impetus as predictor of total surface area of octane isomers. Out of the 148 discrete Adriatic indices studied in 2010, the ISI index finds its place in the list of twenty indices selected as significant predictors.

We now state the formal definitions of some of the topological indices that we have used in our study.

First Zagreb index: $M_1(G) = \sum_{u \in V(G)} (d_G(u))^2 = M_1(G) = \sum_{uv \in E(G)} (d_G(u) + d_G(v))$.

Inverse degree index: $ID(G) = \sum_{u \in V(G)} \frac{1}{d_G(u)}$.

Harmonic index: $H(G) = \sum_{uv \in E(G)} \frac{2}{d_G(u)+d_G(v)}$.

ISI index [4]: $ISI(G) = \sum_{uv \in E(G)} \frac{1}{\frac{1}{d_G(u)} + \frac{1}{d_G(v)}} = \sum_{uv \in E(G)} \frac{d_G(u)d_G(v)}{d_G(u)+d_G(v)}$.

The twenty-first century has seen many notable works based on the ISI index of graphs. Pattabiraman [4, 5] in his paper presents upper and lower bounds on the ISI index in terms of some molecular structural parameters and relates this index to various well-known molecular descriptors. Some recent contributions related to the ISI index can be found in [5–7]. However, unlike other classical topological indices, limited literature has been found for the ISI index of graph operations. There are several papers found in the literature reporting works on Zagreb and harmonic index on operations of graphs. Some recent contributions in this context are [8–11].

In this work, we compute the ISI index of edge-semitotal graphs, total graphs, Q-sums and T-sums. The rest of the paper is organised as follows. In Sect. 2, we study the ISI index of edge-semitotal graphs and total graphs and obtain upper bounds for them. In Sect. 3, we propose upper bounds for Q-sums and T-sums, respectively. Finally, in Sect. 4, conclusions are made.

2 Bounds for the ISI Index for Edge-Semitotal and Total Graphs

It is to be noted that $d_{Q(G)}(u) = d_G(u)$ for all $u \in V(G)$ and $d_{Q(G)}(y) = d_G(u) + d_G(v) = d_{L(G)}(y) + 2$ for all $y \in V(Q(G)) \backslash V(G)$, where y is inserted into the edge uv in G.

Let $G(n_i, m_j)$be the set of all graphs of order n_i and size m_j.

Theorem 1.1 Let $G \in G(n, m)$.*Then,*

$$\mathrm{ISI}(Q(G)) < \frac{9}{8}M_1(G) - \frac{3}{4}m + \frac{1}{16}M_2(L(G)) + \frac{1}{8}M_1(L(G)) + \frac{1}{2}H(L(G)) + \frac{1}{4}\mathrm{ISI}(L(G)).$$

Proof

$$\mathrm{ISI}(Q(G)) = \sum_{uv \in E(G)} \left(\frac{d_{Q(G)}(u)d_{Q(G)}(x)}{d_{Q(G)}(u) + d_{Q(G)}(x)} + \frac{d_{Q(G)}(x)d_{Q(G)}(v)}{d_{Q(G)}(x) + d_{Q(G)}(v)} \right) + \sum_{yy' \in E(L(G))} \left(\frac{d_{Q(G)}(y)d_{Q(G)}(y')}{d_{Q(G)}(y) + d_{Q(G)}(y')} \right)$$

(where x is the vertex inserted into the edge uv of G.)

$$= \sum_{uv \in E(G)} \left(\frac{d_G(u)(d_G(u) + d_G(v))}{d_G(u) + (d_G(u) + d_G(v))} + \frac{(d_G(u) + d_G(v))d_G(v)}{(d_G(u) + d_G(v)) + d_G(v)} \right)$$

$$+\sum_{yy'\in E(L(G)}\left(\frac{(2+d_{L(G)}(y))(2+d_{L(G)}(y'))}{(2+d_{L(G)}(y))+(2+d_{L(G)}(y'))}\right)$$
$$=\sum_{uv\in E(G)}\left(\frac{d_G(u)(d_G(u)+d_G(v))}{d_G(u)+(d_G(u)+d_G(v))}+\frac{(d_G(u)+d_G(v))d_G(v)}{(d_G(u)+d_G(v))+d_G(v)}\right)$$
$$+\sum_{yy'\in E(L(G)}\left(\frac{(2+d_{L(G)}(y))(2+d_{L(G)}(y'))}{(2+d_{L(G)}(y))+(2+d_{L(G)}(y'))}\right)$$
$$=\sum 1+\sum 2.$$

Using Jensen's inequality, for every $uv \in E(G)$, we have

$$\frac{d_G(u)(d_G(u)+d_G(v))}{d_G(u)+(d_G(u)+d_G(v))}\leq\frac{(d_G(u)+d_G(v))+d_G(u)}{4},$$
$$\frac{(d_G(u)+d_G(v))d_G(v)}{(d_G(u)+d_G(v))+d_G(v)}\leq\frac{d_G(v)+(d_G(u)+d_G(v))}{4}.$$

Therefore,

$$\sum 1<\frac{3\sum_{uv\in E(G)}(d_G(u)+d_G(v))}{4}=\frac{3}{4}M_1(G).$$

Similarly, for every $yy' \in E(L(G))$,

$$\frac{(2+d_{L(G)}(y))(2+d_{L(G)}(y'))}{4+(d_{L(G)}(y)+d_{L(G)}(y'))}\leq\frac{3}{4}+\frac{d_{L(G)}(y)d_{L(G)}(y')}{16}+\frac{(d_{L(G)}(y)+d_{L(G)}(y'))}{8}$$
$$+\frac{1}{2}\times\frac{2}{(d_{L(G)}(y)+d_{L(G)}(y'))}+\frac{d_{L(G)}(y)d_{L(G)}(y')}{4(d_{L(G)}(y)+d_{L(G)}(y'))}$$

$$\sum 2\leq\frac{3}{4}|E(L(G))|+\frac{M_2(L(G))}{16}+\frac{M_1(L(G))}{8}+\frac{H(L(G))}{2}+\frac{\mathrm{ISI}(L(G))}{4}$$
$$=\frac{3}{4}\frac{(M_1(G)-m)}{2}+\frac{M_2(L(G))}{16}+\frac{M_1(L(G))}{8}+\frac{H(L(G))}{2}+\frac{\mathrm{ISI}(L(G))}{4}$$
$$=\frac{3M_1(G)}{8}-\frac{3m}{4}+\frac{M_2(L(G))}{16}+\frac{M_1(L(G))}{8}+\frac{H(L(G))}{2}+\frac{\mathrm{ISI}(L(G))}{4}.$$

Hence,

$$\mathrm{ISI}(Q(G))<\frac{9M_1(G)}{8}-\frac{3m}{4}+\frac{M_2(L(G))}{16}+\frac{M_1(L(G))}{8}+\frac{H(L(G))}{2}+\frac{\mathrm{ISI}(L(G))}{4}$$

Example 1 For any $\boldsymbol{n \geq 4}$,

$$\mathrm{ISI}(Q(P_n))=\frac{39}{10}+2(n-3)\frac{4}{3}+\frac{24}{7}+4(n-4)=\frac{513}{70}+\frac{2(n-3)}{3}+4(n-4).$$

We have $d_{T(G)}(u) = 2d_G(u)$ for all $u \in V(G)$ and $d_{T(G)}(y) = d_G(u) + d_G(v) = d_{L(G)}(y) + 2$ for all $y \in V(Q(G))\backslash V(G)$, where vertex y is inserted in uv in G.

Theorem 1.2 Let $G \in \mathcal{G}(n, m)$. *Then,*

$$\mathrm{ISI}(T(G)) \leq 2\mathrm{ISI}(G) + \frac{11}{8}M_1(G) - \frac{3}{4}m + \frac{1}{16}M_2(L(G)) + \frac{1}{8}M_1(L(G)) + \frac{1}{2}H(L(G)) + \frac{1}{4}\mathrm{ISI}(L(G))$$

with equality being obtained for a two-regular graph.

Proof By definition,

$$\begin{aligned}
\mathrm{ISI}(T(G)) &= \sum_{uv\in E(G)} \left(\frac{d_{T(G)}(u)d_{T(G)}(x)}{d_{T(G)}(u) + d_{T(G)}(x)} + \frac{d_{T(G)}(x)d_{T(G)}(v)}{d_{T(G)}(x) + d_{T(G)}(v)} \right) + \\
&+ \sum_{yy'\in E(L(G))} \left(\frac{d_{T(G)}(y)d_{T(G)}(y')}{d_{T(G)}(y) + d_{T(G)}(y')} \right) + \sum_{uv\in E(G)} (\frac{d_{T(G)}(u)d_{T(G)}(v)}{d_{T(G)}(u) + d_{T(G)}(v)} \\
&\text{(where } x \text{ is the vertex inserted into the edge } uv \text{ if } G.) \\
&= \sum_{uv\in E(G)} \left(2\frac{d_G(u)(d_G(u) + d_G(v))}{2d_G(u) + (d_G(u) + d_G(v))} \right) + \frac{(d_G(u) + d_G(v))2d_G(v)}{(d_G(u) + d_G(v)) + 2d_G(v)} \\
&+ \sum_{yy'\in E(L(G))} \left(\frac{(2 + d_{L(G)}(y))(2 + d_{L(G)}(y'))}{(2 + d_{L(G)}(y)) + (2 + d_{L(G)}(y'))} \right) \sum_{uv\in E(G)} \left(\frac{2d_G(u)2d_G(v)}{2d_G(u) + 2d_G(v)} \right) \\
&= \sum_{uv\in E(G)} \left(2\frac{d_G(u)(d_G(u) + d_G(v))}{2d_G(u) + (d_G(u) + d_G(v))} \right) + \frac{(d_G(u) + d_G(v))2d_G(v)}{(d_G(u) + d_G(v)) + 2d_G(v)} \\
&+ \sum_{yy'\in E(L(G))} \left(\frac{(2 + d_{L(G)}(y))(2 + d_{L(G)}(y'))}{(2 + d_{L(G)}(y)) + (2 + d_{L(G)}(y'))} \right) + 2\mathrm{ISI}(G) \\
&= 2\mathrm{ISI}(G) + \sum 1 + \sum 2.
\end{aligned}$$

From Jensen's inequality, for every $uv \in E(G)$, we have

$$\frac{2d_G(u)(d_G(u) + d_G(v))}{2d_G(u) + (d_G(u) + d_G(v))} \leq \frac{(d_G(u) + d_G(v))}{4} + \frac{d_G(u)}{2},$$

with equality obtained if and only if $d_G(u) = d_G(v)$.

$$\frac{(d_G(u) + d_G(v))2d_G(v)}{(d_G(u) + d_G(v)) + 2d_G(v)} \leq \frac{(d_G(u) + d_G(v))}{4} + \frac{d_G(v)}{2},$$

with equality obtained if and only if $d_G(u) = d_G(v)$

Therefore,

$$\sum 1 \leq \sum_{uv\in E(G)} (d_G(u) + d_G(v))$$

$$= M_1(G).$$

Similarly, for every $yy' \in E(L(G))$,

$$\frac{(2 + d_{L(G)}(y))(2 + d_{L(G)}(y'))}{4 + (d_{L(G)}(y) + d_{L(G)}(y'))}$$
$$\leq \frac{3}{4} + \frac{d_{L(G)}(y)}{16} + \frac{d_{L(G)}(y) + d_{L(G)}(y')}{8}$$
$$+ \frac{1}{2}\frac{2}{d_{L(G)}(y) + d_{L(G)}(y')} + \frac{d_{L(G)}(y)d_{L(G)}(y')}{d_{L(G)}(y) + d_{L(G)}(y')},$$

with equality obtained if $d_G(u) = d_G(v) = 2$.

Therefore,

$$\sum_2 \leq \frac{3}{4}|E(L(G))| + \frac{1}{16}M_2(L(G)) + \frac{1}{8}M_1(L(G)) + \frac{1}{2}H(L(G)) + \frac{1}{4}\mathrm{ISI}(L(G))$$
$$= \frac{3}{4}\left(\frac{1}{2}M_1(G) - m\right) + \frac{1}{16}M_2(L(G)) + \frac{1}{8}M_1(L(G)) + \frac{1}{2}H(L(G)) + \frac{1}{4}\mathrm{ISI}(L(G))$$
$$= \frac{3}{8}M_1(G) - \frac{3}{4}m + \frac{1}{16}M_2(L(G)) + \frac{1}{8}M_1(L(G)) + \frac{1}{2}H(L(G)) + \frac{1}{4}\mathrm{ISI}(L(G))$$

Hence,

$$\mathrm{ISI}(T(G)) \leq 2\mathrm{ISI}(G) + \frac{11}{8}M_1(G) - \frac{3}{4}m + \frac{1}{16}M_2(L(G))$$
$$+ \frac{1}{8}M_1(L(G) + \frac{1}{2}H(L(G)) + \frac{1}{4}\mathrm{ISI}(L(G)).$$

Example 2 For any $\boldsymbol{n \geq 4}$,

$$\mathrm{ISI}(T(P_n)) = \frac{8}{3} + 2(n-3) + 2\left(\frac{6}{5} + \frac{12}{7}\right) + 4(n-3) + \frac{24}{7} + 4(n-4).$$
$$= \frac{1252}{105} + 6(n-3) + 4(n-4)$$

3 The ISI Indices of Q-Sums and T-Sums

In this section, some upper bounds are proposed for the ISI index of $G_1 +_Q G_2$, $G_1 +_T G_2$ in terms of $M_1(G_1)$, $M_1(G_2)$, $ID(G_1)$, $H(G_1)$ and $M_1(L(G_1))$.

Theorem 2.1 Let $G_1 \in G(n_1, m_1)$ *and* $G_2 \in G(n_2, m_2)$. *Then,*

$$\mathrm{ISI}(G_1 +_Q G_2) < \frac{3n_2M_1(G_1)}{2} + \frac{n_1M_1(G_2)}{4} + \frac{n_2M_1(Q(G_1))}{4} + \frac{3n_2M_1(L(G_1))}{4} + m_1(2m_2 - 3n_2).$$

Proof

$$\begin{aligned}\mathrm{ISI}(G_1 +_Q G_2) &= \sum_{u\in V(G_1)} \sum_{v_1v_2\in E(G_2)} \left(\frac{d(u,v_1)d(u,v_2)}{d(u,v_1)+d(u,v_2)}\right)\\ &+ \sum_{v\in V(G_2)} \sum_{u_1u_2\in E(Q(G_1))} \left(\frac{d(u_1,v)d(u_2,v)}{d(u_1,v)+d(u_2,v)}\right)\\ &= \sum 1 + \sum 2\end{aligned}$$

Now,

$$\sum 1 = \sum_{u\in V(G_1)} \sum_{v_1v_2\in E(G_2)} \left(\frac{d_{Q(G_1)}(u) + d_{G_2}(v_1)d_{Q(G_1)}(u) + d_{G_2}(v_2)}{2d_{Q(G_1)}(u) + \left(d_{G_2}(v_1) + d_{G_2}(v_2)\right)}\right)$$

For each $u \in V(G_1)$ and each $v_1v_2 \in E(G_2)$, by Jensen's inequality, we have

$$\frac{d_{Q(G_1)}(u) + d_{G_2}(v_1)d_{Q(G_1)}(u) + d_{G_2}(v_2)}{d_{Q(G_1)}(u) + d_{G_2}(v_1) + d_{Q(G_1)}(u) + d_{G_2}(v_2)} \le \frac{d_{G_1}(u)}{2} + \frac{d_{G_2}(v_1) + d_{G_2}(v_2)}{4}$$

with equality holding if and only if G_2 being regular.

Therefore,

$$\begin{aligned}\sum 1 &\le \sum_{u\in V(G_1)} \sum_{v_1v_2\in E(G_2)} \left[\frac{d_{G_1}(u)}{2} + \frac{d_{G_2}(v_1) + d_{G_2}(v_2)}{4}\right]\\ &= \frac{m_2}{2} \sum_{u\in V(G_1)} d_{G_1} + \frac{1}{4} \sum_{u\in V(G_1)} \sum_{v_1v_2\in E(G_2)} d_{G_2}(v_1) + d_{G_2}(v_2)\\ &= \frac{2m_1m_2}{2} + \frac{n_1M_1(G_2)}{4} = m_1m_2 + \frac{n_1M_1(G_2)}{4}\end{aligned}$$

Also,

$$\begin{aligned}\sum 2 = &\sum_{v\in V(G_2)} \sum_{\substack{u_1u_2 \in E(Q(G_1))\\ u_1 \in V(G_1),\, u_2 \in V(Q(G_1))\setminus V(G_1)}} \left(\frac{\left(d_{Q(G_1)}(u_1) + d_{G_2}(v)\right)\left(d_{Q(G_1)}(u_2) + d_{G_2}(v)\right)}{\left(d_{Q(G_1)}(u_1) + d_{G_2}(v)\right) + \left(d_{Q(G_1)}(u_2) + d_{G_2}(v)\right)}\right)\\ + &\sum_{v\in V(G_2)} \sum_{\substack{u_1u_2 \in E(Q(G_1))\\ u_1, u_2 \in V(Q(G_1))\setminus V(G_1)}} \left(\frac{\left(d_{Q(G_1)}(u_1) + d_{G_2}(v)\right)\left(d_{Q(G_1)}(u_2) + d_{G_2}(v)\right)}{\left(d_{Q(G_1)}(u_1) + d_{G_2}(v)\right) + \left(d_{Q(G_1)}(u_2) + d_{G_2}(v)\right)}\right)\end{aligned}$$

$$= \sum_{v \in V(G_2)} \sum_{\substack{u_1u_2 \in E(Q(G_1)) \\ u_1 \in V(G_1), u_2 \in V(Q(G_1))\setminus V(G_1)}} \left(\frac{\left(d_{Q(G_1)}(u_1) + d_{G_2}(v)\right) d_{Q(G_1)}(u_2)}{\left(d_{Q(G_1)}(u_1) + d_{G_2}(v)\right) + d_{Q(G_1)}(u_2)} \right)$$

$$+ \sum_{v \in V(G_2)} \sum_{\substack{u_1u_2 \in E(Q(G_1)) \\ u_1, u_2 \in V(Q(G_1))\setminus V(G_1)}} \left(\frac{d_{Q(G_1)}(u_1) d_{Q(G_1)}(u_2)}{d_{Q(G_1)}(u_1) + d_{Q(G_1)}(u_2)} \right)$$

For each $v \in V(G_2)$ and each $u_1u_2 \in E(Q(G_1))$ with $u_1 \in V(G_1)$ and $u_2 \in V(Q(G_1))\setminus V(G_1)$, by Jensen's inequality, we have

$$\frac{\left(d_{Q(G_1)}(u_1) + d_{G_2}(v)\right) d_{Q(G_1)}(u_2)}{\left(d_{Q(G_1)}(u_1) + d_{G_2}(v)\right) + d_{Q(G_1)}(u_2)} \leq \frac{\left(d_{Q(G_1)}(u_1) + d_{Q(G_1)}(u_2)\right) + d_{G_2}(v)}{4},$$

with equality being valid if and only if $Q(G_1)$ is regular and degree of any vertex from G_2 is zero which is not possible as we have studied only connected graphs here.

Again,

$$\frac{d_{Q(G_1)}(u_1) d_{Q(G_1)}(u_2)}{d_{Q(G_1)}(u_1) + d_{Q(G_1)}(u_2)} \leq \frac{\left(d_{Q(G_1)}(u_1) + d_{Q(G_1)}(u_2)\right)}{2},$$

where equality holds if and only if $Q(G_1)$ is regular.

Therefore,

$$\sum 2 \leq \frac{1}{4} \sum_{v \in V(G_2)} \sum_{\substack{u_1u_2 \in E(Q(G_1)) \\ u_1 \in V(G_1), u_2 \in V(Q(G_1))\setminus V(G_1)}} \left(d_{Q(G_1)}(u_1) + d_{Q(G_1)}(u_2)\right)$$

$$+ \frac{1}{2} \sum_{v \in V(G_2)} \sum_{\substack{u_1u_2 \in E(Q(G_1)) \\ u_1, u_2 \in V(Q(G_1))\setminus V(G_1)}} \left(d_{Q(G_1)}(u_1) + d_{Q(G_1)}(u_2)\right)$$

$$+ \frac{1}{4} \sum_{\substack{u_1u_2 \in E(Q(G_1)) \\ u_1 \in V(G_1), u_2 \in V(Q(G_1))\setminus V(G_1)}} \sum_{v \in V(G_2)} d_{G_2}(v)$$

We have,

$$\sum_{v \in V(G_2)} \sum_{\substack{u_1u_2 \in E(Q(G_1)) \\ u_1 \in V(G_1), u_2 \in V(Q(G_1))\setminus V(G_1)}} (d_{Q(G_1)}(u_1) + d_{Q(G_1)}(u_2)$$

$$= \sum_{v \in V(G_2)} \sum_{u_1 u_{1'} \in E(G_2)} (d_{Q(G_1)}(u_1) + d_{Q(G_1)}(u_2) + d_{Q(G_1)}(u_2) + d_{Q(G_1)}(u_{1'}))$$

(where $u_2$is the vertex inserted into the edge $u_1 u_{1'}$of G_1.)

$$= \sum_{v \in V(G_2)} [M_1(Q(G_1) - \sum_{yy' \in E(L(G_1))} (d_{Q(G_1)}(y) + d_{Q(G_1)}(y'))]$$

And,

$$\sum_{v \in V(G_2)} \sum_{\substack{u_1 u_2 \in E(Q(G_1)) \\ u_1, u_2 \in V(Q(G_1)) \backslash V(G_1)}} (d_{Q(G_1)}(u_1) + d_{Q(G_1)}(u_2))$$

$$= \sum_{v \in V(G_2)} \sum_{u_1 u_2 \in E(L(G_1))} (4 + d_{L(G_1)}(u_1) + d_{L(G_1)}(u_2))$$

$$= 2n_2 M_1(G_1) - 4m_1 n_2 + n_2 M_1(L(G_1))$$

$$\sum_{\substack{u_1 u_2 \in E(Q(G_1)) \\ u_1 \in V(G_1), u_2 \in V(Q(G_1)) \backslash V(G_1)}} \sum_{v \in V(G_2)} d_{G_2}(v)$$

$$= \sum_{\substack{u_1 u_2 \in E(Q(G_1)) \\ u_1 \in V(G_1), u_2 \in V(Q(G_1)) \backslash V(G_1)}} (2m_2) = (2m_1)(2m_2) = 4m_1 m_2$$

Therefore,

$$\sum 2 \leq \frac{3n_2 M_1(G_1)}{2} + \frac{3n_2 M_1(L(G_1))}{4} + \frac{n_2 M_1(Q(G_1))}{4} - 3m_1 n_2 + m_1 m_2.$$

Hence,

$$\begin{aligned} \mathrm{ISI}(G_1 +_Q G_2) &< m_1 m_2 + \frac{n_1 M_1(G_2)}{4} + \frac{3n_2 M_1(G_1)}{2} + \frac{3n_2 M_1(L(G_1))}{4} \\ &\quad + \frac{n_2 M_1(Q(G_1))}{4} - 3m_1 n_2 + m_1 m_2 \\ &= \frac{3n_2 M_1(G_1)}{2} + \frac{n_1 M_1(G_2)}{4} + \frac{n_2 M_1(Q(G_1))}{4} + \frac{3n_2 M_1(L(G_1))}{4} \\ &\quad + m_1(2m_2 - 3n_2). \end{aligned}$$

Theorem 2.2 Let $G_1 \in \mathcal{G}(n_1, m_1)$ *and* $G_2 \in \mathcal{G}(n_2, m_2)$. *Then,*

$$\mathrm{ISI}(G_1 +_T G_2) < n_2 M_1(G_1) + \frac{n_1 M_1(G_2)}{4} + \frac{n_2 M_1(T(G_1))}{4} + 2m_1(2m_2 - n_2)$$

Proof

$$\begin{aligned}\mathrm{ISI}(G_1 +_T G_2) &= \sum_{u\in V(G_1)} \sum_{v_1v_2\in E(G_2)} \left(\frac{d(u,v_1)d(u,v_2)}{d(u,v_1)+d(u,v_2)}\right)\\ &+ \sum_{v\in V(G_2)} \sum_{u_1u_2\in E(Q(G_1))} \left(\frac{d(u_1,v)d(u_2,v)}{d(u_1,v)+d(u_2,v)}\right)\\ &= \sum 1 + \sum 2\end{aligned}$$

Now,

$$\sum 1 = \sum_{u\in V(G_1)} \sum_{v_1v_2\in E(G_2)} \left(\frac{\left(d_{T(G_1)}(u)+d_{G_2}(v_1)\right)\left(d_{T(G_1)}(u)+d_{G_2}(v_2)\right)}{2d_{T(G_1)}(u)+\left(d_{G_2}(v_1)+d_{G_2}(v_2)\right)}\right)$$

Therefore,

$$\sum 1 \le 2m_1m_2 + \frac{n_1M_1(G_2)}{4},$$

where equality holds if and only if G_2 is regular.

Also,

$$\begin{aligned}\sum 2 = &\sum_{v\in V(G_2)} \sum_{\substack{u_1u_2\in E(T(G_1))\\ u_1,u_2\in V(G_1)}} \sum_{v\in V(G_2)}\\ &\sum_{\substack{u_1u_2\in E(T(G_1))\\ u_1\in V(G_1),\,u_2\in V(T(G_1))\setminus V(G_1)}} \left(\frac{\left(d_{T(G_1)}(u_1)+d_{G_2}(v)\right)\left(d_{T(G_1)}(u_2)+d_{G_2}(v)\right)}{\left(d_{T(G_1)}(u_1)+d_{G_2}(v)\right)+\left(d_{T(G_1)}(u_2)+d_{G_2}(v)\right)}\right)\\ &+ \sum_{v\in V(G_2)} \sum_{\substack{u_1u_2\in E(T(G_1))\\ u_1,u_2\in V(T(G_1))\setminus V(G_1)}} \left(\frac{\left(d_{T(G_1)}(u_1)+d_{G_2}(v)\right)\left(d_{T(G_1)}(u_2)+d_{G_2}(v)\right)}{\left(d_{T(G_1)}(u_1)+d_{G_2}(v)\right)+\left(d_{T(G_1)}(u_2)+d_{G_2}(v)\right)}\right)\\ = &\sum_{v\in V(G_2)} \sum_{\substack{u_1u_2\in E(T(G_1))\\ u_1,u_2\in V(G_1)}} \left(\frac{\left(d_{T(G_1)}(u_1)+d_{G_2}(v)\right)\left(d_{T(G_1)}(u_2)+d_{G_2}(v)\right)}{\left(d_{T(G_1)}(u_1)+d_{G_2}(v)\right)+(d_{T(G_1)+d_{G_2}(v))}(u_2)}\right)\\ &+ \sum_{v\in V(G_2)} \sum_{\substack{u_1u_2\in E(T(G_1))\\ u_1\in V(G_1),\,u_2\in V(T(G_1))\setminus V(G_1)}} \left(\frac{\left(d_{T(G_1)}(u_1)+d_{G_2}(v)\right)d_{T(G_1)}(u_2)}{\left(d_{T(G_1)}(u_1)+d_{G_2}(v)\right)+d_{T(G_1)}(u_2)}\right)\\ &+ \sum_{v\in V(G_2)} \sum_{\substack{u_1u_2\in E(T(G_1))\\ u_1,u_2\in V(T(G_1))\setminus V(G_1)}} \left(\frac{d_{T(G_1)}(u_1)d_{T(G_1)}(u_2)}{d_{T(G_1)}(u_1)+d_{T(G_1)}(u_2)}\right).\end{aligned}$$

For each $v \in V(G_2)$ and each $u_1u_2 \in E(T(G_1))$ with $u_1, u_2 \in V(G_1)$, Jensen's inequality gives

$$\frac{\left(d_{T(G_1)}(u_1)+d_{G_2}(v)\right)\left(d_{T(G_1)}(u_2)+d_{G_2}(v)\right)}{\left(d_{T(G_1)}(u_1)+d_{G_2}(v)\right)+\left(d_{T(G_1)}(u_2)+d_{G_2}(v)\right)} \le \frac{\left(\left(d_{T(G_1)}(u_1)+d_{T(G_1)}(u_2)\right)+2d_{G_2}(v)\right)}{4},$$

with equality being valid when $T(G_1)$ is regular.

Therefore,

$$\sum_{v\in V(G_2)} \sum_{\substack{u_1u_2 \in E(T(G_1)) \\ u_1, u_2 \in V(G_1)}} \left(\frac{\left(d_{T(G_1)}(u_1)+d_{G_2}(v)\right)\left(d_{T(G_1)}(u_2)+d_{G_2}(v)\right)}{\left(d_{T(G_1)}(u_1)+d_{G_2}(v)\right)+\left(d_{T(G_1)}(u_2)+d_{G_2}(v)\right)}\right) \le \frac{n_2M_1(G_1)}{2} + m_1m_2$$

Following the same procedure as in the previous theorem, we have

$$\sum_{v\in V(G_2)} \sum_{\substack{u_1u_2 \in E(T(G_1)) \\ u_1 \in V(G_1),\, u_2 \in V(T(G_1))\setminus V(G_1)}} \left(\frac{\left(d_{T(G_1)}(u_1)+d_{G_2}(v)\right)d_{T(G_1)}(u_2)}{\left(d_{T(G_1)}(u_1)+d_{G_2}(v)\right)+d_{T(G_1)}(u_2)}\right)$$
$$\le \frac{n_2M_1(T(G_1))}{4} - \frac{n_2M_1(G_1)}{2} - \frac{n_2M_1(L(G_1))}{4} - m_1n_2 + m_1m_2,$$

where equality holds when the degree of any vertex in G_2 is zero which is not possible in our case as we have considered connected graphs only.

And,

$$\sum_{v\in V(G_2)} \sum_{\substack{u_1u_2 \in E(T(G_1)) \\ u_1, u_2 \in V(T(G_1))\setminus V(G_1)}} \left(\frac{d_{T(G_1)}(u_1)d_{T(G_1)}(u_2)}{d_{T(G_1)}(u_1)+d_{T(G_1)}(u_2)}\right) \le \frac{n_2M_1(G_1)}{2} - m_1n_2 + \frac{n_2M_1(L(G_1))}{4}$$

with equality holding if and only if $T(G_1)$ is regular.

Finally, we have,

$$\text{ISI}(G_1 +_T G_2) < n_2M_1(G_1) + \frac{n_1M_1(G_2)}{4} + \frac{n_2M_1(T(G_1))}{4} + 2m_1(2m_2 - n_2)$$

4 Conclusion

There is relatively limited study of the ISI index for various operations of graphs in the literature. In this paper, we compute the ISI index of edge-semitotal graphs and total graphs and propose upper bounds for them. We also establish bounds for the ISI index of Q-sums and T-sums. The extremal cases are also taken up and studied in each of the bounds. The study of the ISI index for other graph operations can be an interesting prospect for future study.

References

1. Eliasi, M., Taeri, D.: Four new sums of graphs and their Wiener indices. Discret. Appl. Math. **157**, 794–803 (2009)
2. Hammack, R., Imrich, W., Klavžar, S.: Handbook of Product Graphs, Discrete Mathematics and Application, 2nd edn, CRC Press (2011)
3. Gutman, I.: Degree-based topological indices. Croat. Chem. Acta **86**(4), 351–361 (2013)
4. Pattabiraman, K.: Inverse sum indeg index of graphs. AKCE Int. J. Graphs Comb. **15**, 155–167 (2018)
5. Chen, H., Deng, H.: The inverse sum indeg index of graphs with some given parameters. Discret. Math. Algorithms Appl. **10**(1), 1850006 (2018)
6. Jamil, M.K., Javed, A., Farahani, M.R.: Inverse sum indeg index (ISI) of the line graphs of subdivision graphs of some chemical structures. UPB Sci. Bull., Series B: Chem. Mater. Sci. **80**(3), 97–104 (2018)
7. Lokesha, V., Deepika, T., Cangul, I.N.: Symmetric division deg and inverse sum indeg indices of polycyclic aromatic hydrocarbons (PAHs) and polyhex nanotubes. Southeast Asian Bull. Math. **41**(5), 707–715 (2017)
8. Onagh, B.N.: The harmonic index of subdivision graphs. Trans. Comb. **6**(4), 15–27 (2017)
9. Onagh, B.N.: The harmonic index of product graphs. Math. Sci. **11**(3), 203–209 (2017)
10. Onagh, B.N.: The harmonic index of edge-semitotal graphs, total graphs and related sums. Kragujevac Journal of Mathematics **42**(2), 217–228 (2018)
11. Shwetha, B.S., Lokesha, V., Ranjini, P.S.: On the harmonic index of graph operations. Trans. Comb. **4**(4), 5–14 (2015)

Four New Operations of Graphs Related to Tensor Product and Zagreb Indices

J. Buragohain, A. Bharali and A. Mahanta

Abstract The intermolecular forces of a chemical compound exist not only in between the atoms but also between the atoms and the molecular bonds. The *F*-sums of graphs, namely subdivision graph, vertex-semi-total graph, edge-semi-total graph, and total graph of a graph which are popularly denoted by *S*, *Q*, *R*, and *T*, respectively, can capture this property of chemical compound. In this paper, we present four operations of graphs based on tensor product of graphs and establish explicit expressions of Zagreb indices of the newly defined graph operations.

Keywords Degree of vertex · Zagreb indices · Operations of graphs

AMS Classification 05C76 · 05C07

1 Introduction

In this work, we consider only finite graphs which are simple (i.e., without loops or multiple edges) and undirected. Let G be any graph with $V(G)$ and $E(G)$ be its vertex set and the edge set, respectively. The degree of a vertex a in G, which we denote as $\delta_G(a)$ or simply as $\delta(a)$, is the cardinality of the set of first neighboring vertices of a. If there is a direct connection between two vertices a and b of G, then we write it as $ab \in E(G)$.

In chemical graph theory, a topological index (TI) is a mathematical quantity which can be computed for any molecular compound. Topological indices are calculated based on the graph theoretical representation of a molecule which is known as the molecular graph. A molecular graph consists of vertices corresponding to atoms

---

J. Buragohain (✉) · A. Bharali · A. Mahanta
Department of Mathematics, Dibrugarh University, Dibrugarh, Assam 786004, India
e-mail: j.bgohain75@yahoo.com

A. Bharali
e-mail: a.bharali@dibru.ac.in

A. Mahanta
e-mail: am02dib@gmail.com

S. Bhattacharyya et al. (eds.), *Mathematical Modeling and Computational Tools*, Springer Proceedings in Mathematics & Statistics 320,
https://doi.org/10.1007/978-981-15-3615-1_29

and edges are defined based on various chemical bonds between the atoms in the molecule. These TIs are also known as molecular graph-based structure descriptors and are generally graph invariants, i.e., topological indices are invariants under graph isomorphism. Topological index (also known as connectivity index) can be helpful in predicting various physicochemical properties of a chemical compound, and hence, they find importance in QSPR and QSAR studies. This kind of prediction eliminates the constraints in laboratory experiments which are not desirable to perform due to high risk or high cost. For example, the first genuine topological index, i.e., Randić index, is utilized in drug designing, and the atom–bond connectivity index (or ABC index) is utilized in modeling information about heat of formation of alkanes are to name a few. Numerous TIs are defined based on degree, distance, eccentricity, eigenvalue, and other graph theoretic notions. Some of these degree-based TIs may be found in [1].

Among all the degree-based structure descriptors that exist in literature, the Zagreb indices are historically oldest which are introduced by Gutman and Trinajstić in connection with the total π-electron energy of a molecule [2]. But these are considered as topological indices only after their inception which possibly because of their intended purpose of utility. The first Zagreb index of a graph G is defined as

$$M_1(G) = \sum_{a \in V(G)} (\delta_G(a))^2,$$

which can also be written as $M_1(G) = \sum_{ab \in E(G)} (\delta_G(a) + \delta_G(b))$, and the second Zagreb index is defined as

$$M_2(G) = \sum_{ab \in E(G)} \delta_G(a)\delta_G(b).$$

"Zagreb group indices" and "Zagreb group parameters" are also the names devoted to Zagreb indices. Zagreb indices can provide information about the molecular branching as they have the power to discriminate the isomers [1]. Using basic ideas of adjacency matrix, $A(G) = [A_{ij}]$, one can define the Zagreb indices of a graph G as follows [3]:

$$M_1(G) = \sum_{\text{vertices}} (A^2)_{ii}(A^2)_{ii} \text{ and } M_2(G) = \sum_{\text{edges}} (A^2)_{ii}(A^2)_{jj}.$$

The general first Zagreb index M_α of a graph G is defined as [4]:

$$M_1^\alpha(G) = \sum_{a \in V(G)} (\delta_G(a))^\alpha = \sum_{ab \in E(G)} \left((\delta_G(a))^{\alpha-1} + (\delta_G(b))^{\alpha-1}\right),$$

where α is a real number.

The tensor product of two graphs G_1 and G_2, denoted by $G_1 \otimes G_2$, gives a new graph with vertex set $V(G_1 \otimes G_2) = V(G_1) \times V(G_2)$ and edge set $E(G_1 \otimes G_2) = \{(a,b)(c,d)|ac \in E(G_1)$ and $bd \in E(G_2)\}$. The details of this operation may be found in [5, 6]. This operation is also studied in connection with various TIs. The study of Zagreb indices of tensor product of graphs may be found in [7].

For a connected graph G, there are four related graphs $S(G)$, $R(G)$, $Q(G)$ and $T(G)$. These graphs are called subdivision graph, vertex-semi-total graph, edge-semi-total, and total graph, respectively. These operations are defined as below:

- $S(G)$ is the graph obtained by replacing each edge of G by a path of length 2.
- $R(G)$ is obtained from G by adding a path of length 2 parallel to each of the edges of G.
- $Q(G)$ is obtained from G by replacing each edge by path of length 2, then joining with edge those pairs of new vertices on adjacent edges of G.
- $T(G)$ has as its vertices the edges and vertices of G. Adjacency in $T(G)$ is defined as adjacency or incidence for the corresponding elements of G.

For details of these four graph operations, see [8]. Different graph operations based on these four graphs have been defined and studied in connection with Wiener indices and Zagreb indices [9–13]. The reason behind the extensive studies of these four graph operations lies in the fact that they can capture the intermolecular forces that exist between the atoms and the bonds of a molecule along with the conventional atom–atom interactions.

In this communication, we propose four new operations of graphs based on the tensor product of graphs and establish explicit expressions for Zagreb indices of these new operations. The rest of the paper is organized as follows. In Sect. 2, the new sums are introduced. In Sect. 3, formulae for the Zagreb indices of the new graphs are obtained, and in Sect. 4, conclusions are made.

2 New F-Sums of Graphs

Let G_1 and G_2 be simple connected graphs, and let F be any one of S, R, Q and T. Then, we define $G_1 \otimes_F G_2$ as a binary operation of graphs G_1 and G_2 which produces a graph by the tensor product of $F(G_1)$ and G_2. The vertex set and the edge set of this new operation are given as:

$$V(G_1 \otimes_F G_2) = \{(a,b)|a \in V(F(G_1)) \text{ and } b \in V(G_2)\} \text{ and}$$
$$E(G_1 \otimes_F G_2) = \{(a,b)(c,d)|ac \in E(F(G_1)) \text{ and } bd \in E(G_2)\}.$$

There are $(|V(G_1)| + |E(G_1)|)|V(G_2)|$ number of vertices in $G_1 \otimes_F G_2$, and there is an edge between (a,b) and (c,d) in $G_1 \otimes_F G_2$ if and only if ac is an edge in $F(G_1)$ and bd is an edge in G_2. As for example, $P_3 \otimes_S P_3$, $P_3 \otimes_R P_3$, $P_3 \otimes_Q P_3$ and $P_3 \otimes_T P_3$ are shown in Fig. 1.

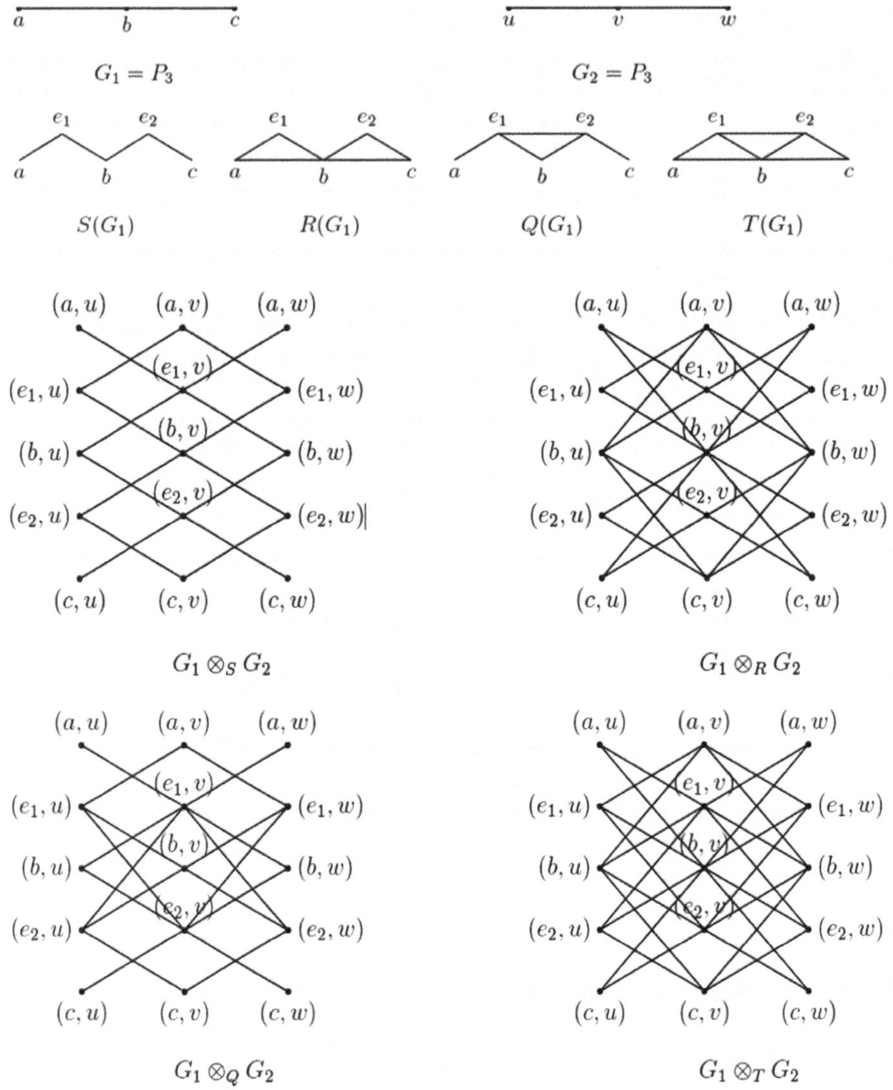

Fig. 1 Four new operations of graphs based on tensor product of graphs

It is not difficult to establish the following relations between the degree of vertices of newly defined graphs and the participating graphs.

Lemma 2.1 *Let G_1 and G_2 be two graphs. Then,*

(a) $\delta_{G_1 \otimes_S G_2}(a, b) = \begin{cases} \delta_{G_1}(a)\delta_{G_2}(b) & \text{if } a \in V(G_1) \\ 2\delta_{G_2}(b) & \text{if } a \in V(S(G_1)) \backslash V(G_1). \end{cases}$

(b) $\delta_{G_1 \otimes_R G_2}(a,b) = \begin{cases} 2\delta_{G_1}(a)\delta_{G_2}(b) & \text{if } a \in V(G_1) \\ 2\delta_{G_2}(b) & \text{if } a \in V(R(G_1)) \backslash V(G_1). \end{cases}$

(c) $\delta_{G_1 \otimes_Q G_2}(a,b) = \begin{cases} \delta_{G_1}(a)\delta_{G_2}(b) & \text{if } a \in V(G_1) \\ \left(\delta_{G_1}(w) + \delta_{G_2}(w')\right)\delta_{G_2}(b) & \text{if } a \in V(Q(G_1)) \backslash V(G_1), \end{cases}$

where in the second case, a is inserted into the edge $ww' \in E(G_1)$.

(d) $\delta_{G_1 \otimes_T G_2}(a,b) = \begin{cases} 2\delta_{G_1}(a)\delta_{G_2}(b) & \text{if } a \in V(G_1) \\ \left(\delta_{G_1}(w) + \delta_{G_2}(w')\right)\delta_{G_2}(b) & \text{if } a \in V(T(G_1)) \backslash V(G_1), \end{cases}$

where in the second case, a is inserted into the edge $ww' \in E(G_1)$.

3 Main Results

In this section, we give explicit expression for Zagreb indices of the newly defined graphs.

3.1 The First Zagreb Index of $G_1 \otimes_F G_2$

Theorem 3.1 *Let G_1 and G_2 be two finite graphs with $|E(G_1)| = m_1$. Then,*

$$M_1(G_1 \otimes_S G_2) = M_1(G_1)M_1(G_2) + 4m_1M_1(G_2).$$

Proof

$$\begin{aligned} M_1(G_1 \otimes_S G_2) &= \sum_{(a,b)\in V(G_1 \otimes_S G_2)} (\delta(a,b))^2 \\ &= \sum_{a\in V(G_1)} \sum_{b\in V(G_2)} \left(\delta_{G_1}(a)\delta_{G_2}(b)\right)^2 + \sum_{a\in V(S(G_1))\backslash V(G_1)} \sum_{v\in V(G_2)} \left(2\delta_{G_2}(b)\right)^2 \\ &= M_1(G_1)M_1(G_2) + 4m_1M_1(G_2). \end{aligned}$$

Hence proved. □

Theorem 3.2 *Let G_1 and G_2 be two finite graphs and $E(G_1) = m_1$. Then,*

$$M_1(G_1 \otimes_R G_2) = 4M_1(G_1)M_1(G_2) + 4m_1M_1(G_2).$$

Proof

$$M_1(G_1 \otimes_R G_2) = \sum_{(a,b)\in V(G_1 \otimes_R G_2)} (\delta(a,b))^2$$
$$= \sum_{a\in V(G_1)} \sum_{b\in V(G_2)} \left(2\delta_{G_1}(a)\delta_{G_2}(b)\right)^2 + \sum_{a\in V(R(G_1))\setminus V(G_1)} \sum_{b\in V(G_2)} \left(2\delta_{G_2}(b)\right)^2$$
$$= 4M_1(G_1)M_1(G_2) + 4m_1 M_1(G_2). \square$$

Theorem 3.3 *Let G_1 and G_2 be two finite graphs. Then,*

$$M_1\big(G_1 \otimes_Q G_2\big) = \big(M_1(G_1) + 2M_2(G_1) + M_1^3(G_1)M_1(G_2)\big).$$

Proof We can divide the set of vertices into two categories.

$$M_1\big(G_1 \otimes_Q G_2\big) = \sum_{(a,b)\in V(G_1 \otimes_Q G_2)} (\delta(a,b))^2$$
$$= \left(\sum_1 + \sum_2\right)(\delta(a,b))^2$$
$$\sum_1 (\delta(a,b))^2 = \sum_{a\in V(G_1)} \sum_{b\in V(G_2)} \left(\delta_{G_1}(a)\delta_{G_2}(b)\right)^2$$
$$= \sum_{a\in V(G_1)} \left(\delta_{G_1}(a)\right)^2 \sum_{b\in V(G_2)} \left(\delta_{G_2}(b)\right)^2$$
$$= M_1(G_1)M_1(G_2).$$

and

$$\sum_2 (\delta(a,b))^2 = \sum_{a\in V(Q(G_1))\setminus V(G_1)} \sum_{b\in V(G_2)} \left(\left(\delta_{G_1}(w) + \delta_{G_1}(w')\right)\delta_{G_2}(b)\right)^2$$
$$= \sum_{ww'\in E(G_1)} \left(\delta_{G_1}(w) + \delta_{G_2}(w')\right)^2 \sum_{b\in V(G_2)} \left(\delta_{G_2}(b)\right)^2$$
$$= \big(M_1^3(G_1) + 2M_2(G_1)\big)M_1(G_2).$$

In the second sum, a is assumed to be inserted in $ww' \in E(G_1)$. Hence, $M_1\big(G_1 \otimes_Q G_2\big) = \big(M_1(G_1) + 2M_2(G_1) + M_1^3(G_1)\big)M_1(G_2)$. $\square$

Theorem 3.4 *Let G_1 and G_2 be two finite graphs. Then,*

$$M_1(G_1 \otimes_T G_2) = \big(4M_1(G_1) + 2M_2(G_1) + M_1^3(G_1)\big)M_1(G_2).$$

The proof of Theorem 3.4 is similar to the proof of Theorem 3.3.

3.2 Second Zagreb Index of $G_1 \otimes_F G_2$

Theorem 3.5 *Let G_1 and G_2 be two simple finite graphs. Then,*

$$M_2(G_1 \otimes_S G_2) = 4M_1(G_1)M_2(G_2).$$

Proof According to the definition of the second Zagreb index, we have

$$\begin{aligned} M_2(G_1 \otimes_S G_2) &= \sum_{(a,b)(c,d)\in E(G_1 \otimes_S G_2)} \delta(a,b)\delta(c,d) \\ &= 2\sum_{ac\in E(G_1)} \sum_{bd\in E(G_2)} \delta_{G_1}(a)\delta_{G_2}(b)2\delta_{G_2}(d) \\ &= 4\sum_{ac\in E(G_1)} \delta_{G_1}(a) \sum_{bd\in E(G_2)} \delta_{G_2}(b)\delta_{G_2}(d) \\ &= 4M_1(G_1)M_2(G_2).\square \end{aligned}$$

Theorem 3.6 *Let G_1 and G_2 be two simple finite graphs. Then,*

$$M_2(G_1 \otimes_R G_2) = 8(M_1(G_1) + M_2(G_1))M_2(G_2).$$

Proof From the definition of the second Zagreb index,

$$M_2(G_1 \otimes_R G_2) = \sum_{(a,b)(c,d)\in E(G_1 \otimes_R G_2)} \delta(a,b)\delta(c,d).$$

The edges of $G_1 \otimes_R G_2$ can be categorized into the following cases.

Case I: $(a,b)(c,d) \in E(G_1 \otimes_R G_2)$ such that $a, c \in V(G_1)$. Then,

$$\begin{aligned} \sum_{(a,b)(c,d)\in E(G_1 \otimes_R G_2)} \delta(a,b)\delta(c,d) &= 2\sum_{ac\in E(R(G_1))} \sum_{bd\in E(G_2)} 2\delta_{G_1}(a)\delta_{G_1}(b)2\delta_{G_2}(c)\delta_{G_2}(d) \\ &= 8\sum_{ac\in E(G_1)} \delta_{G_1}(a)\delta_{G_1}(c) \sum_{bd\in E(G_2)} \delta_{G_2}(b)\delta_{G_2}(d) \\ &= 8M_2(G_1)M_2(G_2). \end{aligned}$$

Case II: $(a,b)(c,d) \in E(G_1 \otimes_R G_2)$ such that $a \in V(G_1)$ and $c \in V(R(G_1))\backslash V(G_1)$. Then,

$$\begin{aligned} \sum_{(a,b)(c,d)\in E(G_1 \otimes_R G_2)} \delta(a,b)\delta(c,d) &= 2\sum_{ac\in E(R(G_1))} \sum_{bd\in E(G_2)} 2\delta_{G_1}(a)\delta_{G_2}(b)2\delta_{G_2}(d) \\ &= 8\sum_{ac\in E(R(G_1))} \delta_{G_1}(a) \sum_{bd\in E(G_2)} \delta_{G_2}(b)\delta_{G_2}(d) \end{aligned}$$

$$= 8M_1(G_1)M_2(G_2).$$

Therefore, $M_2(G_1 \otimes_R G_2) = 8M_2(G_1)M_2(G_2) + 8M_1(G_1)M_2(G_2)$. Hence proved. □

Theorem 3.7 *Let G_1 and G_2 be two simple graphs. Then, we have the following result:*

$$M_2(G_1 \otimes_Q G_2) = \Bigg[2M_2(G_1) + M_1^3(G_1) + M_1^4(G_1) + 2\sum_{w,w'' \in V(G_1)} \gamma_{ww''}\delta_{G_1}(w)\delta_{G_1}(w'') \\ +2\sum_{w' \in V(G_1)} \left(\delta_{G_1}(w')\right)^2 \sum_{w \in V(G_1) s.t. ww' \in E(G_1)} \delta_{G_1}(w)\Bigg] M_2(G_2),$$

where $\gamma_{ww''}$ is the number of common vertices of w and w''.

Proof We have

$$M_2(G_1 \otimes_Q G_2) = \sum_{(a,b)(c,d) \in E(G_1 \otimes_Q G_2)} \delta(a,b)\delta(c,d).$$

The above sum over the edges of $G_1 \otimes_Q G_2$ can be classified in the following ways:

Case I: $(a,b)(c,d) \in E(G_1 \otimes_Q G_2)$ such that $a \in V(G_1)$, $c \in V(Q(G_1)) \backslash V(G_1)$ and let c be inserted in $aa' \in E(G_1)$. Then,

$$\begin{aligned} &\sum_{(a,b)(c,d) \in E(G_1 \otimes_Q G_2)} \delta(a,b)\delta(c,d) \\ &= 2\sum_{ac \in E(Q(G_1)), bd \in E(G_2)} \delta_{G_1}(a)\delta_{G_2}(b)\left(\delta_{G_1}(a) + \delta_{G_1}(a')\right)\delta_{G_2}(d) \\ &= 2\sum_{aa' \in E(G_1)} \left(\delta_{G_1}(a) + \delta_{G_1}(a')\right)^2 \sum_{bd \in E(G_2)} \delta_{G_2}(b)\delta_{G_2}(d) \\ &= 2\left(M_1^3(G_1) + 2M_2(G_1)\right)M_2(G_2). \end{aligned}$$

Case II: $(a,b)(c,d) \in E(G_1 \otimes_Q G_2)$ such that $a, c \in V(Q(G_1)) \backslash V(G_1)$. Let a and c be inserted in ww' and $w'w''$ of $E(G_1)$, respectively. Then,

$$\sum_{(a,b)(c,d) \in E(G_1 \otimes_Q G_2)} \delta(a,b)\delta(c,d)$$

$$= 2 \sum_{ac \in E(Q(G_1)), bd \in E(G_2)} (\delta_{G_1}(w) + \delta_{G_1}(w'))\delta_{G_2}(b)(\delta_{G_1}(w') + \delta_{G_1}(w''))\delta_{G_2}(d)$$

$$= 2 \sum_{ww', w'w'' \in E(G_1)} (\delta_{G_1}(w) + \delta_{G_1}(w'))(\delta_{G_1}(w') + \delta_{G_1}(w'')) \sum_{bd \in E(G_2)} \delta_{G_2}(b)\delta_{G_2}(d)$$

$$= 2\left\{ \sum_{w' \in V(G_1)} \delta_{G_1}(w')(\delta_{G_1}(w') - 1) \sum_{w \in V(G_1) s.t. ww' \in E(G_1)} \delta_{G_1}(w) \right.$$

$$\left. + \sum_{w' \in V(G_1)} \binom{\delta_{G_1}(w')}{2} (\delta_{G_1}(w'))^2 + \sum_{w, w'' \in V(G_1)} \gamma_{ww''}\delta_{G_1}(w)\delta_{G_1}(w'') \right\} M_2(G_2)$$

$$= 2\left\{ \sum_{w' \in V(G_1)} (\delta_{G_1}(w'))^2 \sum_{w \in V(G_1) s.t. ww' \in E(G_1)} \delta_{G_1}(w) - M_2(G_1) \right.$$

$$\left. + \frac{1}{2}(M_1^4(G_1) - M_1^3(G_1)) + \sum_{w, w'' \in V(G_1)} \gamma_{ww''}\delta_{G_1}(w)\delta_{G_1}(w'') \right\} M_2(G_2).$$

Now by combining the above two cases, we get the result. □

Theorem 3.8 *Let* G_1 and G_2 *be any two simple graphs. Then, the second Zagreb index of* $G_1 \otimes_T G_2$ *is given as follows:*

$$M_2(G_1 \otimes_T G_2) = \left\{ 14M_2(G_1) + 3M_1^3(G_1) + M_1^4(G_1) + 2\left(\sum_{w, w' \in V(G_1)} \gamma_{ww'}\delta_{G_1}(w)\delta_{G_1}(w') \right.\right.$$

$$\left.\left. + \sum_{w' \in V(G_1)} (\delta_{G_1}(w'))^2 \sum_{w \in V(G_1) \; s.t. \; ww' \in E(G_1)} \delta_{G_1}(w) \right) \right\} M_2(G_2),$$

where $\gamma_{ww'}$ *is the number of common neighbors of* w *and* w' *in* G_1.

4 Conclusion

In this paper, we first propose four new operations of graphs based on tensor product of graphs, and then, we study the Zagreb indices of these operations of graphs. This study is motivated by similar considerations based on other graph operations like Cartesian product, join and lexicographic product [10, 12, 13]. As an immediate extension of this study, we can compute other topological indices of these new graphs. It will be also interesting to study the spectral property of these newly defined operations.

References

1. Gutman, I.: Degree-based topological indices. Croat. Chem. Acta **86**(4), 351–361 (2013)
2. Gutman, I., Trinajstić, N.: Graph theory and molecular orbitals. Total π-electron energy of alternate hydrocarbons. Chem. Phy. Lett. **74**(4), 535–538 (1992)
3. Nikolić, S., Kovačević, G., Miličević, A., Trinajstić, N.: The Zagreb indices 30 years after. Croat. Chem. Acta **76**(2), 113–124 (2003)
4. Li, X., Zhao, H.: Trees with the first three smallest and largest generalized topological index. MATCH Commun. Math. Comput. Chem. **50**, 57–62 (2004)
5. Hammack, R., Imrich, W., Klavžar, S.: Handbook of Product Graphs. CRC Press (2011)
6. Sirous, M.: A note on tensor product of graphs. Iran. J. Math. Sci. Inform. **7**(1), 73–81 (2012)
7. Yarahmadi, Z.: Computing some topological indices of tensor product of graphs. Iran. J. Math. Chem. **2**(1), 109–118 (2011)
8. Cvetkocić, D.M., Doob, M., Sachs, H.: Spectra of Graphs: Theory and Application. Academic Press, New York (1980)
9. Khalifeh, M., Yousefi-Azari, H., Ashrafi, A.R.: The first and second Zagreb indices of some graph operations. Discrete Appl. Math. **157**(4), 804–811 (2009)
10. Deng, H., Sarala, D., Ayyaswamy, S., Balachandran, K.: The Zagreb indices of four operations of graphs. Appl. Math. Comput. **275**, 422–431 (2016)
11. Eliasi, M., Taeri, D.: Four new sums of graphs and their Wiener indices. Discrete Appl. Math. **157**, 794–803 (2009)
12. Sarala, D., Deng, H., Ayyaswamy, S.K., Balachandran, S.: The Zagreb indices of graphs based on four operations related to the lexicographic product. Appl. Math. Comput. **309**, 156–169 (2017)
13. Sarkar, P., De, N., Pal, A.: The Zagreb indies of graphs based on new operations related to the join of graphs. J. Int. Math. Virtual Inst. **7**, 181–209 (2017)

Some Oscillatory Results for Nonlinear Equation on Time Scales

Shekhar Singh Negi, Syed Abbas and Muslim Malik

Abstract This manuscript provides some oscillatory results of a dynamic equation with variable coefficients, in which a Riccati transformation technique is used. Besides, we obtain the Kamenev-type and Philos-type oscillation criteria for our dynamic equation. Finally, we present an example in the last section.

Keywords Time scale · Oscillation · Delay dynamic equation · Riccati technique

1 Introduction

The thesis work "Unified approach to continuous and discrete calculus" by the "Stephan Hilger" (see 1988 [14]) has recently been received much attention. The advantage of this theory is to avoid the twice analysis, that is, to harmonize discrete and continuous analyses. Basically, a non-empty closed subset of R will be called a time scale ($T \subseteq R$), see, for instance, closed intervals, integers (Z), natural numbers (N), $q^Z \cup \{0\}$, $q > 1$ and $T = \bigcup_{n \in Z}[2k, 2k+1]$, etc. For this, we suggest the researchers to see the excellent monograph [7] by Bohner and Peterson. This theory has a vital role in various research areas. Several applications can be found in various fields, and it can be seen in [6, 8] and references cited therein. For the lack of confusion, we denote $z^\sigma(t) = z(\sigma(t))$ and $[a\ \infty)_T = [a\ \infty) \bigcap T$ for $a \in T$. For more notation, the notation k "$t \in [t_*, \infty)_T$," will be read as "$t_* \leq t$."

In the present manuscript, we will look for a oscillatory solutions of the equation below:

S. S. Negi (✉) · S. Abbas · M. Malik
School of Basic Sciences, Indian Institute of Technology Mandi,
Kamand, H.P. 175005, India
e-mail: shekharsinghnegi2017@gmail.com

S. Bhattacharyya et al. (eds.), *Mathematical Modeling and Computational Tools*,
Springer Proceedings in Mathematics & Statistics 320,
https://doi.org/10.1007/978-981-15-3615-1_30

$$(\emptyset(t)B^{\Delta}(t))^{\Delta}+\sum_{i=1}^{m}\theta_i(t)W_i\left(t,B(t),B^{\Delta}(t),B(K_1(s,B(s))\right)+sgn(B(t))\lambda(t)$$
$$+\int_{-\infty}^{t}g(s)F(s,B(s))\Delta s$$
$$=\sum_{j=1}^{n}\Im_j(t)G_j\left(t,B(t),B^{\Delta}(\sigma(t)),B^{\sigma}(K_2(t,B^{\sigma}(s)))\right)$$

$$+B(t,B(t),|B^{\Delta}(\sigma(t))|) \tag{1}$$

where $\sup\{T\}=\infty$;

$$K_1(t,B(t))=l_1(t,B(l_2(t,\cdots,B(l_m(t,B(t)))\cdots)));$$

and

$$K_2(t,B^{\sigma}(t))=L_1(t,B^{\sigma}(L_2(t,\cdots,B^{\sigma}(L_n(t,B^{\sigma}(t)))\cdots))).$$

Furthermore, $\theta_i,\Im_j,g,r,\lambda:T\to R,\ W_i,G_j:T\times R^3\to R;\ B:T\times R^2\to R$ and $F:T\times R\to R$. It is straightforward to see that Eq. (1) contains a differential equation as well as a difference equations of different choice of time scale T.

Remark 1 Let us consider $T=R$, then Eq. (1) will be reduced in the form:

$$((t)B'(t))'+\sum_{i=1}^{m}\theta_i(t)W_i\left(t,B(t),B'(t),B(K_1(s,B(s)))\right)+sgn(B(t))\lambda(t)$$
$$+\int_{-\infty}^{t}g(s)F(s,B(s))ds$$
$$=\sum_{j=1}^{n}\Im_j(t)G_j\left(t,B(t),B'(t),B(K_2(t,B(s)))\right)$$

$$+B(t,B(t),|B'(t)|) \tag{2}$$

where $\sigma(t)=t,\ \mu(t)=0,\ g^{\Delta}(t)=g'(t)$ and $\int_a^b g(t)\Delta t=\int_a^b g(t)dt.$

Remark 2 If we consider a time scale $T = Z$, then Eq. (1) has a form :

$$\Delta(\emptyset(t)\Delta B'(t)) + \sum_{i=1}^{m} \theta_i(t) W_i\,(t, B(t), \Delta B(t), B(K_1(s, B(s)))) + sgn(B(t))\lambda(t)$$
$$+ \int_{-\infty}^{t} g(s)F(s, B(s))\Delta s$$
$$= \sum_{j=1}^{n} \Im_j(t) G_j\,(t, B(t), \Delta B(\sigma(t)), B^{\sigma}(K_2(t, B^{\sigma}(s))))$$
$$+ B(t, B(t), |\Delta B(\sigma(t))|)$$

where $\sigma(t) = t + 1,\ \mu(t) = 1,\ g^{\Delta}(t) = \Delta g(t)$ and

$$\int_a^b g(t)\Delta t = \sum_{t=a}^{b-1} g(t)\mu(t) = \sum_{t=a}^{b-1} g(t).$$

Remark 3 If $T = \xi' Z,\ \xi' > 0$, then Eq. (1) as follows

$$\Delta_{\xi'}(\emptyset(t)\Delta_{\xi'}B(t)) + \sum_{i=1}^{m} \theta_i(t) W_i \left(t, B(t), \Delta_{\xi'}B(t), B(K_1(s, B(s)))\right) + sgn(B(t))\lambda(t)$$
$$+ \int_{-\infty}^{t} g(s)F(s, B(s))\Delta_{\xi'}s$$
$$= \sum_{j=1}^{n} \Im_j(t) G_j \left(t, B(t), \Delta_{\xi'}B(\sigma(t)), B^{\sigma}(K_2(t, B^{\sigma}(s)))\right)$$
$$+ B(t, B(t), |\Delta_{\xi'}B(\sigma(t))|)$$

where we have $\sigma(t) = t + \xi',\ \mu(t) = \xi',\ f^{\Delta}(t) = \Delta_{\xi'}f(t)$ and

$$\int_a^b f(t)\Delta t = \sum_{l=\frac{a}{\xi'}}^{\frac{b}{\xi'}-1} f(l\xi')\xi'.$$

This paper concerns the oscillatory solutions of Eq. (1) and also discusses two well-known Philos-type and Kamenev-type oscillation criteria. We recall that a non-trivial solution $x(t)$ of Eq. (1) such that $x(t) \in C_{rd}^{\Delta^2}([t_x, \infty)_T)$ for $t_x \geq t_0$. That is, there is a real sequence $\{h_n\}$ with $h_n \to \infty$ as $n \to \infty$ and $y(h_n) = 0\ \forall n \in N$. Besides, we are looking such solutions which are exist on the half-line $[t_y, \infty)_T$ with $\sup\{|y(t)| : t > t_*\} \neq 0$ for any $t_y \leq t_*$ and $\sup T = \infty$.

In order to give the motivation of our study, we present a list of well-known excellent results which affined with our analysis. We start with Kamenev's result which can be seen in the paper [16] by Kamenev. He has studied some necessary conditions of oscillation for the given dynamic equation :

$$\big(W(t)B'(t)\big)' + W^*(t)B(t) = 0. \tag{3}$$

Thereafter, the technique used by the author Kamenev in the paper [16] for the oscillatory solutions of Eq. (3) has been a rapidly growing attention. Several authors have taken an interest on Kamenev-type oscillation criteria, and some of them extended it to the more general criteria. For instance, in 1989, Philos [23] has improved the well-known Kamenev's oscillation criteria by introducing the functions $\sharp(t, s)$ provided that the following assumptions must hold:

$$\sharp : D^* = \{(t, s) : t_0 \leq s \leq t\} \to R$$

defined as continuous function such that

$$\sharp(t, t) = 0 \text{ for } t_0 \leq t, \quad \sharp(t, s) > 0 \text{ for } t_0 \leq s < t \text{ and } \frac{\partial \sharp(t, s)}{\partial s} < 0 \text{ on } D,$$

where $\frac{\partial \sharp(t,s)}{\partial s}$ is continuous on D. In addition, a continuous function $h : D \to R$ is defined by

$$\frac{\partial \sharp(t, s)}{\partial s} = -\sharp(t, s)\sqrt{\sharp(t, s)}, \quad \text{for all } (t, s) \in D.$$

After that, many results of these criteria have been studied for the dynamic equations on time scales. Over the last few decades, some excellent results on oscillation/non-oscillation for the different order ordinary dynamic equations on time scales have been established. Furthermore, the Philos-type and Kamenev-type oscillation criteria have also been studied. We requested the interested readers to take a look on the papers related to periodic and oscillatory solutions [1–4, 9–11, 13, 17, 18, 20, 24, 25, 27–29] and references cited therein. In addition, there is a very recent publication on oscillation [22] by Negi et al. and it contains some oscillatory studies of a first-order neutral dynamic equation on time scale:

$$(B(\sigma(t)) - W(t)x^{\xi}(t - \eta))^{\Delta} + W^*(t)\prod_{j=1}^{n}|G_j'(B(t - \tau_j))|^{\alpha_j(t)} sign(B(t - \tau_j)) = 0,$$

$\forall t \in [t_*, \infty)_T$. Furthermore, in [19], Negi, et. al. have discussed the oscillatory results of the following:

$$B^{\Delta^2}(t) + \beta B^{\Delta}(t) = W(t)B(t) + W_*^{\Delta}\left(t, B(t), \int_{-\infty}^{t} \mathcal{W}_{**}(t - s)\mathcal{W}_{***}(s, B(s))\Delta s\right)$$

Apart from that, the oscillatory results of the singular second-order nonlinear dynamic equation on time scales can be seen in [21]. Motivated by the above literature, we impose a generalized Riccati technique to analyze various studies on time scale for Eq. (1).

We provide some crucial assumptions for our results:

(G_1) $r, b, \aleph_i, \bar{C}_j, \theta_i, Q_i : [t_0, \infty)_T \to (0.\infty)_R$ and $\lambda, g : [0, \infty)_T \to [0, \infty)_R$ all are rd-continuous functions for each $i = 1, 2, \cdots, m, j = 1, 2, \cdots, n$, such that

$$\sum_{i=1}^{m} \theta_i(t)\aleph_i(t) > \sum_{j=1}^{n} \Im_j(t)\bar{C}_j(t) + b(t)$$

for $t_0 \leq t$.

(G_2) $G_j, W_i : [t_0, \infty)_T \times R^3 \to R$, $B : [t_0, \infty)_T \times R^2 \to R$ and $F : [t_0, \infty)_T \times R \to R$ all are rd-continuous functions and satisfy the following:

$$|W_i(t, u, v, B)| \geq \aleph_i(t)|u|, |B^*(t, u, |v^*|)| \leq b(t)|u|$$

and

$$|G_j(t, u, v^*, X)| \leq \bar{C}_j(t)|u|$$

such that $uF > 0, uG_j > 0, uB > 0$ and $uW_i > 0$, for $i = 1, 2, \cdots, m, j = 1, 2, \cdots, n$, $n \neq m$, and $v, v^*, w, X, B, 0 \neq u \in R$.

(G_3) $\int_{t_0}^{\infty} \frac{1}{\emptyset(s)} \Delta s = \infty.$

We set our paper as follows: Some basic definitions and important lemmas are given in Sect. 2. Next section contains some sufficient conditions of oscillation of Eq. (1) that are investigated in the next section. Apart from that, the Kamenev-type and Philos-type oscillation criteria are also discussed. Finally in Sect. 4, results are illustrated by providing an example.

2 Preliminaries

This section provides some predefined definitions, basic theorems, notion of time scales, and important remarks. Besides, we derive some lemmas which will be used in our sequel.

Definition 1 [7]. Define a operator $\sigma : T \to T$ by $\sigma(x) := inf\{s \in T : s > x\}$, which is known as forward jump operator for $x \in T$. Similarly, define a operator $\rho : T \to T$ by $\rho(x) := sup\{s \in T : s < x\}$, which is known as backward jump operator for $x \in T$.

Moreover, we define a graininess operator $\mu : T \to [0, \infty)$ by $\mu(x) = \sigma(x) - x$.

Remark 4 We take $\inf \emptyset = \sup T$ and $\sup \emptyset = \inf T$, where $\emptyset$ is a null set.

Furthermore,

$$C_{rd}(T, R) = \{g : g : T \to R \text{ is rd-continuous function on } T\}.$$

We define $T^{\kappa} = T - \{\omega\}$, if T has a left-scattered maximum ω, and $T^{\kappa} = T$ otherwise.

Definition 2 [7]. A function $B : T \to R$ and $x \in T^{\kappa}$, then $B^{\Delta}(x)$ (if it exists) with for any given $\epsilon_* > 0$, $\exists$ a neighborhood $\mathcal{W}_* = (x - \delta_*, x + \delta_*) \bigcap T$ where some $\delta_* > 0$ such that

$$\left|[B(\sigma(x)) - B(y)] - B^{\Delta}(x)[\sigma(x) - y]\right| \le \epsilon_* |\sigma(x) - y| \ \ \forall y \in \mathcal{W}_*.$$

Thus, we will say $B^{\Delta}(x)$ a Δ or Hilger derivative of B at the point x.

Theorem 1 *[7]. For $B, A : T \to R$ and x be an arbitrary element of T^{κ}. Then:*

1. *B is continuous at x provided that B must differentiable at x;*
2. *B is Δ- derivative at x and has form $B^{\Delta}(x) = \frac{B(\sigma(x)) - B(x)}{\mu(x)}$ provided that B must be continuous at x and x is right−scattered.*
3. *B is differentiable at $x \Leftrightarrow B^{\Delta}(x) = \lim\limits_{y \to x} \frac{B(x) - B(y)}{x - y}$ exists and finite value provided that x is right-dense;*
4. *$B^{\sigma} = B(\sigma(x)) = B(x) + \mu(x)B^{\Delta}(x)$ provided that B is differentiable at x.*
5. *A product $BA : T \to R$ is differentiable at x and*

$$(BA)^{\Delta}(x) = B^{\Delta}(x)Q(x) + B(\sigma(x))A^{\Delta}(x) = B(x)A^{\Delta}(x) + B^{\Delta}(x)A(\sigma(x))$$

provided that B and A are Δ-differentiable at x. Then by this, for $x \in T$ such that x is lying between α and β for all values of α and β in T. We should have

$$\int_{\alpha}^{\beta} B^{\sigma}(y)A^{\Delta}(y)\Delta y = B(\beta)A(\beta) - B(\alpha)A(\alpha) - \int_{\alpha}^{\beta} B^{\Delta}(y)A(y)\Delta y \qquad (4)$$

$$\int_{\alpha}^{\beta} B(y)A^{\Delta}(y)\Delta y = B(\beta)A(\beta) - B(\alpha)A(\alpha) - \int_{\alpha}^{\beta} P^{\Delta}(y)A^{\sigma}(y)\Delta y; \qquad (5)$$

6. *A function $\frac{B}{A}$ is differentiable at x and*

$$\left(\frac{B}{A}\right)^{\Delta}(x) = \frac{B^{\Delta}(x)A(x) - B(x)A^{\Delta}(x)}{A(x)A(\sigma(x))}$$

provided that $A(x)B(\sigma(x)) \neq 0$.

We denote

$$R = \{F : F : T \to R \text{ such that } 1 + F(x)\mu(x) \neq 0\}$$

the collection of all regressive functions. In particular,

$$R^{+} = \{F : F : T \to R \text{ such that } 1 + F(x)\mu(x) > 0\}.$$

For more details, see [7].

Definition 3 [7]. Define

$$e_{w}(t,s) = exp\left(\int_{s}^{t} \eta_{\mu(\xi)}\left(w(\xi)\right) \Delta\xi\right), \quad \forall t \in T, \ s \in T^{\kappa},$$

for each $w \in R$ and $\eta_h(v)$ is defined as follows

$$\eta_h(\xi) = \begin{cases} \frac{\log(1+hv)}{h}, & : h \neq 0, \\ v, & : h = 0. \end{cases}$$

Definition 4 [7]. If an anti-derivative $J^{\Delta}(t) = J(t)$ $\forall t \in T$ where $J, J^{*} : T \to R$. Then for $\alpha, \beta \in T$ such that $\alpha \leq \beta$, we have

$$\int_{\alpha}^{\beta} J(s)\Delta(s) = J(\beta) - J(\alpha) \tag{6}$$

is Cauchy's integral.

Definition 5 [15] Consider $T = \overline{q^{Z}}$, then $J^{\Delta}(t) = D_q J(t)$, where

$$D_q J(t) = \begin{cases} \frac{J(qt) - J(t)}{t(q-1)} & : t \neq 0 \\ \lim\limits_{n\to\infty} \frac{J(q^n) - J(0)}{q^n} & : t = 0, \end{cases} \tag{7}$$

is the $q-$difference operator.

Remark 5 It is easy to observe that Eq. (6) cannot be hold for any T because if we talk about the q-calculus, then it will not give the correct form as Eq. (6). That is, $\int_{\alpha}^{\beta} D_q J(t) d_q t = J(\beta) - J(\alpha)$ (details are in page 12 of [5]).

Two necessary lemmas are derived which have the significant role in our results.

Lemma 1 *If Eq. (1) is not oscillates and assumptions* $(\mathbf{G_1}) - (\mathbf{G_3})$ *hold. Furthermore, if the condition* $\emptyset^{\Delta}(t) \geq 0$ *holds, then* $\exists\, \eta \in T$ *along with* $t_0 \leq \eta < t$, *we have*

$$B(t) > 0, \ \ B^{\Delta}(t) > 0 \ \ and \ \ B^{\Delta\Delta}(t) < 0 \tag{8}$$

Proof If we consider a positive solution of Eq. (1) over a time scale interval $[t_0, \infty)_T$ for $t_0 \in T$, then from Eq. (1) and $(\mathbf{G_1}) - (\mathbf{G_3})$, we obtain

$$(\emptyset(t)B^{\Delta}(t))^{\Delta} \leq -\left(\sum_{i=1}^{m} \theta_i(t)\aleph_i(t) - \sum_{j=1}^{n} Q_i(t)|barC_j(t) - b(t)\right) y(t). \tag{9}$$

Easy to have

$$(\emptyset(t)B^{\Delta}(t))^{\Delta} < 0$$

for $t_0 \leq t$, by this, $\emptyset(t)B^{\Delta}(t)$ is decreasing function on $[t_0, \infty)_T$. And thus, it is either

$$\emptyset(t)B^{\Delta}(t) < 0$$

or

$$\emptyset(t)B^{\Delta}(t) > 0$$

on $[t_0, \infty)_T$. Our assertion that $\emptyset(t)B^{\Delta}(t) < 0$ on $[t_0, \infty)_T$. Therefore, $\exists \eta \in T$ along with $\eta \leq t$ for each $t \in T$, and for any constant k such that

$$\emptyset(t)B^{\Delta}(t) \leq k < 0, \text{ for all } \eta \leq t, \tag{10}$$

integrating from η to t, reach to

$$B(t) \leq B(\eta) + C\int_{\eta}^{t} \frac{1}{\emptyset(s)} \Delta s,$$

for large t, we arrive to contradiction as the condition $(\mathbf{C_3})$. Hence, we have the following relation

$$B(t) > 0,\ B^{\Delta}(t) > 0 \text{ and } B^{\Delta\Delta}(t) < 0, \quad \text{for } \eta \leq t \tag{11}$$

Lemma 2 *If Eq. (8) holds, then for* $t \neq \eta$, *we have the following inequality*

$$0 < \Xi(t) \leq \frac{B(t)}{B^{\sigma}(t)} \leq 1, \tag{12}$$

where $\Xi(t) := \frac{t-\eta}{t-\eta+\mu(t)}$.

Proof From Eq. (8), we obtain

$$B(t) > B(t) - B(\eta) = \int_{\eta}^{t} B^{\Delta}(s)\Delta s > B^{\Delta}(t)(t-\eta). \tag{13}$$

From Eq. (13) and using the following $B^{\sigma}(t) = B(t) + \mu(t)B^{\Delta}(t)$, yields

$$0 < \frac{t-\eta}{t-\eta+\mu(t)} := \Xi(t) \leq \frac{B(t)}{B^{\sigma}(t)} \leq 1.$$

All essential lemmas are proved, so we turn to our main section.

3 Oscillation Criteria

Here, we look for some sufficient conditions of oscillation of Eq. (1).

Theorem 2 *If* $(\mathbf{G_1}) - (\mathbf{G_3})$ *and* $\emptyset^{\Delta}(t) \geq 0$ *hold. Furthermore,* $\exists\Delta$*-derivative function* $\Pi(t)$ *is positive and* $\eta \in T$ *such that* $\eta \leq t$*, respectively. Also, with the following relation,*

$$\limsup_{t\to\infty} \int_{\eta}^{t} \Pi^{\sigma}(s)\Xi(s)\left\{\left(\sum_{i=1}^{m}\theta_i(s)\aleph_i(s) - \sum_{j=1}^{n}\Im_j(s)\bar{C}_j(s)\right) - b(s) - \emptyset(s)\left(\frac{\Pi^{\Delta}(s)}{2\Pi^{\sigma}(s)\Xi(s)}\right)^2\right\}\Delta s = \infty,$$

then Eq. (1) contains oscillatory solutions on $[t_0\ \infty)_T$.

Proof Using the contradictory approach, we start with the assumption that Eq. (1) has no oscillatory solutions, say $B(t)$. Then, there is no doubt $B(t)$ is positive (eventually), i.e., $\exists\ t_0 \leq \eta < t$ such that $B(t)$ is positive for all $t \in [\eta\ \infty)_T$. Similarly, we will do for negative (eventually) case. Now, the Riccati transformation function

$$\$(t) = \Pi(t)\frac{\emptyset(t)B^{\Delta}(t)}{B(t)}, \quad \eta < t. \tag{14}$$

Differentiate Eq. (14) with respect to the vriable t, we obtain

$$\$^{\Delta}(t) = \Pi^{\Delta}(t)\frac{\emptyset(t)B^{\Delta}(t)}{B(t)} + \Pi^{\sigma}(t)\left(\frac{(\emptyset(t)B^{\Delta}(t))^{\Delta}B(t) - \emptyset(t)(B^{\Delta}(t))^2}{B(t)B^{\sigma}(t)}\right) \tag{15}$$

$$\leq \frac{\Pi^{\Delta}(t)}{\Pi(t)}\$(t) - \frac{\Pi^{\sigma}(t)B(t)}{\emptyset(t)\Pi^2(t)B^{\sigma}(t)}\$^2(t) + \frac{\Pi^{\sigma}(t)}{B^{\sigma}(t)}(\emptyset(t)B^{\Delta}(t))^{\Delta}. \tag{16}$$

From lemma (2) and Eq. (16), we get

$$\$^{\Delta}(t) \leq \frac{\Pi^{\Delta}(t)}{\Pi(t)}\$(t) - \frac{\Pi^{\sigma}(t)\Xi(t)}{\emptyset(t)\Pi^2(t)}\$^2(t) + \frac{\Pi^{\sigma}(t)}{B^{\sigma}(t)}(\emptyset(t)B^{\Delta}(t))^{\Delta}. \tag{17}$$

From Eq. (9) and using relation $\frac{\Pi^{\sigma}(t)}{B^{\sigma}(t)}(\emptyset(t)B^{\Delta}(t))^{\Delta}$ in the above equation, we must have

$$\frac{\Pi^{\sigma}(t)}{B^{\sigma}(t)}(\emptyset(t)B^{\Delta}(t))^{\Delta} \leq -\left[\left(\sum_{i=1}^{m}(\theta_i(t)\aleph_i(t) - \sum_{j=1}^{n}\Im_j(t)\bar{C}_j(t))\right) - b(t)\right]\frac{B(t)\Pi^{\sigma}(t)}{B^{\sigma}(t)}$$

$$\leq -\left[\left(\sum_{i=1}^{m}(\theta_i(t)\aleph_i(t) - \sum_{j=1}^{n}\Im_j(t)\bar{C}_j(t))\right) - b(t)\right]\Xi(t)\Pi^{\sigma}(t). \quad (18)$$

From Eq. (17) and (18), we get

$$\$^{\Delta}(t) \leq \frac{\Pi^{\Delta}(t)}{\Pi(t)}\$(t) - \frac{\Pi^{\sigma}(t)\Xi(t)}{\emptyset(t)\Pi^2(t)}\$^2(t)$$

$$-\left[\left(\sum_{i=1}^{m}(\theta_i(t)\aleph_i(t) - \sum_{j=1}^{n}\Im_j(t)\bar{C}_j(t))\right) - b(t)\right]\Xi(t)\Pi^{\sigma}(t). \quad (19)$$

$$-\left[\left(\sum_{i=1}^{m}(\theta_i(t)\aleph_i(t) - \sum_{j=1}^{n}\Im_j(t)\bar{C}_j(t))\right) - b(t)\right]\Xi(t)\Pi^{\sigma}(t) \quad (20)$$

$$-\left(\frac{1}{\Pi(t)}\sqrt{\frac{\Pi^{\sigma}(t)\Xi(t)}{\emptyset(t)}}w(t) - \frac{\Pi^{\Delta}(t)}{2}\sqrt{\frac{\emptyset(t)}{\Pi^{\sigma}(t)\Xi(t)}}\right)^2 \times \frac{(\Pi^{\Delta}(t))^2\emptyset(t)}{4\Pi^{\sigma}(t)\Xi(t)}, \quad (21)$$

which implies that

$$\$^{\Delta}(t) \leq -\left[\left(\sum_{i=1}^{m}(\theta_i(t)\aleph_i(t) - \sum_{j=1}^{n}\Im_j(t)\bar{C}_j(t))\right) - b(t)\right]\Xi(t)\Pi^{\sigma}(t)$$

$$+\frac{(\Pi^{\Delta}(t))^2\emptyset(t)}{4\Pi^{\sigma}(t)\Xi(t)}. \quad (22)$$

Integrating above equation from η to t, yields

$$\int_{\eta}^{t} \Pi^{\sigma}(s)\Xi(s)\left\{\left(\sum_{i=1}^{m}\theta_i(s)\aleph_i(s)-\sum_{j=1}^{n}\Im_j(s)\bar{C}_j(s)\right)-b(s)\right.$$

$$\left.-\O(s)\left(\frac{\Pi^{\Delta}(s)}{2\Pi^{\sigma}(s)\Xi(s)}\right)^{2}\right\}\Delta s \le \$(\eta) < \infty, \tag{23}$$

for large t, we conclude a contradiction to (14). Thus, we reach to the desire result.

From Theorem (3.1), some corollaries are carried out which can be found in below.

Corollary 1 *If the assumptions* $(\mathbf{G_1})-(\mathbf{G_3})$ *and* $\O^{\Delta}(t)\ge 0$ *are hold. Furthermore, if* $\exists$ *a* Δ*-derivative function* $\Pi(t)>0$ *and* $\eta\in T;\ \eta\le t$*, respectively. In addition, the relations must be hold*

$$\limsup_{t\to\infty}\int_{\eta}^{t}\Pi^{\sigma}(s)\Xi(s)\left[\left(\sum_{i=1}^{m}\theta_i(s)\aleph_i(s)-\sum_{j=1}^{n}\Im_j(s)\bar{C}_j(s)\right)-b(s)\right]\Delta s=\infty, \tag{24}$$

and

$$\limsup_{t\to\infty}\int_{\eta}^{t}\frac{(s)(\Pi^{\Delta}(s))^{2}}{4\Pi^{\sigma}(s)\Xi(s)}\Delta s<\infty, \tag{25}$$

then, Eq. (1) has an oscillatory solution on $[t_0\ \infty)_T$.

We immediately obtain the following results by using Theorem (3.1).

Corollary 2 *If* $(\mathbf{G_1})-(\mathbf{G_3})$, $\O^{\Delta}(t)\ge 0$ *are hold. Also, if* $\exists$ *a* Δ*-derivative function* $\Pi(t)>0$ *and* $\eta\in T;\ \eta\le t$ *respectively. Along with*

$$\limsup_{t\to\infty}\int_{\eta}^{t}\Pi^{\sigma}(s)\Xi(s)\left(\sum_{i=1}^{m}\theta_i(s)\aleph_i(s)-\sum_{j=1}^{n}\Im_j(s)\bar{C}_j(s)\right)\Delta s=\infty, \tag{26}$$

and

$$\limsup_{t\to\infty}\int_{\eta}^{t}\left(\frac{\O(s)(\Pi^{\Delta}(s))^{2}}{4\Pi^{\sigma}(s)\Xi(s)}+b(s)\right)\Delta s<\infty, \tag{27}$$

are hold. Then, the solution of Eq. (1) must be oscillates on $[t_0\ \infty)_T$.

Corollary 3 *If the conditions* $(\mathbf{G_1})-(\mathbf{G_3})$ *and* $\emptyset^{\Delta}(t)\geq 0$ *are hold. Furthermore,* $\exists$ *a* Δ*-derivative function* $\Pi(t)>0$ *and* $\eta\in T;\ \eta\leq t$ *respectively. Also, the following relations are satisfied*

$$\limsup_{t\to\infty}\int_{\eta}^{t}\Pi^{\sigma}(s)\Xi(s)\sum_{i=1}^{m}\theta_i(s)\aleph_i(s)\Delta s=\infty, \tag{28}$$

and

$$\limsup_{t\to\infty}\int_{\eta}^{t}\left(\frac{\emptyset(s)(\Pi^{\Delta}(s))^2}{4\Pi^{\sigma}(s)\Xi(s)}+b(s)+\sum_{j=1}^{n}\Im_j(s)\bar{C}_j(s)\right)\Delta s<\infty, \tag{29}$$

then the solution will be oscillates of Eq. (1) on $[t_0\ \infty)_T$.

Before going to establish Kamenev-type oscillation criteria, we need the following result [26]. For $\mathcal{L}>1$ and $\sigma(s)\leq t$.

$$((t-s)^{\mathcal{L}})^{\Delta_s}\leq-\mathcal{L}(t-\sigma(s))^{\mathcal{L}-1}\leq 0. \tag{30}$$

Theorem 3 *If the conditions* $(\mathbf{G_1})-(\mathbf{G_3})$ *and* $\emptyset^{\Delta}(t)\geq 0$ *are hold and* $\exists$ Δ*-derivative function* $\Pi(t)>0$ *and* $\mathcal{L}>1$*. Also, for all sufficient large* $\eta\in T$ *such that* $\eta\leq t$*, the following relation holds;*

$$\limsup_{t\to\infty}\frac{1}{t^{\mathcal{L}}}\int_{\eta}^{t}(t-s)^{\mathcal{L}}\Pi^{\sigma}(s)\Xi(s)\left\{\left(\sum_{i=1}^{m}\theta_i(s)\aleph_i(s)-\sum_{j=1}^{n}\Im_j(s)\bar{C}_j(s)\right)-b(s)\right.$$
$$\left.-\emptyset(s)\left(\frac{\Pi^{\Delta}(s)}{2\Pi^{\sigma}(s)\Xi(s)}\right)^2\right\}\Delta s=\infty, \tag{31}$$

then, Eq. (1) oscillates on $[t_0\ \infty)_T$.

Proof Using the contradictory approach, we start with the assumption that Eq. (1) has no oscillatory solutions, say $B(t)$. Then, there is no doubt $B(t)$ is positive (eventually), i.e., $\exists\ t_0\leq\eta<t$ such that $B(t)$ is positive for all $t\in[\eta\ \infty)_T$. Similarly, we will do for negative (eventually) case. Thus, from (22), we must have

$$\left[\left(\sum_{i=1}^{m}(\theta_i(t)\aleph_i(t)-\sum_{j=1}^{n}\Im_j(t)\bar{C}_j(t))\right)-b(t)\right]\Xi(t)\Pi^{\sigma}(t)$$
$$-\frac{(\Pi^{\Delta}(t))^2\theta(t)}{4\Pi^{\sigma}(t)\Xi(t)}\leq-\$^{\Delta}(t). \tag{32}$$

Multiplying Eq. (32) by $(t-s)^{\mathcal{L}}$ and then integrating from η to t, we obtain

$$\int_{\eta}^{t}(t-s)^{\mathcal{L}}\Pi^{\sigma}(s)\Xi(s)\left\{\left(\sum_{i=1}^{m}\theta_i(s)\aleph_i(s)-\sum_{j=1}^{n}\Im_j(s)\bar{C}_j(s)\right)-b(s)\right.$$

$$\left.-\emptyset(s)\left(\frac{\Pi^{\Delta}(s)}{2\Pi^{\sigma}(s)\Xi(s)}\right)^2\right\}\Delta s\leq-\int_{\eta}^{t}(t-s)^{\mathcal{L}}\$^{\Delta}(s)\Delta s. \tag{33}$$

From Eqs. (5) and (33), yields

$$\int_{\eta}^{t}(t-s)^{\mathcal{L}}\Pi^{\sigma}(s)\Xi(s)\left\{\left(\sum_{i=1}^{m}\theta_i(s)\aleph_i(s)-\sum_{j=1}^{n}\Im_j(s)\bar{C}_j(s)\right)-b(s)\right.$$

$$\left.-\emptyset(s)\left(\frac{\Pi^{\Delta}(s)}{2\Pi^{\sigma}(s)\Xi(s)}\right)^2\right\}\Delta s\leq(t-\eta)^{\mathcal{L}}\$(\eta)+\int_{\eta}^{t}((t-s)^{\mathcal{L}})^{\Delta_s}\$^{\sigma}(s)\Delta s.$$

From Eqs. (30) and above equation, we get

$$\int_{\eta}^{t}(t-s)^{\mathcal{L}}\Pi^{\sigma}(s)\Xi(s)\left\{\left(\sum_{i=1}^{m}\theta_i(s)\aleph_i(s)-\sum_{j=1}^{n}\Im_j(s)\bar{C}_j(s)\right)-b(s)\right.$$

$$\left.-\bar{C}(s)\left(\frac{\Pi^{\Delta}(s)}{2\Pi^{\sigma}(s)\Xi(s)}\right)^2\right\}\Delta s\leq(t-\eta)^{\mathcal{L}}\$(\eta). \tag{34}$$

Thus, we have

$$\frac{1}{t^{\mathcal{L}}}\int_{\eta}^{t}(t-s)^{\mathcal{L}}\Pi^{\sigma}(s)\Xi(s)\left\{\left(\sum_{i=1}^{m}\theta_i(s)\aleph_i(s)-\sum_{j=1}^{n}\Im_j(s)\bar{C}_j(s)\right)-b(s)\right.$$

$$\left.-\emptyset(s)\left(\frac{\Pi^{\Delta}(s)}{2\Pi^{\sigma}(s)\Xi(s)}\right)^2\right\}\Delta s\leq\frac{(t-\eta)^{\mathcal{L}}}{t^{\mathcal{L}}}\$(\eta)\ \text{ for }\eta\leq t. \tag{35}$$

Taking lim sup as $t \to \infty$, we arrive at

$$\limsup_{t\to\infty} \frac{1}{t^{\mathcal{L}}} \int_{\eta}^{t} (t-s)^{\mathcal{L}} \Pi^{\sigma}(s)\Xi(s) \left\{ \left(\sum_{i=1}^{m} \theta_i(s)\aleph_i(s) - \sum_{j=1}^{n} \Im_j(s)\bar{C}_j(s) \right) - b(s) \right.$$

$$\left. -\emptyset(s) \left(\frac{\Pi^{\Delta}(s)}{2\Pi^{\sigma}(s)\Xi(s)} \right)^2 \right\} \Delta s < \infty, \tag{36}$$

Thus, we derive a contradiction to (31). Thus, we proved.

By observing Theorem (3.5), we easily establish new results which are given below.

Corollary 4 *Assume that* $(\mathbf{G_1}) - (\mathbf{G_3})$ *and* $\emptyset^{\Delta}(t) \geq 0$ *hold. Moreover, if* $\exists$ *a* Δ*-derivative function* $\Pi(t) > 0$ *and* $\eta \in T;\ \eta \leq t$*, respectively. Assume that*

$$\limsup_{t\to\infty} \frac{1}{t^{\mathcal{L}}} \int_{\eta}^{t} (t-s)^{\mathcal{L}} \Pi^{\sigma}(s)\Xi(s) \left[\left(\sum_{i=1}^{m} \theta_i(s)\aleph_i(s) - \sum_{j=1}^{n} \Im_j(s)\bar{C}_j(s) \right) - b(s) \right] \Delta s$$

$$= \infty, \tag{37}$$

and

$$\limsup_{t\to\infty} \frac{1}{t^{\mathcal{L}}} \int_{\eta}^{t} (t-s)^{\mathcal{L}} \frac{\bar{\emptyset}(s)(\Pi^{\Delta}(s))^2}{4\Pi^{\sigma}(s)\Xi(s)} \Delta s < \infty, \tag{38}$$

then, the solutions of Eq. (1) will be oscillate on $[t_0\ \infty)_T$.

Corollary 5 *If the conditions* $(\mathbf{G_1}) - (\mathbf{G_3})$ *and* $\emptyset^{\Delta}(t) \geq 0$ *are hold. Furthermore,* $\exists$ *a* Δ*-derivative function* $\Pi(t) > 0$ *and* $\eta \in T;\ t \geq \eta$*, respectively. In addition, the following conditions are satisfied*

$$\limsup_{t\to\infty} \frac{1}{t^{\mathcal{L}}} \int_{\eta}^{t} (t-s)^{\mathcal{L}} \Pi^{\sigma}(s)\Xi(s) \left(\sum_{i=1}^{m} \theta_i(s)\aleph_i(s) - \sum_{j=1}^{n} \Im_j(s)\bar{C}_j(s) \right) \Delta s = \infty, \tag{39}$$

and

$$\limsup_{t\to\infty} \frac{1}{t^{\mathcal{L}}} \int_{\eta}^{t} (t-s)^{\mathcal{L}} \left(\frac{\emptyset(s)(\Pi^{\Delta}(s))^2}{4\Pi^{\sigma}(s)\Xi(s)} + b(s) \right) \Delta s < \infty, \tag{40}$$

then, Eq. (1) has an oscillatory solutions on $[t_0\ \infty)_T$.

Corollary 6 *If the conditions* $(\mathbf{G_1}) - (\mathbf{G_3})$ *and* $\emptyset^{\Delta}(t) \geq 0$ *are hold, and* $\exists$ *a* Δ-*derivative function* $\Pi(t) > 0$ *and* $\eta \in T;\ t \geq \eta$, *respectively. Furthermore, we will assume the following are hold:*

$$\limsup_{t\to\infty} \frac{1}{t^{\mathcal{L}}} \int_{\eta}^{t} (t-s)^{\mathcal{L}} \Pi^{\sigma}(s)\Xi(s) \sum_{i=1}^{m} \theta_i(s)\aleph_i(s)\Delta s = \infty, \tag{41}$$

and

$$\limsup_{t\to\infty} \frac{1}{t^{\mathcal{L}}} \int_{\eta}^{t} (t-s)^{\mathcal{L}} \left(\frac{\emptyset(s)(\Pi^{\Delta}(s))^2}{4\Pi^{\sigma}(s)\Xi(s)} + b(s) + \sum_{j=1}^{n} \Im_j(s)\bar{C}_j(s) \right) \Delta s < \infty, \tag{42}$$

then, Eq. (1) has an oscillatory solution on $[t_0\ \infty)_T$.

Next we need to have the following assumptions (due to Philos-type oscillation criteria):

For any number $\mu \in R$, define its expression, μ_+ and μ_-, respectively, of μ by $\mu_+ := \max\{0,\ \mu\}$ and $\mu_- := \max\{0,\ -\mu\}$. In addition, we will assume the functions $\sharp, D : D^* \to R$ to be rd-continuous along with $D^* = \{(t, s);\ t_0 \leq \eta \leq t\}$ such that

$$\sharp(t,t) = 0,\ t_0 \leq t \text{ and } \sharp(t,s) > 0 \text{ and } \sharp^{\Delta_s}(t,s) < 0.\ t_0 \leq s < t \tag{43}$$

and $\sharp^{\Delta_s}(t,s)$ is rd-continuous function.

Theorem 4 *If* $(\mathbf{G_1}) - (\mathbf{G_3})$, *(43) and* $\emptyset^{\Delta}(t) \geq 0$ *are hold and* $\exists$ *a* Δ-*derivative function* $\Pi(t) > 0$ *and* $\eta \in T;\ \eta \leq t$, *respectively. Furthermore, the following are hold*

$$\sharp^{\Delta_s}(\sigma(t), s) + \frac{\sharp^{\sigma}(\sigma(t), s)\Pi^{\Delta}(t)}{\Pi(t)} = -\frac{D(t,s)}{\Pi(t)}\sqrt{\sharp^{\sigma}(\sigma(t), s)} \tag{44}$$

and

$$\limsup_{t\to\infty} \frac{1}{\sharp(\sigma(t),\eta)} \int_{\eta}^{\sigma(t)} \left\{ \sharp^{\sigma}(\sigma(t), s)\mathcal{V}(s)\Xi(s)\Pi^{\sigma}(s) - \frac{\emptyset(s)(D_-(t,s))^2}{4\Pi^{\sigma}(s)\Xi(s)} \right\} \Delta s = \infty, \tag{45}$$

where

$$\mathcal{V}(t) = \left(\sum_{i=1}^{m} \theta_i(t)\aleph_i(t) - \sum_{j=1}^{n} \Im_j(t)\bar{C}_j(t)) \right) - b(t), \tag{46}$$

then, the solution of Eq. (1) satisfies the oscillatory property over $[t_0\ \infty)_T$.

Proof Using the contradictory approach, we start with the assumption that Eq. (1) has no oscillatory solutions, say $B(t)$. Then, there is no doubt $B(t)$ is positive (eventually), i.e., $\exists\ t_0 \leq \eta < t$ such that $B(t)$ is positive for all $t \in [\eta\ \infty)_T$. Similarly, we will do for negative (eventually) case. Now, from (19), we should have

$$\left[\left(\sum_{i=1}^{m}(\theta_i(t)\aleph_i(t) - \sum_{j=1}^{n}\Im_j(t)\bar{C}_j(t))\right) - b(t)\right]\Xi(t)\Pi^\sigma(t) \leq -\$^\Delta(t) + \frac{\Pi^\Delta(t)}{\Pi(t)}\$(t) - \frac{\Pi^\sigma(t)\Xi(t)}{\emptyset(t)\Pi^2(t)}\$^2(t).$$

Multiplying Eq. (47) by $U(\sigma(t), \sigma(s))$, and then integrating from η to $\sigma(t)$, we obtain the following relation

$$\int_\eta^{\sigma(t)} \sharp^\sigma(\sigma(t), s)\left[\left(\sum_{i=1}^{m}(\theta_i(s)\aleph_i(s) - \sum_{j=1}^{n}\Im_j(s)\bar{C}_j(s))\right) - b(s)\right]\Xi(s)\Pi^\sigma(s)\Delta s$$

$$\leq -\int_\eta^{\sigma(t)} \sharp^\sigma(\sigma(t), s)\$^\Delta(s)\Delta s$$

$$+\int_\eta^{\sigma(t)} \sharp^\sigma(\sigma(t), s)\left(\frac{\Pi^\Delta(s)}{\Pi(s)}\$(s) - \frac{\Pi^\sigma(s)\Xi(s)}{\emptyset(s)\Pi^2(s)}\$^2(s)\right)\Delta s. \tag{47}$$

From Eq. (4) along with Eq. (47), yields

$$\int_\eta^{\sigma(t)} \sharp^\sigma(\sigma(t), s)\left[\left(\sum_{i=1}^{m}(\theta_i(s)\aleph_i(s) - \sum_{j=1}^{n}\Im_j(s)\bar{C}_j(s))\right) - b(s)\right]$$

$$\Xi(s)\Pi^\sigma(s)\Delta s \leq \sharp(\sigma(t), \eta)\$(\eta) + \int_\eta^{\sigma(t)}\left[\sharp^{\Delta_s}(\sigma(t), s) + \frac{\sharp^\sigma(\sigma(t), s)\Pi^\Delta(s)}{\Pi(s)}\right]\$(s)\Delta s$$

$$-\int_\eta^{\sigma(t)} \sharp^\sigma(\sigma(t), s)\frac{\Pi^\sigma(s)\Xi(s)}{\emptyset(s)\Pi^2(s)}\$^2(s)\Delta s. \tag{48}$$

Substituting (44) into (48), it follows that

$$\int_{\eta}^{\sigma(t)} \sharp^{\sigma}(\sigma(t), s)\left[\left(\sum_{i=1}^{m}(\theta_i(s)\aleph_i(s) - \sum_{j=1}^{n}\Im_j(s)\bar{C}_j(s))\right) - b(s)\right]\Xi(s)\Pi^{\sigma}(s)\Delta s$$

$$\leq \sharp(\sigma(t),)\$(\eta) + \int_{\eta}^{\sigma(t)}\left(\frac{D_{-}(t,s)\sqrt{\sharp^{\sigma}(\sigma(t),s)}}{\Pi(s)}\$(s)\right.$$

$$\left. -\sharp^{\sigma}(\sigma(t), s)\frac{\Pi^{\sigma}(s)}{\emptyset(s)\Pi^2(s)}\Xi(s)\$^2(s)\right)\Delta s. \tag{49}$$

Implies that

$$\int_{\eta}^{\sigma(t)} \sharp^{\sigma}(\sigma(t), s)\left[\left(\sum_{i=1}^{m}(\theta_i(s)\aleph_i(s) - \sum_{j=1}^{n}\Im_j(s)\bar{C}_j(s))\right) - b(s)\right]\theta(s)\Pi^{\sigma}(s)\Delta s$$

$$\leq \sharp(\sigma(t), \eta)\$(\eta) + \int_{\eta}^{\sigma(t)}\frac{\emptyset(s)(D_{-}(t,s))^2}{4\Pi^{\sigma}(s)\theta(s)}\Delta s.$$

which is equivalent to

$$\frac{1}{\sharp(\sigma(t), \eta)}\int_{\eta}^{\sigma(t)}\left\{\sharp^{\sigma}(\sigma(t), s)\left[\left(\sum_{i=1}^{m}(\theta_i(s)\aleph_i(s) - \sum_{j=1}^{n}\Im_j(s)\bar{C}_j(s))\right) - b(s)\right]\right.$$

$$\left. -\theta(s)\Pi^{\sigma}(s) - \frac{\emptyset(s)(D_{-}(t,s))^2}{4\Pi^{\sigma}(s)\theta(s)}\right\}\Delta s \leq \$(\eta) < \infty. \tag{50}$$

Taking large t, we get a contradiction to fact that Eq. (45). Hence, proof is done.

Corollary 7 *If the assumptions* $(\mathbf{G_1}) - (\mathbf{G_3})$, *(43) and* $\emptyset^{\Delta}(t) \geq 0$ *are hold. In addition,* $\exists$ *a* Δ*-derivative function* $\Pi(t) > 0$ *and* $\eta \in T;\ t \geq \eta$*, respectively, and assume that*

$$\sharp^{\Delta_s}(\sigma(t), s) + \frac{\sharp^{\sigma}(\sigma(t), s)\Pi^{\Delta}(t)}{\Pi(t)} = -\frac{D(t, s)}{\Pi(t)}\sqrt{\sharp^{\sigma}(\sigma(t), s)}, \tag{51}$$

$$\limsup_{t\to\infty} \frac{1}{\sharp(\sigma(t), \eta)} \int_{\eta}^{\sigma(t)} \sharp^{\sigma}(\sigma(t), s)\mathcal{V}(s)\theta(s)\Pi^{\sigma}(s)\Delta s = \infty \tag{52}$$

and (53)

$$\limsup_{t\to\infty} \frac{1}{\sharp(\sigma(t), \eta)} \int_{\eta}^{\sigma(t)} \frac{\emptyset(s)(D_{-}(t, s))^2}{4\Pi^{\sigma}(s)\theta(t)}\Delta s < \infty. \tag{54}$$

where $\mathcal{V}(t)$ in (46), then the solution of Eq. (1) satisfies the oscillatory property over $[t_0\ \infty)_T$.

Corollary 8 *If the assumption* $(\mathbf{G_1}) - (\mathbf{G_3})$, *(43) and* $\emptyset^{\Delta}(t) \geq 0$ *are hold. Furthermore,* $\exists$ *a* Δ*-derivative function* $\Pi(t)$ *which is positive and* $\eta \in T$; $t \geq \eta$ *respectively, and assume that*

$$\sharp^{\Delta_s}(\sigma(t), s) + \frac{\sharp^{\sigma}(\sigma(t), s)\Pi^{\Delta}(t)}{\Pi(t)} = -\frac{D(t, s)}{\Pi(t)}\sqrt{\sharp^{\sigma}(\sigma(t), s)}, \tag{55}$$

$$\limsup_{t\to\infty} \frac{1}{\sharp(\sigma(t), \eta)} \int_{\eta}^{\sigma(t)} \sharp^{\sigma}(\sigma(t), s)\theta(s)\Pi^{\sigma}(s)\sum_{i=1}^{m}\theta_i(t)\aleph_i(t)\,\Delta s = \infty, \tag{56}$$

and (57)

$$\limsup_{t\to\infty} \frac{1}{\sharp(\sigma(t), \eta)} \int_{\eta}^{\sigma(t)} \left(\sum_{j=1}^{n}\Im_j(t)\bar{C}_j(t)) + b(t) + \frac{\emptyset(s)(D_{-}(t, s))^2}{4\Pi^{\sigma}(s)\theta(t)}\right)\Delta s < \infty. \tag{58}$$

then, all the solutions of Eq. (1) oscillate, which is defined over $[t_0\ \infty)_T$.

Next, we give an example which illustrates our result.

4 Example

Here, we take the following nonlinear equation on T:

$$\left(7B^{\Delta}(t)\right)^{\Delta} + \sum_{i=1}^{3} 2^i \frac{\sqrt{t^2+1}}{\sqrt{t^2+5}}B(t) + sgn(B(t))5^{t^8+44} - \frac{B(t)}{2^t} - \sum_{j=1}^{2}\frac{1}{j}x(t)$$

$$+ \int_1^t (s-1)^2 sgn(B(s))e^{B^{\Delta}(s)} + B(s)\Delta s = 0, \tag{59}$$

here, $\emptyset(t) = 7, \Pi(t) = 4,\ b(t) = \frac{1}{2^t},\ \theta_i(t) = 2^i\sqrt{t^2+1},\ \aleph_i(t) = 2^i\sqrt{t^2+5},\ \Im_j(t) = e_j(t,1),\ \bar{C}_j(t) = \frac{1}{je_j(t,1)},$ for $i = 1, 2, 3$ and $j = 1, 2,\ \lambda(t) = 5^{t^8+44},\ g(t) = (t-1)^2,$ for $t > 1$ otherwise zero.

Also, we take $G_j(\cdot,\cdot,\cdot,\cdot,\cdot) = \frac{1}{je_j(t,1)}x(t),\ W_i(\cdot,\cdot,\cdot,\cdot) = 2^i\sqrt{t^2+5},\ B(\cdot,\cdot,\cdot) = \frac{B(t)}{2^t},\ F(\cdot,\cdot) = sgn(B(t))e^{B^\Delta(t)+B(t)}$. Thus, it is clear that for $\eta = 4$ the following relations hold

$$\liminf_{t\to\infty} \int_4^t 4.5^{t^8+44}\left\{\frac{25}{2} - \frac{1}{2^t}\right\}\Delta s = \infty, \tag{60}$$

and

$$\int_4^\infty \frac{1}{\emptyset(t)}\Delta t = \infty. \tag{61}$$

Thus, all conditions $(\mathbf{G_1}) - (\mathbf{G_3})$ hold. Thus, by Theorem (3.1), we have a oscillatory solution of Eq. (59) on $[1,\infty)_T$.

Acknowledgements The work of Shekhar Singh Negi was supported by the University Grants Commission of India (UGC India) under Sr.No. 2061440966, Ref. No. 22/06/2014(i)EU-V.

References

1. Agarwal, R.P., O'Regan, D., Saker, S.H.: Oscillation criteria for nonlinear perturbed dynamic equation of second-order on time scales. J. Appl. Math. Comput. **20**(1-2), 133–147 (2006)
2. Agarwal, R.P., O'Regan, D., Saker, S.H.: Oscillation criteria for second-order nonlinear neutral delay dynamic equations. J. Math. Anal. App. **300**(1), 203–217 (2004)
3. Agarwal, R.P., Zhang, C., Li, T.: New Kamenev-type oscillation criteria for second-order nonlinear advanced dynamic equations. Appl. Math. Comput. **225**, 822–828 (2013)
4. Agarwal, R.P., Bohner, M., Li, T., Zhang, C.: A Philos-type theorem for third-order nonlinear retarded dynamic equations. Appl. Math. Comput. **249**, 527–531 (2014)
5. Annaby, M.H., Mansour, Z.S.: $q-$Fractional Calculus and Equations. Springer, Berlin (2012)
6. Atici, F.M., Biles, D.C., Lebedinsky, A.: An application of time scales to economics. Math. Comput. Model. **43**(7), 718–726 (2006)
7. Bohner, M., Peterson, A.: Advances in Dynamic Equations on Time Scales. Birkhuser, Boston (2003)
8. Christiansen, F.B., Fenchel, T.M. : Theories of Populations in Biological Communities, Lecture Notes in Ecological Studies, vol. 20, pp. 1-36. Springer, Berlin (1977)
9. Del Medico, A., Kong, Q.: New Kamenev-type oscillation criteria for second-order differential equations on a measure chain. Comput. Math. Appl. **50**(8–9), 1211–1230 (2005)
10. Del Medico, A., Kong, Q.: Kamenev-type and interval oscillation criteria for second-order linear differential equations on a measure chain. J. Math. Anal. Appl. **294**(2), 621–643 (2014)
11. Erbe, L., Peterson, A., Saker, S.H.: Oscillation criteria for second-order nonlinear dynamic equations on time scales. J. Lond. Math. Soc. **67**(3), 701–714 (2003)
12. Erbe, L., Peterson, A., Saker, S.H.: Oscillation criteria for second-order nonlinear delay dynamic equations. J. Math. Anal. Appl. **333**(1), 505–522 (2007)
13. Erbe, L., Karpuz, B., Peterson, A.: Kamenev-type oscillation criteria for higher-order neutral delay dynamic equations. Int. J. Difference Equ. **6**(1), 1–16 (2011)

14. Hilger, S.: Analysis on measure chains-a unified approach to continuous and discrete calculus. Results Math. **18**(1), 18–56 (1990)
15. Jafari, H., Haghbina, A., Johnstonb, S.J., Baleanucd, D.: A new algorithm for solving dynamic equations on a time scale. J. Comput. Appl. Math. **312**, 167–173 (2017)
16. Kamenev, I.V.: An integral criterion for oscillation of nonlinear differential equations of second order. Mat. Zametki. **23**, 249–251 (1978)
17. Negi, S.S., Abbas, S., Malik, M., Grace, S.R.: Study for a new oscillation criteria of a p-Laplacian dynamic equation on time scale. Rocky Mt. J. Math. 1–11 (2019)
18. Negi, S.S., Abbas, S., Malik, M.: Periodic solutions of the N-preys and M-predators model with variable rates on time scale order non linear dynamic equation on time scales. Indian J. Pure Appl. Math. (2019). (Accepted)
19. Negi, S.S., Abbas, S., Malik, M.: Oscillation criteria of second-order non-linear dynamic equations with integro forcing term on time scales. Bull. SUSU. MMCS. **10**(1), 35–47 (2017)
20. Negi, S.S., Abbas, S., Malik, M., Xia, Y.H.: Oscillation criteria of special type second-order delayed dynamic equations on time scales. Math. Sci. **12**(1), 25–39 (2018)
21. Negi, S.S., Abbas, S., Malik, M.: Oscillation criteria of singular initial-value problem for second order non linear dynamic equation on time scales. Nonauton. Dyn. Syst. **5**(1), 102–112 (2018)
22. Negi, S.S., Abbas, S., Malik, M.: Oscillation for a nonlinear neutral dynamic equation on time scale with variable exponents. Math. Methods Appl. Sci. **42**(12), 4146–4169 (2019)
23. Philos, ChG: Oscillation theorems for linear differential equations of second order. Arch. Math. **53**, 482–492 (1989)
24. Qiu, Y.C., Wang, Q.R. : New oscillation results of second-order damped dynamic equations with p-Laplacian on time scales. Discrete Dyn. Nat. Soc. 2015. Art. ID 709242 (2015)
25. Saker, S.H.: Oscillation criteria of second-order half-linear dynamic equations on time scales. J. Comput. Appl. Math. **177**(2), 375–387 (2005)
26. Saker, S.H.: Oscillation of second-order nonlinear neutral delay dynamic equations on time scales. J. Comput. Appl. Math. **187**(2), 123–141 (2006)
27. Saker, S.H., Agarwal, R.P., O'Regan, D.: Oscillation of second-order damped dynamic equations on time scales. J. Math. Anal. Appl. **330**, 1317–1337 (2007)
28. Sun, Y.G.: New Kamenev-type oscillation criteria for second-order nonlinear differential equations with damping. J. Math. Anal. Appl. **291**(1), 341–351 (2004)
29. Wong, J.S.: On Kamenev-type oscillation theorems for second-order differential equations with damping. J. Math. Anal. Appl. **258**(1), 244–257 (2001)

Optimal Investment Decision Model Based on Simplex Algorithm with Variable Optimal Value Evaluation Process

Sanyam Gupta and L. N. Das

Abstract An investment is the current commitment of money or other resources with the expectation of reaping future benefits [1]. Also, investment is a long-term planning at least one year, with low or moderate risks having low or moderate of return. In case planning is short term (few days or months), risk is high with high rates of return. Investment decisions are influenced by hearsay, market psychology and resort to borrowed funds. Market psychology depends on investment analytic descriptions or abstract terms such as purpose, time risks, tools, financial data monitor and adjustment. Each financial product or investment program has rules restrictions, time commitment and cost associate with it. Establishing a time frame for each purpose or goal allows us to make better choices about the tools we use to achieve the purpose. In this paper, the introduction describes a brief literature defining investment decision support technical terms such as expected return or risks, portfolio and steps in decision process of investment analysis. In the second section, we discuss types of investment and investment calculation attributes. The third section contains the formulation of a constrained linear programming modeled investment problem and calculates the optimal decision variable values using simplex algorithm solver MATLAB [2] and TORA [3] tools. In the fourth section, we discuss the application of binary integer program to decide optimum profitable investment projects from a set of listed investment project outcome values.

Keywords Simplex algorithm · Binary integer program · Linear programming

S. Gupta (✉) · L. N. Das
Department of Applied Mathematics, Delhi Technological University, Delhi 110042, India
e-mail: sanyam_phd2k18@dtu.ac.in

L. N. Das
e-mail: lndas@dce.ac.in

S. Bhattacharyya et al. (eds.), *Mathematical Modeling and Computational Tools*, Springer Proceedings in Mathematics & Statistics 320,
https://doi.org/10.1007/978-981-15-3615-1_31

1 Introduction

A proper investment decision process helps the service provider and service availing people happier. The banks and nation's finance servicing units calculate effective investment policies before execution a financial or infrastructure development projects [4, 5]. Government's people welfare schemes are also needed proper financial studies prior to implement the scheme. Each financial product or investment program has certain rules, restrictions, time commitments and cost associates with it. Establishing a time frame for each purpose and goal fulfillment, it allows us to make better choices about the tools.

The insurance company policies and participating people have a certain type of investments, namely CD, bonds, stock, real estate and commodities. The investments are transacting through banks. The programmable investment calculator helps in determining effective set of variables concerning investment with a fixed rate of return. There are four crucial elements such as return rate, starting amount, investment length and additional contribution usually calculated through programmable investment calculators.

2 Literature Defining Investment Decision Support Technical Terms

Expected return and risks: Realized returns meaning actual return might be more or less than the expected return. In case, the actual return is less than the expected return is called the risk.

Steps in decision process: These are the security analysis and portfolio management. The value of the security is a function of future earnings from the security and the risk attached. After securities have been analyzed and valued, the portfolio is selected and security is made.

Portfolio management: These are either passive investment strategy or active investment strategy. In passive strategy, the investors make few changes in the portfolio, so that transaction costs, time and search costs are minimum. In active strategies, investors believe that they can earn better returns by actively making changes in the portfolio.

In the next section, we formulate a bank's annual investment strategy using past years' interest rate, NPA and corresponding constraints in the form of a linear programming algebraic model problem [6]. We use the numerical values to write constraint inequalities for solving the problem using simplex algorithm through MATLAB and TORA [7, 8].

3 A Constrained Linear Programming Modeled Investment Problem and the Optimal Decision Variable Calculation

A bank is devising the loan with the maximum total fund 4652 crore the following table provides the numerical data about the available types of loans. The numerical data consist of interest rate, and NPA meaning non-performing assets. The NPAs are unrecoverable and produce no interest revenue.

S. no.	Type of loans	Interest rate	NPA
1.	Home	8.65	1.3462
2.	Vehicle	11.55	0.212
3.	Education	10.55	0.1749
4.	LAP	11.45	0.2624
5.	Personal	12.55	0.0712
6.	Other	12.90	0.583
7.	SMF	1.9	4.1745
8.	Agriculture	2.65	2.7255
9.	Industry	1.25	5.3450
10.	Service	1.25	12.2950

The bank manager follows the following strategies and restrictions to provide bank loan.

1. Total funds should not exceed 4652 crores.
2. NPA should not exceed 16%.
3. Home, Vehicle, Education, LAP, Personal and Other loans should not exceed 400 crores.
4. SMF and Agriculture loans should not exceed 600 crores.
5. Industry and Service loans should not exceed 3500 crores.
6. Home, Vehicle, Education, LAP, Personal and Other loans should equal to at least 8% of all loans.
7. SMF and Agriculture loans should equal to at least 11% of all loans.
8. Industry and Service loans should equal to at least 60% of all loans.
9. Home, Vehicle, Education, LAP, Personal and Other loans should equal to at least 73% of SMF and Agriculture loans.
10. SMF and Agriculture loans should equal to at least 14% of Industry and Service loans.

The bank manager wants to determine the quantity of loans in each category so that NPA should be minimum and revenue is maximum.

Mathematical models for variable and constraint determination:

Let us assign the variable for loan quantities in crores

x_1 Home loans
x_2 Vehicle loan
x_3 Education loan
x_4 LAP loan
x_5 Personal loan
x_6 Other loans
x_7 SMF loans
x_8 Agriculture loans
x_9 Industry loan
x_{10} Service loan.

The objective of the bank manager is to maximize the difference of interest revenue and NPA. Since 1.3462% of Home loan is non-performing asset, the bank will receive interest on only 98.6538% of the home loan. Thus, the revenue from Home loan will be $0.0865 \times 0.986538x_1$. In this way, the total interest is

$$\begin{aligned} f(x_1, x_2, \ldots, x_{10}) = {} & 0.0865 \times 0.986538x_1 + 0.1155 \times 0.99788x_2 \\ & + 0.1055 \times 0.998251x_3 + 0.1145 \times 0.997376x_4 \\ & + 0.1255 \times 0.99288x_5 + 0.1290 \times 0.99417x_6 \\ & + 0.019 \times 0.958255x_7 + 0.0265 \times 0.972745x_8 \\ & + 0.0125 \times 0.94655x_9 + 0.0125 \times 0.87705x_{10} \end{aligned}$$

$$\begin{aligned} f(x_1, x_2, \ldots, x_{10}) = {} & 0.085335537x_1 + 0.11525514x_2 + 0.1053154805x_3 \\ & + 0.114199552x_4 + 0.125410644x_5 + 0.12824793x_6 \\ & + 0.018206845x_7 + 0.0257777425x_8 + 0.011831875x_9 \\ & + 0.010963125x_{10} \end{aligned}$$

$$\begin{aligned} \text{Total NPA} = {} & 0.013462x_1 + 0.00212x_2 + 0.001749x_3 + 0.002624x_4 + 0.000712x_5 \\ & + 0.00583x_6 + 0.041745x_7 + 0.027255x_8 + 0.05345x_9 + 0.12295x_{10} \end{aligned}$$

$$\text{Maximize Z} = \text{Total interest} - \text{Total NPA}$$

$$\begin{aligned} \text{Maximize Z} = {} & 0.071873537x_1 + 0.11313514x_2 + 0.1035664805x_3 \\ & + 0.111575552x_4 + 0.124698644x_5 + 0.12241793x_6 \\ & - 0.023538155x_7 - 0.0014772575x_8 - 0.041618125x_9 \\ & - 0.111986875x_{10} \end{aligned}$$

The constraints are determined from the investment strategies mentioned in the problem description.

1. Total funds should not exceed 4652 crores.

$$x_1 + x_2 + x_3 + x_4 + x_5 + x_6 + x_7 + x_8 + x_9 + x_{10} \le 4652$$

2. NPA should not exceed 16%.

$$\begin{aligned}&0.013462x_1 + 0.00212x_2 + 0.001749x_3 + 0.002624x_4 + 0.000712x_5\\&\quad + 0.00583x_6 + 0.041745x_7 + 0.027255x_8 + 0.05345x_9 + 0.12295x_{10}\\&\quad \le 0.16(x_1 + x_2 + x_3 + x_4 + x_5 + x_6 + x_7 + x_8 + x_9 + x_{10})\end{aligned}$$

Or

$$\begin{aligned}&-0.146538x_1 - 0.15788x_2 - 0.158251x_3 - 0.157376x_4 - 0.159288x_5\\&-0.15417x_6 - 0.118255x_7 - 0.132745x_8 - 0.10655x_9 - 0.03705x_{10} \le 0\end{aligned}$$

3. Home, Vehicle, Education, LAP, Personal and Other loans should not exceed 400 crores.

$$x_1 + x_2 + x_3 + x_4 + x_5 + x_6 \le 400$$

4. SMF and Other Agriculture loans should not exceed 600 crores.

$$x_7 + x_8 \le 600$$

5. Industry and Service loans should not exceed 3500 crores

$$x_9 + x_{10} \le 3500$$

6. Home, Vehicle, Education, LAP, Personal and Other loans should equal to at least 8% of all loans.

$$\begin{aligned}x_1 + x_2 + x_3 + x_4 + x_5 + x_6 \ge 0.08(&x_1 + x_2 + x_3 + x_4 + x_5\\&+ x_6 + x_7 + x_8 + x_9 + x_{10})\end{aligned}$$

Or

$$\begin{aligned}&-0.92x_1 - 0.92x_2 - 0.92x_3 - 0.92x_4 - 0.92x_5 - 0.92x_6\\&\quad +0.08x_7 + 0.08x_8 + 0.08x_9 + 0.08x_{10} \le 0\end{aligned}$$

7. SMF and Other Agriculture loans should equal to at least 11% of all loans.

$$x_7 + x_8 \ge 0.11(x_1 + x_2 + x_3 + x_4 + x_5 + x_6 + x_7 + x_8 + x_9 + x_{10})$$

Or

$$0.11x_1 + 0.11x_2 + 0.11x_3 + 0.11x_4 + 0.11x_5 + 0.11x_6 - 0.89x_7 \\ -0.89x_8 + 0.11x_9 + 0.11x_10 \leq 0$$

8. Industry and Service loans should equal to at least 60% of all loans.

$$x_9 + x_{10} \geq 0.60(x_1 + x_2 + x_3 + x_4 + x_5 + x_6 + x_7 + x_8 + x_9 + x_{10})$$

Or

$$0.60x_1 + 0.60x_2 + 0.60x_3 + 0.60x_4 + 0.60x_5 \\ +0.60x_6 + 0.60x_7 + 0.60x_8 - 0.4x_9 0.4x_{10} \leq 0$$

9. Home, Vehicle, Education, LAP, Personal and Other loans should equal to at least 73% of SMF and Other Agriculture loans.

$$x_1 + x_2 + x_3 + x_4 + x_5 + x_6 \geq 0.73(x_7 + x_8)$$

Or

$$-x_1 - x_2 - x_3 - x_4 - x_5 - x_6 + 0.73x_7 + 0.73x_8 \leq 0$$

10. SMF and Other Agriculture loans should equal to at least 14% of Industry and Service loans.

$$x_7 + x_8 \geq 0.14(x_9 + x_{10})$$

Or

$$-x_7 - x_8 + 0.14x_9 + 0.14x_{10} \leq 0$$

11. Non-negativity.

$$x_1 \geq 0, x_2 \geq 0, x_3 \geq 0, x_4 \geq 0, x_5 \geq 0, x_6 \geq 0, \\ x_7 \geq 0, x_8 \geq 0, x_9 \geq 0, x_{10} \geq 0$$

Output using MATLAB Version R2017a:
LPP

f = 0.0719 0.1131 0.1036 0.1116 0.1247 0.1224
−0.0235 − 0.0015 − 0.0416 − 0.1120

A =													
1.0000		1.0000	1.0000	1.0000		1.0000		1.0000		1.0000	1.0000	1.0000	1.0000
−0.1465		−0.1579	−0.1583	−0.1574		−0.1593		−0.1542		−0.1183	−0.1327	−0.1066	−0.0371
1.0000		1.0000	1.0000	1.0000		1.0000		1.0000		0	0	0	0
0		0	0	0		0		0		1.0000	1.0000	0	0
0		0	0	0		0		0		0	0	1.0000	1.0000
−0.9200		−0.9200	−0.9200	−0.9200		−0.9200		−0.9200		0.0800	0.0800	0.0800	0.0800
0.1100		0.1100	0.1100	0.1100		0.1100		0.1100		−0.8900	−0.8900	0.1100	0.1100
0.6000		0.6000	0.6000	0.6000		0.6000		0.6000		0.6000	0.6000	−0.4000	−0.4000
−1.0000		−1.0000	−1.0000	−1.0000		−1.0000		−1.0000		0.7300	0.7300	0	0
0		0	0	0		0		0		−1.0000	−1.0000	0.1400	0.1400
b =													
4652	0	400	600	3500	0	0	0	0	0				

Aeq =
[]
Beq =
[]
lb =
0 0 0 0 0 0 0 0 0 0
b =
[]
Optimal solution found.
x =
$1.0e * 03*$
0.3577
0
0
0
0
0
0.4900
0
0
3.5000
Z =
−377.7786
ans =
377.7786

In order to get an authentication about the values of the solution, we use the same LPP and solved using TORA [3]. The TORA output is mentioned in the following table.

Output using TORA Version 2.00

SIMPLEX TABLEAU - (Starting All-Slack Method)

Title: New Problem2 (Maximize)

Steps for generating NEXT tableau from CURRENT one:

1. ENTERING variable: Click a NONBASIC variable (if correct, column turns green)
2. LEAVING variable: Click a BASIC variable (if correct, row turns red)
3. Click command button NEXT ITERATION (or ALL ITERATIONS) – This step may be executed without Steps 1 and/or 2.

Next Iteration | All Iterations | Write to Printer

x10	0.0000	1.0000	1.0000	0.0000	0.0000	0.0000	0.0000	0.0000	0.0000	-297.7963	0.0000	-32.7576	241.1257	0.0000
x1	0.0000	0.0000	0.0000	0.0000	0.0000	0.0000	0.0000	0.0000	0.0000	-30.4348	0.0000	-4.3478	23.9130	0.0000
sx18	0.0000	0.0000	0.0000	0.0000	0.0000	0.0000	0.0000	0.0000	0.0000	-75.8428	1.0000	-7.7427	62.4479	0.0000
x7	1.0000	0.0000	0.0000	0.0000	0.0000	0.0000	0.0000	0.0000	0.0000	-41.6915	0.0000	-4.5861	32.7576	0.0000
sx16	0.0000	0.0000	0.0000	0.0000	0.0000	0.0000	0.0000	0.0000	1.0000	-0.8410	0.0000	-1.0125	0.0893	0.0000
Lower Bound	0.0000	0.0000	0.0000											
Upper Bound	infinity	infinity	infinity											
Unrestr'd (y/n)?	n	n	n											
Iteration 6	Oth. Agri.	Industry	Service											
Basic	x8	x9	x10	sx11	sx12	sx13	sx14	sx15	sx16	sx17	sx18	sx19	sx20	Solution
z (max)	0.0221	0.0704	0.0000	0.0000	0.0000	0.0000	0.0000	0.1079	0.0000	0.0000	0.0000	0.0719	0.0289	377.7786
sx11	0.0000	0.0000	0.0000	1.0000	0.0000	0.0000	0.0000	-1.2422	0.0000	0.0000	0.0000	1.0000	1.7300	304.3000
sx12	-0.0145	-0.0688	0.0000	0.0000	1.0000	0.0000	0.0000	0.0692	0.0000	0.0000	0.0000	-0.1465	-0.2252	242.3291
sx13	0.0000	0.0000	0.0000	0.0000	0.0000	1.0000	0.0000	-0.1022	0.0000	0.0000	0.0000	1.0000	0.7300	42.3000
sx14	0.0000	0.0000	0.0000	0.0000	0.0000	0.0000	1.0000	-0.1400	0.0000	0.0000	0.0000	0.0000	1.0000	110.0000
sx17	0.0000	0.0000	0.0000	0.0000	0.0000	0.0000	0.0000	0.0034	0.0000	1.0000	0.0000	0.1100	-0.8097	11.7530
x10	0.0000	1.0000	1.0000	0.0000	0.0000	0.0000	0.0000	1.0000	0.0000	0.0000	0.0000	0.0000	0.0000	3500.0000
x1	0.0000	0.0000	0.0000	0.0000	0.0000	0.0000	0.0000	0.1022	0.0000	0.0000	0.0000	-1.0000	-0.7300	357.7000
sx18	0.0000	0.0000	0.0000	0.0000	0.0000	0.0000	0.0000	0.2547	0.0000	0.0000	1.0000	0.6000	1.0380	891.3800
x7	1.0000	0.0000	0.0000	0.0000	0.0000	0.0000	0.0000	0.1400	0.0000	0.0000	0.0000	0.0000	-1.0000	490.0000
sx16	0.0000	0.0000	0.0000	0.0000	0.0000	0.0000	0.0000	0.0028	1.0000	0.0000	0.0000	-0.9200	-0.5916	9.8840
Lower Bound	0.0000	0.0000	0.0000											
Upper Bound	infinity	infinity	infinity											
Unrestr'd (y/n)?	n	n	n											

* This is the last 6th iteration of TORA.

4 Bank Loan Policy Decision by Using Binary Integer Program

A bank is devising a loan policy by observing the NPA of five quarters of a financial year. The aim of the bank manager is to decide which category of loan should be preferred in the coming quarter to reduce the NPA. The numerical data are provided in the following table. Based on this, we determine a LPP and solve it using binary integer program to decide which category loans to be provided in the next quarter in a preference.

Loan/months	Mar-17	June-17	Dec-17	Mar-18	June-18	Return
Retail	3.12	2.65	2.33	2.11	2.65	48,638.26,415,094,340
Agriculture	5.10	7.98	6.06	6.05	6.09	42,097.39130434780
Micro and small	8.92	9.56	11.02	11.99	12.03	42,398.17622610140
Medium and large	15.21	17.36	18.15	23.34	23.25	134,456.09677419300

Non-performing assists (NPAs) are unrecoverable and produce no interest revenue.

Strategies to distribution of loan by the bank:

1. Total NPA of month Mar-17 should not exceed 11.17.
2. Total NPA of month June-17 should not exceed 12.63.
3. Total NPA of month Dec-17 should not exceed 13.03.
4. Total NPA of month Mar-18 should not exceed 15.73.
5. Total NPA of month June-18 should not exceed 16.00.

Mathematical models for variable and constraint determination:

Let us assign the variable for loan quantities in crores,

x_1 Retail,
x_2 Agriculture,
x_3 Micro and small,
x_4 Medium and large.

The objective of the bank manager is to maximize return.

$$\begin{aligned}\text{Maximize Z} = {} & 48638.26415094340x_1 + 42097.39130434780x_2 \\ & + 42398.17622610140x_3 + 134456.09677419300x_4\end{aligned}$$

The constraints are determined from the investment strategies mentioned in the problem description.

1. Total NPA of month Mar-17 should not exceed 11.17.

$$3.12x_1 + 5.10x_2 + 8.92x_3 + 15.21x_4 \leq 11.17$$

2. Total NPA of month June-17 should not exceed 12.63.

$$2.65x_1 + 7.98x_2 + 9.56x_3 + 17.36x_4 \leq 12.63$$

3. Total NPA of month Dec-17 should not exceed 13.03.

$$2.33x_1 + 6.06x_2 + 11.02x_3 + 18.15x_4 \leq 13.03$$

4. Total NPA of month Mar-18 should not exceed 15.73.

$$2.11x_1 + 6.05x_2 + 11.99x_3 + 23.34x_4 \leq 15.73$$

5. Total NPA of month June-18 should not exceed 16.00.

$$2.65x_1 + 6.90x_2 + 12.03x_3 + 23.25x_4 \leq 16.00$$

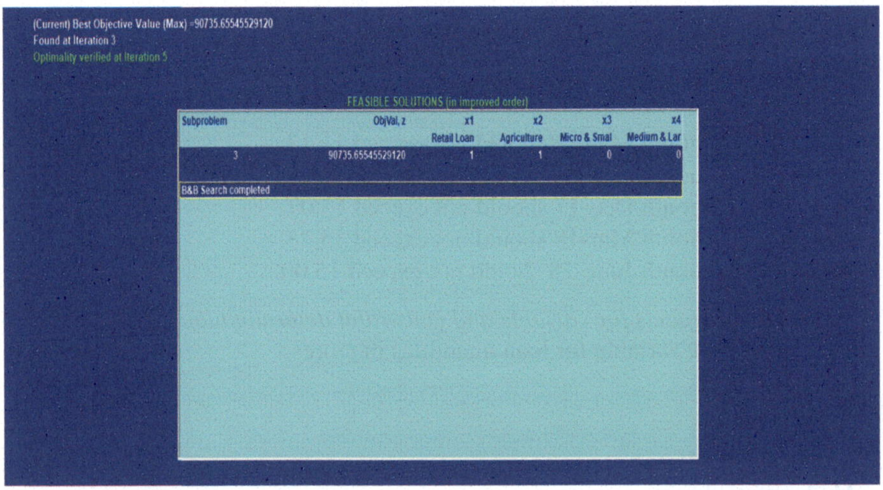

5 Conclusion

The numerical data used in the formulation of LPP problems mentioned in Sects. 3 and 4 are taken from the Web site of the financial year 2017–2018, Union Bank of India [9, 10]. In Sect. 3, the LPP solution is $x_1 = 357.7, x_7 = 490.0, x_{10} = 3500.0$ and $x_2, x_3, x_4, x_5, x_6, x_8, x_9 = 0$. The objective value is $z = 377.7786$ crores. In Sect. 4, binary integer LPP solution more emphasizes the bank investment category of the Retail and Agriculture and lesser emphasizes Micro–small and Medium–large-scale investment.

References

1. www.slideshare.net/linashuja/investment-decision-process
2. MATLAB with version R (2017)
3. TORA with version 2.00, Feb (2016)
4. Hillier, F.S., Liberman, G.J.: Introduction to Operations Research. Seventh Edition, McGraw-Hill (2017)
5. Chandra, S.: Jayadeva and Aparna Mehra. Narosa Publishing House, Numerical Optimization with Applications (2011)
6. Taha, H.A.: Operations Research an Introduction. Eighth Edition, Pearson Education Inc. (2007)
7. Mishra, S.K., Ram, B.: Introduction to Linear Programming with MATLAB. CRC Press (2018)
8. Lopez, C.P.: MATLAB Optimization Techniques, Apress (2014)
9. Financial Results Q4/FY 18 and FY 2017-18, Union Bank of India (UBI)
10. Financial Results Q1/FY 19, Aug 10, 2018, Union Bank of India (UBI)

Stochastic Modelling and Machine Learning

Asymptotic Theory of Bayes Factor in Stochastic Differential Equations with Increasing Number of Individuals

Trisha Maitra and Sourabh Bhattacharya

Abstract Research on asymptotic model selection in the context of stochastic differential equations (*SDE*s) is almost nonexistent in the literature. In particular, when a collection of *SDE*s is considered, the problem of asymptotic model selection has not been hitherto investigated. Indeed, even though the diffusion coefficients may be considered known, questions on appropriate choice of the drift functions constitute a non-trivial model selection problem. In this article, we develop the asymptotic theory for comparisons between collections of *SDE*s with respect to the choice of drift functions using Bayes factors when the number of equations (individuals) in the collection of *SDE*s tends to infinity while the time domains remain bounded for each equation. Our asymptotic theory covers situations when the observed processes associated with the *SDE*s are independently and identically distributed (*iid*), as well as when they are independently but not identically distributed (non-*iid*). In particular, we allow incorporation of available time-dependent covariate information into each *SDE* through a multiplicative factor of the drift function; we also permit different initial values and domains of observations for the *SDE*s. Our model selection problem thus encompasses selection of a set of appropriate time-dependent covariates from a set of available time-dependent covariates, besides selection of the part of the drift function free of covariates. For both *iid* and non-*iid* set-ups, we establish almost sure exponential convergence of the Bayes factor. Furthermore, we demonstrate with simulation studies that even in non-asymptotic scenarios Bayes factor successfully captures the right set of covariates.

Electronic supplementary material The online version of this chapter (https://doi.org/10.1007/978-981-15-3615-1_32) contains supplementary material, which is available to authorized users.

T. Maitra (✉)
Prasanta Chandra Mahalanobis Mahavidyalaya, 111/3 B.T. Road (Bonhooghly), Kolkata 700108, India
e-mail: trishamaitra@yahoo.com

S. Bhattacharya
Indian Statistical Institute, 203 B. T. Road, Kolkata 700108, India
e-mail: sourabh@isical.ac.in

S. Bhattacharyya et al. (eds.), *Mathematical Modeling and Computational Tools*, Springer Proceedings in Mathematics & Statistics 320,
https://doi.org/10.1007/978-981-15-3615-1_32

Keywords Bayes factor consistency · Kullback–Leibler divergence · Martingale · Stochastic differential equations · Time-dependent covariates · Variable selection

1 Introduction

In statistical applications where "within" subject variability is caused by some random component varying continuously in time, stochastic differential equations (*SDE*s) have important roles to play for modeling the temporal component of each individual. The inferential abilities of the *SDE*s can be enhanced by incorporating covariate information available for the subjects. In these time-dependent situations, it is only natural that the available covariates are also continuously varying with time. Examples of statistical applications of *SDE*-based models with time-dependent covariates are Oravecz et al. [14], Overgaard et al. [15], Leander et al. [8], the first one also considering the hierarchical Bayesian paradigm.

Unfortunately, asymptotic inference in systems of *SDE*-based models consisting of time-varying covariates seems to be rare in the statistical literature, in spite of their importance. So far, random effect *SDE* models have been considered for asymptotic inference, without covariates. We refer to Delattre et al. [3] for a brief review, who also undertake theoretical and classical asymptotic investigation of a class of random effect models based on *SDE*s. Specifically, they model the ith individual by

$$dX_i(t) = b(X_i(t), \phi_i)dt + \sigma(X_i(t))dW_i(t), \tag{1.1}$$

where, for $i = 1, \ldots, n$, $X_i(0) = x^i$ is the initial value of the stochastic process $X_i(t)$, which is assumed to be continuously observed on the time interval $[0, T_i]$; $T_i > 0$ is assumed to be known. The function $b(x, \varphi)$, which is the drift function, is a known, real-valued function on $\mathbb{R} \times \mathbb{R}^d$ ($\mathbb{R}$ is the real line, and d is the dimension), and the function $\sigma : \mathbb{R} \mapsto \mathbb{R}$ is the known diffusion coefficient. The *SDE*s given by (1.1) are driven by independent standard Wiener processes $\{W_i(\cdot);\ i = 1, \ldots, n\}$ and $\{\phi_i;\ i = 1, \ldots, n\}$, which are to be interpreted as the random effect parameters associated with the n individuals, which are assumed by Delattre et al. [3] to be independent of the Brownian motions and independently and identically distributed (*iid*) random variables with some common distribution. For the sake of convenience, Delattre et al. [3] (see also Maitra and Bhattacharya [10, 11]) assume $b(x, \phi_i) = \phi_i b(x)$. Thus, the random effect is a multiplicative factor of the drift function. In this article, we generalize the multiplicative factor to include time-dependent covariates.

In the case of *SDE*-based models, proper specification of the drift function and the associated prior distributions demand serious attention, and this falls within the purview of model selection. Moreover, when (time-varying) covariate information is available, there arises the problem of variable selection; that is, the most appropriate subset from the set of many available covariates needs to be chosen. As is well known (see, e.g., Kass and Raftery [7]), the Bayes factor (Jeffreys [6]) is a strong candidate for dealing with complex model selection problems. Hence, it is natural to consider this criterion for model selection in *SDE* set-ups. However, dealing with Bayes factors directly in *SDE* set-ups is usually infeasible due to unavailability of closed-form expressions, and hence various numerical approximations based on Markov chain Monte Carlo, as well as related criteria such as Akaike information criterion (Akaike [1]) and Bayes information criterion (Schwarz [18]), are generally employed (see, e.g., Fuchs [4] and Iacus [5]). But quite importantly, although Bayes factor and its variations find use in general *SDE* models, in our knowledge covariate selection in *SDE* set-ups has not been addressed so far.

Moreover, asymptotic theory of Bayes factors in *SDE* contexts, with or without covariates, is still lacking (but see Sivaganesan and Lingham [19] who asymptotically compare three specific diffusion models in single equation set-ups using intrinsic and fractional Bayes factors). In this paper, our goal is to develop an asymptotic theory of Bayes factors for comparing different sets of *SDE* models. Our asymptotic theory simultaneously involves time-dependent covariate selection associated with a multiplicative part of the drift function, in addition to selection of the part of the drift function free of covariates. The asymptotic framework of this paper assumes that the number of individuals tends to infinity, while their domains of observations remain bounded.

It is important to clarify that the diffusion coefficient is not associated with the question of model selection. Indeed, it is already known from Roberts and Stramer [17] that when the associated continuous process is completely observed, the diffusion coefficient of the relevant *SDE* can be calculated directly. Moreover, two diffusion processes with different diffusion coefficients are orthogonal. Consequently, we assume throughout that the diffusion coefficient of the *SDE*s is known.

We first develop the model selection theory using Bayes factor in general *SDE*-based *iid* set-up; note that the *iid* set-up ensues when there is no covariate associated with the model and when the initial values and the domains of observations are the same for every individual. The model selection problem in *iid* cases is essentially associated with the choice of the drift functions with no involvement of covariate selection. We then extend our theory to the non-*iid* set-up, consisting of time-varying covariates and different initial values and domains of observations. Here, model selection involves not only selection of the part of the drift functions free of the covariates, but also the subset of important covariates from a set of available covariates.

Specifically, we prove almost sure exponential convergence of the relevant Bayes factors in our set-ups. Assuming the *iid* set-up, we develop our asymptotic theory based on a general result already existing in the literature. However, for the non-*iid* situation we first develop a general theorem which may perhaps be of independent interest, and prove almost sure exponential convergence of the Bayes factor in our non-*iid* *SDE* set-up as a special case of our theorem.

It is important to note that (which we also clarify subsequently in Sect. 2.6), in the asymptotic framework of this paper, where the domains of observations remain bounded for the individuals, incorporation of random effects does not make sense from the asymptotic perspective. For this reason, we include random effects in our paper Maitra and Bhattacharya [12], where we assume that even the domains of observations are allowed to increase indefinitely.

The rest of our article is structured as follows. In Sect. 2, we formalize the problem of model selection in our aforementioned asymptotic framework. We then present the necessary assumptions and results in Sect. 3. In Sect. 4, we investigate convergence of the Bayes factor when the *SDE* models being compared form an *iid* system of equations. In Sect. 5, we develop a general asymptotic theory of Bayes factors in the non-*iid* situation, and then in Sect. 6 we investigate exponential convergence of the Bayes factor when the system of *SDE*s is non-*iid*. In Sect. 7, we demonstrate with simulation studies that Bayes factor yields the correct covariate combination for our *SDE* models even in non-asymptotic cases. We provide a brief summary of this article and make concluding remarks in Sect. 8.

The proofs of our lemmas and theorems are provided in the supplementary document whose sections will be referred to in this article by the prefix "S-".

2 Formalization of the Model Selection Problem in the *SDE* Set-Up

Our assumptions (H2′) in Sect. 3 ensure that our considered systems are well defined and we are able to compute the exact likelihood. We consider the filtration $(\mathcal{F}_t^W, t \geq 0)$, where $\mathcal{F}_t^W = \sigma(W_i(s), s \leq t)$. Each process W_i is a $(\mathcal{F}_t^W, t \geq 0)$-adapted Brownian motion.

In connection with model selection, we must analyze the same data set with respect to two different models. So, although the distribution of the underlying stochastic process under the two models is different, to avoid notational complexity we denote the process by $X_i(t)$ under both the models, keeping in mind that the distinction becomes clear from the context and also by the model-specific parameters.

2.1 *The Structure of the SDE Models to Be Compared*

Now, let us consider the following two systems of *SDE* models for $i = 1, 2, \ldots, n$:

$$dX_i(t) = \phi_{i,\xi_0}(t) b_{\beta_0}(X_i(t))dt + \sigma(X_i(t))dW_i(t) \tag{2.1}$$

and

$$dX_i(t) = \phi_{i,\xi_1}(t) b_{\beta_1}(X_i(t))dt + \sigma(X_i(t))dW_i(t) \tag{2.2}$$

where $X_i(0) = x^i$ is the initial value of the stochastic process $X_i(t)$, which is assumed to be continuously observed on the time interval $[0, T_i]$; $T_i > 0$ for all i and assumed to be known. We assume that (2.1) represents the true model and (2.2) is any other model. In the above equations, for $j = 0, 1$, $\boldsymbol{\xi}_j$ and $\boldsymbol{\beta}_j$ denote the sets of parameters associated with the true model and the other model.

2.2 Incorporation of Time-Varying Covariates

We model $\phi_{i,\xi_j}(t)$ for $j = 0, 1$, as

$$\phi_{i,\xi_j}(t) = \phi_{i,\xi_j}(z_i(t)) = \xi_{0j} + \xi_{1j}g_1(z_{i1}(t)) + \xi_{2j}g_2(z_{i2}(t)) + \cdots + \xi_{pj}g_p(z_{ip}(t)), \tag{2.3}$$

where $\boldsymbol{\xi}_j = (\xi_{0j}, \xi_{1j}, \ldots, \xi_{pj})$ is a set of real constants for $j = 0, 1$, and $z_i(t) = (z_{i1}(t), z_{i2}(t), \ldots, z_{ip}(t))$ is the set of available covariate information corresponding to the ith individual, depending upon time t. We assume $z_i(t)$ is continuous in t, $z_{il}(t) \in \mathbf{Z}_l$ where $\mathbf{Z}_l$ is compact and $g_l : \mathbf{Z}_l \to \mathbb{R}$ is continuous, for $l = 1, \ldots, p$. We let $\boldsymbol{\mathcal{Z}} = \mathbf{Z}_1 \times \cdots \times \mathbf{Z}_p$, and $\mathfrak{Z} = \{z(t) \in \boldsymbol{\mathcal{Z}} : t \in [0, \infty)$ such that $z(t)$ is continuous in $t\}$. Hence, $z_i \in \mathfrak{Z}$ for all i. The functions $b_{\boldsymbol{\beta}_j}$ are multiplicative parts of the drift functions free of the covariates.

2.3 Model Selection with Respect to the Drift Function and the Covariates

We accommodate the possibility that the dimensions of $\boldsymbol{\beta}_0, \boldsymbol{\beta}_1$, associated with the drift functions, may be different. In reality, $b_{\boldsymbol{\beta}_0}$ may be piecewise linear or convex combinations of linear functions, where the number of linear functions involved (and hence, the number of associated intercept and slope parameters) may be unknown. That is, not only the values of the components of the parameter $\boldsymbol{\beta}_0$, but also the number of the components of $\boldsymbol{\beta}_0$ may be unknown in reality. In general, $b_{\boldsymbol{\beta}_0}$ may be any function, linear or nonlinear, satisfying some desirable conditions. Linearity assumptions may be convenient, but need not necessarily be unquestionable. In other words, modeling $b_{\boldsymbol{\beta}_0}$ in the *SDE* context is a challenging exercise, and hence the issue of model selection in this context must play an important role in the *SDE* set-up.

We also accommodate the possibility that $\boldsymbol{\xi}_0$ and $\boldsymbol{\xi}_1$, associated with ϕ_{i,ξ_0} and ϕ_{i,ξ_1}, may be coefficients associated with different subsets of the available set of p covariates. This has an important implication from the viewpoint of variable selection. Indeed, in a set of p time-dependent covariates, all the covariates are unlikely to be significant, particularly if p is large. Thus, some (perhaps, many) of the coefficients ξ_{l0} associated with the true model must be zero. This means that only a specific subset of the p covariates is associated with the true model. If a different set of covariates, associated with $\boldsymbol{\xi}_1$, is selected for actually modeling the data, then the Bayes factor is expected to favor the true set of covariates associated with $\boldsymbol{\xi}_0$.

If two different models are compared by the Bayes factor, none of which may be the true model, then the Bayes factor is expected to favor that model which is closest to the true model in terms of the Kullback–Leibler divergence.

2.4 Form of the Bayes Factor

For $j = 0, 1$, letting $\boldsymbol{\theta}_j = (\boldsymbol{\beta}_j, \boldsymbol{\xi}_j)$, we first define the following quantities:

$$U_{i,\boldsymbol{\theta}_j} = \int_0^{T_i} \frac{\phi_{i,\boldsymbol{\xi}_j}(s) b_{\boldsymbol{\beta}_j}(X_i(s))}{\sigma^2(X_i(s))} dX_i(s), \qquad V_{i,\boldsymbol{\theta}_j} = \int_0^{T_i} \frac{\phi_{i,\boldsymbol{\xi}_j}^2(s) b_{\boldsymbol{\beta}_j}^2(X_i(s))}{\sigma^2(X_i(s))} ds \quad (2.4)$$

for $j = 0, 1$ and $i = 1, \ldots, n$.

Let $\boldsymbol{C}_{T_i}$ denote the space of real continuous functions $(x(t), t \in [0, T_i])$ defined on $[0, T_i]$, endowed with the σ-field $\mathcal{C}_{T_i}$ associated with the topology of uniform convergence on $[0, T_i]$. We consider the distribution $P_j^{x_i, T_i, z_i}$ on $(C_{T_i}, \mathcal{C}_{T_i})$ of $(X_i(t), t \in [0, T_i])$ given by (2.1) and (2.2) for $j = 0, 1$. We choose the dominating measure P_i as the distribution of (2.1) and (2.2) with null drift. So, for $j = 0, 1$,

$$\frac{dP_j^{x_i, T_i, z_i}}{dP_i} = f_{i,\boldsymbol{\theta}_j}(X_i) = \exp\left(U_{i,\boldsymbol{\theta}_j} - \frac{V_{i,\boldsymbol{\theta}_j}}{2}\right), \quad (2.5)$$

where $f_{i,\boldsymbol{\theta}_0}(X_i)$ denotes the true density and $f_{i,\boldsymbol{\theta}_1}(X_i)$ stands for the other density associated with the modeled *SDE*.

Let $\boldsymbol{\Theta} = \mathfrak{B} \times \boldsymbol{\Gamma}$ be the parameter space on which a prior probability measure of $\boldsymbol{\theta}_1$, which we denote by $\pi(\boldsymbol{\theta}_1)$, is proposed. In the set-up where $n \to \infty$ and T_i are given, we are interested in asymptotic properties of the Bayes factor, given by, $I_0 \equiv 1$ and for $n \geq 1$,

$$I_n = \int_{\boldsymbol{\Theta}} R_n(\boldsymbol{\theta}_1) \pi(d\boldsymbol{\theta}_1), \quad (2.6)$$

as $n \to \infty$, where

$$R_n(\boldsymbol{\theta}_1) = \prod_{i=1}^{n} \frac{f_{i,\boldsymbol{\theta}_1}(X_i)}{f_{i,\boldsymbol{\theta}_0}(X_i)}.$$

2.5 The iid and the Non-iid Set-Ups

Note that, for *iid* set-up $\boldsymbol{\theta}_j = (\boldsymbol{\beta}_j, \xi_{0j})$, along with $x^i = x$ and $T_i = T$ for all i. Since, for the *iid* set-up $\boldsymbol{\xi}_j = \xi_{0j}$, so in this case $\boldsymbol{\Gamma} = \mathbb{R}$. Thus, here the problem of model selection reduces to comparing $\xi_{00} b_{\boldsymbol{\beta}_0}$ with $\xi_{01} b_{\boldsymbol{\beta}_1}$ using Bayes factor.

In the non-*iid* set-up, we relax the assumptions $\xi_{1j} = \xi_{2j} = \cdots = \xi_{pj} = 0$ and $x^i = x$, $T_i = T$ for each i. Hence, in this case, the model selection problem involves variable selection as well as comparison between different drift functions.

2.6 No Random Effects When T_i Are Given

It is important to perceive that when the T_i are fixed constants, it is not possible to allow random effects into the model and still achieve consistency of the Bayes factor. This is because in that case the *SDE* set-up would simply reduce to n-independent models, each with independent sets of parameters, leaving no scope for asymptotics since T_i are held constants. In Maitra and Bhattacharya [12], we consider random effects when $T_i \to \infty$ along with $n \to \infty$.

2.7 A Key Relation Between U_{i,θ_j} and V_{i,θ_j} in the Context of Model Selection Using Bayes Factors

A useful relation between U_{i,θ_j} and V_{i,θ_j} which we will often make use of in this paper is as follows.

$$
\begin{aligned}
U_{i,\theta_j} &= \int_0^{T_i} \frac{\phi_{i,\xi_j}(s) b_{\beta_j}(X_i(s))}{\sigma^2(X_i(s))} dX_i(s) \\
&= \int_0^{T_i} \frac{\phi_{i,\xi_j}(s) b_{\beta_j}(X_i(s))}{\sigma^2(X_i(s))} \left[\phi_{i,\xi_0}(s) b_{\beta_0}(X_i(s))\, ds + \sigma(X_i(s))\, dW_i(s)\right] \\
&= \int_0^{T_i} \frac{\phi_{i,\xi_j}(s)\phi_{i,\xi_0}(s) b_{\beta_j}(X_i(s))\, b_{\beta_0}(X_i(s))}{\sigma^2(X_i(s))} ds \\
&\quad + \int_0^{T_i} \frac{\phi_{i,\xi_j}(s) b_{\beta_j}(X_i(s))}{\sigma(X_i(s))} dW_i(s) \\
&= V_{i,\theta_0,\theta_j} + \int_0^{T_i} \frac{\phi_{i,\xi_j}(s) b_{\beta_j}(X_i(s))}{\sigma(X_i(s))} dW_i(s),
\end{aligned} \tag{2.7}
$$

with

$$
V_{i,\theta_0,\theta_j} = \int_0^{T_i} \frac{\phi_{i,\xi_j}(s)\phi_{i,\xi_0}(s) b_{\beta_j}(X_i(s))\, b_{\beta_0}(X_i(s))}{\sigma^2(X_i(s))} ds. \tag{2.8}
$$

Note that $V_{i,\theta_0} = V_{i,\theta_0,\theta_0}$ and $V_{i,\theta_1} = V_{i,\theta_1,\theta_1}$. Also note that, for $j = 0, 1$, for each i,

$$
E_{\theta_0}\left[\int_0^{T_i} \frac{\phi_{i,\xi_j}(s) b_{\beta_j}(X_i(s))}{\sigma(X_i(s))} dW_i(s)\right] = 0, \tag{2.9}
$$

so that $E_{\theta_0}\left(U_{i,\theta_j}\right) = E_{\theta_0}\left(V_{i,\theta_0,\theta_j}\right)$.

3 Requisite Assumptions and Results for the Asymptotic Theory of Bayes Factor When $n \to \infty$ but T_i Are Constants for Every i

We assume the following conditions:

(H1′) The parameter space $\boldsymbol{\Theta} = \mathfrak{B} \times \boldsymbol{\Gamma}$ such that $\mathfrak{B}$ and $\boldsymbol{\Gamma}$ are compact.

(H2′) For $j = 0, 1$, $b_{\boldsymbol{\beta}_j}(\cdot)$ and $\sigma(\cdot)$ are C^1 on $\mathbb{R}$ and satisfy $b^2_{\boldsymbol{\beta}_j}(x) \leq K_1(1 + x^2 + \|\boldsymbol{\beta}_j\|^2)$ and $\sigma^2(x) \leq K_2(1 + x^2)$ for all $x \in \mathbb{R}$, for some $K_1, K_2 > 0$. Now, due to (H1′) the latter boils down to assuming $b^2_{\boldsymbol{\beta}_j}(x) \leq K(1 + x^2)$ and $\sigma^2(x) \leq K(1 + x^2)$ for all $x \in \mathbb{R}$, for some $K > 0$.

Because of (H2′), it follows from Theorem 4.4 of Mao [13], p. 61, that for all $T_i > 0$, and any $k \geq 2$,

$$E\left(\sup_{s\in[0,T_i]} |X_i(s)|^k\right) \leq \left(1 + 3^{k-1}E|X_i(0)|^k\right) \exp\left(\tilde{\vartheta} T_i\right), \tag{3.1}$$

where

$$\tilde{\vartheta} = \frac{1}{6}(18K)^{\frac{k}{2}} T_i^{\frac{k-2}{2}} \left[T_i^{\frac{k}{2}} + \left(\frac{k^3}{2(k-1)}\right)^{\frac{k}{2}}\right].$$

We further assume:

(H3′) For every x, $b_{\boldsymbol{\beta}_j}(x)$ is continuous in $\boldsymbol{\beta}_j$, for $j = 0, 1$.

(H4′) For $j = 0, 1$,

$$\frac{b^2_{\boldsymbol{\beta}_j}(x)}{\sigma^2(x)} \leq K_{\boldsymbol{\beta}_j}\left(1 + x^2 + \|\boldsymbol{\beta}_j\|^2\right), \tag{3.2}$$

where $K_{\boldsymbol{\beta}_j}$ is continuous in $\boldsymbol{\beta}_j$.

(H5′) (i) Let $\boldsymbol{\mathcal{Z}} = \mathbf{Z}_1 \times \mathbf{Z}_2 \times \cdots \times \mathbf{Z}_p$ be the space of covariates where $\mathbf{Z}_l$ is compact for $l = 1, \ldots, p$ and $z_i(t) = (z_{i1}(t), z_{i2}(t), \ldots, z_{ip}(t)) \in \boldsymbol{\mathcal{Z}}$ for every $i = 1, \ldots, n$ and $t \in [0, T_i]$. Moreover, $z_i(t)$ are continuous in t, so that $z_i \in \mathfrak{Z}$ for every i.

(ii) For $j = 0, 1$, the vector of covariates $z_i(t)$ is related to the ith *SDE* of the jth model via

$$\phi_{i,\xi_j}(t) = \phi_{\xi_j}(z_i(t)) = \xi_{0j} + \sum_{l=1}^{p} \xi_{lj} g_l(z_i(t)),$$

where, for $l = 1, \ldots, p$, $g_l : \mathbf{Z}_l \to \mathbb{R}$ is continuous. Notationally, for a given $z(t)$, we denote $\phi_{\xi_j}(t) = \phi_{\xi_j}(z(t)) = \xi_{0j} + \sum_{l=1}^{p} \xi_{lj} g_l(z(t))$.

(iii) For $l = 1, \ldots, p$, and for $t \in [0, T_i]$,

$$\frac{1}{n}\sum_{i=1}^{n} g_l(z_{il}(t)) \rightarrow c_l(t); \tag{3.3}$$

and for $l, m = 1, \ldots, p$; $t \in [0, T_i]$,

$$\frac{1}{n}\sum_{i=1}^{n} g_l(z_{il}(t))g_m(z_{im}(t)) \rightarrow c_l(t)c_m(t), \tag{3.4}$$

as $n \rightarrow \infty$, where $c_l(t)$ are real constants.

Note that, given l and t, had $z_{il}(t)$ been random and *iid* with respect to i, then (3.3) would hold almost surely by the strong law of large numbers. Additionally, if $z_{il}(t)$ and $z_{im}(t)$ were independent, then (3.4) would hold almost surely as well. Hence, in this paper, one may assume that for $i = 1, \ldots, n$, and $l = 1, \ldots, p$, the covariates z_{il} are observed realizations of stochastic processes that are *iid* for $i = 1, \ldots, n$, for all $l = 1, \ldots, p$, and that for $l \neq m$, the processes generating z_{il} and z_{im} are independent. Thus, in essence, we assume here that for $l \neq m$, $g_l(z_{il}(t))$ and $g_m(z_{im}(t))$ are uncorrelated.

We then have the following lemma, which will be useful for proving our main results.

Lemma 1 *Assume (H1′)–(H4′). Then for all $\boldsymbol{\theta}_1 \in \mathfrak{B} \times \boldsymbol{\Gamma}$, for $k \geq 1$,*

$$E_{\boldsymbol{\theta}_0}\left[U_{i,\boldsymbol{\theta}_j}\right]^k < \infty; \quad j = 0, 1, \tag{3.5}$$

$$E_{\boldsymbol{\theta}_0}\left[V_{i,\boldsymbol{\theta}_1}\right]^k < \infty, \tag{3.6}$$

$$E_{\boldsymbol{\theta}_0}\left[V_{i,\boldsymbol{\theta}_0,\boldsymbol{\theta}_j}\right]^k < \infty; \quad j = 0, 1. \tag{3.7}$$

Moreover, for $j = 1$, the above expectations are continuous in $\boldsymbol{\theta}_1$.

4 Convergence of Bayes Factor in the *SDE*-Based *iid* Set-Up

We first consider the *iid* set-up; in other words, we assume that $x^i = x$, $T_i = T$ for $i = 1, \ldots, n$, and $j = 0, 1$. In this case, $\boldsymbol{\theta}_j = (\boldsymbol{\beta}_j, \xi_{0j})$ for $j = 0, 1$. We shall relax these assumptions subsequently when we take up the non-*iid* (that is, independent, but nonidentical) case.

4.1 A General Result on Consistency of Bayes Factor in the iid Set-Up

To investigate consistency of the Bayes factor, we resort to a general result in the *iid* set-up developed by Walker [20] (see also Walker et al. [21]). To state the result, we first define some relevant notation which applies to both parametric and nonparametric problems. For any x in the appropriate domain, let

$$\hat{f}_n(x) = \int f(x)\pi_n(df)$$

be the posterior predictive density, where π_n stands for the posterior of f, given by

$$\pi_n(A) = \frac{\int_A \prod_{i=1}^n f(X_i)\pi(df)}{\int \prod_{i=1}^n f(X_i)\pi(df)}$$

and let

$$\hat{f}_{nA}(x) = \int f(x)\pi_{nA}(df)$$

be the posterior predictive density restricted to the set A, that is, for the prior probability $\pi(A) > 0$,

$$\pi_{nA}(df) = \frac{\boldsymbol{I}_A(f)\pi_n(df)}{\int_A \pi_n(df)},$$

where $\boldsymbol{I}_A$ denotes the indicator function of the set A.

Clearly, the above set-up is in accordance with the *iid* situation. The following theorem of Walker [20] is appropriate for our *iid* set-up.

Theorem 1 (Walker *[20])* *Let* f_0 *be the density of the true data-generating distribution and* f *be the density of the modeled distribution. Also, let* $\mathcal{K}(f_0, f) = \int f_0(x) \log\left(\frac{f_0(x)}{f(x)}\right) dP_0$ *denote the Kullback–Leibler divergence between* f_0 *and* f*, where* P_0 *is the appropriate dominating measure associated with* f_0*. Assume that*

$$\pi\left(f : \mathcal{K}(f_0, f) < c_1\right) > 0, \tag{4.1}$$

only for, and for all $c_1 > \delta$*, for some* $\delta \geq 0$*, and that for all* $\epsilon > 0$*,*

$$\liminf_n \mathcal{K}\left(f_0, \hat{f}_{nA(\epsilon)}\right) \geq \epsilon, \tag{4.2}$$

when $A(\epsilon) = \{f : \mathcal{K}(f_0, f) > \epsilon\}$*. Property (4.1) is the Kullback–Leibler property, and (4.2) has been referred to as the* Q^* *property by Walker [20]. Assume further that*

$$\sup_n Var\left(\frac{I_{n+1}}{I_n}\right) < \infty. \tag{4.3}$$

Then,

$$n^{-1}\log(I_n) \to -\delta, \tag{4.4}$$

almost surely.

The following corollary provides the result on asymptotic comparison between two models using Bayes factors, in the *iid* case.

Corollary 1 (Walker *[20]) Let* $R_n(f) = \prod_{i=1}^{n} \frac{f(X_i)}{f_0(X_i)}$. *For* $j = 1, 2$, *let*

$$I_{jn} = \int R_n(f)\pi_j(df),$$

where π_1 *and* π_2 *are two different priors on* f. *Let* $B_n = I_{1n}/I_{2n}$ *denote the Bayes factor for comparing the two models associated with* π_1 *and* π_2. *If* π_1 *and* π_2 *have the Kullback–Leibler property (4.1) with* $\delta = \delta_1$ *and* $\delta = \delta_2$, *respectively, and satisfy the* Q^* *property (4.2) and (4.3) with* $I_n = I_{jn}$, *for* $j = 1, 2$, *then*

$$n^{-1}\log B_n \to \delta_2 - \delta_1,$$

almost surely.

Remark 1 In Walker [20], the densities are assumed to be dominated by the Lebesgue measure. However, this is not necessary. The results remain true if the densities are with respect to any valid measure; see, for example, Barron et al. [2] for related concepts and results (Lemma 4 in particular) with respect to general measures. As such, in our *SDE*-based situation, although the densities are not dominated by the Lebesgue measure [see (2.5)], all our results still remain valid.

We exploit Theorem 1 to prove the following theorem in the *SDE*-based *iid* set-up. The detailed verification of Theorem 1 is provided in Section S-2.

Theorem 2 *Assume the iid case of the SDE-based set-up and conditions (H1′)–(H4′). Then (4.4) holds.*

The following corollary in the *iid SDE* context is motivated by Corollary 1.

Corollary 2 *For* $j = 1, 2$, *let* $R_{jn}(\boldsymbol{\theta}_j) = \prod_{i=1}^{n} \frac{f_{\boldsymbol{\theta}_j}(X_i)}{f_{\boldsymbol{\theta}_0}(X_i)}$, *where* $\boldsymbol{\theta}_1$ *and* $\boldsymbol{\theta}_2$ *are two different finite sets of parameters, perhaps with different dimensionalities, associated with the two models to be compared. For* $j = 1, 2$, *let*

$$I_{jn} = \int R_{jn}(\boldsymbol{\theta}_j)\pi_j(d\boldsymbol{\theta}_j),$$

where π_j is the prior on $\boldsymbol{\theta}_j$. Let $B_n = I_{1n}/I_{2n}$ as before. Assume the iid case of the SDE-based set-up, and suppose that both the models satisfy conditions (H1′)–(H4′) and have the Kullback–Leibler property with $\delta = \delta_1$ and $\delta = \delta_2$, respectively. Then,

$$n^{-1}\log B_n \to \delta_2 - \delta_1,$$

almost surely.

5 General Asymptotic Theory of Bayes Factor in the Non-*iid* Set-Up

In this section, we first develop a general asymptotic theory of Bayes factors in the non-*iid* set-up and then obtain the result for the non-*iid* *SDE* set-up as a special case of our general theory.

5.1 The Basic Set-Up

We assume that for $i = 1, \ldots, n$, $X_i \sim f_{0i}$, that is, the true density function corresponding to the ith individual is f_{0i}. Considering another arbitrary density f_i for individual X_i, we investigate consistency of the Bayes factor in this general non-*iid* set-up. For our purpose, we introduce the following two properties:

1. Kullback–Leibler (δ) property in the non-*iid* set-up:

We denote the Kullback–Leibler divergence measure between f_{0i} and f_i by $\mathcal{K}(f_{0i}, f_i)$ and assume that the limit

$$\mathcal{K}^{\infty}(f_0, f) = \lim_{n\to\infty}\frac{1}{n}\sum_{i=1}^{n} E\left[\log\frac{f_{0i}(X_i)}{f_i(X_i)}\right] = \lim_{n\to\infty}\frac{1}{n}\sum_{i=1}^{n}\mathcal{K}(f_{0i}, f_i) \tag{5.1}$$

exists almost surely with respect to the prior π on f. Let the prior distribution π satisfy

$$\pi\left(f : \inf_i \mathcal{K}(f_{0i}, f_i) \geq \delta\right) = 1, \tag{5.2}$$

for some $\delta \geq 0$. Then, we say that π has the Kullback–Leibler (δ) property if, for any $c > 0$,

$$\pi\left(f : \delta \leq \mathcal{K}^{\infty}(f_0, f) \leq \delta + c\right) > 0. \tag{5.3}$$

2. Q^* property in the non-*iid* set-up:

Let us denote the posterior distribution corresponding to n observations by π_n. We denote $\pi(df_1, df_2, \ldots, df_n)$ by $\pi(\tilde{df})$. For any set A,

$$\pi_n(A) = \frac{\int_A \prod_{i=1}^n f_i(X_i)\pi(\tilde{df})}{\int \prod_{i=1}^n f_i(X_i)\pi(\tilde{df})}$$

denotes the posterior probability of A. Let

$$R_n(f_1, f_2, \ldots, f_n) = \prod_{i=1}^n \frac{f_i(X_i)}{f_{0i}(X_i)}.$$

Let us define the posterior predictive density by

$$\hat{f}_n(X_n) = \int f_n(X_n)\pi_n(df_n),$$

and

$$\hat{f}_{nA}(X_n) = \int f_n(X_n)\pi_{nA}(df_n)$$

to be the posterior predictive density with posterior restricted to the set A, that is, for $\pi(A) > 0$,

$$\pi_{nA}(df_n) = \frac{I_A(f_n)\pi_n(df_n)}{\int_A \pi_n(df_n)}.$$

Then, we say that the prior has the *property Q^* in the non-iid set-up* if the following holds for any $\epsilon > 0$:

$$\liminf_n \mathcal{K}(f_{0n}, \hat{f}_{n,A_n(\epsilon)}) \geq \epsilon, \tag{5.4}$$

when

$$A_n(\epsilon) = \{f_n : \mathcal{K}(f_{0n}, f_n) \geq \epsilon\}. \tag{5.5}$$

Let $I_0 \equiv 1$, and for $n \geq 1$, let us define

$$I_n = \int R_n(f_1, f_2, \ldots, f_n)\pi(\tilde{df}), \tag{5.6}$$

which is relevant to the study of the Bayes factors. Regarding convergence of I_n, we formulate the following theorem.

Theorem 3 *Assume the non-iid set-up and that the limit (5.1) exists almost surely with respect to the prior π. Also, assume that the prior π satisfies (5.2) and has* *the Kullback–Leibler* (δ) *and* Q^* *properties given by (5.3) and (5.4), respectively. Assume further that*

$$\sup_i E\left[\log\frac{f_{0i}(X_i)}{f_i(X_i)}\right]^2 < \infty \tag{5.7}$$

and

$$\sup_n E\left[\log\frac{I_n}{I_{n-1}}\right]^2 < \infty. \tag{5.8}$$

Then,

$$n^{-1}\log I_n \to -\delta, \tag{5.9}$$

almost surely as $n \to \infty$.

Corollary 3 *For* $j = 1, 2$, *let*

$$I_{jn} = \int R_n(f_1, \ldots, f_n)\pi_j(d\tilde{f}),$$

where π_1 *and* π_2 *are two different priors on* f. *Let* $B_n = I_{1n}/I_{2n}$ *denote the Bayes factor for comparing the two models associated with* π_1 *and* π_2. *If both the models satisfy the conditions of Theorem 3 and satisfy the Kullback–Leibler property with* $\delta = \delta_1$ *and* $\delta = \delta_2$, *respectively, then*

$$n^{-1}\log B_n \to \delta_2 - \delta_1,$$

almost surely.

6 Specialization of Non-*iid* Asymptotic Theory of Bayes Factors to Non-*iid SDE* Set-Up Where T_i Are Constants for Every i but $n \to \infty$

In this section, we relax the restrictions $T_i = T$ and $x^i = x$ for $i = 1, \ldots, n$. In other words, here we deal with the set-up where the processes $X_i(\cdot)$; $i = 1, \ldots, n$, are independently, but not identically distributed. Following Maitra and Bhattacharya [10, 11], we assume the following:

(H6′) The sequences $\{T_1, T_2, \ldots\}$ and $\{x^1, x^2, \ldots\}$ are sequences in compact sets $\mathfrak{T}$ and $\mathfrak{X}$, respectively, so that there exist convergent subsequences with limits in $\mathfrak{T}$ and $\mathfrak{X}$. For notational convenience, we continue to denote the convergent subsequences as $\{T_1, T_2, \ldots\}$ and $\{x^1, x^2, \ldots\}$. Let us denote the limits by T^∞ and x^∞, where $T^\infty \in \mathfrak{T}$ and $x^\infty \in \mathfrak{X}$.

Remark 2 Note that the choices of the convergent subsequences $\{T_1, T_2, \ldots\}$ and $\{x^1, x^2, \ldots\}$ are not unique. However, this non-uniqueness does not affect asymptotic selection of the correct model via Bayes factor. Indeed, as will be evident from our proof, for any choice of convergent subsequence, the Bayes factor almost surely converges exponentially to the correct quantity. The reason for this is that we actually need to deal with the infimum of the Kullback–Leibler distance over $\mathfrak{X}$ and $\mathfrak{T}$, which is of course independent of the choices of subsequences; see Section S-6.1 for the details.

Following Maitra and Bhattacharya [11], we denote the process associated with the initial value x and time point t as $X(t, x)$, so that $X(t, x^i) = X_i(t)$, and $X_i = \{X_i(t);\ t \in [0, T_i]\}$.

Let $\boldsymbol{\theta}_j = (\boldsymbol{\beta}_j, \boldsymbol{\xi}_j)$ for $j = 0, 1$ denote the set of finite number of parameters, where $\boldsymbol{\beta}_j$ and $\boldsymbol{\xi}_j$ have the same interpretation as in the *iid* set-up. As before, $z_i(t) = (z_{i1}(t), z_{i2}(t), \ldots, z_{ip}(t))$ is the set of covariate information corresponding to ith individual at time point t. For $x^i \in \mathfrak{X}$, $T_i \in \mathfrak{T}$, $z_i(t) \in \boldsymbol{\mathcal{Z}}$ and $\boldsymbol{\theta}_j \in \boldsymbol{\Theta}$, let

$$U_{x^i,T_i,z_i,\boldsymbol{\theta}_j} = \int_0^{T_i} \frac{\phi_{i,\boldsymbol{\xi}_j}(s) b_{\boldsymbol{\beta}_j}(X_i(s, x^i))}{\sigma^2(X_i(s, x^i))} dX_i(s, x^i); \tag{6.1}$$

$$V_{x^i,T_i,z_i,\boldsymbol{\theta}_0,\boldsymbol{\theta}_j} = \int_0^{T_i} \frac{\phi_{i,\boldsymbol{\xi}_j}(s)\phi_{i,\boldsymbol{\xi}_0}(s) b_{\boldsymbol{\beta}_j}(X_i(s, x^i)) b_{\boldsymbol{\beta}_0}(X_i(s, x^i))}{\sigma^2(X_i(s, x^i))} ds. \tag{6.2}$$

As before, $V_{x^i,T_i,z_i,\boldsymbol{\theta}_0} = V_{x^i,T_i,z_i,\boldsymbol{\theta}_0,\boldsymbol{\theta}_0}$ and $V_{x^i,T_i,z_i,\boldsymbol{\theta}_1} = V_{x^i,T_i,z_i,\boldsymbol{\theta}_1,\boldsymbol{\theta}_1}$.

In this non-*iid* set-up, $f_{0i} = f_{\boldsymbol{\theta}_0,x^i,T_i,z_i}$ and $f_i = f_{\boldsymbol{\theta}_1,x^i,T_i,z_i}$. An extension of Lemma 1 incorporating x, T and z shows that moments of $U_{x,T,z,\boldsymbol{\theta}_j}$, $V_{x,T,z,\boldsymbol{\theta}_j}$, $V_{x,T,z,\boldsymbol{\theta}_0,\boldsymbol{\theta}_j}$ of all orders exist and are continuous in x, T, z, $\boldsymbol{\theta}_1$. Formally, we have the following lemma.

Lemma 2 *Assume (H1′)–(H6′). Then for all $x \in \mathfrak{X}$, $T \in \mathfrak{T}$, $z \in \boldsymbol{\mathcal{Z}}$ and $\boldsymbol{\theta}_1 \in \boldsymbol{\Theta}$, for $k \geq 1$,*

$$E_{\boldsymbol{\theta}_0}\left[U_{x,T,z,\boldsymbol{\theta}_j}\right]^k < \infty; \quad j = 0, 1, \tag{6.3}$$

$$E_{\boldsymbol{\theta}_0}\left[V_{x,T,z,\boldsymbol{\theta}_1}\right]^k < \infty, \tag{6.4}$$

$$E_{\boldsymbol{\theta}_0}\left[V_{x,T,z,\boldsymbol{\theta}_0,\boldsymbol{\theta}_j}\right]^k < \infty; \quad j = 0, 1. \tag{6.5}$$

Moreover, the above expectations are continuous in $(x, T, z, \boldsymbol{\theta}_1)$.

In particular, the Kullback–Leibler distance is continuous in x, T, z and $\boldsymbol{\theta}_1$. The following lemma asserts that the average of the Kullback–Leibler distance is also a Kullback–Leibler distance in the limit.

Lemma 3 *The limiting average $\lim\limits_{n\to\infty} \frac{1}{n}\sum_{k=1}^{n} \mathcal{K}(f_{\boldsymbol{\theta}_0,x^k,T_k,z_k}, f_{\boldsymbol{\theta}_1,x^k,T_k,z_k})$ is also a Kullback–Leibler distance.*

Even in this non-*iid* context, the Bayes factor is of the same form as (2.6); however, for $j = 0, 1$, $U_{x^i,T_i,z_i,\boldsymbol{\beta}_j,\boldsymbol{\xi}_j}$ and $V_{x^i,T_i,z_i,\boldsymbol{\beta}_j,\boldsymbol{\xi}_j}$ are not identically distributed for

$i = 1, \ldots, n$. Next, we establish strong consistency of Bayes factor in the non-*iid SDE* set-up by verifying the sufficient conditions of Theorem 3.

We verify the conditions of Theorem 3 to obtain the following theorem in our non-*iid SDE* set-up.

Theorem 4 *Assume the non-iid SDE set-up and conditions (H1′)–(H6′). Then (5.9) holds.*

As in the previous cases, the following corollary provides asymptotic comparison between two models using Bayes factor in the non-*iid SDE* set-up.

Corollary 4 *For $j = 1, 2$, let $R_{jn}(\boldsymbol{\theta}_j) = \prod_{i=1}^{n} \frac{f_{\boldsymbol{\theta}_j, x^i, T_i, z_i}(X_i)}{f_{\boldsymbol{\theta}_0, x^i, T_i, z_i}(X_i)}$, where $\boldsymbol{\theta}_1$ and $\boldsymbol{\theta}_2$ are two different finite sets of parameters, perhaps with different dimensionalities, associated with the two models to be compared. For $j = 1, 2$, let*

$$I_{jn} = \int R_{jn}(\boldsymbol{\theta}_j)\pi_j(d\boldsymbol{\theta}_j),$$

where π_j is the prior on $\boldsymbol{\theta}_j$. Let $B_n = I_{1n}/I_{2n}$ as before. Assume the non-iid SDE set-up, and suppose that both the models satisfy (H1′)–(H6′) and have the Kullback–Leibler property with $\delta = \delta_1$ and $\delta = \delta_2$, respectively. Then,

$$n^{-1} \log B_n \to \delta_2 - \delta_1,$$

almost surely.

7 Simulation Studies

7.1 Covariate Selection When n = 15, T = 1

We demonstrate with simulation study the finite sample analogue of Bayes factor analysis as $n \to \infty$ and T is fixed. In this regard, we consider $n = 15$ individuals, where the ith one is modeled by

$$dX_i(t) = (\xi_1 + \xi_2 z_1(t) + \xi_3 z_2(t) + \xi_4 z_3(t))(\xi_5 + \xi_6 X_i(t))dt + \sigma_i dW_i(t), \quad (7.1)$$

for $i = 1, \ldots, 15$. We fix our diffusion coefficients as $\sigma_{i+1} = \sigma_i + 5$ for $i = 1, \ldots, 14$ where $\sigma_1 = 10$. We consider the initial value $X(0) = 0$ and the time interval $[0, T]$ with $T = 1$.

To achieve numerical stability of the marginal likelihood corresponding to each data, we choose the true values of ξ_i; $i = 1, \ldots, 6$ as follows: $\xi_i \overset{iid}{\sim} N(\mu_i, 0.001^2)$, where $\mu_i \overset{iid}{\sim} N(0, 1)$. This is not to be interpreted as the prior; this is just a means to set the true values of the parameters of the data-generating model.

We assume that the time-dependent covariates $z_i(t)$ satisfy the following *SDE*s

$$\begin{aligned} dz_1(t) =&(\tilde{\theta}_1 + \tilde{\theta}_2 z_1(t))dt + dW_1(t) \\ dz_2(t) =&\tilde{\theta}_3 dt + dW_2(t) \\ dz_3(t) =&\tilde{\theta}_4 z_3(t))dt + dW_3(t), \end{aligned} \tag{7.2}$$

where $W_i(\cdot)$, $i = 1, 2, 3$, are independent Wiener processes and $\tilde{\theta}_i \overset{iid}{\sim} N(0, 0.01^2)$ for $i = 1, \ldots, 4$.

We obtain the covariates by first simulating $\tilde{\theta}_i \overset{iid}{\sim} N(0, 0.01^2)$ for $i = 1, \ldots, 4$, fixing the values and then by simulating the covariates using the *SDE*s (7.2) by discretizing the time interval [0, 1] into 500 equispaced time points. In all our applications, we have standardized the covariates over time so that they have zero means and unit variances.

Once the covariates are thus obtained, we assume that the data are generated from the (true) model where all the covariates are present. For the true values of the parameters, we simulated $(\xi_1, \ldots, \xi_6)$ from the prior and treated the obtained values as the true set of parameters $\boldsymbol{\theta}_0$. We then generated the data using (7.1) by discretizing the time interval [0, 1] into 500 equispaced time points.

As we have three covariates, we will have $2^3 = 8$ different models. Denoting a model by the presence and absence of the respective covariates, it then is the case that (1, 1, 1) is the true, data-generating model, while (0, 0, 0), (0, 0, 1), (0, 1, 0), (0, 1, 1), (1, 0, 0), (1, 0, 1) and (1, 1, 0) are the other 7 possible models.

Case 1: The true parameter set $\boldsymbol{\theta}_0$ is fixed Prior on $\boldsymbol{\theta}$

For the prior π on $\boldsymbol{\theta}$, we first obtain the maximum likelihood estimator (*MLE*) of $\boldsymbol{\theta}$ using simulated annealing (see, e.g., Liu [9], Robert and Casella [16]) and consider a normal prior where the mean is the *MLE* of ξ_i for $i = 1, \ldots, 6$ and the variance is $0.8^2\mathbb{I}_6$, $\mathbb{I}_6$ being the six-dimensional identity matrix. As will be seen, this results in consistent model selection using Bayes factor.

Form of the Bayes Factor

In this case, the related Bayes factor has the form

$$I_n = \int \prod_{i=1}^{n} \frac{f_{i,\boldsymbol{\theta}_1}(X_i)}{f_{i,\boldsymbol{\theta}_0}(X_i)} \pi(d\boldsymbol{\theta}_1),$$

where $\boldsymbol{\theta}_0 = (\xi_{0,1}, \xi_{0,2}, \xi_{0,3}, \xi_{0,4}, \xi_{0,5}, \xi_{0,6})$ is the true parameter set and $\boldsymbol{\theta}_1 = (\xi_1, \xi_2, \xi_3, \xi_4, \xi_5, \xi_6)$ is the unknown set of parameters corresponding to any other model. Table 1 describes the results of our Bayes factor analyses. It is clear from the 7 values of the table that the correct model (1, 1, 1) is always preferred.

Table 1 Bayes factor results

Model	$\frac{1}{15}\log I_{15}$
(0, 0, 0)	−3.25214
(0, 0, 1)	−1.39209
(0, 1, 0)	−3.31954
(0, 1, 1)	−1.11729
(1, 0, 0)	−3.40378
(1, 0, 1)	−1.22529
(1, 1, 0)	−3.46790

Table 2 Values of $\frac{1}{15}\times$ marginal log-likelihoods

Model	ℓ_i
(0, 0, 0)	2.42430
(0, 0, 1)	4.29608
(0, 1, 0)	1.75213
(0, 1, 1)	4.84717
(1, 0, 0)	1.56242
(1, 0, 1)	4.92628
(1, 1, 0)	0.47111
(1, 1, 1)	5.84665 (true model)

Case 2: The parameter set $\boldsymbol{\theta}_0$ is random and has the prior distribution π

We consider the same form of the prior π as in Sect. 7.1, but with variance $0.1^2\mathbb{I}_6$. The smaller variance compared to that in Case 1 attempts to somewhat compensate, in essence, for the lack of precise information about the true parameter values.

In this case, we calculate the marginal log-likelihood of the 8 possible models as

$$\ell_i = \frac{1}{15}\log\int\prod_{i=1}^{n} f_{i,\boldsymbol{\theta}_1}(X_i)\pi(d\boldsymbol{\theta}_1); \quad i = 1, \ldots, 8,$$

with ℓ_8 corresponding to the true model. Table 2 shows that ℓ_8 is the highest. This clearly implies that the Bayes factor consistently selects the correct set of covariates even though the parameters of the true model are not fixed.

8 Summary and Conclusion

In this article, we have investigated the asymptotic theory of Bayes factors when the models are associated with systems of *SDE*s consisting of sets of time-dependent covariates. The model selection problem we consider encompasses appropriate selection of a subset of covariates, as well as appropriate selection of the part of the drift function that does not involve covariates. Such an undertaking, according to our knowledge, is a first-time effort which did not hitherto take place in the literature.

We have established almost sure exponential convergence of the Bayes factor when the time domains remain bounded but the number of individuals tends to infinity, in both *iid* and non-*iid* cases. In the non-*iid* context, we proposed and proved general results on Bayes factor asymptotics, which should be of independent interest.

Our simulation studies demonstrate that Bayes factor is a reliable criterion even in non-asymptotic situations for capturing the correct set of covariates in our *SDE* set-ups.

Note that our theory for non-*iid* situations readily extends to model comparison problems when one of the models is associated with an *iid* system of *SDE*s and another with a non-*iid* system of *SDE*s. For instance, if the true model is associated with an *iid* system, then $f_{0i} \equiv f_0 \equiv f_{\theta_0}$, and the rest of the theory remains the same as our non-*iid* theory of Bayes factors. The case when the other model is associated with an *iid* system is analogous.

Acknowledgements The first author gratefully acknowledges her NBHM Fellowship, Government of India.

References

1. Akaike, H.: Information theory and an extension of the maximum likelihood principle. In: Petrov B.N., Csaki, F. (eds.) *Second International Symposium on Information Theory*, pp. 267–281, Budapest. Academiai Kiado (1992). Reprinted in Kotz, S., Johnson, N.L. (eds.) *Breakthroughs in Statistics Volume I: Foundations and Basic Theory*, pp. 610–624. Springer (1973)
2. Barron, A., Schervish, M.J., Wasserman, L.: The consistency of posterior distributions in nonparametric problems. Ann. Stat. **27**, 536–561 (1999)
3. Delattre, M., Genon-Catalot, V., Samson, A.: Maximum likelihood estimation for stochastic differential equations with random effects. Scand. J. Stat. **40**, 322–343 (2013)
4. Fuchs, C.: Inference for Diffusion Processes: With Applications in Life Sciences. Springer, New York (2013)
5. Iacus, S.M.: Simulation and Inference for Stochastic Differential Equations: With R Examples. Springer, New York (2008)
6. Jeffreys, H.: Theory of Probability, 3rd edn. Oxford University Press, Oxford (1961)
7. Kass, R.E., Raftery, R.E.: Bayes factors. J. Am. Stat. Assoc. **90**(430), 773–795 (1995)
8. Leander, J., Almquist, J., Ahlström, C., Gabrielsson, J., Jirstrand, M.: Mixed effects modeling using stochastic differential equations: illustrated by pharmacokinetic data of nicotinic acid in obese zucker rats. AAPS J. **17**, 586–596 (2015)
9. Liu, J.: Monte Carlo Strategies in Scientific Computing. Springer, New York (2001)
10. Maitra, T., Bhattacharya, S.: On Bayesian asymptotics in stochastic differential equations with random effects. Stat. Prob. Lett. **103**, 148–159. Also available at http://arxiv.org/abs/1407.3971 (2015)
11. Maitra, T., Bhattacharya, S.: On asymptotics related to classical inference in stochastic differential equations with random effects. Stat. Probab. Lett. **110**, 278–288. Also available at http://arxiv.org/abs/1407.3968 (2016)

12. Maitra, T., Bhattacharya, S.: Asymptotic Theory of Bayes Factor in Stochastic Differential Equations: Part II. ArXiv preprint (2018)
13. Mao, X.: Stochastic Differential Equations and Applications. Woodhead Publishing India Private Limited, New Delhi, India (2011)
14. Oravecz, Z., Tuerlinckx, F., Vandekerckhove, J.: A hierarchical latent stochastic differential equation model for affective dynamics. Psychol. Methods **16**, 468–490 (2011)
15. Overgaard, R.V., Jonsson, N., Tornœ, C.W., Madsen, H.: Non-linear mixed-effects models with stochastic differential equations: implementation of an estimation algorithm. J. Pharmacokinet. Pharmacodyn. **32**, 85–107 (2005)
16. Robert, C.P., Casella, G.: Monte Carlo Statistical Methods. Springer, New York (2004)
17. Roberts, G., Stramer, O.: On inference for partially observed nonlinear diffusion models using the metropolis-hastings algorithm. Biometrika **88**, 603–621 (2001)
18. Schwarz, G.: Estimating the dimension of a model. Ann. Stat. **6**, 461–464 (1978)
19. Sivaganesan, S., Lingham, R.T.: On the asymptotic of the intrinsic and fractional Bayes factors for testing some diffusion models. Ann. Inst. Stat. Math. **54**, 500–516 (2002)
20. Walker, S.G.: Modern Bayesian asymptotics. Stat. Sci. **19**, 111–117 (2004)
21. Walker, S.G., Damien, P., Lenk, P.: On priors with a Kullback-Leibler property. J. Am. Stat. Assoc. **99**, 404–408 (2004)

Text Detection Based on Text Shape Feature Analysis with Intelligent Grouping in Natural Scene Images

D. Kavitha and V. Radha

Abstract Developing an assistive system for visually impaired people using computer vision is an active area of research. The proposed assistive system is developed in an aim to be implemented in Braille e-book reader which facilitates visually impaired persons to recognize the text through tactile or speech output. Examples for such facilities include recognizing text in medicine pills, traffic sign detection, automatic mobile robot navigation, etc. This paper presents an automated system to recognize text in an image based on structural features like size, orientation, and distance between the successive region of interest (ROI). The system is based on two stages, the first performs text localization and the second performs the text detection. In the first stage, the localizing of text area is done by intelligent grouping algorithm. In the second stage, text detection is done based on text shape structural features. Our proposed system achieved an average of 76.26% precision rate, 75.8% of recall/sensitivity rate, and 76.03% of F-measure rate. The advantage of such a simple and lightweight model is that it can be deployed rapidly in any single-board microprocessors like Raspberry Pi and can be made to run effortlessly to produce quality results in real time.

Keywords Text detection · Intelligent grouping · Text shape structure analysis

1 Introduction

An estimated 253 million people live with vision impairment: 36 million are visually impaired and 217 million have moderate to severe vision impairment, 81% of people who are visually impaired or have moderate or severe vision impairment are aged 50 years and above. Globally, chronic eye diseases are the main cause of

Supported by DST-Women Scientist Scheme(A).

D. Kavitha (✉) · V. Radha
Avinashilingam Institute For Home Science and Higher Education For Women, Coimbatore, Tamilnadu, India
e-mail: kavitha.ravindran2@gmail.com

S. Bhattacharyya et al. (eds.), *Mathematical Modeling and Computational Tools*, Springer Proceedings in Mathematics & Statistics 320,
https://doi.org/10.1007/978-981-15-3615-1_33

vision loss. The vision impairment is caused by uncorrected refractive errors and unoperated cataract. In the low and middle developed countries, the second case is the main reason. The prevalence of infectious eye diseases, such as trachoma and onchocerciasis, has reduced significantly over the last 25 years. Over 80% of all vision impairment can be prevented or cured [1]. Hence, developing an assistive system is very important for such a huge numbered population.

In the modern urban environment, the text was an inseparable feature. From city streets to washrooms, the text is present everywhere, to name a few, to label something, to convey an instruction, to alert about something, to provide live data, and much more. Gathering this text to convert them into meaningful information is vital in the modern world for equipping visually challenged to assist their urban living, developing automated systems, navigation, etc. Even though the humans effortlessly decipher the text to information, automated systems in computer vision face tough challenges. There is a huge difference between detecting text in a constrained and controlled environment like scans of a document and detecting text from natural scene images. Text detection gains its applications in various fields like assisting visually impaired peoples [2] in face recognition [3], traveling aid [4], traffic sign detection [5], medical pill recognition [6], video text analysis [7], document analysis [8], and detecting text in natural scene images [9].

Detecting text from scanned document images almost achieved 100 % performance. With natural scene images, there is a need to deal with challenges like noise [10], blur, multi-scale edges [11], font size [12], angle view distortions [13], lighting conditions [14], non-planar text surface [15], bounding layouts [16], colors [17], styles, etc. Some of the natural scene images with textual information and with some of the above said challenges are shown in Fig. 1. These complexities can be summed up to diversity of text styles and complexity of the background which contains the text region. In the recent past, text detection in natural scene images have triggered a lot of interest among researchers in the field of computer vision, mainly because of smartphone revolution. Text detecting algorithms starting from local operators-based methods to complex DNN classifiers are furnished in the past. Even today, the researchers are actively developing text detection methodologies, because there is no unified method to tackle all the different scenarios.

The common architecture of text detection and extraction falls into following steps: (1) text detection is the process of finding text area in the image, (2) text localization is a way to generate bounding boxes around the text location, (3) text segmentation means isolating text regions from the background, and (4) text extraction is the process of recognizing text contents. We explore the first two stages and the flowchart of our proposed method as shown in Fig. 2.

Our proposed work of text detection is based on an intelligent grouping algorithm, which localizes and groups individual text characters in a text region, is presented. This algorithm group's text is of similar size, equally spaced and in a common orientation.

The grouped candidate ROI which have more probability to have text are classified by analyzing the straight lines and curves present in the text shape structure. This is based on the concept that there will be strong presence of lines and curves in the center

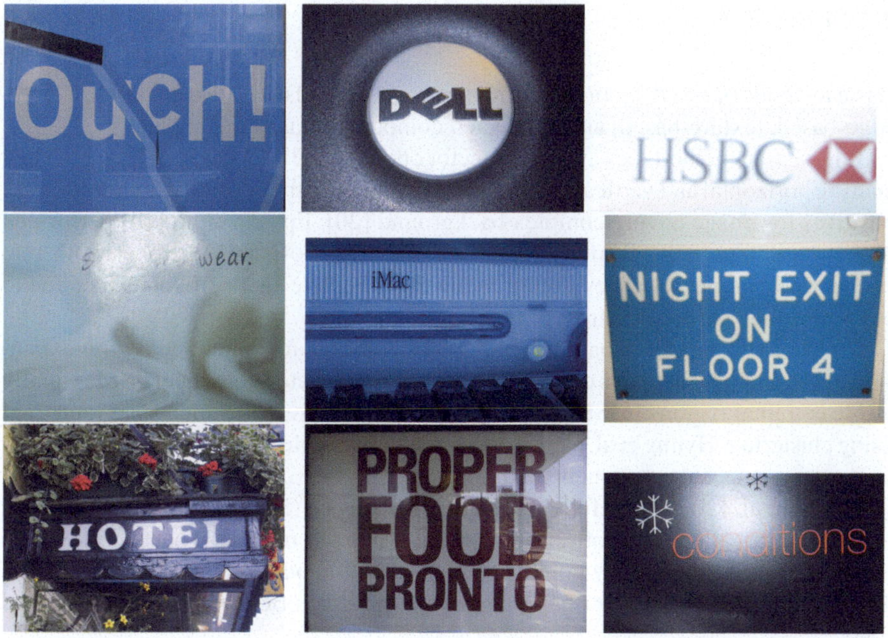

Fig. 1 Natural scene text images of ICDAR 2015 dataset with variations like size, lighting, blur, distortion, orientation, etc

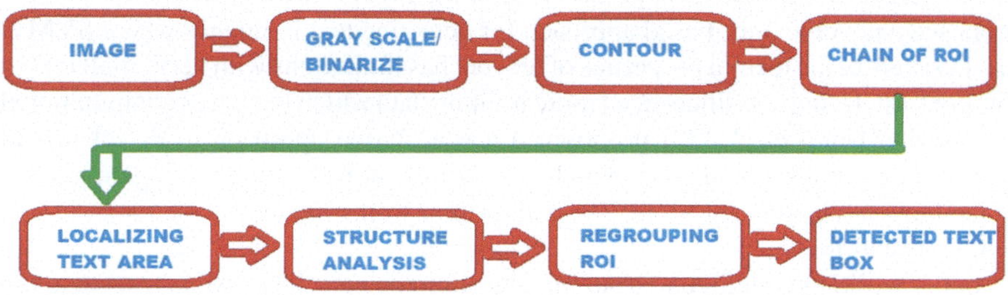

Fig. 2 Flowchart of text detection

region of a candidate ROI than in the cluttered background. As both the operators are local and do not require additional trained models for their computation, the overall computational resource required, is heavily reduced. The advantage of such a simple and lightweight model is that it can be deployed rapidly in any single-board microprocessors like Raspberry Pi and can be made to run effortlessly to produce quality results in real time.

2 State-of-Art

Basic methods of text detection in an image mainly based on three categories, namely edge-based, texture-based, and connected component-based methods.

Edge-based method uses an edge detector operator to detect edges of images. They analyze horizontal and vertical profiles of edge map. But they produce numerous false positives for image having complex background [20]. Epstein et al. [18] performed bottom-up integration of information, merging pixels of similar stroke width into connected components. They do not retain the complete shape of characters due to color bleeding and low contrast of text lines.

Connected component-based method uses color quantization and region expansion to group adjacent pixels of similar colors into connected components. Maximally stable extremal regions (MSERs) are a type of CC where components are identified using clustering. Hyung et al. [19] used a maximally stable extremal region algorithm to extract connected components in images.

Zhang et al. [20] built a fully convolutions network (FCN) model that is trained to predict the salient map of text regions in a holistic manner. Then, the text line hypotheses are estimated by combining the salient map and character components. The framework is general for handling text in multiple orientations, languages, and fonts.

Texture-based defines textural properties and divides the text regions as contours or texture. It distinguishes the text better and produces satisfactory results. In our work, we use texture-based approach to find the region of interest. Kim et al. [21] proposed a novel texture-based approach for detecting text in images where SVM is used to analyze the textual properties of text but has limitations with very small text or low contrast. Using classifiers need more training data which increases computational complexity. Hanif et al. [22] proposed a texture-based approach to detect text in gray-level natural scene images which is a part of project called intelligent glasses to facilitate navigation for blind. Their algorithm well suits for a wide range of text font sizes and fonts.

In our work, the intelligent grouping algorithm detects the possible text region in an image followed by a text shape structure verification algorithm which localizes individual characters in the previously detected image area and checks each character for the presence of lines and curves and classifies the text from false positives.

3 Proposed System

3.1 Pre-processing

The original image Fig. 3a is loaded and then it is converted from RGB to grayscale image Fig. 3b. Deblurring is done for noise removal by adaptive Gaussian threshold method to segment objects from a cluttered background. If the pixel value is greater

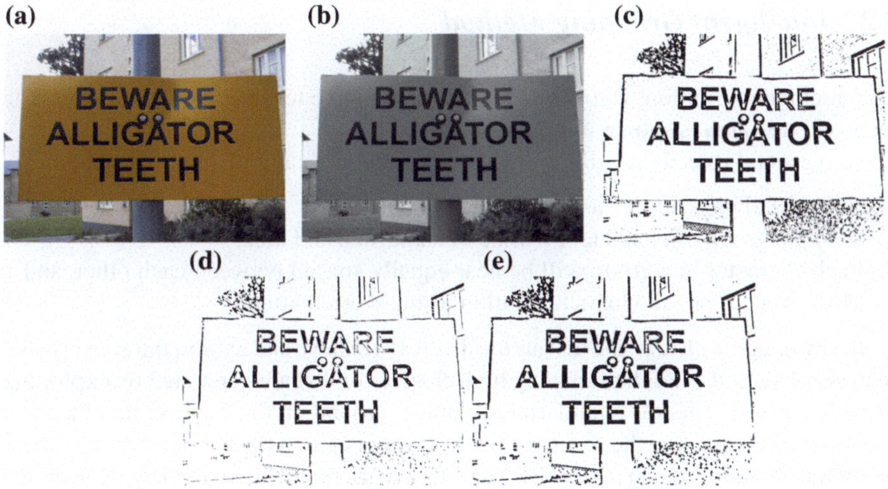

Fig. 3 **a** Original image, **b** grayscale image, **c** binarized image, **d** eroded image, and **e** dilated image

than the threshold value which is set to be 0.20, then is assigned one value (white), else it is assigned another value (black). The resulting binarized Fig. 3c image is less sensitive to noise.

Laplacian method is used for edge detection by determining a threshold based on local values. The Laplacian $L(x, y)$ of an image with pixel intensity values $I(x, y)$ is calculated by:

$$L(x, y) = \frac{\partial^2 I}{\partial x^x} + \frac{\partial^2 I}{\partial y^2}$$

Two morphological operators, namely Erode and Dilate are used, one to remove the unwanted background noise by discarding the pixels near the boundary depending on the size of the kernel and the other to enhance the object of interest by increasing its size. For this, we use the luminosity method which is more sophisticated version of the average method. The algorithm gives more weight to green since humans are more sensitive to green than the other two colors. The resulting eroded and dilated image is as shown in Fig. 3d, e.

After smoothing the image, our proposed approach has two phases of processing. In the first phase, the intelligent grouping algorithm detects the possible text region in an image, and in the second phase, the text shape structure verification algorithm localizes individual characters in the previously detected image area and checks each character for the presence of lines and curves and classifies the text from false positives.

3.2 Intelligent Grouping Method

The intelligent grouping algorithm detects the possible text region in an image. The localized text area is shown in Fig. 4 .

As a general rule, there will be always some unique features for text in any image.

1. Text will always appear as groups of characters,
2. A single group of characters will be of same size and area,
3. Each character in a group will be near equally spaced between each other, and
4. Most of the time, all characters fall in a single orientation.

In any image with text, the text area will always behave and exhibit the above-listed features. The ROI candidates having high chances of text are generated by exploiting these features. Perimeter boundaries are drawn around all the foreground objects in the fostered image, and the resulting list of contours are extracted to a NumPy array. Minimum bonding rectangle (MBR) and its center points are calculated for all list of contours and are finally grouped according to their area. A k-d tree is formed out of grouped MBR and queried to find all pairs of points within a specified distance.

These paired points are further grouped based on their orientation. These grouped pairs of points are finally converted into a chain of interlinked points which hypothetically represents a chain of characters. These operations will result in '*n*' number of character chains along with false positives. Some odd-shaped clutters present near the background of a text region might also be grouped as candidate text ROI. Sometimes, a single character in a group of characters will be bigger or smaller than the rest and will have different distances from the adjacent character.

It is found that sometimes a few characters are left out while grouping, based on the area of bounding rectangle because, for example, there is a huge variation in area between the bounding box for character '*I*' and character '*w*'. Also, it is found that there is no uniform ratio for distance between adjacent characters and their MBR area. Because of these limitations, a few characters in a given area group/chain are left out are grouped randomly with other area groups/chains.

To regroup the missed out characters belonging to a particular family, a bounding box across the image is drawn for every chain and the character candidate ROI inside this bounding box are grouped to form the final chain.

3.3 Text Shape Structure Analysis

The resulting chain of characters has a good chance to have false positives among their chains. To filter out these false positives, the text shape is analyzed inside every

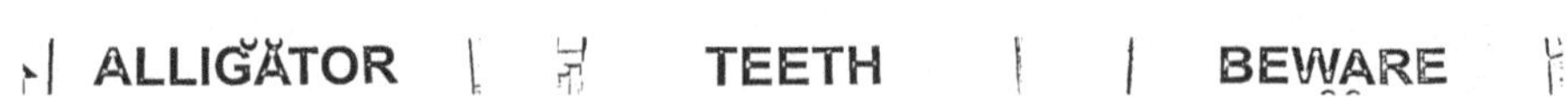

Fig. 4 Localized text area

candidate ROI. This is based on the fact that the probability of having lines and smooth curves in the shape of text character is more than the ROI from cluttered background. To extract these features from the candidate ROI, Fig. 5a, the eroded and dilated ROI is blurred with Gaussian blur operator. This results in a smooth foreground text shape. Medial axis Fig. 5b of this blurred image is generated and converted it into a NumPy array.

Presence of straight lines in the resulted median axis is checked by houghlines (r) operator Fig. 5c. It simply returns an array of (r, θ) values. r is measured in pixels and θ is measured in radians. A line can be represented as

$$y = mx + c \tag{1}$$

or in parametric form, as

$$r = x\cos\theta + y\sin\theta \tag{2}$$

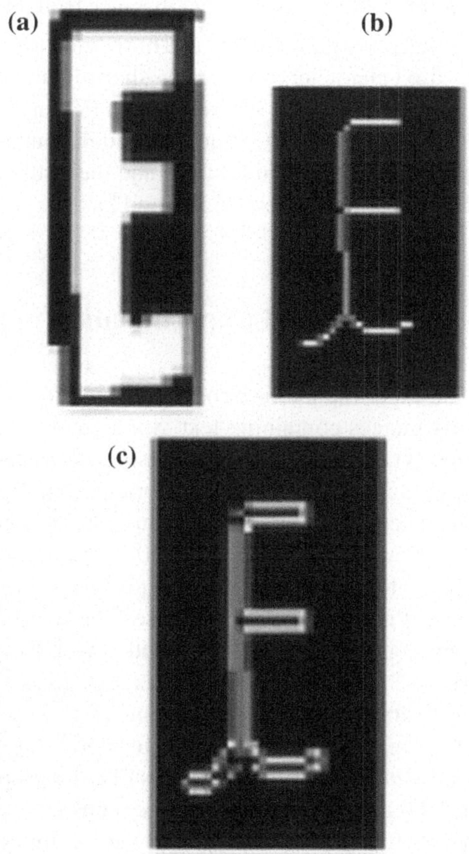

Fig. 5 **a** Localized individual text, **b** skeletonized image after a series of image enhancement, and **c** generation of houghlines on the skeletonized image

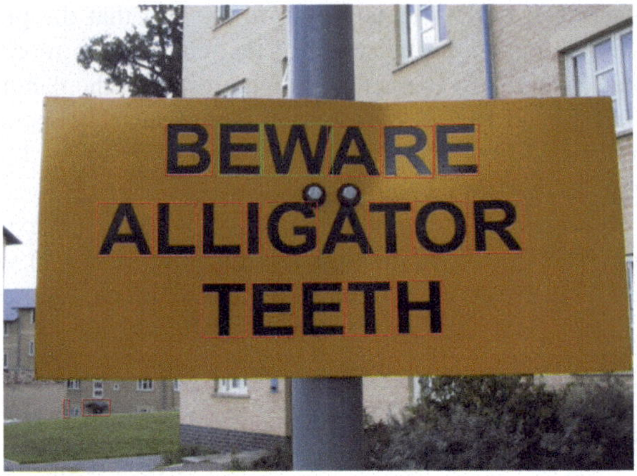

Fig. 6 Text detection after text shape analysis

where r is the perpendicular distance from origin to the line, and θ is the angle formed by this perpendicular line and horizontal axis measured in counter-clockwise (Fig. 6).

Text characters will have a shape in an organized way while background clutters have random lines all over the ROI. Total number of straight lines present in the central region of ROI and the total distance of prominent lines are measured. If the total number of straight lines and their sum of distance is above a certain threshold, it is classified as text (Figs. 6 and 7).

4 Dataset and Experiments

The experiments were conducted over focused text dataset [23] of ICDAR 2015 with 464 images containing text. Some of the images with bounding boxes created over the text region Fig. 6 in good resolution images are always 100% using our algorithm. As practically, the character orientation may be of multi-scale, our algorithm was designed based on this assumption. However, during the experiments, characters found with orientation up to 30° were detected efficiently Fig. 9c.

As this algorithm was designed to run in a single-board microprocessor like Raspberry Pi, we made sure that it uses minimum computational power and memory. While running text detection in live video with Raspberry Pi 3 and LogiTech HD720p camera, we found near real-time text detection Fig. 9a, b, if 2–3 lines of text area present in the frame. We achieved around 2.5 FPS for practical scenario. In desktop computer, we achieved around 4–5 FPS for normal text detection in live 720 p video.

In addition to the above results, the proposed algorithm was compared Fig. 8 to EAST: an efficient and accurate scene text detector [24], which uses TensorFlow and DNN for classification which can be implemented in low processing devices like

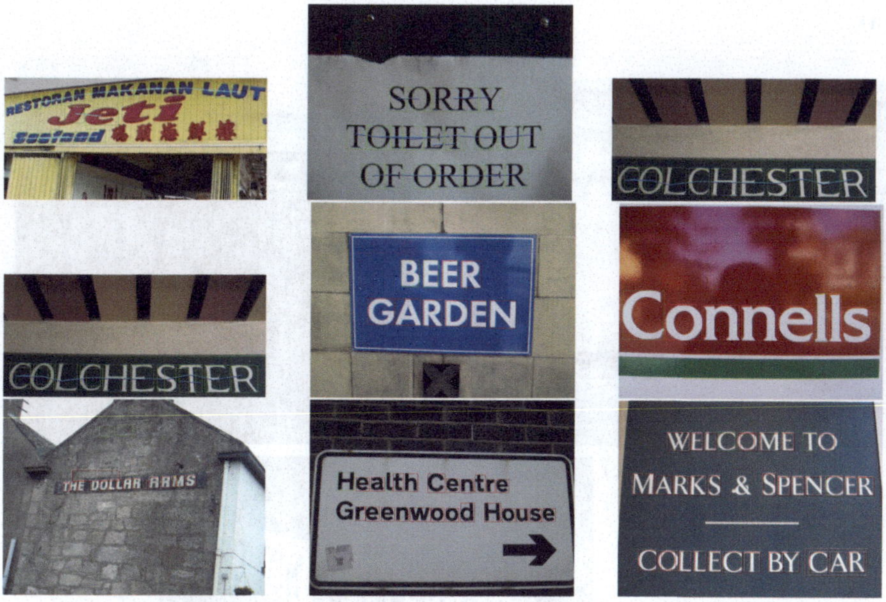

Fig. 7 Text detection shown in bounding boxes

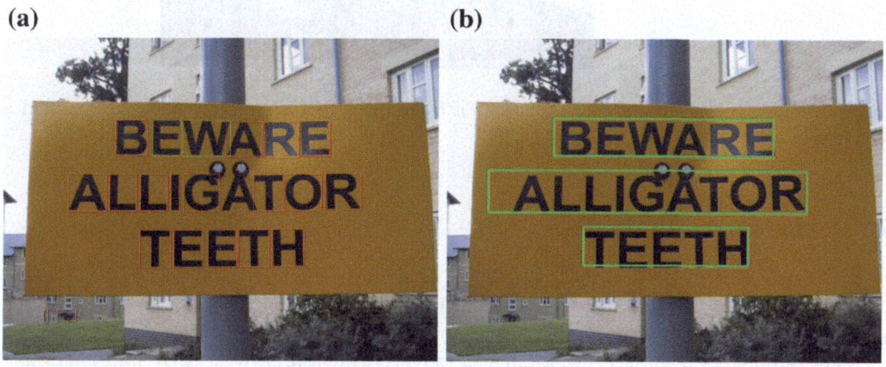

Fig. 8 Comparision **a** proposed algorithm, **b** text detection by EAST

Raspberry Pi. It is found that the proposed algorithm yielded 4–5 FPS while EAST yielded 1.0–1.5 FPS for text detection. While the bounding boxes generated by the proposed algorithm are more precise and extract individual text from the text region, EAST generates an overall rectangle for the entire text region while our proposed method draws rectangle over each character. EAST was more accurate to detect the presence of text when proposed algorithm produces false positives in low resolution images.

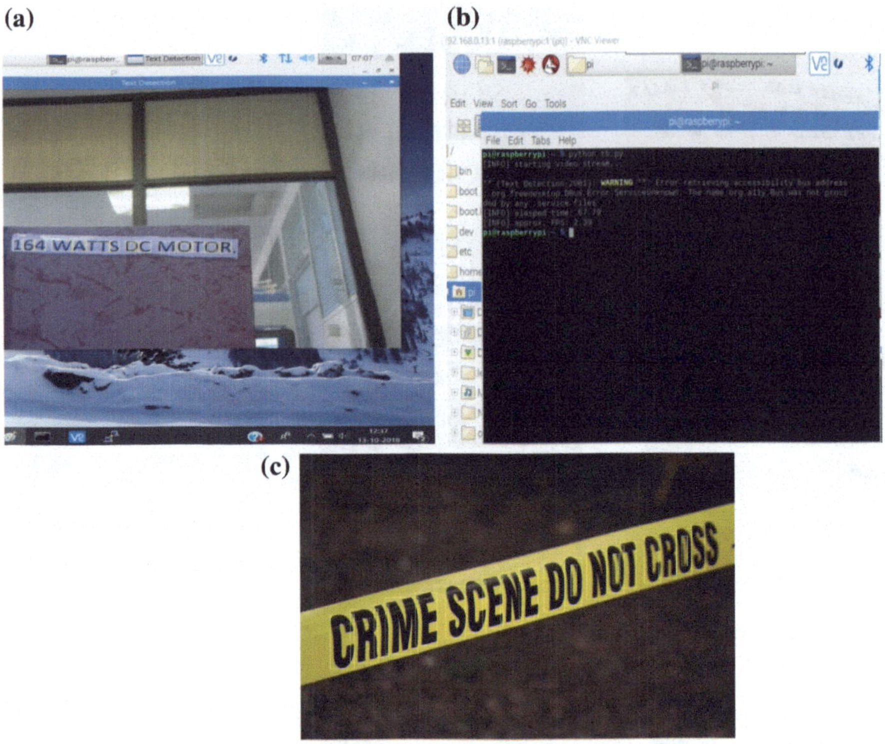

Fig. 9 **a** Video text detection in Raspberry Pi, **b** Raspberry Pi experiment performance, and **c** detection of angular aligned text

5 Performance Metrics

The performance metrics used are precision, recall, and F-measure. To evaluate our performance, the following protocol has been chosen. Three classes are defined for each detected block: (i) true positives (TP) (ii) false positives (FP), and (iii) false negative (FN). Precision (P) is the ratio of correctly predicted positive observations to the total predicted positive observations. Recall (R) is the ratio of correctly predicted positive observations to the all observations in actual class. F-measure (F) score is the weighted average of precision and recall. Therefore, this score takes both false positives and false negatives into account.

To make a fair comparison with other existing approaches, we have followed the standard evaluation scheme given in the ICDAR 2015 robust reading competition. For comparison, we have used the four existing methods described in Table: 1 (i) Pan et al. [25] used the hybrid approach to localize texts in natural scene images, (ii) Yan et al. [26] used color clustering and connected component method to obtain candidate regions, (iii) Tian et al. [27] proposed a novel connectionist text proposal network which localizes text in natural scene images. The same parameter values are used

Table 1 Comparision between various methods over ICDAR 2015

Method	Precision	Recall	F-measure
Pan et al.	67.4	69.7	68.5
Yan et al.	74.6	73.9	74.25
Tian et al.	74	52	61
Hyan et al.	51.88	47.52	49.60
TSFA (proposed)	76.26	75.8	76.03

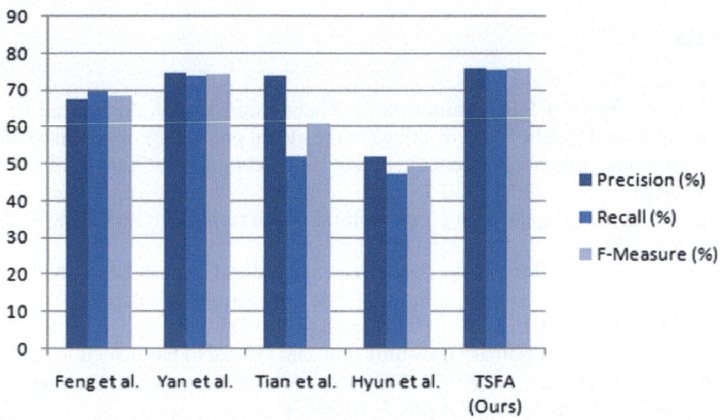

Fig. 10 Comparision between various methods over ICDAR 2015

for all of the experiments. ICDAR 2015 dataset was used by the above works and performs well for text localization but needs more accuracy in terms of measures like precision, recall, and F-measure. When compared with all other discussed methods, our proposed algorithm performed well in terms of the following measures Fig. 10. Which is formulated as

$$\text{Precision(P)} = \text{TP}/\text{TP} + \text{FP}$$
$$\text{Recall(R)}/\text{Sensitivity} = \text{TP}/\text{TP} + \text{FN}$$
$$\text{F} - \text{measure(F)} = 2 * \text{Precision} * \text{Recall}/(\text{Precision} + \text{Recall})$$

6 Conclusion

Text detection is a field of study that can be used for the development of assistive devices for visually impaired. It can be useful for them to guide in text detection in pills, traffic signs, natural scene images, etc. Our algorithm performs well in detecting text in natural scene images. Also, it is capable to produce the quality results even in low power devices like Raspberry Pi. The proposed algorithm is capable of producing better to near equivalent results when compared to the best present text detectors. There are certain scenarios where our text detector could not pick up text, like more vertically oriented text, low resolution texts, very small texts, and designer texts. The algorithm slows down if more text is present in a single frame. Our future work would optimize the code to run faster and to improve the algorithm so that it works in all practical scenarios.

References

1. Bourne, R.R.A., Flaxman, S.R., Braithwaite, T., Cicinelli, M.V., Das, A., Jonas, J.B., Keeffe, J.: Magnitude, temporal trends, and projections of the global prevalence of blindness and distance and near vision impairment: a systematic review and meta-analysis. Lancet Glob Health **5**(9), 888–897 (2017)
2. Maddala, K.T., et al.: Adaptable ring for vision-based measurements and shape analysis. IEEE Trans. Instrum. Meas. **66**(4), 746–756 (2017)
3. Islam, K.T., Raj, R.G., Al-Murad, A.: Performance of SVM, CNN, and ANN with BoW, HOG, and image pixels in face recognition. In: 2017 2nd International Conference on Electrical and Electronic Engineering (ICEEE), Rajshahi, pp. 1–4 (2017)
4. Pan, H., Yi, C., Tian, Y.: A primary travelling assistant system of bus detection and recognition for visually impaired people. In: 2013 IEEE International Conference on Multimedia and Expo Workshops (ICMEW), San Jose, CA, pp. 1–6 (2013)
5. Islam, K.T., Ram, R.G, Mujtaba, G.: Recognition of traffic sign based on bag-of-words and artificial neural network. Symmetry. **9** (2017). https://doi.org/10.3390/sym9080138
6. Hartl, A.: Computer-vision based pharmaceutical pill recognition on mobile phones (2012)
7. Cai, M., Song, J., Lyu, M.R.: A new approach for video text detection. In: Proceedings. International Conference on Image Processing, Rochester, NY, USA, pp. I–I (2002)
8. Forczmański, P., Smolinski, A., Nowosielski, A., Małecki, K.: Segmentation of scanned documents using deep-learning approach (2020). https://doi.org/10.1007/978-3-030-19738-40-15
9. Cho, H., Sung, M., Jun, B.: Canny text detector: fast and robust scene text localization algorithm. In: 2016 IEEE Conference on Computer Vision and Pattern Recognition (CVPR), Las Vegas, NV, pp. 3566–3573 (2016)
10. Fan, K.-C., Wang, Y.-K., Lay, T.-R.: Marginal noise removal of document images. Pattern Recognit. **35**(11), 2593–2611 (2002)
11. Liu, X., Jagath, S.: Multiscale edge-based text extraction from complex images. In: 2006 IEEE International Conference on Multimedia and Expo. IEEE (2006)
12. Slimane, F., et al.: A study on font-family and font-size recognition applied to Arabic word images at ultra-low resolution. Pattern Recognit. Lett. **34**(2), 209–218 (2013)
13. Yin, X-C., et al.: Multi-orientation scene text detection with adaptive clustering. IEEE Trans. Pattern Anal. Mach. Intell. **37**(9), 1930–1937 (2015)
14. Gao, J., Jie, Y.: An adaptive algorithm for text detection from natural scenes. In: Proceedings of the 2001 IEEE Computer Society Conference on Computer Vision and Pattern Recognition. CVPR 2001. Vol. 2. IEEE (2001)
15. Jung, K., Kim, K.I., Han, J.: Text extraction in real scene images on planar planes. In: Object Recognition Supported by User Interaction for Service Robots. vol. 3. IEEE (2002)
16. Alshameri, A., Abdou, S., Mostafa, K.: A combined algorithm for layout analysis of Arabic document images and text lines extraction. Int. J. Comput. Appl. **49**(23) (2012)
17. Shivakumara, P., Phan, T.Q., Tan, C.L.: New Fourier-statistical features in RGB space for video text detection. IEEE Trans. Circuits Syst. Video Technol. **20**(11), 1520–1532 (2010)

18. Epshtein, B., Ofek, E., Wexler, Y.: Detecting text in natural scenes with stroke width transform. In: 2010 IEEE Computer Society Conference on Computer Vision and Pattern Recognition. IEEE (2010)
19. Koo, H.I., Kim, D.H.: Scene text detection via connected component clustering and nontext filtering. IEEE Trans. Image Process. **22**(6), 2296–2305 (2013)
20. Zhang, Z., et al.: Multi-oriented text detection with fully convolutional networks. In: Proceedings of the IEEE Conference on Computer Vision and Pattern Recognition (2016)
21. Kim, K.I., Jung, K., Kim, J.H.: Texture-based approach for text detection in images using support vector machines and continuously adaptive mean shift algorithm. IEEE Trans. Pattern Anal. Mach. Intell. **25**(12), 1631–1639 (2003)
22. Hanif, S.M., Prevost, L.: Texture based Text Detection in Natural Scene Images-A Help to Blind and Visually Impaired Persons. CVHI (2007)
23. https://rrc.cvc.uab.es/?ch=2&com=downloads
24. Zhou, X., et al.: EAST: an efficient and accurate scene text detector. In: Proceedings of the IEEE conference on Computer Vision and Pattern Recognition (2017)
25. Pan, Y.-F., Hou, X., Liu, C.-L.: A hybrid approach to detect and localize texts in natural scene images. IEEE Trans. Image Process. **20**(3), 800–813 (2010)
26. Yan, J., Gao, X.: Detection and recognition of text superimposed in images base on layered method. Neurocomputing **134**, 3–14 (2014)
27. Tian, Z., et al.: Detecting text in natural image with connectionist text proposal network. In: European Conference on Computer Vision. Springer, Cham (2016)

Anthrophilia* Algorithm

Sujoy Seal

Abstract Optimization nowadays is not a choice. We need a system of check and balance in any dynamic system. For this, we must have a general system of equations, some mathematical model, some much generalized yet fundamentally strong algorithm having large domain of applications. We need to understand all the visible constraints which presently cannot be ignored. Simultaneously, we must realize the demand of the situation and the limitations of the present algorithms. By algorithms, we mean those who definitely reach out to global optima in finite time. Such techniques are lagging in situations where the goal is to achieve states which are, in general, functions bounded by variable constraints (Krumke in Wireless networks 7(6):575–584, [1]). Hence, this is the time when we look for an algorithm which is multidimensional, recursive and is expected to reason fastest to the solution when several variable boundaries are on the line.

Keywords Artificial intelligence · Swarm · Genetic algorithm · Multidimensional · Optimization

1 Introduction

We, as scientists, look up for automation in space as well as marine research both of which interest our thirst for knowledge. Imagine traveling along some curve for space research. It may be necessary to send some satellite along some optimum conic from one planet to some other planets. As no planet is stationary in space, the time algorithm which governs their motion needs to be dynamic. We must recall here that if such algorithms are incorporated in systems which can never learn nor be trained, it then becomes the sole task of the algorithm to take decisions [2] as a function of time. So we need an algorithm which is intelligent enough to modify itself with time by itself. Hence at this point of time, we understand that we do need unsupervised

S. Seal (✉)
Department of Computer Science and Engineering, Institute of Engineering and Management Kolkata, Kolkata, India
e-mail: sujoyseal11@gmail.com

S. Bhattacharyya et al. (eds.), *Mathematical Modeling and Computational Tools*, Springer Proceedings in Mathematics & Statistics 320,
https://doi.org/10.1007/978-981-15-3615-1_34

machine learning which will be done by another machine having intelligent systems. By intelligent systems, we do not necessarily mean hash tables or systems using memorization to the utmost. What we mean is to have some dynamic responsive system that will specify the range for each constraint. Obviously for entirely new set of constrained equations, we need to some amount of prior knowledge because starting with no information is not possible in a variable multidimensional space–time graphical plot with as many possibilities as we think. Keeping difficulties and challenges in mind our idea will be to approach and create this generalized system of equations. We hence have throughout the paper focused on the numerical method, the technique rather than on the coding. The algorithm is a "*" algorithm and to demand so we have given a theoretical proof at the end of the paper. One key feature is to cover all key domains under exploring graphs and bounding possibly all constraints which may generate in any dimension recursively and reinforcibly in some sense.

2 Literature Review

We shall here glance at the problems of present algorithms [3] which are taught under artificial intelligence. To start with, we take up blind (non-directional) algorithms: Breadth-First Search (BFS), Depth-First Search (DFS), Depth-First-Iterartive-Deepening (DFID) which have no sense of directionality of a possible solution. These algorithms hence waste a lot of time and space and are totally irrelevant in dynamic situations. Next, we take up directional algorithms fundamentally all of which are improvements over the hill climbing algorithm. There are several versions like heuristic search and so on, all of whom share a common problem. They all get stuck up in local optima. Scientists therefore have come up with Tabu search [4], simulated annealing [5], genetic algorithms (GA) [6], A* [7], IDA*, RBFS [8], DCBFS [9], some of which have major improvements over the earlier algorithms. The purpose of making a new algorithm is to clarify that the earlier algorithms have drawbacks and may not succeed in cases of dynamic environment and constraint change and when situations are multidimensional in some sense.

The ant colony optimization algorithm [10] makes use of randomized methods. With time, path to goal becomes very definite and hence the algorithm reaches the goal node. Idea here is an analogy to motion of ants depositing pheromone on their trail. This trail becomes strong once one of the random nodes coincides with the actual optima. The trail hence becomes stronger with time, and at some point of time, when pheromone from all other paths have disappeared, all trails vanish and a single path in the search tree is identified we terminate and the path so developed is termed as the optimum path. Here, ants represent functions and search algorithms.

However, the ant colony algorithm [11] (which is complete in some sense) suffers some major drawbacks in real life. In an analogous sense, if we surround the goal of ants by fire, the ants will never reach their goal which corresponds to a state of no solution. However, the solution would have easily existed if we would have used bees instead of ants once we feel the effect of fire. Now consider that in the motion of bees and ants, there is a system of poisonous atmosphere so that only possible way of reaching the goal is to manage underground. The whole idea is to project the fact that an army of different search algorithms (insects) is better than one single individual search engine [12]. Consider a ground having rings of fire. So we can just have to call ants and bees repeatedly and recursively. Also realize that choice of insect is based on three factors, namely probability of succeeding, dynamic hindrance factor and dimensionality [13] of space. We will visit details in the numerical section, but now we want to draw attention in three aspects, namely creation of environment, taking input and displaying output, space and time complexities of the algorithm. Environment will be created as a system of multidimensional arrays which would be made of several cells each of whom will be a structure (node). Their states will be mentioned with respect to the start state. Output and input is still a part of our research, and work is still in progress. Space and time complexities will depend on the nature of evaluation function which empirically is large. This is necessary because this algorithm differs from all other algorithms by one major clause that no need to reset the compiler for new situations because that is inbuilt.

3 Creation of Search Space

Search space here means an entire graph of nodes in r dimensions. We explain the search space here. We say here that r is a variable which can take values as $\alpha < r < \beta$ where α, β are non-negative integer constants that depend on which state solution space algorithm is in. However, we need to first generate N-dimensional environment for the algorithm to work on. This is achieved by creating a system of N-dimensional arrays (actually tree of linked lists) which are made of cells. Such cells are structures which have in them several parameters. Some of them are *check( )* function, heuristic value and system of pointers p[]. Now, we will consider the parameters individually. So, looking at the diagrams below, we follow the explanation.

In Fig. 1, we have defined our search space. In this specific figure, we have defined our space in three dimensions, and presently to understand N dimensions, we visualize things in three dimensions. Realize that by dimension we mean constraint and this terminology will be followed throughout the entire paper. Hence, N-dimensional space represents N different constraints. The big cuboid represents the entire search space, and the search cannot go beyond the boundaries of this cuboid. When we encounter any of the terminal surfaces, we terminate and the algorithm calls for recursive backtracking. The condition for termination is: (if *surface( ) == leaf surface*) OR (*present state == goal state*). The smaller cuboids denote states each having their own set of properties. What we do essentially is match those properties with that of the goal state. If those set of properties match at some particular time, we say that solution is available at that time. We have said that each cell has various parameters. One of these parameters is called checkbox which is like a flag denoting whether or not some search engine has visited this cell earlier or not. This is necessary since we don't appreciate loops and want the search to finish in finite time if possible. Cells

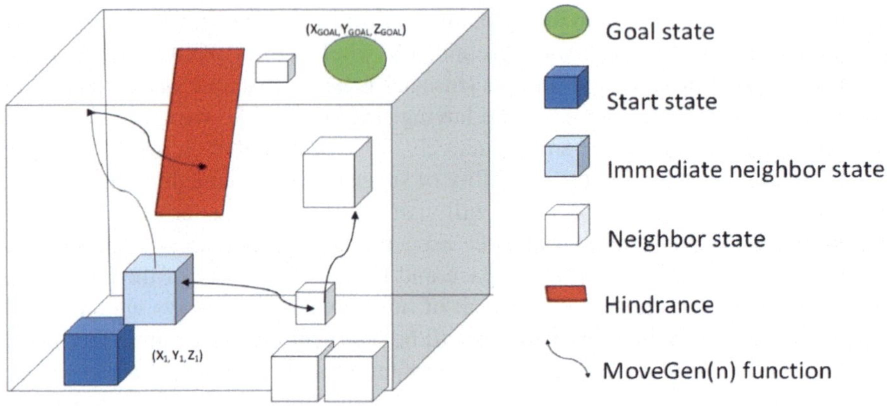

Fig. 1 N-dimensional constrained solution space

not visited are by default have their checkbox set to −1 by the algorithm. Even if some cells are having some different values, the algorithm by itself changes their state of checkbox, something which we will discuss in detail in the dynamic manipulation section. Cells which are visited are set to zero, and the goal is set to some value ∞. This ∞ represents that in the worst case, we may not be able to find the goal node. It seems that this algorithm assumes that there is no path to the solution node before actually beginning the search process. The arrows represent *movegen( )* [14] function. The decision taking will be based on probabilistic approach. After the *movegen(current node)* has generated neighboring nodes, we will apply *test( )* function to go to the next node. The green oval represents to the goal state. The red plane represents hindrances, and there is system of pointers which we will connect to all cells once we realize that visiting such cells is impossible from our current state. For this, we give to them a value μ, where μ represents some tabu parameter. Notice, the index for Fig. 2 is same as Fig. 1.

We shift our attention to Fig. 2: In Fig. 2, firstly we have shown that we visit cells in a one-to-many bi-directional approach. To extend this idea, we have shown that bi-directional means that the search algorithm has backtracking abilities, so that search can proceed in both ways. Finally, we have shown that the entire search space is dynamic and cells shift their positions in space and time. The hindrance planes also shift their positions which mean that constraints change with time.

4 Methodology

At first, we have a system of network in a network web as shown below. Each of the nodes in that web network has guide value ∂ attached to them. This ∂ represents the maximum number of times a search engine can be applied to a node before it is modified. They are in some sense heuristic values which guides the search. Three

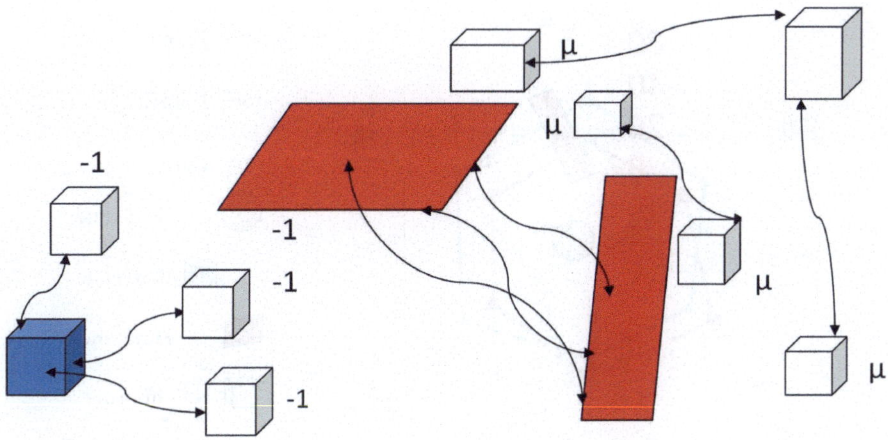

Fig. 2 Dynamicity and flagging concept in the algorithm

possible paths along the direction of search are shown in the diagram below. Such paths as we have said are generated in r-dimensional space and in each step we move closer to the goal. The goal in the diagram is the center, and the idea is to show that we need to overcome all the local optima. While we do this, we do somewhat similar to the variable neighborhood descent [15] algorithm. We use a system of equations to reach somewhat closer to the solution. Then, we change the system and again and use this new system to come further closer to the solution. We may need to use the earlier system (old insect called by the new insect) as and when the algorithm judges so. We need to recursion at several sub-stages of the journey. So we need to maintain the system of pointers accurately so that we can reconstruct the path easily once we reach the global optima. Now we have been talking of finding the optima for some time. How does the Anthrophilia* algorithm fade out all local optima and reach out to global optima? This is done by using some system of values whose absolute magnitude change with time. If going along any sub-tree of a root node (node with respect to which we are currently optimizing), we find stronger trails and greater probability of succeeding (we will take this up in details), the earlier system of values are updated having greater value systems. We do the inverse, while we find lesser chances of succeeding. Randomized methods are used here, and each time the search engine looks up for stronger value system marked cells (Fig. 3).

4.1 Stages and Dynamics

There are several principal sections but firstly we focus using the probabilistic method (In the subsequent sections we shall focus on statistical method):

If $(p_i > k_i)$: make move else don't make move. $P_i \equiv$ probability factor $(0 \leq p \leq 1) k_i$ $\equiv$ dynamic randomized factor k is a random number whose value is generated by

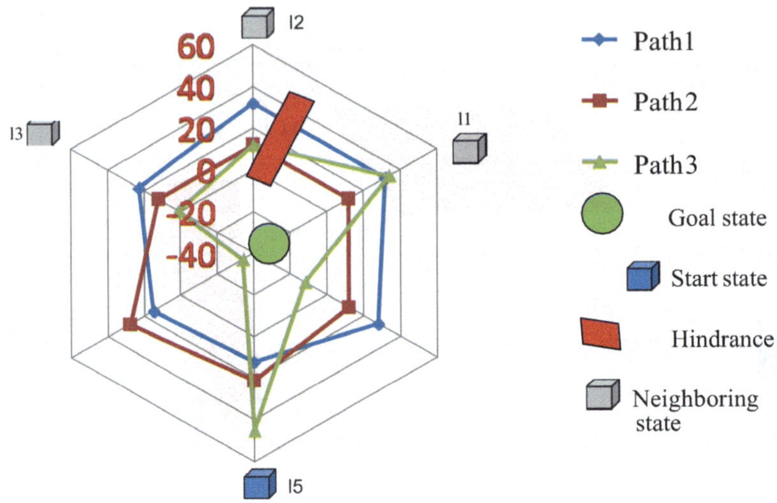

Fig. 3 Recursive steps to eliminate local optima

the system dynamically with change in situation. k acts like a threshold parameter. Notice that, $0 \leq k \leq 1$ (Fig. 4).

Randomized methods used are based on the fact that insects (search engines) in general when not having any trail (sense of direction) can choose any direction of their choice. However, when they have a sense of direction, then they have a greater chance of following the trail than ignoring the trail. This "k" is of course different for different insects. In the analogical sense, this means that employing different search engines accounts for having different extent of randomization. This is essential since in different constrained situations, insects (engines) should have different tendency of randomization. This is particularly useful since we need to have varying space and time complexities at different stages of the particular partial solution.

$$P(\text{AT ANY STEP}) = \text{MAXTERM IN SERIES}\left(\left(\sum_{k=0}^{n} \alpha[t_{ij}]^{\alpha}[\acute{\eta}_{ij}]^{\beta}[\omega_{ij}]^{\gamma}\right)\right) \tag{1}$$

Fig. 4 Generating and using randomized methods for exploration

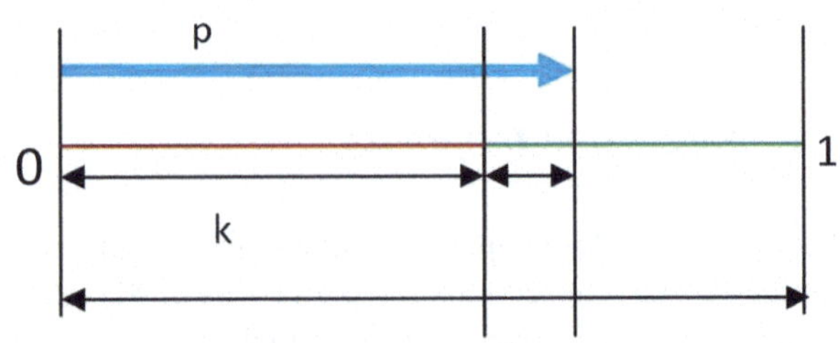

α, β, γ constants generated by algorithm
t_{ij} amount of pheromone
$\acute{\eta}_{ij}$ visibility
ω_{ij} recursive factor
P tendency of moving.

Tendency of making the move is given by P. α, β, γ are constants generated by the algorithm. Σ has only to do with expanding (1) in a series. Practically, we have nothing to do with the sum in (1). t_{ij} is the amount of pheromone on the ijth edge. $\acute{\eta}_{ij}$ is called the visibility factor, and it depends inversely on the cost of that edge. ω_{ij} is called the recursive factor, and its value depends on a parameter called heuristic factor. The update in the heuristic factor is again based on the probabilistic approach. We can see that tendency of making the move is directly proportional to all the earlier parameters.

$$\sum t_{ij}(t+n) = \sum \prod_{r=1}^{r=n} (1 - \lambda_{ij}, \ldots, r) t_{ij}(t) + \sum \delta t_{ij}(t+n) \tag{2}$$

λ_{ij} evaporation rate between vertices i and j.

The above formula is called the randomization formula. This is used to make the system dynamic and update the checkbox system. Σ here again is used to shorten the series. We are not interested in figuring total time. We only want to figure evaporation in pheromone. From Eq. (2), we compare corresponding terms on both sides of the equation. Term at ith position in L.H.S is equated to ith position in R.H.S. We have said about this parameter (flagging aspect) in the graph of cells shown earlier. The pheromone along each dimension needs to be updated with time, and the evaporation factor λ is used as a fraction which represents fraction of pheromone (heuristic value) disappearing each cycle of search. Here, we will actually realize that there is no single heuristic value in a particular cell. Each cell maintains a single dimension array which stores heuristic values over a range of dimensions. Hence, the algorithm says, if we are in the kth dimension and the search engine prefers to send r insects (r search trees in r dimensions; 1 in each), we have in the kth cell of that dimension a array of size r, indices labeled 0, 1, 2, 3, …, $(r-1)$. Each index of this array stores value (heuristic parameter) to go from any one dimension to "r" possible dimensions. So we have a system of $\lambda_1, \lambda_2, \lambda_3, \lambda_4, \lambda_5, \ldots, \lambda_r$. Here notice that, these heuristic values will now help in creating evolutionary systems. Now, here comes the concept of recursive genetics. What we mean here that till now we had $h_1(n), h_2(n), h_3(n), \ldots, h_r(n)$ for all r dimensions. Where n is the current representation of node. These r heuristic values will be genetically crossover and mutated after some constant steps say χ. After χ steps, we will have fitter cells than that we had earlier. In this entirely evolved search, we shall again look for the fittest insect ($h(n)$ with highest probability) to start off with. Then again insects (search functions) will be modified and we will again repeat. The entire system is put under a loop with the condition of termination described earlier. So principally, what we are doing is searching dynamically in r dimensions (recursively in r sub-trees with each having a root which is chosen by the algorithm based on test( ) function), backtracking to find local optima, and repeating this for χ steps as described earlier. Then, we modify the entire search space to fit in new conditions, again repeat for χ steps and this goes on indefinitely, till we reach some conclusion. Note that, here we are doing somewhat similar to VND algorithm but that neither accounted for r-dimensional space nor backtracking. Hence essentially, we have figured out all local optima. We will have a storage system for all such paths, and from there, we shall find out the global path. Realize here that the algorithm hence has the capacity to find global optima as a function of time as well because of the system of χ steps described earlier. So we have described the complete algorithm in the earlier lines. We will again come back here in the section of implementation as data structure section. However presently, I will again go back to the point of how decisions are made in N-dimensional space recursively. For that, however, I need implementation systems, but we will look at the equations first, the principal one given below.

$$P = \prod_{h=1}^{h=n} \frac{\left[t_{ij}\right]^{\propto}\left[\eta_{ij}\right]^{\beta}}{\left[t_{ih}\right]^{\propto}\left[\eta_{ih}\right]^{\beta}} \tag{3}$$

where h is the total no. of states. Other symbols carry their usual meaning as discussed earlier.

This equation is called probability equation. This equation is used as a decision-making parameter of whether or not we shall move from one cell to a different cell. If P is maximum for a pair of cells say cell i and cell j, we shall go from i to j and update the system of checkboxes. Now, we need to calculate the probability of moving from rth dimension to the kth dimension. For this, we take up each of rth dimension, and we use this system of probability [16] as the heuristic function. Notice that it is not necessary we go from r_i dimension to r_j dimension directly. If we need to halt at a system r_k where k is $\{i+1, i+2, \ldots, j-2, j-1\}$, it is perfectly fine.

Recall here that we said k can take integer values only. So for each such r_i, r_k pair we have a system of p_i, p_k. So we have a system of multiplications denoted as $p(1).p(2).p(3) \ldots p(r)$. To satisfy completeness and theory of total probability, we have the following equation to be valid.

$$-\oint_{h=n}^{h=1} P(h)n(h)\mathrm{d}h = 1 \tag{4}$$

Negative sign has a special significance in (4). We start initially optimizing N boundaries and then reduce to 1 where we stop. Recall, however, that:

$$\int_a^b f(x)\mathrm{d}x = -\int_b^a f(x)\mathrm{d}x \tag{5}$$

To calculate the probability, we have just divided the present tendency with the total no. of allowed choices represented by the state h. By allowed choice what we mean is that we don't appreciate loops and the states already examined are banished from h. So initially value of h is: $\lim_{\text{time}\to 0} h \to n$ and at subsequent stages of the algorithm value of h decreases. Where N denotes total no. of states. Dynamic equation of h is hence given as

$$\bigcup_{r=k}^{r=n}\{h\} = \bigcup_{r=0}^{r=n}\{h(\text{Total})\} - \bigcup_{r=0}^{r=k}\{h(\text{flagged})\} \tag{6}$$

So by now we are already familiar with what we mean by flagged and unflagged. What we mean by the earlier equation is that we need to update our search space with time. So from the total search space we need to remove those cells which we have already inspected before.

4.2 Implementation

Till now we have made it quite clear that the algorithm is recursive and multidimensional. We will in short while visit the evolutionary nature of the algorithm. We will now take up the implementations of the earlier equations by means of data structures. But before that we will look at a diagram which not only will make the dynamic of the algorithm clear but also give us an insight on the time and space complexities of the algorithm.

Look carefully at the figure given below. What we have tried to explain is the number of states considered at a time in a system of r dimensions. This approach is called as k-ply approach, and we consider those nodes which are inside this k-ply tree. The value of this k is also judged by this algorithm. We have k which is a measure of P.

All states are in different dimensions. And the edges in the graph represent the movegen(n) function. The red state represents that all paths which are through red state can never be included in solution set of local optima described earlier. Variable μ is like a Tabu parameter and this is what keeps the search engine updated with the recent changes coming as a function of time. Next, we move on to the space and time complexities [17] of the algorithm. We use a system of k-ply to decrease the space and time complexity of the algorithm.

The curved line connecting the red state with that of other states represents that the red state forces other states connected to it to be red as well. By this, we mean that heuristic values [18] can change very rapidly with time so as to force the algorithm to work backward and find a new path (Fig. 5).

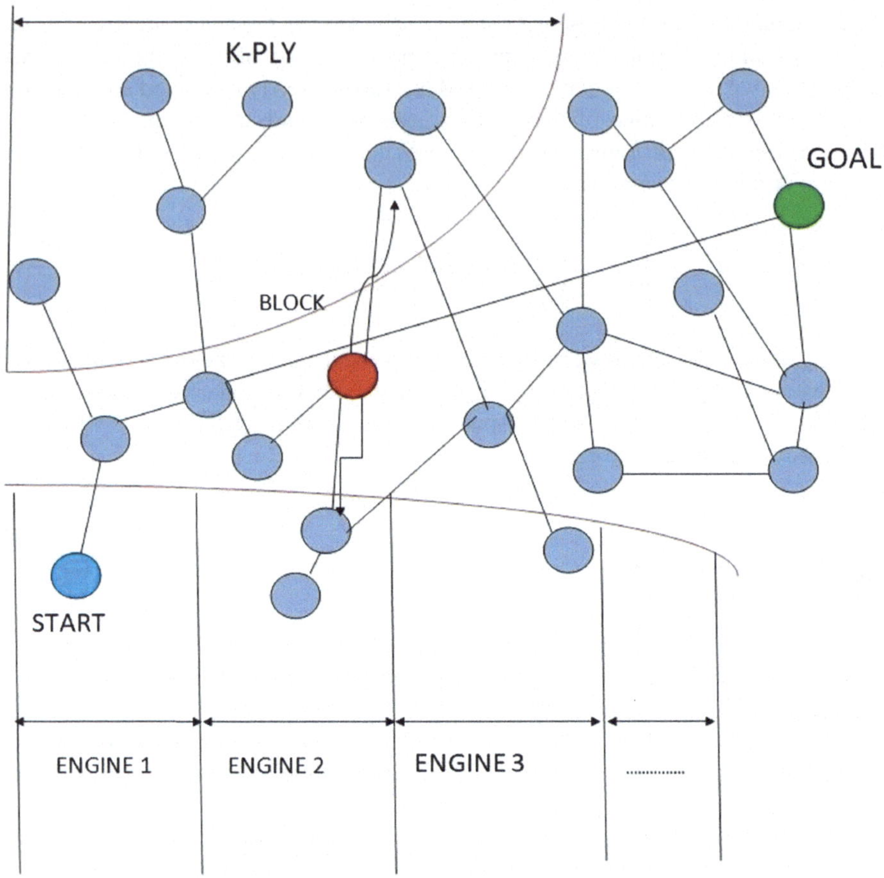

Fig. 5 Reducing the complexities using variable heuristics by different engines

5 Evolutionary Nature (Threaded Data Structures)

Each small cell represents a different search engine (insect) in a different dimension (forest). The entire cycle happens after every χ times search. The bars are linked lists and not arrays. The system of pointers is used to reconstruct the path. The system is someting like "linlist of linklist of linklist…". We can think it as tree of link list [19] since the system of pointers never forms a loop. Calling a node from a linklist twice or more than twice is an obvious possibility and that represents the recursive nature of the algorithm. Recall again that we are talking about N-dimensional space so calling a node more than once represents calling the same insect (function) in a different forest (new dynamic search space). This is why what we are doing is recursion and not iteration. This is the reason the search proceeds in a tree [20] and never has any cycle if we take properties of N dimensions into account (Fig. 6).

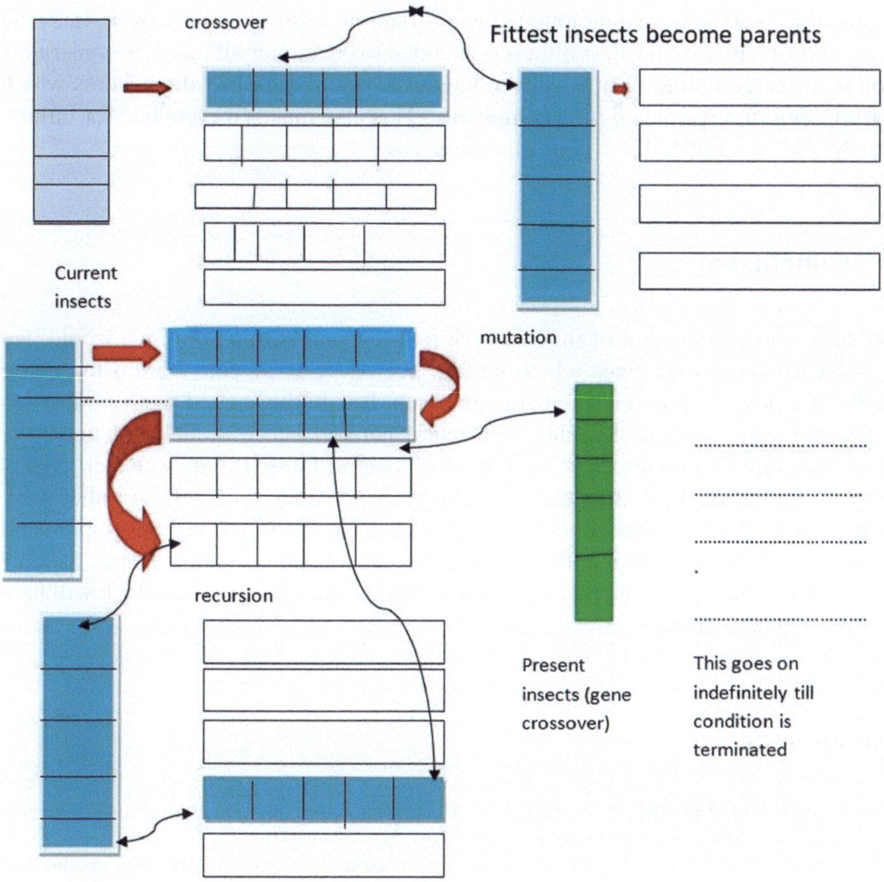

Fig. 6 Use of threaded N-ary trees for evolution (genetic steps)

6 Completeness

In this final section, we shall prove (rather demand) that the algorithm is indeed complete and for this we argue as follows. Consider that there are "*a*" number of local optima. Because the algorithm is genetic, one of the new insect "genetically evolved" [21] will indeed crossout all the local optima and reach out to global optima because pheromone to all local optima will fade with the λ factor for all paths, where λ is called as evaporation factor. Next, we had the trouble of unidimensionality. Since for each dimension we have a probability factor *P*, best *r* out of *k* dimensions will always be chosen one of which will coincide with the global optima at some point of time. Next, we needed dynamicity for which we have this χ factor which updates the search engine (genetically evolves the insect) according to the scenario every χ cycles. This ensures the new insect has those genes of the parents which is still required as well as has some mutated genes (sub-algorithms) which overcomes the present problem. So, the algorithm is demanded to encounter all possible constraints and is hence complete [22]. It is even having *K*-ply in each of r dimensions which ensure optimum space and time complexity. This also makes it complete for infinite graphs. So, in a nutshell the algorithm deserves *.

7 Conclusion

We have come to the end of this research journey, and at this point, we would like to refer to those milestones which we did not cover as of yet. We did the entire technique assuming the probabilistic approach. It is highly hoped that training this algorithm with machine learning and neural networks to a model will make the algorithm function better. Next, coding of this algorithm will require expert coders since formulae are difficult in codes. Coding is hence under progress. Another work needed is to think of how input and output shall be fed to the system. Inputs and outputs are N-dimensional and constraints are exponential in some sense. So how shall our machinery handle this. It is also needed to think of systems which will help to give dynamic outputs.

References

1. Krumke, S.O., Marathe, M.V., Ravi, S.S.: Models and approximation algorithms for channel assignment in radio networks. Wirel. Netw. **7**(6), 575–584 (2001)
2. Schmid, H.: Probabilistic part-of-speech tagging using decision trees. In: New methods in language processing, p. 154 (2013)
3. Mannila, H., Toivonen, H., Verkamo, A.I.: E cient algorithms for discovering association rules. In: KDD-94: AAAI workshop on Knowledge Discovery in Databases (pp. 181–192) ((1994, July).)
4. Barbarosoglu, G., Ozgur, D.: A tabu search algorithm for the vehicle routing problem. Comput. Oper. Res. **26**(3), 255–270 (1999)
5. Corana, A., Marchesi, M., Martini, C., Ridella, S.: Minimizing multimodal functions of continuous variables with the "simulated annealing" algorithm Corrigenda for this article is available here. ACM Transactions on Mathematical Software (TOMS) **13**(3), 262–280 (1987)
6. Jones, G., Willett, P., Glen, R.C., Leach, A.R., Taylor, R.: Development and validation of a genetic algorithm for flexible docking. J. Mol. Biol. **267**(3), 727–748 (1997)
7. Walker, M.A., Prince, E.F.: a Centering Algorithm. Reference and referent accessibility **38**, 291 (1996)
8. Delimata, P., Suraj, Z.: Feature selection algorithm for multiple classifier systems: a hybrid approach. Fundamenta Informaticae **85**(1–4), 97–110 (2008)
9. Ye, X., Lin, A., Han, S.P.: Searching for Shortest Path in A Large. A Successive Mixed Bidirectional Search Method, Sparse Graph under Memory Limitation (2007)
10. Merkle, D., Middendorf, M.: Ant colony optimization with global pheromone evaluation for scheduling a single machine. Applied Intelligence **18**(1), 105–111 (2003)
11. Stutzle, T., Dorigo, M.: A short convergence proof for a class of ant colony optimization algorithms. IEEE Trans. Evol. Comput. **6**(4), 358–365 (2002)

12. Blum, C., & Li, X. (2008). Swarm intelligence in optimization. In *Swarm Intelligence* (pp. 43–85). Springer, Berlin, Heidelberg
13. . Gilmour, A. R., Thompson, R., & Cullis, B. R. (1995). Average information REML: an efficient algorithm for variance parameter estimation in linear mixed models. *Biometrics*, 1440– 1450
14. Oren, N., & Norman, T. J. (2009, May). Arguing using opponent models. In *International Workshop on Argumentation in Multi-Agent Systems* (pp. 160–174). Springer, Berlin, Heidelberg
15. Hansen, P., Mladenović, N., Pérez, J.A.M.: Variable neighbourhood search: methods and applications. Ann. Oper. Res. **175**(1), 367–407 (2010)
16. Yates, R. D., & Goodman, D. J. (2014). *Probability and stochastic processes: a friendly introduction for electrical and computer engineers*. John Wiley & Sons
17. Damen, O., Chkeif, A., Belfiore, J.C.: Lattice code decoder for space-time codes. IEEE Commun. Lett. **4**(5), 161–163 (2000)
18. Hart, P.E., Nilsson, N.J., Raphael, B.: A formal basis for the heuristic determination of minimum cost paths. IEEE transactions on Systems Science and Cybernetics **4**(2), 100–107 (1968)
19. Dolev, D., Mokryn, O., Shavitt, Y.: On multicast trees: structure and size estimation. IEEE/ACM Transactions on Networking (TON) **14**(3), 557–567 (2006)
20. Bentley, J.L.: Multidimensional binary search trees used for associative searching. Commun. ACM **18**(9), 509–517 (1975)
21. Deb, K., Pratap, A., Agarwal, S., Meyarivan, T.A.M.T.: A fast and elitist multiobjective genetic algorithm: NSGA-II. IEEE Trans. Evol. Comput. **6**(2), 182–197 (2002)
22. Wu, Y., Fahmy, S., Shroff, N. B.: On the construction of a maximum-lifetime data gathering tree in sensor networks: NP-completeness and approximation algorithm. In: INFOCOM 2008. The 27th conference on computer communications. IEEE (pp. 356–360)(2008)

Stochastic Modeling of Earthquake Interevent Counts (Natural Times) in Northwest Himalaya and Adjoining Regions

Sumanta Pasari

Abstract In the driven nonlinear complex dynamical earthquake system in which the event occurrences are distributed along a frequency-magnitude spectrum, "natural time" statistics can be utilized to evaluate the contemporary state of earthquake hazards in a region. The natural times, in contrary to the clock/calendar times, are nothing but the interspersed number of small magnitude counts between successive large earthquake events in a fixed area. Natural times are positive and often random in nature. In this paper, our aim is to investigate the best-fit probability distribution in order to develop natural time statistics in the seismogenic northwest Himalayan orogen including some part of north-central India, east-northeast Pakistan and its contiguous regions. We consider eight continuous probability distributions to fit the observed natural time data. We use maximum likelihood strategy for model parameter estimation and several goodness-of-fit measures for model prioritization. Results based on the natural times corresponding to $M \geq 3$ events between $M \geq 6$ events reveal that the exponential, exponentiated exponential, Weibull and exponentiated Weibull distributions provide the best fit to the observed natural times in the study area. In addition, assuming that the seismicity statistics of larger northwest Himalaya region is indifferent from the "local" regions (e.g., cities) embedded in the larger area, we calculate "nowcast" values for a number of cities, namely Jammu, Ludhiana, Chandigarh, Shimla, Dehradun and New Delhi, to assess the current state of earthquake hazards in these cities. It is found that their earthquake potential scores (%) are 99, 89, 86, 87, 83 and 58, respectively. From these results, we argue that the concept of natural times and thereby nowcasting technique provide a rapid, alternative and effective way to analyze earthquake hazards in a seismic region.

Keywords Natural times · Northwest Himalaya · Earthquake hazards

S. Pasari (✉)
Department of Mathematics, Birla Institute of Technology and Science, Pilani Campus, Pilani, Rajasthan 333031, India
e-mail: sumanta.pasari@pilani.bits-pilani.ac.in

S. Bhattacharyya et al. (eds.), *Mathematical Modeling and Computational Tools*, Springer Proceedings in Mathematics & Statistics 320,
https://doi.org/10.1007/978-981-15-3615-1_35

1 Introduction

Statistical seismology has become an increasingly important tool for estimating seismic hazards and associated earthquake risks in seismic-prone areas [1]. With physical reasoning such as crustal velocity field distribution, geodetic slip rate estimation, strain partitioning and geophysical imaging in a tectonically active region, the stochastic models aim to reduce the misalignment between statistics-based and physics-based models [1–3]. Thus far, the common statistical approach in earthquake hazard assessment has focused on estimating earthquake interoccurrence time and conditional probability of large earthquakes based on some limited historical and instrumental catalog [1–11]. These earthquake data (main shocks), after removal of seismic swarms, foreshocks or aftershocks, are then fitted to some potential probability distributions for future seismicity projection [2]. An important assumption in this empirical approach is that the data points of interevent times (between subsequent earthquakes) in a selected region must constitute a random sample [1–11]. In other words, the seismic interoccurrence times are assumed to be independent and identically distributed. When such assumption applies, we not only discard the possible interaction among earthquakes, but also neglect the developing problem of co-seismic physical changes of fault dynamics and fault patterns on complex fault zones. In addition, the contribution from dependent events, such as destruction due to large aftershocks or partial release of accumulated stress, is not accounted in these studies. As a result, such a program of empirical interevent time analysis although provides an estimation of future earthquake hazards, the current state of earthquake hazard due to events of all magnitudes (small, moderate, to great earthquakes) in a large tectonic area remains elusive [11–16]. To address this existing gap, in this paper, we carry out stochastic modeling of earthquake interevent counts (natural times) in the densely populated northwest Himalaya and its adjacent regions including some part of north-central India, east-northeast Pakistan and adjoining regions. Our goal is to formulate the entire problem statistically and investigate the potential probability model to develop natural time statistics for the present-day risk assessment of the study area. At the end of experimental design, we also perform some sensitivity analysis to the threshold values of small earthquake magnitude and city radius to determine their effect on the best-fit models and associated nowcast values.

2 Formulation of Natural Time Statistics

Concept of natural time ("NT") is based on the idea of using interevent counts of "small" earthquakes (say, $3 \leq M < 6$) between "large" earthquakes (say, $M \geq 6$) [12–14]. Varotsos et al. [17] first introduced this term followed by many (e.g., [11–18]) in their respective analyses of earthquakes. The concept of NT has numerous benefits in seismology in comparison with the perception of traditional interevent times that are based on clock/calendar time. First, the statistics of NT does not depend on the background seismicity level (a) in a selected region, as long as the b-value in the classical Gutenberg–Richter frequency-magnitude relation turns out to be a constant [14]. As a consequence, the natural time statistics is valid throughout smaller and larger geographical areas of interest as long as there are sufficient (~20 or more) number of large earthquake cycles in the region to develop a statistical model [12–16]. Another key advantage of using NT statistics over usual interevent times is that neither declustering of seismic catalog nor homogeneity in event magnitude is mandatory [14].

The NT, by construction, is discrete in nature. It considers nonnegative random values [17, 18]. However, if modeled properly, the NT statistics can provide significant information of the present status of a fault system through the elapsed number of small event counts at time t (calendar time) after the last significant earthquake in the region. The modeling of NT is grounded on two important assumptions. First, it formulates NT statistics from a wider geographical area and then utilizes the identical statistics to smaller spatial regions of interest, such as city or towns [11–18]. The physics-based ergodicity property in earthquakes lays the foundation of such hypothesis [12–18]. Second, the random variable of NT, say X, is considered to be a continuous random variate [11, 12]. This assumption is driven by the reality that small seismic events in a wider active region seem to occur continuously [11–14]. To identify the underlying "theoretical" distribution, we fit eight probability models, namely exponential, exponentiated exponential, gamma, lognormal, Weibull, inverse Weibull (Frechet), exponentiated Weibull and inverse Gaussian (Brownian Passage Time) distributions [11, 12].

3 Study Area and Earthquake Data

The study region, defined in 26° N to 36° N latitude and 72° E to 84° E longitude (Fig. 1), marks one of the most active orogenic regions in the southeast Asia as an effect of the ongoing tectonic collision between Indian plate and Eurasian plate at an average rate of about 40 mm/year [8, 19]. The crustal deformation in these areas is associated with several active thrust fault systems, such as Karakorum fault zone, the Main Central Thrust (MCT) zone, Main Boundary Thrust (MBT) and Himalayan Frontal Thrust (HFT), along with the structures of different geological ages [8]. The region comprises Himalayan foothills and fertile alluvial plains including a number of developing cities (e.g., Lahore, Amritsar, Jammu-Srinagar, Patiala, Ludhiana, Chandigarh, Dehradun, New Delhi, Agra, Lucknow and Jaipur). The present seismic catalog of $M \geq 3$ events is adopted from the Advanced National Seismic System (ANSS) composite catalog (1963–2012) and the International Seismological Centre (ISC) catalog (2013–2018). We rely only on the instrumental catalog and consider focal depths up to 200 km [11–16]. Between March 6, 1963, and November 14, 2018, we found 3251 small events in the study region, among which there are 27 large earthquakes. As there are two large events on January 19, 1975, without experiencing any small earthquakes between them, we obtain 25 natural times for modeling.

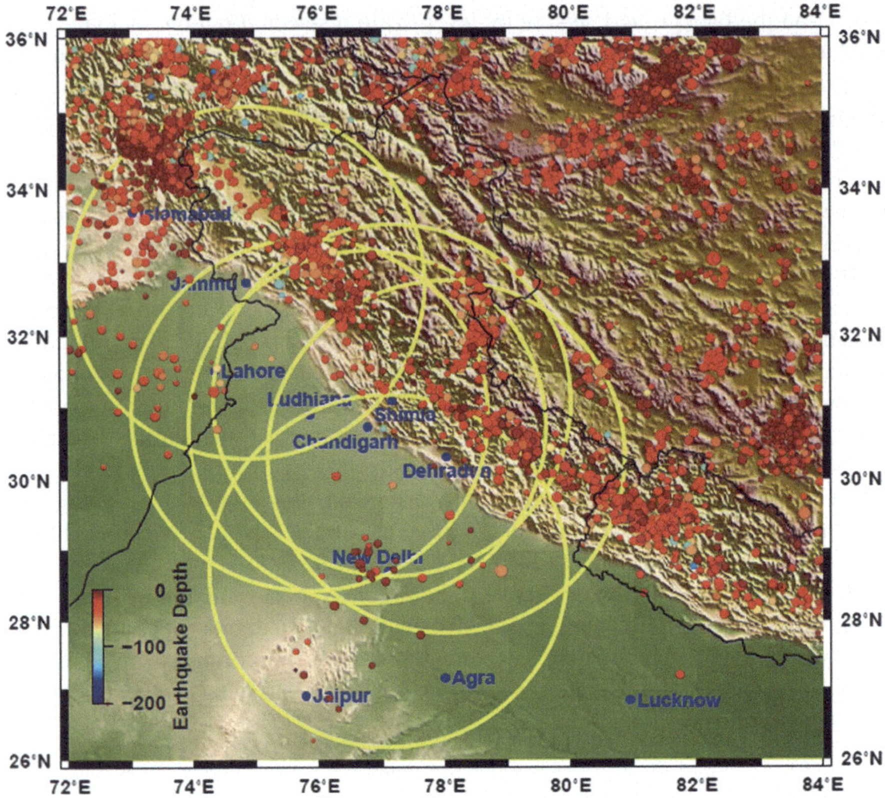

Fig. 1 Seismicity in the study area of northwest Himalaya; selected circular city regions are highlighted in yellow

4 Methodology, Results and Conclusions

Prior to the development of the NT statistics based on the observed data, we compute some descriptive statistical measures. The observed NT data values lie between 2 and 695 having sample mean 120.2, standard deviation 144.3, mode 64, median 83 and skewness 2.84. The dataset is highly asymmetric with a long tail to the right of the peak. We fit eight continuous probability distributions to these observations. The MLE estimated model parameters and the goodness of fit measures from the AIC and K-S tests are presented in Table 1.

Table 1 suggests that the exponential, Weibull and the exponentiated models provide the best representation. In particular, the exponential model offers the most economical fit (lowest AIC value), whereas the exponentiated Weibull model provides the best representation in terms of the least separation to the empirical distribution function (EDF) of the observed data [20].

Table 1 Estimated parameter values and model prioritization

Distribution	Parameter estimation		Model priority	
			AIC	K-S
Exponential	$\hat{\alpha}$	120.20	291.46	0.116
Gamma	$\hat{\alpha}$	158.82	293.61	0.115
	$\hat{\beta}$	0.76		
Lognormal	$\hat{\alpha}$	4.13	295.90	0.153
	$\hat{\beta}$	1.34		
Weibull	$\hat{\alpha}$	114.96	293.09	0.102
	$\hat{\beta}$	0.91		
Inverse Gaussian	$\hat{\alpha}$	120.20	304.75	0.301
	$\hat{\beta}$	24.37		
Inverse Weibull	$\hat{\alpha}$	30.35	304.81	0.205
	$\hat{\beta}$	0.66		
Exponentiated exponential	$\hat{\alpha}$	129.99	293.25	0.111
	$\hat{\beta}$	0.89		
Exponentiated Weibull	$\hat{\alpha}$	75.02	293.94	0.093
	$\hat{\beta}$	0.77		
	$\hat{\gamma}$	1.56		

Developing the NT statistics, we now compute nowcast values (Table 2) to appraise how far a particular city has progressed to its next large earthquake. The nowcast value for a circular (say, a radius of 300 km) city region is expressed in terms of its earthquake potential score (EPS) calculated from cumulative probability $P\{X \leq n(t)\}$; $n(t)$ is the present number of small ($3 \leq M < 6$) events in the region [14–16]. From the nowcast scores (as on November 14, 2018) in Table 2, we intuitively infer that New Delhi is somewhere in the middle of its earthquake cycle, whereas Jammu has crossed about 99% of the way through its cycle. Large earthquake in Jammu region thus is overdue. The nowcast values for the other cities are

Table 2 Nowcast scores of selected cities

City	City center		EPS (%)	Current count
	Lat	Long		
Jammu	32.727	74.857	99	941
Ludhiana	30.901	75.857	89	271
Chandigarh	30.733	76.779	86	238
Shimla	31.105	77.173	87	248
Dehradun	30.317	78.032	83	217
New Delhi	28.704	77.103	58	99

also significantly high. Now, in order to determine the effect of the small magnitude threshold and the circular city radius on the nowcast scores, we vary the magnitude threshold of small events from 3.0 to 4.0 and circular city radius from 300 to 350 km. The sensitivity results (available on request), as on November 14, 2018, reveals a consistent ranking of EPS scores.

The nowcast values as a proxy to the physical modeling serve a number of practical purposes, such as the relative ranking of cities as to their current hazard level, revising insurance premiums and safety consideration for engineering planning. It is believed that the nowcasting approach that determines the current state of a regional fault system may significantly contribute to improve the earthquake forecasting for future seismicity analysis [11–16].

In summary, the present study has successfully formulated the problem of stochastic earthquake interevent count (natural times) modeling in the northwest Himalaya. The nowcast scores obtained through the best-fit probability model provide a fast, alternative and effective way to assess earthquake hazards in a seismic region.

References

1. Vere-Jones, D., Ben-Zion, Y., Zuniga, R.: Statistical seismology. Pure Appl. Geophys. **162**, 1023–1026 (2005)
2. Utsu, T.: Estimation of parameters for recurrence models of earthquakes. Bull. Earthq. Res. Inst., Univ. Tokyo **59**, 53–66 (1984)
3. Pasari, S., Dikshit, O.: Impact of three-parameter Weibull models in probabilistic assessment of earthquake hazards. Pure appl. Geophys. **171**(7), 1251–1281 (2014)
4. Pasari, S., Dikshit, O.: Three-parameter generalized exponential distribution in earthquake recurrence interval estimation. Nat. Hazards **73**, 639–656 (2014)
5. Pasari, S., Dikshit, O.: Distribution of earthquake interevent times in northeast India and adjoining regions. Pure appl. Geophys. **172**(10), 2533–2544 (2015)
6. Pasari, S., Dikshit, O.: Earthquake interevent time distribution in Kachchh, northwestern India. Earth, Planets Space **67**, 129 (2015)
7. Pasari, S., Dikshit, O.: Stochastic earthquake interevent time modelling from exponentiated Weibull distributions. Nat. Hazards **90**(2), 823–842 (2018)
8. Pasari, S.: Understanding Himalayan tectonics from geodetic and stochastic modeling. Ph.D. Thesis, Indian Institute of Technology Kanpur, India, pp. 1–376 (2015)
9. Pasari, S.: Stochastic modeling of earthquake interoccurrence times in northwest Himalaya and adjoining regions. Geomat., Nat. Hazards Risk **9**(1), 568–588 (2018)
10. Pasari, S.: Inverse Gaussian versus lognormal distribution in earthquake forecasting: keys and clues. J. Seism. **23**(3), 537–559 (2019)
11. Bhatia, A., Pasari, S., Mehta, A.: Earthquake forecasting using artificial neural networks. ISPRS-Int. Arch. Photogramm. Remote Sens. Appl. **42**(5), 823–827 (2018)
12. Pasari, S.: Nowcasting earthquakes in the Bay of Bengal region. Pure Appl. Geophys. **176**(4), 1417–1432 (2019)
13. Pasari, S., Mehta, A.: Nowcasting earthquakes in the northwest Himalaya and surrounding regions. ISPRS-Int. Arch. Photogramm, Remote Sens. Appl. **42**(5), 855–859 (2018)
14. Rundle, J.B., Turcotte, D.L., Donnellan, A., Grant-Ludwig, L., Luginbuhl, M., Gong, G.: Nowcasting earthquakes. Earth Space Sci. **3**, 480–486 (2016)
15. Holliday, J.R., Rundle, J.B., Turcotte, D.L., Klein, W., Tiampo, K.F., Donnellan, A.: Using earthquake intensities to forecast earthquake occurrence times. Phys. Rev. Lett. **97**, 238501 (2006)

16. Luginbuhl, M., Rundle, J.B., Hawkins, A., Turcotte, D.L.: Nowcasting earthquakes: a comparison of induced earthquakes in Oklahoma and at the Geysers, California. Pure Appl. Geophys. **175**(1), 49–65 (2018)
17. Varostos, P.A., Sarlis, N.V., Tanaka, H.K., Skordas, E.S.: Some properties of the entropy in natural time. Phys. Rev. E **71**, 032102 (2005)
18. Varostos, P.A., Sarlis, N.V., Skordas, E.S.: Natural Time Analysis: The New View of Time. Springer, Berlin (2011)
19. Sharma, Y., Pasari, S., Dikshit, O., Ching, K.E.: GPS-based monitoring of crustal deformation in Garhwal-Kumaun Himalaya. ISPRS-Int. Arch. Photogramm. Remote Sens. Appl. **42**(5), 451–454 (2018)
20. Johnson, N.L., Kotz, S., Balakrishnan, N.: Continuous Univariate Distributions (pp. 1–761). Wiley-Interscience, New York (1995)

Analysis of Three Major Airline Networks of India: A Complex Network Approach

Dimpee Baruah and A. Bharali

Abstract Air transportation network is one of the most important transport networks in recent time. In the air transportation network, the study of robustness of airlines network plays a key role. Robustness is the ability of a network to continue to perform properly when it is subject to failures or attacks. We adopt a complex network approach to analyze the robustness of three major airlines of India viz. Indigo, Air India, Jet Airways by simulating random attack and targeted attack on the separate airlines networks. Random attack is based on the removal of random airports from the network and targeted attack is based on the removal of important airports based on the node attributes like degree, betweenness.

Keywords Complex network · Network measures · Robustness · Airport network of India (ANI) · Airline networks

1 Introduction

Air transportation network is one of the most important transport networks in recent time. Nowadays, air transportation network is one of the essential elements of our present societies for their high level of mobility. Various countries such as USA [1], China [2], Italy [3], India [4], Australia [5], Brazil [6] air transportation network have been studied to analyze the infrastructure, connectivity, flow of traffic, etc. Due to the increasing dependency on this network, the study of the robustness of the network also plays an important role. Robustness is the ability of a network to continue to perform properly when it is subjected to failures or attacks [7]. Robustness is one of the most anticipated properties of any transportation network. The study of the robustness of a network subjected to different nodes or edge failures can evaluate the

D. Baruah (✉) · A. Bharali
Department of Mathematics, Dibrugarh University, Dibrugarh, Assam 786004, India
e-mail: dimpeebaruah2005@gmail.com

A. Bharali
e-mail: a.bharali@dibru.ac.in

S. Bhattacharyya et al. (eds.), *Mathematical Modeling and Computational Tools*,
Springer Proceedings in Mathematics & Statistics 320,
https://doi.org/10.1007/978-981-15-3615-1_36

level of vulnerability to which the network can expose through random, most central nodes, and link failures [8].

This paper adopts a complex network approach to analyse the robustness of three major airlines networks of India viz. Indigo, Air India, Jet Airways by simulating random attack and targeted attack on the separate airlines networks. Random attack is based on the removal of random airports from the network and targeted attack is based on the removal of important airports based on the node attributes like degree, betweenness, etc. Many papers have been done to analyze airline networks for both structure and robustness perspectives. In [9], Han et al. analyzed the daily network in the busiest week for four different European airlines. They found that all airline networks have scale-free and small-world properties [9]. Also, the works of Reggiani et al. [10] and Reggiani et al. [11] investigated the Lufthansa network (LH) as both the worldwide and European networks; and they found the network is scale-free in both the cases. Again, Lordan et al. [12] analyzed multiple airlines in different alliances and parts of the world. Wijdeveld [13] conducted a study on robustness analysis of 17 European airline networks for both error or random failure and targeted attacks [13].

The rest of the paper is organized as follows: next section includes some popular measures used in complex network analysis. In Sect. 3, an introduction of airport network of India and three airline networks are given and we calculate the values of different metrics of these networks. In Sect. 4, the robustness analysis of three airline networks is given. Conclusions are presented in Sect. 5.

2 Some Measures in Network Analysis

In this section, we formally present the definitions of some measures popularly used in network analysis.

Shortest Path: The shortest path of a network is the path that has the lowest number of hops between the source and destination pairs in the network.

Diameter: Diameter of a network is the longest shortest path between any pair of nodes in the network. If L_{ij} is the shortest path between nodes i and j, then

$$\text{Diameter, } d = \max_{i,j \in V} L_{ij}.$$

Average Shortest-Path Length [14]: The Average shortest-path length (L), also known as the characteristic path length, is defined as

$$L = \frac{1}{N(N-1)} \sum_{i,j=1,i\neq j}^{N} L_{ij},$$

where L_{ij} is the shortest path between the vertex i and j and N is the total number of vertices in the network. For a random network of size, N, and average degree, $< k >$, it is $\frac{\log(N)}{\log(\langle k \rangle)}$.

Network Clustering Coefficient [6]: In a network, if node A is connected to node B and node B is connected to node P, then there is a intensify probability that node A will also be connected to node P. The clustering coefficient of a network is defined as:

$$C = \frac{3 \times \text{ number of triangles in the network}}{\text{number of connected triples of vertices}},$$

where a "connected triple" means a node with edges running to an unordered pair of others. Clustering coefficient is also known as network transitivity. For a random network of size, N, and average degree, $< k >$, it is $\frac{\langle k \rangle}{N}$.

Betweenness [15]: The Betweenness of a node is the number of the shortest path going through the node. The Betweenness η_u of a node u is given by,

$$\eta_u = \sum_{s \neq u \in V} \sum_{t \neq u \in V} \frac{\sigma_{st}(u)}{\sigma_{st}},$$

where σ_{st} is the number of the shortest paths from vertex s to t and $\sigma_{st}(u)$ is the number of the shortest paths from s to t that pass through u.

Similarly, Betweenness of a link (i, j), η_{ij} is the number of shortest path going through (i, j), which is defined as

$$\eta_{ij} = \sum_{s \in V} \sum_{t \in V} \frac{\sigma_{st}(i, j)}{\sigma_{st}},$$

$\sigma_{st}(i, j)$ is the number of shortest paths from s to t that pass through (i, j).

Graph Density [6]: The graph density or network density D is defined as a ratio of the number of edges M to the number of possible edges considering the complete graph or network:

$$D = \frac{2M}{N(N-1)}$$

Reachability [16]: Reachability of a network is the probability of the connectivity between any pair of its nodes, (u, v), which is represented by R, and the reachability of node R_i is as follows:

$$R_i = \frac{\text{number of nodes reachable from node } i}{N - 1}$$

The Reachability(R) of overall network is defined as the average of all R_i, with a fully reachable network achieving 1 and an isolated network with no physical connection (links) between the nodes is always 0.

Network Criticality [17]: The network criticality is defined as

$$\tau = 2N \text{ Trace}\left(L^{+}\right),$$

where N is the number of nodes and L^{+} is the Moore–Penrose inverse [5] of Laplacian matrix L of the network. Smaller the value of τ higher is the robustness of the network.

3 Airport Network of India and Three Airlines Networks

In the airport network of India (ANI), the domestic airports are taken as nodes and two airports are connected by a link if there is at least one direct flight between them per week. The number of such flight per week between the airports (nodes) is the weight of the link in the network. The network measures of ANI are shows in Table 1 [18] where some dummy links were added to make ANI symmetric. In this paper, three major airlines of India, viz. Indigo, Jet Airways and Air India are considered for the robustness analysis of airline networks of India. All the air movement data for the networks are considered for the year 2016, obtained from Airports Authority of India (www.aai.aero).

Similarly, for the construction of airline networks, the domestic destinations (airports) of the airlines are taken as nodes and there is a link between two airports if

Table 1 Network measures of ANI

Network measures	Value
Number of nodes (airports)	79
Directed links (edges)	496
Connected components	1
Diameter	4
Average degree	6.279
Average path length	2.262
Network clustering coefficient	0.605
Network density	0.08
Network criticality	1.1334×10^{3}

Table 2 Network measures of three airline networks

Network measures	Indigo airline	Jet Airways airline	Air India airline
Number of nodes (airports)	37	46	53
Directed links (edges)	264	158	178
Connected components	1	1	1
Network diameter	3	5	5
Average degree	7.135	3.435	3.358
Average path length	1.891	2.44	2.405
Network clustering coefficient	0.738	0.531	0.486
Density	0.198	0.076	0.065
Network criticality	778.4555	2.9715×10^3	3.6996×10^3

there is at least one direct flight of that airline between them per week. The Indigo airline network consists of 37 domestic destinations (airports) and 257 directed links with 6.946 average degree and network diameter 3. The Jet Airways airline network consists of 46 domestic destinations (airports) and 158 directed links. The network has average degree 3.435 and network diameter 5. Also, the Air India airline network consists of 53 domestic destinations (airports) and 178 directed links with average degree 3.358 and network diameter 5. None of these three airline networks is symmetric. Table 2 gives the network measures of the three airline networks under consideration and Table 3 gives top 10 ranks of the nodes (airports) of the networks based on degree and betweenness.

4 Robustness of Airline Networks

Robustness analysis of the airline networks can evaluate the effect of targeted attack (e.g., terrorist attack on an airport) and random attack or failures (e.g., weather inclemency) of the networks. For the analysis, we remove five highest degree nodes (airports) from each airline networks and observe the change in some network measures for targeted attack. Table 4 shows the change of network measures of the three airline networks in percentage after the removal of a key node based on the degree where the negative sign indicates decrement and positive sign indicates the increment of the values.

We also calculate these measures after removal of the nodes sequentially, based on relatively high degree or high betweenness, i.e., in order to assess the network robustness of the airlines networks, in each time a node with high degree or betweenness is isolated (removed) and the centrality measures are calculated again for all the remaining connected nodes (airports). Then from the remaining nodes, the airport with highest centrality is selected for removal in the next step and so on. The process will continue until removal of five airports. Figure 1 shows the change of average

Table 3 Top ten airports of the networks based on degree and betweenness

Rank	ANI		Indigo network		Jet Airways network		Air India network	
	Degree	Betweenness	Degree	Betweenness	Degree	Betweenness	Degree	Betweenness
1	Delhi	Delhi	Delhi	Delhi	Mumbai	Mumbai	Delhi	Delhi
2	Mumbai	Mumbai	Mumbai	Kolkata	Delhi	Delhi	Mumbai	Mumbai
3	Kolkata	Kolkata	Kolkata	Mumbai	Bangalore	Kolkata	Kolkata	Kolkata
4	Bangalore	Bangalore	Bangalore	Bangalore	Kolkata	Chennai	Chennai	Varanasi
5	Chennai	Chennai	Hyderabad	Chennai	Chennai	Bangalore	Hyderabad	Chennai
6	Hyderabad	Varanasi	Chennai	Guwahati	Pune	Guwahati	Bangalore	Hyderabad
7	Guwahati	Hyderabad	Ahmedabad	Hyderabad	Hyderabad	Varanasi	Varanasi	Agra
8	Ahmedabad	Guwahati	Pune	Ahmedabad	Guwahati	Hyderabad	Srinagar	Khajuraho
9	Pune	Kochi	Guwahati	Lucknow	Coimbatore	Pune	Guwahati	Visakhapatnam
10	Goa	Port Blair	Jaipur	Patna	Indore	Rajahmundry	Imphal	Bangalore

Table 4 Changes of network measures after removal of a node based on degree

Airline network	Airport removed	Number of nodes	Number of edges	ΔL (%)	ΔC (%)	$\Delta \tau$ (%)	ΔR (%)
Indigo	Delhi	36	204	9.52	−16.39	35.79	−0.08
	Mumbai	35	214	0.63	−6.36	8.06	−2.86
	Kolkata	35	219	3.49	−0.68	12.56	−5.71
	Bangalore	36	227	1.27	0.54	17.53	−0.08
	Hyderabad	36	234	0.95	−0.68	−0.35	−0.08
Jet Airways	Mumbai	39	106	3.5	−37.85	2.1	−24.84
	Delhi	42	110	0.16	−46.51	0.47	−28.26
	Bangalore	45	134	1.68	−16.76	8.9	0.04
	Chennai	43	140	−1.31	1.69	−5.61	−8.65
	Kolkata	44	139	−8.64	−9.8	−11.54	−2.41
Air India	Delhi	45	116	8.64	−38.48	−2.1	0
	Mumbai	47	131	3.95	−26.95	−2.75	−3.85
	Kolkata	50	148	3.2	−21.39	4.07	−14.78
	Chennai	51	162	0.29	0.41	−2.79	0
	Hyderabad	51	162	−0.04	−3.7	−3.28	0

path length and change of clustering coefficient after consecutive removal of five nodes (airports) based on the degree and betweenness. Figure 2 shows the change of the average path length and clustering coefficient after consecutive removal of random nodes (airports).

In addition, to assess the robustness of the networks, the number of airports removed is compared to the size of the giant component. The giant component is the largest component of the network, which is still connected within the network after removal of a percentage or a number of nodes (airports) from the network. The size of the giant component is the number of nodes (airports) in the giant component. Table 5 gives the size of the giant component after removal of key nodes based on degree from the respective networks. Figure 3 gives the percentage of the giant component after consecutive removal of nodes based on degree and betweenness, respectively. From Fig. 3, it is clear that after consecutive removal of top five nodes (airports) based on degree, the size of the giant component are decreased to almost 8 and 9% in the case of Jet Airways and Air India networks. Whereas the Indigo network does not much affect by it and after the removal, size of the giant component of Indigo network is above 60%. However, in case of betweenness, the size of the giant component of Indigo network decreases to 43%. For random failures, after consecutive removal of random nodes (airports) the size of the giant component presented in Fig. 4.

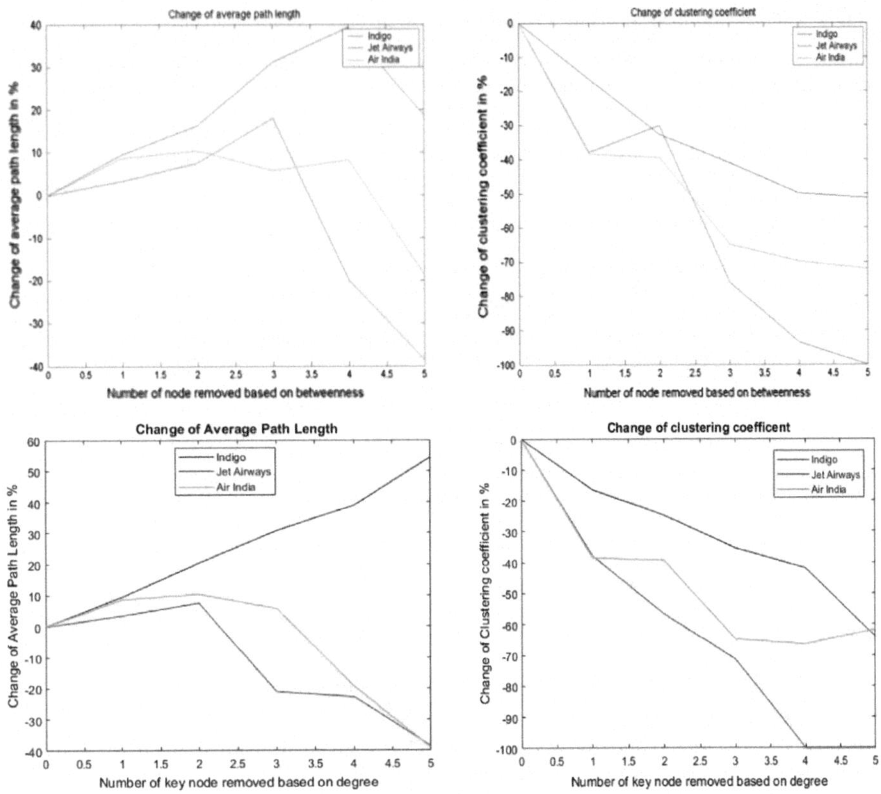

Fig. 1 Change of the average path length and clustering coefficient after consecutive removal of nodes based on degree and betweenness

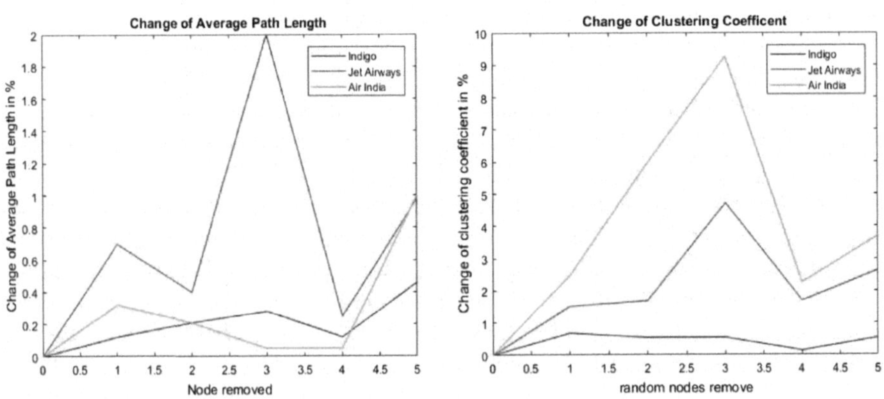

Fig. 2 Change of the average path length and clustering coefficient after consecutive removal of random nodes

Table 5 Size of giant component after isolating the airports based on degree

Rank	Indigo airline		Jet Airways airline		Air India airline	
	Airport removed	Size of giant component	Airport removed	Size of giant component	Airport removed	Size of giant component
1	Delhi	35	Mumbai	39	Delhi	42
2	Mumbai	35	Delhi	38	Mumbai	47
3	Kolkata	34	Bangalore	45	Kolkata	48
4	Bangalore	35	Kolkata	39	Chennai	51
5	Hyderabad	35	Chennai	43	Hyderabad	51
6	Chennai	35	Pune	45	Bangalore	52
7	Ahmedabad	35	Hyderabad	45	Varanasi	50
8	Pune	35	Guwahati	44	Srinagar	52
9	Guwahati	35	Coimbatore	45	Guwahati	52
10	Jaipur	35	Indore	45	Imphal	52

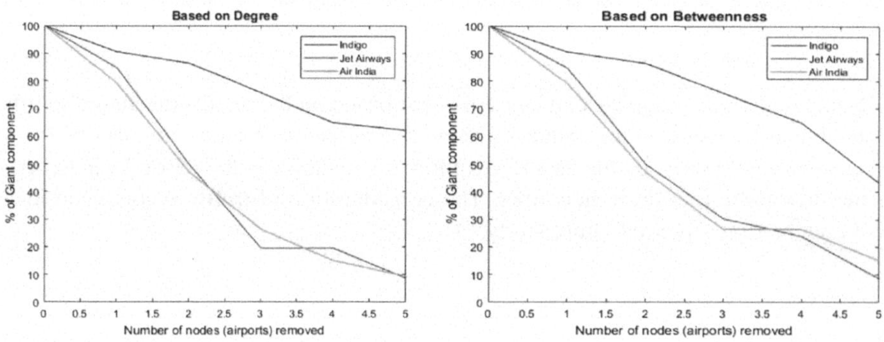

Fig. 3 Percentage of change of giant component after consecutive removal of nodes based on degree and betweenness

5 Conclusion

In this study, we analyze the robustness of the three major airport networks that give a reasonable idea about the robustness of whole ANI. Here, we observed that only Indigo network shows the increment in the average path length after removal of high-degree nodes. However, it is expected that average path lengths should be increased and clustering coefficient should be decreased after the removal of high-degree nodes from the networks. It suggests that Jet Airways and Air India are more robust to targeted attacks than Indigo. In Air India network, there are some key nodes (Khajuraho, Visakhapatnam, Agra) with high betweenness. These nodes can be very important in the study of robustness of the network for targeted attack.

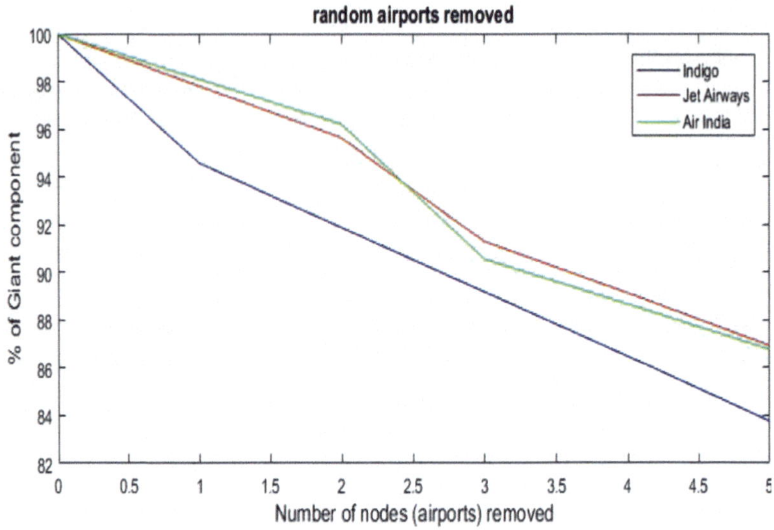

Fig. 4 Percentage of change of giant component after consecutive removal of random nodes (airports)

Some interesting analysis can be performed based on the results discussed in this work. For instance, it is important to know the impact of closing an airport, for a given amount of hours. In this paper, we ignore the dynamic behavior of the networks or the flow pattern in these networks. The consideration of traffic volume can also be an interesting topic for future study.

References

1. Li-Ping, C., Ru, W., Hang, S., Xin-Ping, X., Jin-Song, Z., Wei, L., Xu, C.: Structural properties of US flight network. Chin. Phys. Lett. **20**(8), 1393–1396 (2003)
2. Li, W., Cai, X.: Statistical analysis of airport network of China. Phys. Rev. E **69**(4), 1–6 (2004)
3. Quartieri, J., Guida, M., Guarnaccia, C., D'Ambrosio, S., Guadagnuolo, D.: Topological properties of the Italian airport network studied via multiple addendials and graph theory. Int. J. Math. Model. Methods Appl. Sci. **2**(2), 312–316 (2008)
4. Bagler, G.: Analysis of the airport network of India as a complex weighted network. Phys. A **387**(12), 2972–2980 (2008)
5. Harville, D.A.: Matrix Algebra From a Statistician's Perspective. Springer, New York, NY (1997)
6. Couto, G.S., Couto Da Silva, A.P., Ruiz, L.B., Benevenuto, F.: Structural properties of the Brazilian air transportation network. Ann. Brazil Acad. Sci. **87**(3), 1653–1674 (2015)
7. Gribble, S.: Robustness in complex systems. In: Proceedings of the 8th Workshop on Hot Topics in Operation Systems (Hot OS-VIII) (2001)
8. Albert, R., Jeong, H., Barabási, A.-L.: Error and attack tolerance of complex networks. Nature **406**, 378–382 (2000)
9. Han, D.D., Qian, J.H., Liu, J.G.: Network topology and correlation features affiliated with European airline companies. Physica A **388**(1), 71–81 (2009)

10. Reggiani, A., Signoretti, S., Nijkamp, P., Cento, A.: Network measures in civil air transport: a case study of Lufthansa. In: Naimzada, A.K., Stefani, S., Torriero, A. (eds.) Networks, Topology and Dynamics. Lecture Notes in Economics and Mathematical Systems. Springer, Berlin Heidelberg (2009)
11. Reggiani, A., Nijkamp, P., Cento, A.: Connectivity and concentration in airline networks: a complexity analysis of Lufthansa network. Eur. J. Inf. Syst. **19**(4), 449–461 (2010)
12. Lordan, O., Sallan, J.M., Simo, P., Gonzalez-Prieto, D.: Robustness of airline alliance route networks. Commun. Nonlinear Sci. Numer. Simul. **22**(1–3), 587–595 (2015)
13. Wijdeveld, S. J.: Airline and Alliance Networks Topology and Robustness from a Complex Network Approach. Master Thesis (2015). http://resolver.tudelft.nl/uuid:7bfc759c-e2bc-422e-ae69-3277d31c307f. Last accessed 31 Aug 2019
14. Barabási, A.L., Albert, R.: Emergence of scaling in random networks. Science **286**, 509–512 (1999)
15. Freeman, L.: Centrality in social networks conceptual classification. Soc. Netw. **1**, 215–239 (1978)
16. Hossain, M., Alam, S., Rees, T., Abbass, H.: Australian airport network robustness analysis: a complex network approach. In: Proceedings of Australasian Transport Research Forum, pp. 1–21 (2013)
17. Tizghadam, A., Leon-Garcia, A.: On robust traffic engineering in core networks. In: IEEE GLOBECOM Global Telecommunications Conference, pp. 1–6 (2008)
18. Bharali, A., Baruah, D.: On structure and robustness of airport network of India. Res. Rev. Discret. Math. Struct. **5**(2), 26–33 (2018)

The manufacturer's authorised representative in the EU is Springer Nature Customer Service Centre GmbH, Europaplatz 3, 69115 Heidelberg, Germany. If you have any concerns regarding our products, please contact ProductSafety@springernature.com

Printed and bound by CPI Group (UK) Ltd, Croydon, CR0 4YY
30/09/2026
02225556-0016